W9-BEA-947

# Disorders of Hemostasis

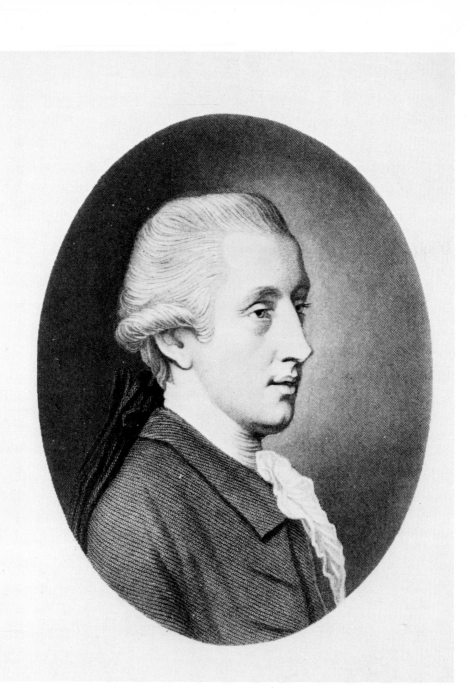

William Hewson (1739–1774), a pioneer in the study of blood coagulation. He recognized that blood, isolated within a segment of vein in the living animal, remained fluid, and localized the clotting process to an alteration in plasma. From The Works of William Hewson, F.R.S., G. Gulliver, edit. The Sydenham Society, London, 1846.

# Disorders of Hemostasis

*Edited by*

## Oscar D. Ratnoff, M.D.

*Professor of Medicine*
*Case Western Reserve University School of Medicine*
*Career Investigator of the American Heart Association*
*Cleveland, Ohio*

## Charles D. Forbes, M.D., F.R.C.P.

*University Department of Medicine*
*Royal Infirmary, Glasgow*
*Senior Lecturer in Medicine*
*University of Glasgow*
*Glasgow, Scotland*

(G&S)

**Grune & Stratton, Inc.**
*(Harcourt Brace Jovanovich, Publishers)*

| | | |
|---|---|---|
| Orlando | San Diego | San Francisco |
| New York | London | Toronto |
| Montreal | Sydney | Tokyo | São Paulo |

**Library of Congress Cataloging in Publication Data**

Main entry under title:
Disorders of hemostasis.

    Includes bibliographical references and index.

    1. Blood—Coagulation, Disorders of. I. Ratnoff,
Oscar D. II. Forbes, C. D. (Charles Douglas),
1938-    . [DNLM: 1. Blood coagulation disorders.
WH 322 D611]
RC647.C55D57   1984      616.1'57      83-22777
ISBN 0-8089-1622-X

© 1984 by Grune & Stratton, Inc.
All rights reserved. No part of this publication
may be reproduced or transmitted in any form or
by any means, electronic or mechanical, including
photocopy, recording, or any information storage
and retrieval system, without permission in
writing from the publisher.

Grune & Stratton, Inc.
Orlando, Florida 32887

*Distributed in the United Kingdom by*
Grune & Stratton, Ltd.
24/28 Oval Road, London NW 1

Library of Congress Catalog Number 83-22777
International Standard Book Number 0-8089-1622
Printed in the United States of America

*This book is dedicated to
Dr. A. Stuart Douglas,
Regius Professor of Medicine,
University of Aberdeen,
Aberdeen, Scotland*

# Contents

# Preface

The last decades have brought about an exponential rise in knowledge about normal and disordered hemostasis and about the complex relationships among such defense mechanisms as coagulation, fibrinolysis, inflammation, and complement. Hematologists and nonspecialists alike have found hemostasis an obscure and challenging area. This volume attempts to bring together current laboratory and clinical knowledge to provide an up-to-date, easily readable text to assist the clinician in his day-to-day work. Emphasis has been placed on diagnosis and treatment, including such vexing problems as hepatitis and the acquired immunodeficiency syndrome that have shattered our complacent view that the burden of hemophilia can be lessened by home therapy programs.

Controversy still exists in many areas. No attempt has been made to reconcile different points of view or to delete redundancy among the chapters of this volume, for each author sees problems in a somewhat different light. Nonetheless, the reader will find more consensus than disagreement among the authors of this volume. We have also not attempted to use a uniform terminology, but instead have provided synonyms whenever they seem helpful.

The editors wish to acknowledge the seminal thoughts of Dr. Colin R. M. Prentice of the University of Glasgow in the design of this work. It goes without saying that we owe an especial debt to our wives, who have endured the long hours needed to assemble this work.

# Contributors

BRUCE BENNETT, M.D., F.R.C.P., M.R.C.PATH., Reader in Medicine, University of Abderdeen; Honorary Consultant Physician, Aberdeen Hospitals, Aberdeen, Scotland

RODGER L. BICK, M.D., Assistant Professor of Medicine (Division of Hematology/Oncology), University of California, Los Angeles Center for Health Sciences; Medical Director, San Joaquin Hematology/Oncology Medical Group, Bakersfield, California

WALTER E. J. BOWIE, D.M., F.R.C.P. PATH., F.A.C.P., Professor of Medicine and of Laboratory Medicine, Mayo Medical School, Head Section of Hematology Research, Mayo Clinic and Mayo Foundation, Rochester, Minnesota

PETER A. CASTALDI, M.D.(SYD), F.R.A.C.P., F.R.C.P.A., Professor of Medicine, University of Sydney, Westmead Center, Westmead, New South Wales, Australia

BARRY. S. COLLER, M.D., Professor of Medicine and Pathology, State University of New York at Stony Brook School of Medicine, Stony Brook, New York

VIRGINIA H. DONALDSON, M.D., Professor of Pediatrics and Medicine, University of Cincinnati College of Medicine, The Childrens Hospital Research Foundation, Cincinnati, Ohio

A. STUART DOUGLAS, D.SC., M.D., F.R.C.P., F.R.C.PATH., F.A.C.P., Regius Professor of Medicine, University of Aberdeen, Aberdeen, Scotland

CHARLES D. FORBES, M.D., F.R.C.P. (GLAS. EDIN. LOND.), Senior Lecturer, Honorary Consultant Physician, University Department of Medicine, Royal Infirmary, Glasgow, Scotland

GEORGE H. GOLDSMITH, JR., M.D., Associate Professor of Medicine, Case Western Reserve University School of Medicine, Cleveland, Ohio

JACK LEVIN, M.D., Professor of Laboratory Medicine and Medicine, University of California School of Medicine, San Francisco; Chief Hematology Lab/Blood Bank, VA Medical Center, San Francisco, California

GORDON D. O. LOWE, M.B., Ch.B., M.R.C.P., Lecturer in Medicine, Honorary Senior Registrar, University Department of Medicine, Royal Infirmary, Glasgow, Scotland

MICHAEL MACKIE, B (MED) BIOL., M.D., M.R.C.P., M.R.C.PATH., Senior Lecturer and Honorary Consultant Haematologist, University Department of Haematology, University of Liverpool, Liverpool, England

DEREK OGSTON, D.SC., Ph.D., M.D., F.R.C.P. (EDIN. LOND.), Professor, University Department of Medicine, University of Abderdeen, Aberdeen, Scotland

CHARLES OWEN, M.D., PH.D., D.SCI., F.A.C.PATH., Emeritus Professor of Pathology and of Medicine (Medical Research), Mayo Medical School; Emeritus Chairman, Department Biochemistry, Mayo Clinic and Mayo Foundation, Rochester, Minnesota

OSCAR D. RATNOFF, M.D., LLD (HON. ABERDEEN), Professor of Medicine and Career Investigator of the American Heart Association, Case Western Reserve University School of Medicine, Cleveland, Ohio

H. ALISTAIR REID, O.B.E., M.D., F.R.C.P.E., F.R.A.C.P., D.T.M. and H. (Deceased), Emeritus Consultant Physician, Honorary Director, World Health Organisation Collaborative Centre for the Control of Antivenoms, Liverpool School of Tropical Medicine, Liverpool, England

HIDEHIKO SAITO, M.D., Professor of Medicine, Head, Division of Hematology, Saga Medical School, Nabeshima, Saga, Japan

SANDOR S. SHAPIRO, M.D., Professor of Medicine, Cardeza Foundation for Hematologic Research, Jefferson Medical College of Thomas Jefferson University, Philadelphia, Pennsylvania

# Disorders of Hemostasis

Oscar D. Ratnoff

# 1

# The Evolution of Knowledge About Hemostasis

The transformation of fluid blood to a gellike mass when it escapes the body was a source of wonder in ancient times. To Plato[1] and his pupil Aristotle,[2] blood clotted because it cooled upon exposure to the air; as a result its "fibers" congealed, a view later echoed by Galen.[3] Surprisingly, the idea that clots could stem the loss of blood from wounds came only with the beginning of the eighteenth century.[4] That adhesion of platelets to the walls of injured vessels abetted this beneficial effect of clotting was learned only a century ago.[5,6] We are led to ask what other protective devices against exsanguination we are yet blind to.

## THE FORMATION OF FIBRIN

The first major contributor to our understanding of coagulation was Malpighi,[7] who, in mid-seventeenth century, separated the fibers of the clot from blood cells and serum and studied their morphologic characteristics under the microscope. More than a century later, William Hewson,[8] a British surgeon who made many remarkable observations about blood and lymph, demonstrated that the fibers were derived from what we now call plasma. Babington[9] recognized that the fibers, which had acquired the name fibrin, were generated from a precursor in plasma. This precursor, fibrinogen (factor I*), was extensively purified[10] and was quantified with remarkable accuracy[11,12] in the last century.

The earliest clue to the way fibrinogen was changed into the insoluble strands of fibrin was provided by a Scottish physiologist, Buchanan,[13] who reported that hydrocele fluid clotted upon addition of fresh serum. He concluded that clotting reflected the interaction of fibrinogen with something that was present in the serum. How this second agent, later called thrombin, coagulated fibrinogen was disputed well into the present century, but early views that thrombin was an enzyme[10,14,15] have prevailed. We now know that thrombin separates 2 pairs of small polypeptides, designated fibrinopeptides A and B,

---

*Through the stimulus provided by Dr. Irving Wright of New York, an International Committee of Blood Clotting Factors has designated roman numerals to describe most of the blood clotting factors; these have been provided throughout this chapter for clarity.

1

from each molecule of fibrinogen.[16] The shorn fibrinogen, named *fibrin monomer*, then polymerizes until it forms the insoluble fibrin network. Normally, too, the fibrin monomers are bound covalently to each other through the action of another plasma enzyme, fibrin-stabilizing factor (fibrinoligase, factor XIII), providing tensile strength to the clot.[17,18]

## THE FORMATION OF THROMBIN

Alexander Schmidt,[15] whose studies of clotting dominated the second half of the nineteenth century, realized that free thrombin could not be a constituent of normal circulating blood, for otherwise it would clot the fibrinogen in plasma. Rather, he postulated, it must circulate as an inert precursor, for which Pekelharing[19] provided the name prothrombin (factor II). Prothrombin has now been highly purified and its structure elucidated, largely through the pioneer efforts of Dr. Walter Seegers, formerly at Wayne State University in Detroit.[20]

Reflecting a paucity of data, innumerable hypotheses, some of great ingenuity, were devised to explain how prothrombin changed to thrombin when blood was withdrawn from the endothelial-lined blood vessels.[21] One popular view, first expressed by John Hunter,[22] was that the blood vessels exerted a "vital force" that prevented coagulation. A more mechanistic concept was presented by Lord Lister[23] and others, who believed that shed blood clotted because it came into contact with a "foreign" surface such as that of the cup into which it was drawn. This hypothesis assumed that blood itself—indeed, just the plasma—contained all the elements needed for clotting. We now describe the steps that lead to clotting when plasma touches a foreign surface as the *intrinsic pathway of thrombin formation*. Schmidt[15] offered an alternative view, stating that clotting was brought about by contact of blood with injured tissues, a sequence of events now called the *extrinsic pathway of thrombin formation*. Until relatively recently, investigators had a difficult time accepting the possiblity that both of these hypotheses might be correct under different circumstances. Now we have learned not only that this is true, but also that the 2 pathways are intertwined so that the reactions of one influence those of the other.

### The Extrinsic Pathway of Thrombin Formation

In 1819, Thackrah[24] reported that blood clotted more rapidly if it flowed over an exposed tissue surface than if it was carefully collected in a container. That tissues might induce blood clotting was dramatically confirmed a few years later by de Blainville[25] when he infused a suspension of brain into animals. The result, immediately lethal, was occlusion of the recipients' blood vessels with clotted blood. Extending this observation, Schmidt[15] found that blood clotted rapidly upon the addition of tissue suspensions, which he believed contained a "zymoplastic" substance, that is, an agent that could convert prothrombin to enzymatically active thrombin. The active principle, subsequently called *tissue thromboplastin* (factor III), thrombokinase, or tissue factor, appeared to contain phospholipid. Many years later, Howell,[26] Mills,[27] and Chargaff et al.[28] recognized that the phospholipid was bound to a tissue protein that was essential for its function.

At first, Schmidt[25] believed that exposure of prothrombin to tissue thromboplastin was sufficient for the formation of thrombin. When oxalate and citrate solutions were found to inhibit clotting,[29,30] Hammarsten[10] suggested that the action of tissue thromboplastin depended on the presence of calcium ions. These ideas of Schmidt and Hammarsten were crystallized by Fuld and Spiro[31] and Morawitz[32] into what was thereafter called the classic theory of blood coagulation. Clotting took place in two steps, the conversion of prothrombin to thrombin by tissue thromboplastin and the transformation of fibrinogen to fibrin by thrombin. Calcium ions were required for the first but not the second step. Only years later did it become evident that calcium ions, at the concentration present in plasma, also accelerated the polymerization of fibrin.[33,34]

Morawitz's formulation of the mechanism of blood coagulation held sway for many decades, although each investigator had his own explanation of the data he had obtained. Morawitz himself ignored his contemporaries, Nolf[35] and Bordet,[36] who provided evidence that in addition to calcium ions, other plasma agents were needed for the conversion of prothrombin to thrombin by tissue thromboplastin. In the 1930s, new methods for measuring the generation of thrombin confirmed these heterodox views and led to the discovery of additional plasma clotting factors.

Warner, Brinkhous and Smith,[37] members of a group of investigators at the University of Iowa, devised a two-step method for the measurement of prothrombin. In the first step, prothrombin was transformed quantitatively to thrombin through the action of tissue thromboplastin and calcium ions. In the second stage, the thrombin that had evolved was quantified by its ability to clot fibrinogen. Meanwhile, Armand J. Quick,[38] most of whose investigative career was spent at what is now the Medical College of Wisconsin, described a one-stage method that telescoped the 2 phases of fibrin formation. He added tissue thromboplastin and calcium ions to decalcified plasma and measured the clotting time of the mixture. Quick's prothrombin time technique is now universally used in the clinic. A moral is in order: Quick had great difficulty in getting his radical paper accepted for publication.[39]

Soon it became evident that in certain situations the prothrombin content of plasma measured by the 2-step method was greater than that predicted by Quick's one-stage prothrombin time. For example, the one-stage prothrombin time lengthened during prolonged storage of blood,[40] whereas the prothrombin content found by the two-stage technique was relatively stable.[41] This discrepancy suggested that other plasma factors participated in the formation of thrombin, an idea supported by observations of Quick,[42] Owen and Bollman,[43] and others. Three such factors have now been described: proaccelerin (factor V), first discovered by Quick[19] and Owren,[44] factor VII, detected by Alexander et al.[45] and Stuart factor (factor X), recognized by Hougie et al.[46] and Telfer et al.[47] In each case, the existence of these accessory factors was supported by their apparent absence from the plasma of individuals with hereditary hemorrhagic disorders. These are 3 examples of the interplay between clinic and laboratory that has been a major source of new ideas about hemostasis. In brief, factor VII reacts stoichiometrically with tissue thromboplastin, and in this form changes Stuart factor to an active form (factor Xa) that converts prothrombin to thrombin. This transformation is an enzymatic process that is greatly speeded by proaccelerin (factor V).

## The Intrinsic Pathway of Coagulation

The authority of Schmidt and Morawitz retarded an understanding of how blood clots in the absence of tissue thromboplastin. This is all the more remarkable because considerable evidence already existed that such an alternative pathway existed. In 1830, Babington[9] recorded that clotting was retarded when blood was submerged in olive oil, an observation whose significance he did not grasp. Later, in experiments already alluded to, Lister[23] found that venous blood clotted more rapidly in a cup than in an india rubber tube. Lister's conclusion, still valid, was that blood coagulated when it came into contact with surfaces foreign to the body; in this regard, the cup was more foreign than india rubber. Freund[48] refined Lister's experiments in studies reminiscent of those of Babington,[9] demonstrating that clotting was slowed by coating test tubes with oil or petroleum jelly. Bordet and Gengou[49] added that the clot-promoting effect of glass was localized to an effect upon some undefined agent in plasma. The latter observation was made by centrifuging blood in paraffin-lined tubes in the absence of an anticoagulant, using a primitive cold centrifuge. Plasma separated in this way clotted much more rapidly in glass than in the paraffin-lined tubes.

These and similar observations were ignored or rationalized even when Conley et al.,[50] in 1949, confirmed Bordet's observations, using silicone to prevent contact of blood with glass. What finally led to recognition of a mechanism through which blood could clot in the absence of tissue thromboplastin was expansion of knowledge about the hereditary disorders of coagulation.

The first such familial disorder to be described was hemophilia, undoubtedly because its severe and often lethal hemorrhagic symptoms ensured its recognition. In the second century A.D., Rabbi Judah,[51] a distinguished scholar, exempted from circumcision a new-born boy whose brothers had died aften this operation. Individuals who probably had hemophilia were described repeatedly thereafter, but it was not until 1803 that John Otto,[52] who himself never saw a patient with this disease, realized that it was limited to males. He recognized that their asymptomatic female relatives transmitted the bleeding tendency to their sons. Another American physician, John Hay,[53] added that the daughters of hemophiliacs were carriers. Hemophilia, of course, is a prototypic X chromosone-linked disorder, inherited in the manner proposed by Morgan[54] from studies of fruit flies. Delineation of the mode of inheritance of hemophilia was made easier by the chance that Christmas disease, a closely similar familial disorder that will be discussed subsequently, is also X chromosome linked.

In 1819, a British surgeon, Mr. Ward,[55] ascribed the hemorrhagic tendency of a patient who may have had hemophilia to a defect in blood clotting. This suggestion was ignored in favor of other hypotheses until Sir Almroth Wright,[56] at the close of the century, found that the newly described clotting time of whole blood was abnormally long in this disease. A few years later, Thomas Addis[57] suggested that hemophilia was due to the presence of an abnormal prothrombin, a view soon rejected. Less than a half-century ago, Patek,[58,59] building on the work of others, reported that a crude globulin fraction of normal plasma corrected the defective clotting of hemophilic plasma, whereas a similar fraction of hemophilic plasma was inert. The active principle in the normal globulin fraction is now described as antihemophilic factor (factor VIII). Further, Patek reported that transfusion of the globulin fraction of normal plasma into a hemophiliac shortened his clotting time—a modern confirmation of Lane's[60] early report that blood transfusion controlled bleeding in a patient with this disease.

Patek's studies provided the impetus for the use of plasma or plasma fractions rich in antihemophilic factor for the treatment of classic hemophilia. Currently, two types of preparation are used. Pool et al.[61] made the striking discovery that an insoluble residue present in plasma that had been frozen and thawed was rich in antihemophilic factor. Such "cryoprecipitates," preserved in the frozen state or lyophilized, are useful to stanch bleeding in hemophiliacs or as prophylaxis before surgery. Lyophilized antihemophilic factor can also be prepared by precipitating this protein with certain neutral amino acids.[62] The availability of lyophilized preparations has made possible the home treatment of relatively minor bleeding episodes, greatly reducing the need for hospital care.

Patek could not decide whether antihemophilic factor was lacking in hemophilic plasma or was present in an unavailable form. Some years later, Shanberge and Gore[63] published a brief note suggesting that the latter hypothesis was correct; hemophilic plasma appeared to contain a non-functional variant of antihemophilic factor that was recognized by heterologous antiserum. More time was to elapse before the correctness of Shanberge and Gore's hypothesis was established.[64,65] A by-product was an improved technique for the detection of hemophilic carriers.[64,66]

The nature of antihemophilic factor was clarified by studies of patients with another disorder in which this substance was functionally deficient in plasma. In 1926, von Willebrand[67] described an unusual hemorrhagic disorder, inherited in an autosomal dominant manner, in a family residing in the Åland Islands off Finland. He reported that the bleeding time, which had been devised by Hayem[68] and improved by Duke,[69] was prolonged in affected individuals; this test gives normal results in patients with classic hemophilia. Von Willebrand ascribed the hemorrhagic tendency in his patients to a defect of platelets. What was probably the same disorder was described independently by Minot.[70] In 1953, Alexander and Goldstein,[71] and Larrieu and Soulier,[72] and Quick and Hussey[73] each observed a deficiency of antihemophilic factor in the plasma of similar patients; the same deficiency was present in members of von Willebrand's original family.[74]

The nature of von Willebrand's disease became clear from a number of subsequent observations. Patients with this disease proved to be truly deficient in antihemophilic factor, in contrast to those with classic hemophilia, in whom this protein could be detected by the use of heterologous antiserum.[65] Further, Howard and Firkin[75] found that ristocetin, an antibiotic that had been withdrawn from use because it induced thrombocytopenia, agglutinated normal or hemophilic platelets that were suspended in autologous plasma, but not the platelets of patients with von Willebrand's disease suspended in their own plasma. These and other studies suggested that the long bleeding time in von Willebrand's disease could be explained if antihemophilic factor were needed for the adhesion of platelets to injured blood vessel walls; this was soon demonstrated in an animal model by Tschopp et al.[76] Studies of von Willebrand's disease and its variants have thus contributed greatly to our understanding of hemostasis.

At the same time that Wright rediscovered impaired coagulation in hemophilia, Manteuffel,[77] a pupil of Schmidt, demonstrated that hemophilic blood clotted normally upon addition of tissue thromboplastin. The defect in hemophilia thus must reside in a pathway not envisioned by Schmidt; in modern terms, the extrinsic pathway was normal in hemophilia. This disturbing observation did not shake belief in the primacy of Morawitz's classic hypothesis until the 1950s, when the discovery of other hereditary defects in the intrinsic pathway made this view untenable.

The first of the new clotting disorders to be described was Christmas disease (factor IX deficiency). In 1944, Castex, Pavlovsky and Simonetti,[78] three Argentinian investigators, reported the results of some perplexing experiments. Occasionally, a mixture of the blood of two hemophiliacs behaved like normal blood. Further, the transfusion of the blood of one hemophiliac into another shortened the clotting time of blood drawn from the recipient. How this paradox came about was soon explained by Aggeler et al.[79] and Schulman and Smith,[80] who reported simultaneously that some individuals with symptoms typical of hemophilia appeared to be functionally deficient not in antihemophilic factor but rather in another, previously unrecognized plasma protein. This agent was first called plasma thrombo-plastin component (PTC) or plasma factor X (not to be confused with Stuart factor, now designated factor X). Later it was renamed Christmas factor by Biggs and her associates[81] and its functional deficiency, Christmas disease, after the family name of one of her patients. It is easy to understand why classic hemophilia and Christmas disease were not distinguished earlier, for both have the same symptomatology and both are X chromosome-linked disorders. Indeed, in retrospect, one wonders if some of the "hemophiliacs" studied by early investigators did not really have Christmas disease.[57]

Several additional clotting factors that participate in the intrinsic pathway have since been discovered, allowing a tentative delineation of the way blood clots in the absence of tissue thromboplastin. When plasma comes into contact with a foreign surface such as glass, a plasma protein, Hageman factor (factor XII), is changed from an inert to an enzymatically active state. Hageman factor was first recognized by its apparent absence from the plasma of an asymptomatic railroad brakeman, John Hageman, whose clotting time was unusually long.[82] The activated form of Hageman factor then activates plasma thromboplastin antecedent (PTA, factor XI),[83,84] a protein that Rosenthal et al.[85] found to be deficient in the plasma of several related individuals with a mild hemorrhagic tendency.

This simplistic view of the activation of PTA was clouded by experiments of Schiffman and her associates[86] in which activation of PTA could not be detected in mixtures of purified preparations of this agent and Hageman factor. Perhaps, then, something more was needed for the reaction between activated Hageman factor and PTA to proceed. This interpretation was borne out by the discovery of two additional defects in clotting in asymptomatic individuals said to have Fletcher trait[87] and Fitzgerald, Williams, or Flaujeac trait,[88–91] respectively. Activation of PTA requires the presence of Fitzgerald factor (deficient in the plasma in Fitzgerald trait) and is accelerated by Fletcher factor (deficient in the plasma in Fletcher trait). Fitzgerald factor turned out to be identical to a previously recognized plasma protein, high molecular weight kininogen,[90,91] and Fletcher factor proved to be the same as plasma prekallikrein.[92]

Both high molecular weight kininogen and plasma prekallikrein had long been recognized as participants in experimental inflammatory reactions. Plasma prekallikrein can be converted to its enzymatic form, plasma kallikrein, by activated Hageman factor. Plasma kallikrein then releases certain low molecular weight peptides, notably bradykinin, from their precursor in plasma, high molecular weight kininogen.[93] These low molecular weight peptides can then induce some of the phenomena of inflammation. Such observations have led to the view that clotting, inflammation, and certain other defense reactions are closely interwoven phenomena, and that to a large extent their separate study is more a matter of convenience than a true reflection of the way that the body responds to injury.

After PTA has been converted to its catalytic state, it transforms Christmas factor (factor IX) to an enzymatically active form [94,95] that can bring about the activation of Stuart factor (factor X).[96] The subsequent steps of the intrinsic and extrinsic pathways are identical. The physiologic role of antihemophilic factor (factor VIII) is not known, but its presence greatly potentiates the action of Christmas factor.

The observations that hereditary deficiencies of Hageman factor, plasma prekallikrein, and high molecular weight kininogen are entirely asymptomatic, and that PTA deficiency is associated with only a mild bleeding tendency, suggested that in real life some other method must exist by which Christmas factor can be activated. In fact, studies of Østerud and Rapaport[97] reveal that the tissue thromboplastin–factor VII complex of the extrinsic pathway can activate Christmas factor. Conversely, the action of factor VII is augmented by activated Hageman factor and other plasma enzymes.[98] The differentiation between the intrinsic and extrinsic pathways thus is less rigid than was first believed.

## THE ROLE OF VITAMIN K IN THE SYNTHESIS OF CLOTTING FACTORS

In order to study cholesterol metabolism, a Danish investigator, Henrik Dam,[99] fed chicks an ether-extracted diet. The chicks developed a bleeding tendency that could be prevented by feeding the chicks cereals or seeds. Dam concluded that these foods contained a "Koagulations-Vitamin".[100] Almquist[101] isolated vitamin K from alfalfa, and its synthesis was soon accomplished.[102-104] The bleeding diathesis brought about by a deficiency of vitamin K was related to impaired blood coagulation;[105] only later was it realized that this vitamin was needed for the synthesis of prothrombin, Christmas factor (factor IX), Stuart factor (factor X), and factor VII. Recently, too, vitamin K has been implicated in the synthesis of other proteins, including protein C, a plasma inhibitor of clotting that was originally described by Seegers and Ulutin[106] and Stenflo,[107] and proteins in bone[108] and other tissues.

The discovery of vitamin K quickly provided an explanation for the bleeding tendency associated with hemorrhagic disease of the newborn[109] and obstructive jaundice.[110-112] In both of these disorders, Quick's one-stage prothrombin time was abnormally long. The infant with hemorrhagic disease was apparently deficient in vitamin K. In contrast, the patient with obstructive jaundice could not absorb this vitamin from the gut. The obstruction reduced the intestinal concentration of bile salts that are required for the normal absorption of fat-soluble vitamin K.

How vitamin K acts to bring about the synthesis of the proteins dependent upon its presence is an exciting story. Olson et al.[113] and others showed that synthesis takes place in two steps. First, hepatocytes synthesize proteins that are nonfunctional and cannot be converted to their activated state. In the second step, vitamin K changes this "precursor protein" to a biologically competent form. Stenflo et al.[114] found that the role of vitamin K is to insert a second carboxyl group into the $\gamma$–carbon of glutamic acid residues in the precursor proteins. These unique tricarboxylic glutamic acid residues are the sites of attachment for calcium ions, needed for transformation of the vitamin K-dependent factors to their enzymatically active states.

In the winter of 1921–1922, an epidemic of hemorrhagic disease swept through herds of cattle in Canada. Schofield,[115] a veterinarian, related the outbreak to the ingestion of spoiled sweet clover, which appeared to impair blood coagulation. The defect in clotting was identified as a deficiency of prothrombin. Another outbreak in the 1930s, this time in Wisconsin, caused a farmer named Ed Carlson to bring some spoiled sweet clover to the University of Wisconsin, where he induced Karl Paul Link[116] to investigate the problem. Link extracted an agent from the clover, bishydroxycoumarin (Dicumarol), that proved to be responsible for the hypoprothrombinemia. Dicumarol and its congeners, particularly warfarin, quickly found use as a rat poison and, perhaps of equal importance, in the prevention and treatment of thromboembolic disease, first attempted by Butt et al.[117] and Bingham et al.[118] Warfarin is now known to inhibit the regeneration of vitamin K that has been expended to complete the synthesis of the vitamin K-dependent clotting factors.[119]

## FIBRINOLYSIS

That the blood of individuals who die suddenly may be incoagulable was probably recognized by the Hippocratic school[120] and was rediscovered by John Hunter[22] at the end of the eighteenth century. Andral,[12] a pioneer hematologist of the early nineteenth century, recognized that postmortem blood clots sometimes reliquefied. This process of "fibrinolysis" was studied in vitro by Andral's contemporary, Denis,[121] but it was only at the end of the nineteenth century that Denys and Marbaix[122] and Dastre[123] recognized that fibrinolysis was the consequence of proteolysis, and Morawitz[124] linked this process to the liquefation of postmortem clots. Hedin[125] localized the proteolytic properties of serum to a globulin fraction that was later shown to contain the precursor of a protease subsequently named plasmin.[126]

An unheralded observation by Gratia[127] in 1921 was the dissolution of clots by staphylococcal extracts. Then in 1933, Tillett and Garner[128] reported that bacteria-free filtrates of cultures of beta-hemolytic streptococci contained an agent, now called streptokinase, that had a similar effect. Streptokinase is not a bodily constituent, but activators of plasminogen, the precursor of plasmin, are found in many tissues, secretions, and excretions, notably urokinase, an enzyme in urine.[129] Streptokinase and urokinase have been highly purified, and largely through the efforts of Sherry and his collaborators,[130] have received extensive trial for the dissolution of intravascular clots, particularly pulmonary emboli.

As was evident from the earliest observations, blood also appears to have the intrinsic capacity to activate plasminogen. Hunter[22] had reported that the blood of individuals who died as the result of "fits, anger, electricity, or lightning" was incoagulable. In our time, Macfarlane and his colleagues[131,132] refined this observation, noting that fibrin prepared from individuals who had undergone surgery or other stresses reliquefied abnormally rapidly. How this comes about is still uncertain, but Todd[133] and others have suggested that an activator of plasminogen could be released to the bloodstream from venous endothelium. Other pathways for the activation of plasminogen have been related to the initial steps of the intrinsic pathway. Activation of Hageman factor by foreign surfaces leads to the formation of plasma kallikrein and activated PTA; these enzymes can then convert plasminogen to plasmin.[134,135]

The teleologic beauty that plasma contains not only a system designed to clot blood but also to dissolve thrombi is self-evident. Plasmin, however, has the additional capacity to digest many other proteins, and the significance of this property is only beginning to be understood. Perhaps, in the the end, other actions of plasmin may turn out to be as important as the startling dissolution of fibrin.

## PLASMA INHIBITORS OF COAGULATION AND FIBRINOLYSIS

Schmidt,[15] in another of his many contributions to blood coagulation, postulated that plasma has the inherent capacity to inhibit clotting. His ideas were seized upon by Howell[136] and others, who believed that clotting takes place when tissue thromboplastin releases prothrombin from its combination with an inhibitor. This concept persisted for some years, even though Morawitz[32] had proposed that the plasma inhibitor is directed at thrombin rather than prothrombin. Inhibition of thrombin by plasma was more clearly demonstrated by Rettger,[137] and later shown to be due for the most part to a specific plasma protein, designated antithrombin III.[20]

In 1914, Jay MacLean,[138] then a student of Howell, reported that a crude fraction of hepatic tissue inhibited clotting. Howell,[136] who named the agent heparin, showed that it acted only in the presence of an agent in plasma that we now realize is the same as antithrombin III. The effect of antithrombin III, itself a powerful but slow inhibitor of thrombin, is greatly potentiated by the presence of heparin.[139] Largely through the efforts of Yin et al.[140] and Rosenberg,[141] antithrombin III has been found to inhibit other clotting enzymes as well, actions that are also enhanced by heparin. Heparin, a mucopolysaccharide that was highly purified and characterized by Charles and Scott[142] and Jorpes,[143] is in everyday use as an anticoagulant in the prevention and therapy of thromboembolic disease, an idea first tested in 1924, albeit unsuccessfully, by Mason.[144]

A number of other plasma proteins inhibit one or another of the enzymatically active forms of the various clotting factors as well as the plasma proteolytic enzyme, plasmin. $\alpha_2$-plasmin inhibitor, for example, was first isolated by Collen[145] and Moroi and Aoki,[146] although its existence had been postulated many years before by Delezenne and Pozerski.[147] The principal action of this inhibitor is to block the action of plasmin, and its hereditary absence is associated with a severe bleeding tendency.[148] In the test tube, $\alpha_2$-plasmin inhibitor also inhibits the activated form of several clotting enzymes, although this is probably not physiologically significant. Yet another inhibitor of thrombin and plasmin, $\alpha_2$-macroglobulin, seems to provide a backup mechanism;[149] again, evidence for its existence long preceded its isolation. $\alpha_2$-trypsin inhibitor, which in the test tube inhibits plasmin, thrombin,[150] and activated PTA,[151] probably plays no role in hemostasis. Similarly, the inhibitor of the enzymatic form of the first component of complement (C$\bar{1}$-INH) can inhibit plasmin and several other activated clotting factors in the test tube, but its absence is unassociated with defects in hemostasis.

An exciting new development has been the rediscovery of protein C,[107] originally described by Seegers and Ulutin.[106] Protein C is a vitamin K-dependent plasma protein that destroys the clot-promoting properties of two nonenzymatic clotting factors, antihemophilic factor (factor VIII) and proaccelerin (factor V). A rare hereditary disorder of blood coagulation, the combined hereditary deficiency of these two factors, has recently been related to deficiency of a plasma inhibitor of protein C.[152]

## PLATELETS

Platelets serve many biologic functions, including a major role in the hemostatic process. The history of the discovery of platelets has been admirably reviewed by Kemp,[153] Robb-Smith,[154] and Spaet.[155] Alfred Donné[156] is often credited with the discovery of platelets, whose existence he reported in 1842. His contemporaries, George Gulliver[157] and William Addison,[158] however, appear to have been the first to realize that these cells are distinct entities. Robb-Smith[154] points out that, as is so often true, the recognition of platelets came about through the invention of a new technology, the ability to construct achromatic lenses that provided greater resolution for microscopic observation. The platelets were repeatedly described over the next 30 years, but were accepted as unique cells only with the studies of Hayem[159] and William Osler.[160]

The origin of platelets was puzzling. Early hypotheses suggested that they were precipitated from plasma or originated from vascular endothelium.[161] A more popular view was that they were the precursors of erythrocytes;[159] alternatively, perhaps they were derived from leukocytic granules.[161] That they arose from the cytoplasm of megakaryocytes was first recognized by James Homer Wright[162] in 1906, but acceptance of this hypothesis was strangely slow.[163]

The clinical importance of platelets for hemostasis came to be appreciated at the end of the nineteenth century with the discovery that certain patients with purpura had thrombocytopenia.[164–166] In some of these patients, remission of the bleeding tendency occurred after splenectomy, a procedure first proposed for the treatment of idiopathic thrombocytopenic purpura by Kaznelson[167] in 1916. Platelets participate in hemostasis by sealing vascular injuries and by fostering the process of blood coagulation.

Osler,[160] in studies of rat platelets, observed that these cells were ''isolated and single'' in the circulation, but in ''a drop of blood taken from one of these . . . animals, the corpuscles were always to be found accumulated together.'' At about the same time, Ranvier[168] had noted that in shed blood the platelets adhered to the forming fibrin strands, a rediscovery of a similar observation of Addison.[158]

Hayem[169] suggested that the aggregation of platelets that Osler had observed possessed utility, for a puncture wound in the jugular vein of a dog was plugged by a *hemostatic spike* of platelets and fibrin. The same year, Bizzozero[5] added that platelets adhered to the damaged wall of blood vessels and formed clumps that would break off and be swept into the bloodstream, only to be replaced. Shortly thereafter, Eberth and Schimmelbusch[6] noted that the platelets that stuck to injured vessel walls appeared to be swollen and granular, and had become sticky so that other platelets adhered to them. They called this process *viscous metamorphosis,* a term that subsequently underwent various alterations in meaning[170] and is now seldom used. Thus, a century ago the critical role of platelets in hemostasis was recognized, long before the physiologic mechanisms involved began to be understood.

The introduction of electron microscopy has made it evident that platelets do not stick to the damaged endothelial cells, but rather to collagen fibers exposed by vascular injury.[171] This observation is in agreement with studies of Bounameaux and Roskam[172] and Hughes[173] that demonstrated that platelets adhered to connective tissue and in particular to collagen. How antihemophilic factor abets this process[76] is not clear.

The reactions that bring about aggregation of platelets to those adherent to collagen are complicated. Zucker and Borelli[174] observed that connective tissue suspensions and collagen caused platelets to clump; this is presumably one way that aggregation occurs at sites of vascular injury. After Gaarder et al.[175] reported that adenosine diphosphate (ADP) would aggregate platelets, collagen was found to stimulate the release of ADP from platelet granules,[176,177] providing one pathway for the evolution of clumping. Other agents, such as thrombin and epinephrine, also bring about a discharge of the contents of platelets into the surrounding milieu, a process described by Grette[178] as the release reaction.

When they first form, platelet aggregates are loose, but as was early recognized, fibrin strands soon form, binding the platelets together; the formation of fibrin is the consequence of the rapid generation of thrombin at the site of vascular injury.

More recent studies suggest that this formulation is too simple. Aggregation of platelets that have been stimulated with collagen, ADP, and other substances has been related to the generation within these cells of cyclic derivatives of arachidonic acid, the prostaglandins.[179–181] Marcus[182] has reviewed the history of the discovery of these interesting agents. Knowledge of platelet prostaglandins derives from an apparently unrelated observation. In 1930, Kurzrok, a gynecologist, and Lieb, a pharmacologist, observed that different samples of human semen would either contract or relax human uterine strips in vitro[183] Goldblatt[184] attributed the contraction of smooth muscle by human semen to an agent that resisted proteolysis and boiling. This agent was further characterized and named prosta-glandin by von Euler.[185] The structure of the prostaglandins (for there was more than one) was elucidated[186] and their derivation from arachidonic acid demonstrated.[187,188] Arach-idonic acid itself aggregated platelets,[189] presumably by its transformation to prostaglandins. Platelet prostaglandins, however, proved to be only intermediates in the synthesis of the agent ultimately responsible for aggregation, which was identified by Hamberg et al.[190] and named thromboxane $A_2$. A current view is that stimulation of the platelet leads to intracellular release of arachidonic acid from membrane phospholipids[191] and thence to the formation of thromboxane $A_2$.

Almost 40 years ago, Singer[192] proposed that the administration of aspirin increased the frequency of bleeding in the days after tonsillectomy. Later, aspirin was recognized to enhance the hemorrhagic tendency of bleeders[193] and to inhibit platelet aggregation by collagen and ADP.[194–196] It became evident that one role of aspirin was to inhibit one of the enzymes responsible for the formation of thromboxane $A_2$ from arachidonic acid.[197,198]

Many substances other than ADP and prostaglandins are released from stimulated platelets. Worthy of note is serotonin (5-hydroxytryptamine), an agent that is not synthe-sized by platelets but is adsorbed to these cells from plasma. As early as 1907, O'Connor[199] observed that serum, but not plasma, had vasoconstrictor activity. Vasoconstriction was attributed to a substance released from platelets[200,201] that was later identified as serotonin.[202] Discharge of platelet serotonin upon the addition of thrombin was an early example of the release reaction.[203]

Platelets stick not only to collagen but also, as was first reported by Vulpian[204] in 1873, to nonbiological surfaces such as glass. Platelet adhesion to glass was studied in some detail by Wright[205] and Moolten and Vroman,[206] who tried to relate the genesis of thrombosis to a change in these cells that enhanced their ''adhesiveness.'' In a series of experiments that had unexpected implications, Hellem[207] filtered whole blood through col-umns of glass beads; the effluent was partially depleted of platelets. Hellem attributed this result to the release of ADP from erythrocytes, but it was later evident that the source of ADP was the platelets.[208] Our present understanding is that platelets adhere to the glass beads and, as a consequence, ADP is released from platelet granules and induces aggregation of other platelets within the column. What brings about adhesion of the platelets to glass is less obvious, but Salzman,[209] a Boston surgeon, showed that retention of platelets within a column of glass beads was decreased in von Willebrand's disease. This result was later attributed to the deficiency of a critical part of the antihemophilic factor molecule in the plasma of patients with this disorder.[210]

Another function of platelets of great importence, recognized as early as 1877 by William Norris,[211] is their participation in clotting. Hayem,[212] Bizzozero,[5] Morawitz,[32] and Lee and Vincent,[213] among many others, agreed that platelets had an important role in clotting both in vivo and in vitro. Kemp,[153] in a long forgotten work, wrote that ''the break-ing down of the plaque (i.e., the platelets) is intimately connected with the clotting of the blood. The connection between the breakdown of the plaques is . . . chemical, i.e., the plaques appear to give up a soluble substance which is active in coagulation.'' The idea that platelets furnish an agent analogous to tissue thromboplastin persisted despite the evi-dence that plasma has an intrinsic capacity to clot. In fact, Lee and Vincent[213] reported in 1914 that platelets that had been boiled for 15 minutes retained their clot-promoting properties; tissue thromboplastin is heat labile. Lee and Vincent's studies were eventually clarified when Chargaff et al.[214] reported that equine platelets could furnish phospholipids which, as we have seen, are needed for the clotting process. Indeed, as Brinkhous[215] and others showed, the coagulation of plasma is delayed by careful removal of contaminating platelets.

More recently, the clot-promoting properties of platelets, described by van Creveld and Paulssen[216] as platelet factor 3, were localized to the lipoproteins of platelet membrances.[217] They are made available by stimulation of the platelets by such agents as ADP.[218] Platelets also have binding sites for activated Stuart factor (factor Xa) that may enhance the clotting process.[219]

Perhaps as early as the age of Hippocrates, it was recognized that normal blood clots shrink, a process accompanied by extrusion of serum. Shortly after the discovery of platelets, Hayem[212] ascribed the shrinkage of clots to the presence of these cells, and LeSourd and Pagniez[221] suggested that retraction depended upon their integrity. In modern times, clot retraction has been recognized to be dependent upon an active metabolic process that brings about contraction of an actomyosin-like protein.[221] The strands of fibrin adherent to platelets are pulled together by the contraction of these cells without themselves being shortened. The value of clot retraction to the defenses of the body is still not clear. Budtz-Olsen,[222] who reviewed what was known about clot retraction in 1951, believed that this process was without utility. Teleologic reasoning would suggest instead that shrinkage of a clot might help to pull together the edges of small wounds. In agreement with this idea, a familial defect in clot retraction is associated with a hemorrhagic tendency.[223] This disorder, Glanzmann's disease, was the first example of a bleeding diathesis due to a qualitative disorder of platelets.

Additionally, platelets have the property of blocking the action of heparin, an action first described by Conley et al.[224] and soon confirmed by van Creveld and Paulssen.[216]

This brief review of hemostasis has avoided a discussion of the impact of modern techniques on the purification of proteins and the study of their properties upon the knowledge of hemostasis. Powerful tools, such as those used to prepare monoclonal antibodies, are now being exploited vigorously, and one can anticipate a growing appreciation in molecular terms of how the body defends itself against hemorrhage.

## REFERENCES

1. Plato: Timaeus, in Jewett B (ed): The Dialogues of Plato (ed 3), vol. 3. New York, Macmillan, 1892, pp 339–543
2. Aristotle: Meteorologica, Lee HDP (trans), Loeb Classical Library. Cambridge, Mass. Harvard University Press, 1952
3. Galen C: On the Natural Faculties, Brock AJ (trans). Cambridge, Mass, Harvard University Press, 1916
4. Petit JL: Dissertation sur la mannière d'arrester le sang dans les hémorrhagies. Mem Acad Roy Sci 1:85–102, 1731
5. Bizzozero J: Ueber eine neuen Formbestandtheil des Blutes und desen Rolle bei der Thrombose und der Blutgerinnung. Virchows Arch (Pathol Anat) 90:261–332, 1882
6. Eberth JC, Schimmelbusch C: Experimentalle Untersuchungen über Thrombose. Virchows Arch (Pathol Anat) 103:39–87, 1886
7. Malpighi M: De Polypo Cordis, Forester JM (trans). Uppsala, Almquist and Wiksels, 1956
8. Hewson W: The Works of William Hewson, F.R.S., Gulliver G (ed). London, The Sydenham Society, 1846
9. Babington BG: Some considerations with respect to the blood founded on one or two very simple experiments on that fluid. Med Chir Trans 16:293–319, 1830
10. Hammarsten O: A Textbook of Physiological Chemistry (ed 6), Mandel JA (trans). New York, Wiley, 1911

11.  Thackrah CT: An Inquiry into the Nature and Properties of the Blood. London, Cox, 1834

12.  Andral G: Practical Haematology. An Essay on the Blood in Disease, Meigs JF, Stillé A (trans.) Philadelphia, Lea and Blanchard, 1844

13.  Buchanan A: On the coagulation of the blood and other fibriniferous liquids. Lond Med Gaz (ns) 1: 617, 1845; reprinted in J Physiol 2:158–168, 1879–1880

14.  Mellanby J: Thrombase—its preparation and properties. Proc Royal Soc Lond, Sect B 113:93–106, 1933

15.  Schmidt A: Zur Blutlehre. Leipzig, Vogel, 1892

16.  Bailey K, Bettleheim FR, Lorand L, et al: Action of thrombin in the clotting of fibrinogen. Nature 167:233–234,1951

17.  Robbins KD: A study on the conversion of fibrinogen to fibrin. Am J Physiol 142:581–588, 1944

18.  Laki K, Lorand L: On the solubility of fibrin clots. Science 108:280, 1948

19.  Quick AJ: Hemorrhagic Diseases. Philadelphia, Lea and Febiger, 1957

20.  Seegers WH: Prothrombin. Cambridge, Mass, Harvard University Press, 1962

21.  Ratnoff, OD: Why do people bleed?, in Wintrobe MM (ed): Blood, Pure and Eloquent, New York, McGraw-Hill, 1980, pp 600–657

22.  Hunter J: A Treatise on the Blood, Inflammation, and Gun-Shot Wounds. Philadelphia, Webster, 1817

23.  Lister J: On the coagulation of the blood. Proc Royal Soc Lond 12:580–611, 1863

24.  Thackrah CT: An Inquiry into the Nature and Properties of the Blood. London, Cox and Sons, 1819

25.  de Blainville HMD: Injection de matière cerebrale dans les veins. Gaz Med Paris (s 2)2:524, 1834

26.  Howell WH: The nature and action of the thromboplastic (zymoplastic) substance of the tissues. Am J Physiol 31: 1–21, 1912

27.  Mills CA: Chemical nature of tissue coagulins. J Biol Chem 46:135–165, 1921

28.  Chargaff E, Benedich A, Cohen SS: The thromboplastic protein: Structure, properties, disintegration. J Biol Chem 156:161–178, 1944

29.  Arthus M, Pagès C: Nouvelle théorie chimique de la coagulation du sang. Arch Physiol Norm Pathol (5s) 2:739–746, 1890

30.  Sabbatini L: Le calcium-ion dans la coagulation du sang. C R Soc Biol (Paris) 54:716–718, 1902

31.  Fuld E, Spiro K: Der Einfluss einiger gerinnungshemender Agentien auf das Vogelplasma. Beitr Chem Phys Pathol 5:171–190, 1904

32.  Morawitz P: The chemistry of blood coagulation. Ergeb Physiol 4:307–422, 1905. Reprinted in Hartmann RC, Guenther PF (trans), Springfield, Ill, Charles C Thomas, 1958

33.  Lorand L, Konishi K: Activation of the fibrin stabilizing factor of plasma by thrombin. Arch Biochem Biophys 105:58–67, 1964

34.  Boyer MH, Shainoff JR, Ratnoff OD: Acceleration of fibrin polymerization by calcium ions. Blood 39:382–387, 1972

35.  Nolf P: The coagulation of the blood. Medicine (Balt) 17:381–411, 1938

36.  Bordet J: The theories of blood coagulation. Bull Johns Hopkins Hosp 32:213–218, 1921

37.  Warner ED, Brinkhous KM, Smith HP: A quantitative study on blood clotting: Prothrombin fluctuations under experimental conditions. Am J Physiol 114:667–675, 1936

38.  Quick AJ, Stanley-Brown M, Bancroft FW: A study of the coagulation defect in hemophilia and in jaundice. Am J Med Sci 190:501–511, 1935

39.  Quick AJ: The development and use of the prothrombin tests. Circulation 19:92–96, 1959

40.  Rhoads JE, Panzer LM: The prothrombin time of "bank blood." JAMA 112:309–310, 1939

41.  Lord JW Jr, Pastore JB: Plasma prothrombin content of bank blood. JAMA 113:2231–2232, 1939

42.  Quick AJ: On the constitution of prothrombin. Am J Physiol 140:212–220, 1943

43. Owen CA Jr, Bollman JL: Prothrombin conversion factor of Dicumarol plasma. Proc Soc Exp Biol Med 67:231–234, 1948

44. Owren PA: The coagulation of blood. Investigations on a new clotting factor. Acta Med Scand Suppl 194:1–327, 1947

45. Alexander B, Golstein R, Landwehr G, et al: Congenital SPCA deficiency: A hitherto unrecognized coagulation defect with hemorrhage rectified by serum and serum fractions. J Clin Invest 30:596–608, 1951

46. Hougie E, Barrow EM, Graham JB: Stuart clotting defect. I. Segregation of an hereditary hemorrhagic state from the heterogeneous group heretofore called "stable factor" (SPCA, proconvertin, factor VII) deficiency. J Clin Invest 36:485–496, 1957

47. Telfer TP, Denson KW, Wright DR: A "new" coagulation defect. Br J Haematol 2:308–316, 1956

48. Freund E: Ein Beitrag zur Kenntniss der Blutgerinnung. Med Jahrb (Vienna) ns (3)1:46–48, 1886

49. Bordet J, Gengou O: Réchèrches sur la coagulation du sang et les serum anticoagulants. Ann Inst Pasteur 15:129–144, 1901

50. Conley CL, Hartmann RC, Morse WI II: The clotting behavior of human "platelet-free" plasma: Evidence for the existence of a "plasma thromboplastin." J Clin Invest 28:340–352, 1949

51. Epstein I (ed): The Babylonian Talmud, Yebamoth. Sect. 64B, Slotki WI (trans), vol 1. London, Soncino Press, 1936, p 431

52. Otto JC: An account of an hemorrhagic disposition existing in certain families. Med Repository 6:1–4, 1803

53. Hay J: Account of a remarkable haemorrhagic disposition existing in many individuals of the same family. N Engl J Med Surg 2:221–225, 1813

54. Morgan TH: The Theory of the Gene. New York, Haffner, 1964 (reprint of 1929 edition, second printing)

55. Mr. Ward, quoted by Wardrop J: On the Curative Effects of the Abstraction of Blood. Philadelphia, A Waldie, 1837, pp 9–10

56. Wright AE: On the method of determining the condition of blood coagulability for clinical and experimental purposes, and on the effect of the administration of calcium salts in haemophilia and actual or threatened hemorrhage. Br Med J 2:223–225, 1893

57. Addis T: The pathogenesis of hereditary hemophilia. J Pathol Bacteriol 15:427–452, 1911

58. Patek AJ Jr, Stetson RH: Hemophilia. I. The abnormal coagulation of the blood and its relation to the blood platelets. J Clin Invest 15:531–542, 1936

59. Patek AJ Jr, Taylor FHL: Hemophilia. II. Some properties of a substance obtained from normal plasma effective in accelerating the clotting of hemophilic blood. J Clin Invest 16:113–124, 1937

60. Lane S: Hemorrhagic diathesis. Successful transfusion of blood. Lancet 1:185–188, 1840

61. Pool JG, Hershgold EJ, Pappenhagen AR: High-potency antihaemophilic factor concentrate prepared from cryoglobulin precipitate. Nature 203:312, 1964

62. Wagner RH, McLester WD, Smith M, et al: Purification of antihemophilic factor (factor VIII) by amino acid precipitation. Thromb Diath Haemorrh 11:67–74, 1964

63. Shanberge JN, Gore I: Studies on the immunologic and physiologic activites of antihemophilic factor (AHF). J Lab Clin Med 59:954, 1957 (abstract)

64. Bennett E. Heuhns ER: Immunologic differentiation of three types of haemophilia and identification of some female carriers. Lancet 2:956–958, 1970

65. Zimmerman TS, Ratnoff OD, Powell AE: Immunologic differentiation of classic hemophilia (factor VIII deficiency) and von Willebrand's disease, with observations on combined deficiencies of antihemophilic factor and proaccelerin (factor V) and on an acquired circulating anticoagulant against antihemophilic factor. J Clin Invest 50:244–254, 1971

66. Zimmerman TS, Ratnoff OD, Littell AS: Detection of carriers of classic hemophilia using an immunologic assay for antihemophilic factor (factor VIII). J Clin Invest 50:255–258, 1971

67. Willebrand EA von: Über hereditare Pseudohämophilie. Acta Med Scand 76:521–549, 1931

68. Hayem G, quoted by Dreyfuss C: Some Milestones in the History of Hematology. New York, Grune & Stratton, 1956

69. Duke WW: The relation of blood platelets to hemorrhagic disease. Description of a method for determining the bleeding time and coagulation time and report of three cases of hemorrhagic disease relieved by transfusion. JAMA 55:1185–1192, 1910

70. Minot GR: A familial hemorrhagic condition associated with prolongation of the bleeding time. Am J Med Sci 175:301–306, 1928

71. Alexander B, Goldstein R: Dual hemostatic defect in pseudohemophilia. J Clin Invest 32:55, 1953 (abstract)

72. Larrieu M-J, Soulier JP: Deficit en facteur anti-hemophilique chez une fille associé à un trouble de saignement. Rev Hemotal 8:361–370, 1953

73. Quick AJ, Hussey CV: Hemophilic condition in the female. J Lab Clin Med 42:929–930, 1953 (abstract)

74. Jürgens R, Lehmann W, Wegelius O, et al: Mitteilung über den Mangel an antihämophilem Globulin (Faktor VIII) bei der Aaländischen Thrombopathie (v. Willebrand-Jürgens). Thromb Diath Haemorrh 1:257–260, 1957

75. Howard MA, Firkin BG: Ristocetin—a new tool in the investigation of platelet aggregation. Thromb Diath Haemorrah 26:362–369, 1971

76. Tschopp T, Weiss HJ, Baumgartner H: Decreased adhesion of platelets to subendothelium in von Willebrand's disease. J Lab Clin Med 83:296–300, 1974

77. Manteuffel Z v: Bermerkungen zur Blutstillung bei Häemophilie. Dtsch Med Wochenschr 19:665–667, 1893

78. Pavlovsky A: Contribution to the pathogenesis of hemophilia. Blood 2:185–191, 1947

79. Aggeler PM, White SG, Glendenning MB, et al: Plasma thromboplastin component (PTC) deficiency: A new disease resembling hemophilia. Proc Soc Exp Biol Med 79:692–694, 1952

80. Schulman I, Smith CH: Hemorrhagic disease in an infant due to deficiency of a previously undescribed clotting factor. Blood 7:794–807, 1952

81. Biggs R, Douglas AS, Macfarlane RG, et al: Christmas disease: A condition previously mistaken for haemophilia. Br Med J 2:1378–1382, 1952

82. Ratnoff OD, Colopy JE: A familial hemorrhagic trait associated with a deficiency of a clot-promoting fraction of plasma. J Clin Invest 34:602–613, 1955

83. Margolis J: Glass surface and blood coagulation. Nature 178:805–806, 1956

84. Shafrir E, deVries A: Studies on the clot-promoting activity of glass. J Clin Invest 35:1183–1190, 1956

85. Rosenthal RL, Dreskin OH, Rosenthal N: New hemophilia-like disease caused by deficiency of a third plasma thromboplastin factor. Proc Soc Exp Biol Med 82:171–174, 1953

86. Schiffman S, Rapaport SI, Ware AG, et al: Separation of plasma thromboplastin antecedent (PTA) and Hageman factor (HF) from human plasma. Proc Soc Exp Biol Med 105:453–455, 1960

87. Hathaway WE, Belhasen LP, Hathaway HS: Evidence for a new plasma thromboplastin factor. I. Case report, coagulation studies and physicochemical properties. Blood 26:521–532, 1965

88. Waldmann, R, Abraham JP, Rebuck JW, et al: Fitzgerald factor: A hitherto unrecognized clotting factor. Lancet 1:949–950, 1975

89. Colman RW, Bagdasarian A, Talamo RC, et al: Williams trait: Human kininogen deficiency with diminished levels of plasminogen proactivator and prekallikrein associated with abnormalities of the Hageman factor-dependent pathways. J Clin Invest 56:1650–1662, 1975

90. Wuepper KD, Miller DR, Lacombe MJ: Flaujeac trait: Deficiency of human plasma kininogen. J Clin Invest 56:1663–1672, 1975

91. Donaldson VH, Glueck HI, Miller MA, et al: Kininogen deficiency in Fitzgerald trait: Role of high molecular weight kininogen in clotting and fibrinolysis. J Lab Clin Med 87:327–337, 1976

92. Wuepper KD: Biochemistry and biology of components of the plasma kinin-forming system,

in Lepow IH, Ward PA (eds): Inflammation, Mechanisms and Control. New York, Academic Press, 1972, pp 93–117

93. Ratnoff OD: Some relationships among hemostasis, fibrinolytic phenomena, immunity, and the inflammatory response, in Dixon FJ Jr, Kunkel HG (eds): Advances in Immunology, vol. 10, New York, Academic Press, 1969 pp 145–227

94. Bachman F, Duckert F, Fisch U, et al: Der Gerinnungsdefekt beim konigenitalen PTA-mangel. Schweiz Med Wochenschr 88:1037–1044, 1958

95. Soulier JP, Wartelle O, Ménaché D: Caractères differentiels des facteurs Hageman et P.T.A. Rôle du contact dans la phase initiale de la coagulation. Rev Fr Etudes Clin Biol 3:263–267, 1958

96. Bergsagel DE, Hougie C. Intermediate stages in the formation of blood thromboplastin. Br J. Haematol 2:113–129, 1956

97. Østerud B, Rapaport S: Activation of factor IX by the reaction product of tissue factor and factor VII: Additional pathway for initiating blood coagulation. Proc Natl Acad Sci USA 74:5260–5264, 1977

98. Laake K, Østerud B: Activation of purified plasma factor VII by human plasmin, plasma kallikrein, and activated components of the human intrinsic blood coagulation system. Thromb Res 5:759–772, 1974

99. Dam H: Cholesterinstoffwechsel in Hühnereiern und Hühnchen. Biochem Z 215:475–492, 1929

100. Dam H: The antihaemorrhagic vitamin of the chick. Occurrence and chemical nature, letter. Nature 135:652–653,1935

101. Almquist HJ: Purification of the antihemorrhagic vitamin. J Biol Chem 114:241–245, 1936

102. Almquist HJ, Close AA: Synthetic and natural antihemorrhagic compounds. J Am Chem Soc 61:2557–2558, 1939

103. Binkley SB, Cheney LC, Holcomb WF, et al: The constitution and synthesis of vitamin K. J Am Chem Soc 61:2558–2559, 1939

104. Feiser LF: Synthesis of 2-methyl-3-phytyl-1,4-naphthoquinine. J Am Chem Soc 61:2559–2560, 1939

105. Schönheyder F: The antihaemorrhagic vitamin of the chick. Measurement and biological action, letter. Nature 135:653, 1935

106. Seegers WH, Ulutin ON: Autoprothrombin II-anticoagulant (autoprothrombin II-A). Thromb Diath Haemorrh 6:270–281, 1961

107. Stenflo J: A new vitamin K-dependent protein. Purification from bovine plasma and preliminary characterization. J Biol Chem 251:355–363, 1976

108. Hauschka PV, Lian JB, Gallo PPM: Direct identification of calcium-binding amino acid, γ-carboxyglutamate, in mineralized tissue. Proc Natl Acad Sci USA 72:3925–3929, 1975

109. Waddell WW Jr, Guerry DuP III, Bray WE, et al: Possible effects of vitamin K on prothrombin and clotting time in newly-born infants. Proc Soc Exp Biol Med 40:432–434, 1939

110. Butt HR, Snell AM, Osterberg AE: The use of vitamin K and bile in treatment of the hemorrhagic diathesis in cases of jaundice. Proc Staff Meet Mayo Clin 13:74–77, 1939

111. Warner ED, Brinkhous KM, Smith HP: Bleeding tendency of obstructive jaundice: Prothrombin deficiency and dietary factors. Proc Soc Exp Biol Med 37:628–630, 1938

112. Dam H, Glavind J: Vitamin K in human pathology. Lancet 1:720–721, 1938

113. Olson JP, Miller LL, Troup SB: Synthesis of clotting factors by the isolated perfused rat liver. J Clin Invest 45:690–701, 1966

114. Stenflo J, Fernlund P, Egan W, et al: Vitamin K dependent modifications of glutamic acid residues in prothrombin. Proc Natl Acad Sci USA 71:2730–2733, 1974

115. Schofield FW: Damaged sweet clover: The cause of a new disease in cattle simulating hemorrhagic septicemia and black leg. J Am Vet Med Assoc 64:(ns 17):553–575, 1924

116. Link KP: The discovery of Dicumarol and its sequels. Circulation 19:97–107, 1959

117. Butt HR, Allen EV, Bollman JL: A preparation from spoiled sweet clover [3,3′-methylene-bis-

(4-hydroxycoumarin)] which prolongs coagulation and prothrombin time of the blood: Preliminary report of experimental and clinical studies. Proc Staff Meet Mayo Clin 16:388–395, 1941

118. Bingham JB, Meyer OO, Pohle FJ: Studies on the hemorrhagic agent 3,3′methylene bis-(4-hydroxycoumarin). I. The effect on the prothrombin and coagulation time of the blood of dogs and humans. Am J Med Sci 202:563–578, 1941

119. Suttie JW: Oral anticoagulant therapy: The biosynthetic basis. Semin Hematol 14:365–374, 1977

120. Konttinen YP: Fibrinolysis: Chemistry, Physiology, Pathology and Clinics. Tampere, Finland, Cy Star Ab, 1968

121. Denis PS: Essai sur l'Application de la Chemie à l'Étude Physiologique du Sang de l'Homme et à l'Étude Physio-pathologique, Hygiéneque et Thérapeutique des Maladies de Cette Humeur. Paris, Béchet Jeune, 1838

122. Denys J, de Marbaix H: Sur les peptonisations provoqueés par le chloroforme et quelques autre substances. Cellule 5:197–251, 1899

123. Dastre A: Fibrinolyse dans le sang. Arch Physiol Norm Pathol 5:661–663, 1893

124. Morawitz P: Uber einege postmortale Blutveränderungen. Beitr Chem Physiol Pathol Brunschweig 8:1–14, 1906

125. Hedin SG: On the presence of a proteolytic enzyme in the normal serum of the ox. J Physiol 30:195–201, 1904

126. Christensen LR, MacLeod CM: Proteolytic enzyme of serum: Characterization, activation and reaction with inhibitors. J Gen Physiol 23:559–583, 1945

127. Gratia A: Quoted by Kontinnen YP, in Fibrinolysis: Chemistry, Physiology, Pathology and Clinics. Tampere, Finland, Cy Star Ab, 1968

128. Tillett WS, Garner RL: The fibrinolytic activity of hemolytic streptococci. J Exp Med 58:485–502, 1933

129. Williams JRB: The fibrinolytic activity of urine. Br J Exp Pathol 32:530–537, 1951

130. Sherry S, Fletcher A, Alkjaersig N: Fibrinolysis and fibrinolytic activity in man. Physiol Rev 39:343–381, 1959

131. Macfarlane RG: Fibrinolysis after operation. Lancet 1:10–12, 1937

132. Biggs R, Macfarlane RG, Pilling J: Observations on fibrinolysis. Experimental activity produced by exercise or adrenaline. Lancet 1:402–405, 1947

133. Todd AS: The histological localisation of fibrinolysin activator. J Pathol Bacteriol 78:281–283, 1959

134. Laake K, Venneröd AM: Factor XII-induced fibrinolysis: Studies on the separation of prekallikrein, plasminogen proactivator, and factor XI in human plasma. Thromb Res 4:285–302, 1974

135. Mandle RJ Jr, Kaplan AP: Hageman-factor-dependent fibrinolysis: Generation of fibrinolytic activity by the interaction of human activated factor XI aand plasminogen. Blood 54:850–862, 1979

136. Howell WH: Theories of blood coagulation. Physiol Rev 15:435–470, 1935

137. Rettger LA: The coagulation of blood. Am J Physiol 24:406–435, 1909

138. McLean J: The discovery of heparin. Circulation 19:75–78, 1959

139. Seegers WH, Warner ED, Brinkhous KM, et al: Heparin and the antithrombic activity of plasma. Science 96:300–301, 1942

140. Yin ET, Wessler S, Stoll PJ: Biological properties of the naturally occurring plasma inhibitor to activated factor X. J Biol Chem 246:3703–3711, 1971

141. Rosenberg RD: Heparin, antithrombin and abnormal clotting. Ann Rev Med 29:367–378, 1978

142. Charles AF, Scott DA: Studies on heparin IV. Observations on the chemistry of heparin. Biochem J 30:1927–1933, 1936

143. Jorpes E: Heparin in the Treatment of Thrombosis. An Account of its Chemistry, Physiology and Application in Medicine (ed 2). New York, Oxford University Press, 1946

144. Mason EC: Blood coagulation. The production and prevention of thrombosis and pulmonary embolism. Surg Gynecol Obstet 39:421–428, 1924

145. Collen D: Identification and some properties of a new fast-reacting plasmin inhibitor in human plasma. Eur J Biochem 69:209–216, 1976

146. Moroi M, Aoki N: Isolation and characterization of $\alpha_2$-plasmin inhibitor from human plasma. A novel proteinase inhibitor which inhibits activator-induced clot lysis. J Biol Chem 251:5956–5965, 1976

147. Delezenne C, Pozerski E: Action proteolytique du sérum sanguin préalablement traité par le chloroforme. C R Soc Biol 55:690–692, 1903

148. Aoki N, Saito H, Kamiya T, et al: Congenital deficiency of $\alpha_2$-plasmin inhibitor associated with severe hemorrhagic tendency. J Clin Invest 63:877–884, 1979

149. Ganrot PO: Inhibition of plasmin activity by $\alpha_2$-macroglobulin. Clin Chim Acta 16:328–330, 1967

150. Gans H, Tan BH: $\alpha_1$-Antitrypsin, an inhibitor for thrombin and plasmin. Clin Chim Acta 17:111–117, 1967

151. Heck LW, Kaplan AP: Substrates of Hageman factor. I. Isolation and characterization of human factor XI (PTA) and inhibition of the activated enzyme by $\alpha_1$-antitrypsin. J Exp Med 140:1615–1630, 1974

152. Marlar RA, Griffin JH: Deficiency of protein C inhibitor in combined factor V/VIII deficiency disease. J Clin Invest 66:1186–1189, 1980

153. Kemp GT: On the so called "new element" of the blood and its relation to coagulation. Johns Hopkins Univ Biol Lab Studies 3:292–349, 1884

154. Robb-Smith AHT: Why the platelets were discovered. Br J Haematol 13:618–637, 1967

155. Spaet TH: Platelets: The blood dust, In Wintrobe MM (ed): Blood, Pure and Eloquent. New York, McGraw-Hill, 1980, pp 548–571

156. Donné A: De l'origine des globules du sang, de leur mode de formation et leur fin. C R Acad Sci (Paris) 14:366–368, 1842 (abstract)

157. Gulliver G, quoted by Robb-Smith (154)

158. Addison W: On the colourless corpuscles and on the molecules and cytoblasts in the blood. Lond Med Gaz ns 30:144–148, 1841–1842

159. Hayem G: Recherches sur l'évolution des hématies dans le sang de l'homme et des vertébrés. Arch Physiol Norm Pathol 10:692–734, 1878

160. Osler W: An account of certain organisms occurring in the liquor sanguinis. Proc Royal Soc (Lond) 22:391–398, 1874

161. Tocantins LM: The mammalian blood platelet in health and disease. Medicine 17:155–258, 1938

162. Wright JH: Die Entstehung der Blutplättchen. Virchows Arch (Pathol Anat) 186:55–63, 1906

163. Woodcock HM: An introduction to the study of haematophagy. J Royal Army Med Corps 37:321–341, 1921

164. Krauss 1883 Inaug Dis Heidelberg, quoted by Macfarlane RG: Critical review: The mechanism of haemostasis. Q J Med ns 10:1–29, 1941

165. Hayem G: Sur un cas de diathése hémorrhagique. Bull Mem Soc Med Hop Paris 8:389–394, 1891

166. Denys J: Études sur la coagulation du sang. Cellule 3:445–461, 1886

167. Kaznelson P: Verschwinden der hämorrhagischen Diathese bei einem Falle von "essentieller Thrombopenie" (Frank) nach Milzextirpation. Splenogene thrombolytische purpura. Wien Klin Wochenschr 29:1451–1464, 1916

168. Ranvier LA: Du mode de formation de la fibrine dans le sang extrait des vaisseaux. C R Soc Biol 5:46–50, 1873

169. Hayem G: Sur le méchanisme de l'arrêt des hémorrhagies. C R Acad Sci 95:18–21, 1882

170. Wright JH, Minot GR: The viscous metamorphosis of the blood platelets. J Exp Med 26:395–409, 1917

171. Marcus AJ: Platelet function. N Engl J Med 280:1213–1220, 1278–1284, 1330–1335, 1969
172. Bounameaux Y, Roskam J: L'accolement des plaquettes aux fibres sous-endothéliales. C R Soc Biol 153:865–867, 1959
173. Hugues J: Accolement des plaquettes au collagéne. C R Soc Biol 154:866–868, 1960
174. Zucker MG, Borelli J: Platelet clumping produced by connective tissue suspensions and by collagen. Proc Soc Exp Biol Med 109:779–787, 1962
175. Gaarder A, Jonsen J, Laland L, et al: Adenosine diphosphate in red cells as a factor in the adhesiveness of human blood platelets. Nature 192:531–532, 1961
176. Hovig T: Release of a platelet-aggregating substance (adenosine diphosphate) from rabbit blood platelets induced by saline "extract" of tendons. Thromb Diath Haemmorrh 9:264–278, 1973
177. Spaet TH, Zucker MB: Mechanism of platelet plug formation and role of adenosine diphosphate. Am J Physiol 206:1267–1274, 1964
178. Grette K: Studies on the mechanism of thrombin-catalyzed hemostatic reactions in blood platelets. Acta Physiol Scand Suppl 195:1–93, 1962
179. Smith JB, Ingerman C, Kocsis JJ, et al: Formation of prostaglandins during aggregation of human blood platelets. J Clin Invest 52:965–969, 1973
180. Willis AL, Vane FM, Kuhn DC, et al: An endoperoxide aggregator (LASS), formed in platelets in response to thrombotic stimuli. Prostaglandins 8:453–507, 1974
181. Packham MA, Kinlough-Rathbone RL, Reimers JH, et al: Mechanisms of platelet aggregation independent of adenosine diphosphate, in Silver MJ, Smith JB, Kocsis JJ, (eds): Prostaglandins in Hematology. New York, Spectrum Books, 1977 pp 247–276
182. Marcus AJ: The role of prostaglandins in platelet formation, in Brown EB (ed): Progress in Hematology, vol. 11. New York, Grune & Stratton, 1979, pp 147–171
183. Kurzrok R, Lieb CC: Biochemical studies of human semen. II. The action of semen on the human uterus. Proc Soc Exp Biol Med 28:268–272, 1930
184. Goldblatt MW: Properties of human seminal plasma. J Physiol 84:208–218, 1935
185. von Euler US: On the specific vaso-dilating and plain muscle stimulating substances from accessory genital glands in man and certain animals (prostaglandin and vesiglandin). J Physiol 88:213–234, 1936
186. Bergström S, Ryhage R, Samuelsson B, et al: Prostaglandins and related factors. 15. The structure of prostaglandin $E_1$, $F_{1\alpha}$ and $F_{1\beta}$. J Biol Chem 238:3555–3564, 1963
187. Bergström S, Danielsson H, Samuelsson B: The enzymatic formation of prostaglandin $E_2$ from arachidonic acid. Prostaglandins and related factors 32. Biochem Biophys Acta 90:207–210, 1964
188. Dorp DA van, Beerthius RK, Nugteren DH, et al: The biosynthesis of prostaglandins. Biochem Biophys Acta 90:204–207, 1964
189. Silver MJ, Smith JB, Ingerman C, et al: Arachidonic acid-induced human platelet aggregation and prostaglandin formation. Prostaglandins 4:863–875, 1973
190. Hamberg M, Svensson J, Samuelsson B: Thromboxanes: A new group of biologically active components derived from prostaglandin endoperoxides. Proc Natl Acad Sci USA 72:2994–2998, 1975
191. Bills TK, Smith JB, Silver MJ: Selective release of arachidonic acid from the phospholipids of human platelets in response to thrombin. J Clin Invest 60:1–6, 1977
192. Singer R: Acetylsalicylic acid, a probable cause for secondary posttonsillectomy hemorrhage. A preliminary report. Arch Otolaryngol 42:19–20, 1945
193. Quick AJ: Salicylates and bleeding: The aspirin tolerance test. Am J Med Sci 252:265–269, 1966
194. Weiss HJ, Aledort LM: Impaired platelet/connective-tissue reaction after aspirin ingestion. Lancet 2:495–497, 1967
195. O'Brien JR: Effects of salicylates on human platelets. Lancet 1:779–783, 1968

196.  Zucker MG, Peterson J: Inhibition of adenosine diphosphate-induced secondary aggregation and other platelet functions by acetylsalicylic acid ingestion. Proc Soc Exp Biol Med 127: 547–551, 1968

197.  Willis AL, Kuhn DC: A new potential mediator of arterial thrombosis whose biosynthesis is inhibited by aspirin. Prostaglandins 4:127–130, 1973

198.  Roth GJ, Stanford N, Majerus PW: Acetylation of prostaglandin synthetase by aspirin. Proc Natl Acad Sci USA 72:3073–3076, 1975

199.  O'Connor JM: Über den Adrenalingehalt des Blutes. Arch Exp Pathol Pharmacol 67:195–232, 1912

200.  Janeway TC, Richardson HB, Park EA: Experiments on the vasoconstrictor action of blood serum. Arch Intern Med 21:565–603, 1918

201.  Hirose K: Relation between the platelet count of human blood and its vasoconstrictor action after clotting. Arch Intern Med 21:604–612, 1918

202.  Rand M, Reid G: Source of "serotonin" in serum. Nature 168:385, 1951

203.  Zucker MB, Borreli J: Relationship of some blood-clotting factors to serotonin release from washed platelets. J Appl Physiol 7:432–442, 1955

204.  Vulpian: CR Soc Biol 5:49–50, 1873 (no title)

205.  Wright HP: Changes in the adhesiveness of blood platelets following parturition and surgical operations. J Pathol Bacteriol 54:461–468, 1942

206.  Moolten S, Vroman L: The adhesiveness of blood platelets in thrombo-embolism. I. Measurement of platelet adhesiveness by glass-wool filter. Am J Clin Pathol 19:701–709, 1949

207.  Hellem AJ: Platelet adhesiveness. Ser Haematol 1 (2):99–145, 1968

208.  Mustard JF, Packham MA: Factors influencing platelet function: Adhesion, release and aggregation. Pharmacol Rev 22:97–187, 1970

209.  Salzman EW: Measurement of platelet adhesiveness. A simple in vitro technique demonstrating an abnormality in von Willebrand's disease. J Lab Clin Med 62:724–735, 1963

210.  Bouma BN, Wiegerinck Y, Sixma JJ et al: Immunological characterization of purified anti-haemophilic factor A (factor VIII) which corrects abnormal platelet retention in von Willebrand's disease. Nature (New Biol) 236:104–106, 1972

211.  Norris W, quoted by Robb-Smith AHT: Why the platelets were discovered. Br J Haematol 13:618–637, 1967

212.  Hayem G: Du Sang et des Alterations Anatomiques. Paris, Masson, 1889

213.  Lee RI, Vincent B: The coagulation of normal human blood. An experimental study. Arch Intern Med 13:398–425, 1914

214.  Chargaff E, Bancroft FW, Stanley-Brown M: Studies on the chemistry of blood coagulation. III. The chemical constituents of blood and their role in blood clotting, with remarks on the activation of clotting by lipids. J Biol Chem 116:237–251, 1936

215.  Brinkhous KM: Clotting defect in hemophilia: Deficiency in a plasma factor required for platelet utilization. Proc Soc Exp Biol Med 66:117–120, 1947

216.  Creveld S van, Paulssen MMP: Isolation and properties of the third clotting factor in blood platelets. Lancet 1:23–25, 1952

217.  Marcus AJ, Zucker-Franklin D, Safier LB, et al: Studies on human platelet granules and membranes. J Clin Invest 45:14–28, 1966

218.  Mustard JF, Hegardt B, Rowsell HC, et al: Effect of adenosine nucleotides on platelet aggregation and clotting time. J Lab Clin Med 64:548–559, 1964

219.  Miletich JP, Jackson CM, Majerus PW: Interaction of coagulation factor $X_a$ with human platelets. Proc Natl Acad Sci USA 74:4033–4036, 1977

220.  LeSourd L, Pagniez P: Du rôle des hématoblastes dans la rétraction du caillot. Recherches expérimentales. C R Soc Biol 61:109–111, 1906

221.  Bettex-Galland M, Lüscher EF: Extraction of an actomyosin-like protein from human thrombocytes. Nature 184:276–277, 1959

222. Budtz-Olsen OE: Clot Retraction. Springfield, Ill, Charles C Thomas, 1951
223. Glanzmann E: Hereditáre hámorrhagische Thrombasthenie: Ein Beitrag zur Pathologie der Blutplättchen. Jahrbuch Kinderheilkunde 88:113–141, 1918
224. Conley CL, Hartmann, RC, Lalley JS: The relationship of heparin activity to platelet concentration. Proc Soc Exp Biol Med 69:284–287, 1948

Hidehiko Saito

# 2

# Normal Hemostatic Mechanisms

It is not uncommon in everyday life to see bleeding from a nose or a small cut in the skin. In most instances, however, the bleeding appears to stop promptly. This happy outcome results from the action of our normal hemostatic process. Hemostasis, the arrest of hemorrhage at the site of injury, is one of the most basic host defense mechanisms. Without hemostasis, we might exsanguinate from even a trivial trauma. On the other hand, excessive and untimely formation of blood clots inside blood vessels may cut off the blood supply to vital organs. Fortunately, the body has an integrated system of checks and balances that allows both maintenance of blood fluidity and prompt, timely arrest of hemorrhage.

When a blood vessel is disrupted, three major mechanisms operate to control the bleeding: (1) vessel wall contraction, (2) platelet adherence to the injured vessel wall and platelet aggregation, and (3) formation and maintenance of fibrin clots. All three mechanisms are essential for normal hemostasis, and they function in concert rather than at random. Abnormal bleeding (a hemorrhagic tendency) may result from defects in any of these mechanisms, and if two or all three are impaired, very severe bleeding may occur.

For an understanding of hemorrhagic tendency, it is convenient to divide hemostasis into two continuous yet separate stages, primary and secondary. Primary hemostasis, the instantaneous plugging of a hole in the vessel wall, is achieved by a combination of vasoconstriction and platelet adhesion and aggregation. The formation of a fibrin clot is not essential at this stage. Patients with impaired blood coagulation such as hemophiliacs, therefore, have normal primary hemostasis, whereas those with thrombocytopenia show defective primary hemostasis. Primary hemostasis, however, is of temporary benefit. Bleeding may start afresh unless the friable platelet plug is reinforced by a tough fibrin mesh. This secondary hemostasis is accomplished by the formation of fibrin (blood coagulation) and helps to maintain a hemostatic plug until healing is complete. In the process of tissue repair, a fibrin-platelet plug is gradually resolved by fibrinolysis and replaced by organized tissue. Premature lysis of a clot by accelerated fibrinolysis may also lead to rebleeding, suggesting a role for fibrinolysis in normal hemostasis.

For clarity, the following sections deal with each component of the hemostatic mechanisms individually. It cannot, however, be overemphasized that these mechanisms are intimately related and inseparable.

## ROLE OF VESSEL WALL CONTRACTION IN HEMOSTASIS

The immediate control of bleeding from a severed small vessel is accomplished by vasoconstriction. Small arteries and veins contain smooth muscle that can contract powerfully when injured. Capillaries do not have muscle fibers, but the precapillary sphincter may serve to control the bleeding. Vascular contraction reduces the blood flow through an injured area and may be sufficient, at least temporarily, to seal off the defect in small vessels. Vasoconstriction is less effective in preventing blood loss from a large artery or vein.

What initiates and mediates vasoconstriction is only poorly understood. There appear to be two types of responses to injury, neurogenic spasm and myogenic spasm. The first response is a reflex dependent upon an intact nerve supply and lasts for only 10–30 seconds. The second is mediated by a direct local myogenic impulse and continues for as long as one hour. It is interesting to speculate that vasoactive substances such as serotonin (5-hydroxytryptamine) may be liberated from damaged platelets at the site of injury and may contribute to the vascular response. There is no convincing evidence to support this view. In fact, depletion of serotonin by administration of reserpine in man has no effect in hemostasis. Platelets also produce and release a potent vasoconstricter, thromboxane $A_2$, in the process of adhesion and aggregation.

Agents that affect the vessel wall may be generated during blood coagulation. When factor XII (Hageman factor) is activated, it induces the production of small peptides such as bradykinin that increase vascular permeability and cause smooth muscle to contract. Further, a segment of fibrinogen (fibrinopeptide B), released by the action of thrombin, has been shown to induce smooth muscle contraction directly or indirectly. Whether these substances contribute to in vivo hemostasis is not known.

The extent of bleeding is also influenced by the tension of the extravascular supporting tissue. Hemorrhage into muscles or joints is usually limited, as the increased tissue pressure causes small blood vessels to collapse. In contrast, bleeding into the gastrointestinal tract may be difficult to control.

## ROLE OF PLATELETS IN HEMOSTASIS

Platelets are small, round anuclear cells that contain fine, scattered granules and have a diameter about one-third that of red cells. Platelets are produced by megakaryocytes found in adult bone marrow. Platelets circulate for approximately 10 days in the blood. Normal blood contains 200,000–400,000 platelets/μl. Platelets normally circulate as round, disc-shaped cells that do not adhere to normal vascular lining or to each other.

An electron micrograph of the platelet (Fig. 2-1) demonstrates many subcellular granules (dense bodies and α-granules) as well as mitochondria (M). Dense bodies (DB) contain adenosine diphosphate (ADP), adenosine triphosphate (ATP), calcium, and serotonin. The α-granules (G) store, among other substances, fibrinogen, platelet factor 4 (PF 4), β-thromboglobulin, and platelet-derived growth factor. These substances present in granules play a major role in platelet function, as discussed below. Platelets also contain microfilaments and a circumferential band of microtubules (MT). The latter may be involved in maintaining the shape of the platelets and in the contractile phenomena that occur during platelet secretion and clot retraction. The open canalicular system (OCS) represents tortuous channels in the platelet cytoplasm and may facilitate the uptake and transfer of

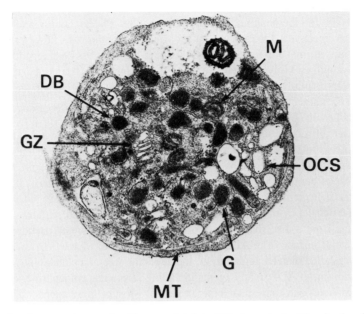

**Fig. 2-1.** An electron micrograph of human platelets. DB: dense body; M: mitochondria; OCS: open canalicular system; G: α-granules; MT: microtobules; GZ: Golgi apparatus. Magnification 26,000 × . (Courtesy of Dr. M. Aikawa, the Institute of Pathology, Case Western Reserve University, School of Medicine)

substances in blood plasma. It may also serve as a conduit for the discharge of stored materials during the platelet release reaction.

The role of platelets in hemostasis is at least twofold. Platelets form a hemostatic plug at the site of injury and provide procoagulant activity including phospholipid for fibrin formation.

## THE FORMATION OF A HEMOSTATIC PLUG

Hemostatic plug formation may be divided into several separate yet interrelated steps. Within seconds after injury, platelets gather at the site of vascular damage and begin to adhere to the surface of the disrupted vessel wall. This is referred as platelet adhesion and is the initial event in platelet plug formation. Platelets do not adhere to normal endothelium. The reason for the lack of reactivity of intact endothelial cells and platelets is not known, but it has been suggested that a potent platelet inhibitor, prostacyclin (PGI$_2$), which is produced by endothelial cells, may prevent platelet adhesion. It is the disruption of the vascular lining and the contact of platelets with subendothelial structures that initiate adhesion. Collagen, basement membrane, and microfibrils are among the substances to which platelets adhere. Platelets have a particularly strong affinity for collagen.

The actual mechanisms of adhesion are not fully understood. There are two hereditary hemorrhagic disorders in which platelet adhesion to the subendothelium is impaired. Both conditions are associated with a prolonged bleeding time. Platelets from patients with von Willebrand's disease do not adhere normally to damaged vascular walls. This abnormality is corrected by a plasma protein present in normal plasma but deficient in that of von Willebrand's disease (von Willebrand factor). This factor is now believed to be part of the factor VIII (antihemophilic factor, AHF) complex. Platelet adhesion to the subendo-thelium is also defective in the Bernard-Soulier syndrome. In this case, however, the patient's plasma contains normal amounts of von Willebrand factor. It has been recently shown that one of the glycoproteins (glycoprotein I) of the platelet membrane is reduced in this syndrome. These observations imply that both von Willebrand factor and platelet membrane glycoprotein are required for interaction of the platelet surface and subendothelium.

After adhesion, platelets undergo a shape change and a secretory process by which certain biologically active substances such as ADP, ATP, and serotonin that are present in platelet granules are actively discharged to the outside of cells (release reaction). This process is analogous to the secretion by endocrine glands and appears to require the participa-tion of a platelet contractile protein, actomyosin. The release reaction is not due to the rupture of the cell membranes; rather, it is a highly selective process since not all sub-stances in the platelet cytoplasm are discharged. The released ADP, in turn, causes plate-lets to change from a disc shape to a more rounded form in which pseudopodia extend from the platelet surface. The ADP induces the adhesion of platelets to each other. This phenomenon, called platelet aggregation, increases the size of a platelet plug at the site of injury. In addition to ADP, many agents including serotonin, epinephrine, collagen, and immune complexes can cause platelet aggregation. Most of these agents appear to act by binding to specific receptors on the platelet surface membrane. How a variety of substances initiates aggregation is not fully understood. It is possible that there is more than one mode of action.

Recent studies suggest that a group of lipids, prostaglandins, play an important role in mediating the platelet release reaction and aggregation. ADP and collagen trigger the activation of one or more phospholipases present in the platelet membrane. The phos-pholipases then hydrolyze membrane phospholipid, releasing arachidonic acid. Once liberated, arachidonic acid is metabolized by an enzyme, cyclooxygenase, to form prosta-glandin endoperoxides that, in turn, are converted to thromboxane $A_2$. Thromboxane $A_2$ is an extremely potent but labile (half-life = 30 seconds) substance that induces platelet aggregation and secretion. Platelet aggregation will not occur in the absence of fibrinogen. This suggests a requirement for fibrinogen, although the exact mechanism is not known. When thrombin is generated via activation of the blood-clotting cascade, it too can induce platelet aggregation, and it brings about the formation of a fibrin mesh around the platelet mass that consolidates the hemostatic plug. It is important to note that all of these reac-tions proceed synergistically and almost simultaneously with each other to promote hemostasis.

The importance of the platelet in hemostasis is well illustrated not only by patients with thrombocytopenia but also by those with qualitative platelet abnormalities. The latter group includes patients with congenital or acquired defects in the secretory process such as storage pool disease and a primary release defect. These patients suffer from a bleeding tendency despite the presence of normal numbers of platelets because ADP is not released normally.

## ROLE OF PLATELETS IN FIBRIN FORMATION

It has long been recognized that besides playing a role in hemostatic plug formation, platelets contribute to blood coagulation. They supply the procoagulant activity known as platelet factor 3 (PF 3). This activity has been attributed to surface membrane lipoproteins.

**Table 2-1**
Glossary of Coagulation Factors

| Factor | Synonyms | Normal Plasma Concentration (mg/dl) |
|---|---|---|
| I | Fibrinogen | 200–400 |
| II | Prothrombin | 10 |
| III | Tissue thromboplastin, tissue factor | 0 |
| IV | Calcium ion | 4–5 |
| V | Proaccelerin, labile factor | 1 |
| VII | Serum prothrombin conversion accelerator (SPCA), stable factor | 0.05 |
| VIII | Antihemophilic factor | 1–2 |
| IX | Christmas factor | 0.3 |
| X | Stuart–Prower factor | 1 |
| XI | Plasma thromboplastin antecedent (PTA) | 0.5 |
| XII | Hageman factor | 3 |
| XIII | Fibrin stabilizing factor (FSF) | 1–2 |
| Prekallikrein | Fletcher factor | 5 |
| High molecular weight kininogen | Fitzgerald, Flaujeac, Williams factor, contact activation cofactor | 6 |

PF 3 is not demonstrable in intact platelets, but it apparently becomes activated or available on the surface of aggregated platelets. PF 3 appears to act at least 2 steps in blood coagulation, the activation of factor X (Stuart factor) and the conversion of prothrombin to thrombin. PF 3 supplies a suitable surface upon which prothrombin or factor X forms a multimolecular complex with their respective enzymes and cofactors.

Recent studies have elucidated some mechanisms by which platelets participate in the activation of prothrombin. Platelets accelerate prothrombin conversion by binding factor V (proaccelerin), which, when activated to factor Va by thrombin, serves as a receptor for factor Xa. The binding of Xa to Va on the platelet's surface dramatically increases prothrombin conversion to thrombin.

Platelets have also been proposed to participate in the earliest phase of blood coagulation, but the significance of this phenomenon has not yet been confirmed.

Some coagulation factors, including fibrinogen, factor V, and factor VIII, are known to be released from platelet granules during the release reaction. The role of this phenomenon in hemostasis, however, is obscure.

A much more complete discussion of platelet physiology and pathology is provided in Chapter 4.

## ROLE OF BLOOD COAGULATION IN HEMOSTASIS

When vasoconstriction and platelet plug formation fail to stop bleeding or to maintain hemostasis, the formation of fibrin clots via blood coagulation serves to ensure hemostasis.

Blood coagulation is the end result of many complex reactions involving various trace plasma proteins named coagulation factors. Table 2-1 lists the well-recognized coagulation factors with their roman numerical designations and synonyms and their normal plasma concentrations. The numerals were assigned in the order of the discovery of the clotting

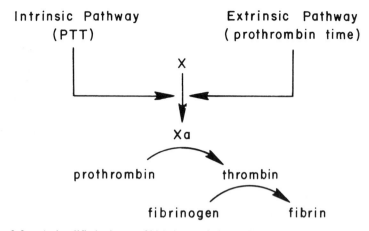

**Fig. 2-2.** A simplified scheme of blood coagulation. PTT: partial thromboplastin time.

factors and do not reflect the sequence of reactions. Factor III originally referred to tissue thromboplastin and factor IV to calcium ions. These terms are, however, seldom used. For the other factors, roman numerals and the descriptive terms are used interchangeably. The majority of clotting factors are present in plasma in an inert precursor form and are converted to their active enzymatic forms during coagulation. When the letter ''a'' accompanies a roman numeral (e.g., factor Xa), this indicates that the factor is in its activated form rather than in its naturally occurring precursor form (factor X).

It is interesting to note that most coagulation factors were originally discovered as agents functionally deficient in the plasmas of patients with certain hereditary bleeding disorders. Factor VIII (antihemophilic factor, AHF) is an agent functionally deficient in plasmas of patients with classic hemophilia, and factor X (Stuart factor) is a factor absent in plasmas of patients with factor X deficiency. Studies of these patients strongly influenced the development of our concept of blood coagulation. Without these hereditary disorders, our understanding of this highly complex reaction would still be in a primitive stage.

During the past 10 years, most of the coagulation factors have been isolated from both human and animal plasma and have been fairly well characterized. We therefore now know more about the biochemical basis of their mode of action. On the other hand, most of our information has been derived from artificial in vitro experiments using purified proteins, and hence is not necessarily applicable to in vivo phenomena. Some of our knowledge has been obtained from studies of bovine clotting factors, but no attempt is made in the following sections to distinguish the species from which the factors were derived.

Blood coagulation results from the conversion of a soluble plasma protein, fibrinogen, into insoluble fibrin. This reaction is catalyzed by an enzyme, thrombin. Thrombin is not normally present in our circulating blood, but exists as an inert precursor, prothrombin. Figure 2-2 illustrates a simplified view of blood coagulation. The generation of thrombin from prothrombin is mediated by at least two separate chains of reactions described as extrinsic and intrinsic pathways. Exposure of blood to injured tissue initiates blood clotting by the extrinsic pathway. We call it extrinsic because tissue thromboplastin (tissue factor) comes from outside the blood. The prothrombin time screens the efficiency of this pathway. When blood is drawn carefully so that it is not contaminated with tissue juice, it still clots in a glass tube. This pathway is called intrinsic since everything required for clotting appears to be present in the blood. The intrinsic pathway is triggered by contact of factor XII (Hageman factor) with foreign surfaces. The partial thromboplastin time (PTT) is a good monitor for this pathway. The difference in the two pathways lies in the way factor X is activated. Both pathways share a common pathway after the activation of factor X. Once it is activated, the steps leading to the formation of thrombin in both pathways consist of a series of proenzyme–enzyme conversions, each enzyme sequentially activating the proenzyme next in line, as will be discussed below. This basic concept, originally proposed in 1964 (the waterfall or cascade hypothesis), still appears to hold, although some minor modifications have been necessary.

The concept of two separate pathways is of practical value, since the results of the prothrombin time and PTT tests usually help to localize an abnormality in the coagulation scheme. Recent studies, however, suggest that there are many links between them. Whether the two pathways are sharply separable in vivo is not known. It is clear from clinical observations that both pathways are essential for normal hemostasis, since deficiencies of factors VII, VIII, and IX all result in bleeding tendencies.

Each step in the blood coagulation mechanism will be described individually in the following sections.


## THE FORMATION OF FIBRIN

Fibrinogen (factor I) is a large plasma protein, (340,000 molecular weight). It is synthesized in hepatic parenchymal cells, and its concentration in normal plasma ranges between 200 and 400 mg/dl. The half-life of fibrinogen in the circulation is about 3 days. How fibrinogen is catabolized is not fully understood, but it appears that the formation of fibrin from fibrinogen plays only a minor role in its catabolism. Fibrinogen is a dimer, each half of which is composed of three nonidentical peptide chains, called $A\alpha$, $B\beta$, and $\gamma$ respectively. The formula for fibrinogen may thus be expressed as $A\alpha_2 B\beta_2 \gamma_2$. The chains and dimer structure are held together by disulfide bonds. Small amounts of carbohydrate are present, but their role in the function of fibrinogen is not known.

The conversion of fibrinogen to fibrin proceeds in three stages (Fig. 2-3). The first step is the cleavage of 4 small peptides (2 fibrinopeptides A and 2 fibrinopeptides B) from the fibrinogen molecule by the action of a proteolytic enzyme, thrombin. Fibrinopeptides A are released from the amino-terminal end of the two $A\alpha$ chains and fibrinopeptides B from that of two $B\beta$ chains. The release of the A peptides occurs much faster than that of the B peptides and seems to be essential for polymerization of the fibrin monomers. Indeed, snake venoms such as Reptilase cleave only the A peptide and are still able to bring about clotting. The $\gamma$-chains are not hydrolyzed during the formation of fibrin and stay intact.

Fibrinogen from which peptides A and B have been severed is called fibrin monomer. The second step is the polymerization of fibrin monomers. These aggregate or polymerize spontaneously, end to end and side to side, to form fibrin polymers (fibrin strands). Fibrin polymer is readily dissolved in denaturing agents such as urea or monochloroacetic acid. It is also very susceptible to attack by a fibrinolytic enzyme, plasmin. The third step of fibrin formation is the production of a tough, insoluble form of this protein and requires the action of factor XIII (fibrin-stabilizing factor) and calcium ions. Factor XIII, activated by thrombin, crosslinks fibrin polymer by covalent bonds. Factor XIIIa catalyzes the formation of intermolecular $\gamma$-glutamyl-$\epsilon$-lysine bridges between the side chains of fibrin molecules. This increases the mechanical rigidity of the clot and renders it insoluble in urea and

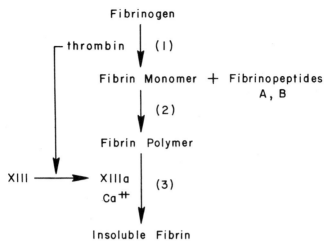

**Fig. 2-3.**  Three steps in the formation of fibrin.

monochloroacetic acid. It has recently been shown that two plasma proteins (fibronectin and $\alpha_2$-plasmin inhibitor) are also covalently crosslinked to fibrin by factor XIIIa and are incorporated into the clot. Increased resistance of the insoluble fibrin to fibrinolysis is probably related to incorporation into the clot of $\alpha_2$-plasmin inhibitor, a potent inhibitor of plasmin.

Factor XIII is present in plasma as an inert precursor (1–2 mg/dl) that consists of two pairs of two different subunits called *a* and *b*. The structure of plasma factor XIII thus may be written as $a_2b_2$. Platelets also contain factor XIII that is composed only of two a subunits ($a_2$). At the time of clotting, factor XIII is converted to its active form (factor XIIIa) by the action of thrombin. Thombin cleaves a small polypeptide from each a subunit. In platelets, factor XIII, activated in this way, has enzymatic activity. In plasma factor XIII, the $a_2b_2$ tetramer then dissociates in the presence of calcium ions into $a_2$ and $b_2$ dimers. This step is apparently required for exposure of the active center. Thrombin thus has two functions in the conversion of fibrinogen to fibrin; it splits fibrinopeptides A and B from the A$\alpha$ and B$\beta$ chains of fibrinogen, respectively, and it activates factor XIII to its enzymatic form (factor XIIIa).

## ACTIVATION OF PROTHROMBIN AND GENERATION OF THROMBIN

Thrombin is generated during blood coagulation by the activation of its inactive precursor, prothrombin. The concentration of prothrombin in normal plasma is approximately 10 mg/dl, and its half-life in the circulation is about 60 hours. Prothrombin (factor II) is a single-chain glycoprotein (70,000 molecular weight) that is produced by hepatic parenchymal cells in the presence of vitamin K. The structure of prothrombin has been studied extensively, and its complete amino acid sequence is now known. Recent evidence suggests that prothrombin and other vitamin K-dependent clotting factors (factors VII, IX, and X) contain unique $\gamma$-carboxylglutamic acid residues. These unusual amino acid residues are apparently incorporated into a polypeptide chain of the vitamin K-dependent clotting factors by the action of a carboxylase in hepatocytes. Vitamin K is an essential cofactor of this reaction; the formation of $\gamma$-carboxylglutamic acid residues are vitamin K

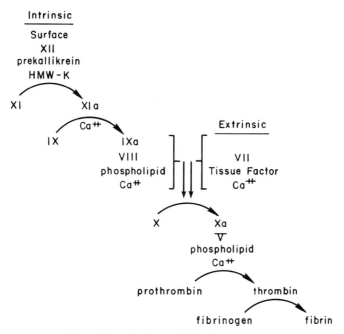

**Fig. 2-4.**   A scheme of blood coagulation.

dependent. The unique amino acid residues bind calcium ions and are essential for the function of vitamin K-dependent clotting factors.

The conversion of prothrombin to thrombin is mediated by the action of activated factor X (factor Xa). Factor Xa splits two peptide bonds in the prothrombin molecule and releases thrombin. Although factor Xa alone is able to activate prothrombin, the speed of the reaction is rather slow. The rate of activation by factor Xa is accelerated several thousandfold by the presence of factor V (proaccelerin), phospholipids (PF 3), and calcium ions (Fig. 2-4). The mechanism of this tremendous enhancement has been recently elucidated. It has been proposed that both factor Xa and prothrombin bind to the phospholipid surface via their γ-carboxylglutamic acid residues and calcium ions. Factor V also binds to phospholipid and prothrombin. The common property of these factors of binding to phospholipids provides a mechanism for bringing together into a highly organized complex these three factors that normally circulate separately. Formation of this multimolecular complex on the phospholipid surface brings molecules of prothrombin (a substrate) and factor Xa (an enzyme) together and increases their chance of interacting. It has also been shown that when factor Xa is associated with phospholipid and factor V, it is protected from inhibition by antithrombin III.

Factor V is a large plasma protein (250,000–300,000 molecular weight) and is present in normal plasma at an average concentration of 1 mg/dl. It is probably produced in the liver. Factor V has no enzymatic activity of its own and participates as a cofactor in the activation of prothrombin by factor Xa. When factor V is altered or activated by a trace amount of thrombin, it is converted to a form that is able to bind to prothrombin. In this state, it enhances prothrombin activation markedly. The nature of the accelerating effect of factor V is poorly understood, but it has been suggested that a conformational change may be induced in prothrombin, making cleavage by factor Xa more efficient.

Several mechanisms appear to control the generation of thrombin from prothrombin.

The interaction of factor V with thrombin not only enhances its reactivity but also brings about its activation. During the initial phase of the reaction, thrombin accelerates the rate of its own production, and at later stages it limits its own formation by inactivating factor V. When sufficient amounts of thrombin have been generated from prothrombin, thrombin can cleave off that part of the prothrombin molecule that contains γ-carboxylglutamic acid residues. Prothrombin altered in this way cannot bind to the phospholipid surfaces and thus can be activated only very slowly. A recently discovered vitamin K-dependent plasma protein, protein C, when activated by thrombin, also inactivates factor V. All of these reactions seem to regulate the rate of thrombin generation very delicately.

Thrombin is a serine protease that contains a serine residue at its active site. Thrombin plays several important roles in hemostasis. It cleaves not only fibrinogen but also factors XIII, V, and VIII, prothrombin, and protein C. Thrombin also aggregates platelets, facilitating the formation of the hemostatic plug.

## THE EXTRINSIC PATHWAY OF FACTOR X ACTIVATION

When blood is exposed to tissue extracts, factor X is rapidly generated via the extrinsic pathway by the interaction of a plasma protein, factor VII, and a tissue lipoprotein, tissue factor (or tissue thromboplastin).

Tissue factor exists in all tissues, including brain, lung, placenta, liver, and kidney. It is localized in these tissues to plasma membranes in various types of cells. Tissue factor is also present in the surface membranes of cells that are normally in contact with blood (leukocytes, vascular endothelial cells, etc.). Tissue factor on these surfaces, however, is usually cryptic (hidden), and cellular damage is required for the full expression of its activity. Tissue factor is composed of 2 parts, a protein and a phospholipid component, both of which are required for its procoagulant activity.

Factor VII (stable factor) is a trace plasma protein (0.05 mg/dl) produced by the liver in the presence of vitamin K. The half-life of factor VII in the circulation is very short (approximately 6 hours), and its concentration decreases first during vitamin K deficiency. The function of factor VII in blood coagulation appears to be limited primarily to the extrinsic pathway. Factor VII is composed of a single polypeptide chain with an approximate molecular weight of 60,000 and is structurally similiar to other vitamin K-dependent clotting factors such as prothrombin, factor IX, and factor X, all of which contain γ-carboxylglutamic acid residues. The activation of factor VII is achieved by the formation of a complex with tissue factor. Factor VII binds to the phospholipid portion of tissue factor via its γ-carboxylglutamic acid residues and calcium ions, and is in this way changed to an active two-chain enzyme. It is this factor VII–tissue factor–calcium complex that activates factor X in the extrinsic pathway. Some studies have suggested that a native single-chain form of factor VII is catalytically active and has weak coagulant activity, but the physiological significance of this enzyme is not certain.

Factor X (Stuart factor) occupies a key position in the sequence of blood clotting at the point at which the intrinsic and extrinsic pathways converge. Factor X is a glycoprotein that, like prothrombin, requires vitamin K during its biosynthesis in the liver for its biological activity. The plasma concentration of factor X is approximately 1 mg/dl, and its half-life in the circulation is about 40 hours. Factor X is composed of two chains held together by disulfide bonds, a heavy (35,000 molecular weight) and a light (17,000 molecular weight) chain. The former contains all of the carbohydrate. The activation of factor X involves cleavage of a peptide bond in the heavy chain, releasing a carbohydrate-rich fragment and unmasking an active serine site on the heavy chain. As described above, factor X is activated by the factor VII–tissue factor–calcium complex in the extrinsic pathway. It is also activated by the intrinsic pathway, by the venom of the Russell's viper, or by trypsin. The mechanism of activation appears to be identical in all three instances.

## THE INTRINSIC PATHWAY OF FACTOR X ACTIVATION

The intrinsic pathway is initiated by contact of blood with a foreign surface, that is, surfaces other than those of normal vascular lining and circulating blood cells. The intrinsic pathway of factor X activation requires the participation of six clotting factors: factors XII (Hageman factor, HF), plasma prekallikrein (Fletcher factor), high molecular weight kininogen (HMW kininogen, Fitzgerald, Flaujeac, or Williams factor, contact activation cofactor), factor XI (plasma thromboplastin antecedent, PTA), factor IX (Christmas factor), and factor VIII (antihemophilic factor, AHF) (Fig. 2-4). The earliest steps in this pathway are called the *contact phase,* since these are triggered by surface contact.

### The Contact Phase and the Activation of Factor XI

Four plasma proteins (HF, prekallikrein, HMW kininogen, and factor XI) are involved in the contact phase. This phase of blood coagulation has some unique characteristics compared to other stages. First, the reactions among these proteins do not require the presence of calcium ions. Second, all of these factors are avidly adsorbed onto certain surfaces, where they can interact with each other. Third, studies performed in vitro have demonstrated that the contact phase appears to participate not only in blood clotting but also in other systems of the host defense mechanisms such as fibrinolysis, kinin generation, and complement activation. The physiological significance of the contact phase, however, is still obscure, since individuals with a deficiency of any of these factors seem to be asymptomatic.

All agents that can trigger or activate the contact phase of blood coagulation are negatively charged. Glass, clay (kaolin), diatomaceous earth (Celite), ellagic acid, and dextran sulfate are some of the substances that initiate the contact phase. A number of possible biological activators have also been identified, including sebum, basement membrane, insoluble collagen, urate crystals, the soaps of saturated fatty acids, and bacterial lipopolysaccharides (endotoxin). These biological substances, however, are much weaker in their ability to initiate the contact reaction compared to glass or kaolin. Certain positively charged agents such as cytochrome C, lysozyme, and protamine sulfate can strongly attach to negatively charged surfaces and inhibit the subsequent activation of the contact phase. Human plasma also contains several unidentified proteins with similar properties. The exact nature of surfaces that have clot-promoting activity is poorly understood. Total surface charge (zeta potential) does not correlate with such activity, and it has been suggested that appropriately spaced foci or clusters of negative charges may be required. A better understanding of the nature of surfaces may be important in the development of nonthrombogenic surfaces for artificial organs.

When factor XII, prekallikrein, HMW kininogen, and factor XI are assembled on a negatively charged surface, factor XI is rapidly activated (Fig. 2-4). The enzyme that is responsible for the conversion of XI to XIa is activated factor XII (factor XIIa). Both prekallikrein and HMW kininogen are required for the optimal activation of factor XI. The exact sequence of events, however, is highly complex and not completely clear. Factor XII is a plasma protein with an approximate molecular weight of 80,000 that consists of a single polypeptide chain. Factor XII is probably produced in the liver, and its concentration in normal plasma is about 3mg/dl. The factor XII molecule is composed of two separate regions that are associated with distinct functions. The amino-terminal portion, of 52,000 molecular weight, is related to its ability to bind to negatively charged surfaces and the carboxy-terminal portion, of 28,000 molecular weight, to its enzymatic activities.

The initial event that triggers the activation of HF is not yet clear, but several hypotheses have been put forward. The adsorption of factor XII to surfaces may induce a conformational change in the molecule that exposes hidden active sites. Factor XII may have a low degree of inherent activity in its single-chain form that may be sufficient to initiate activation. Alternatively, the interaction of factor XII with prekallikrein on a surface may induce its activation. Autoactivation of factor XII has also been suggested as a trigger. In any event, once small amounts of activated factor XII (factor XIIa) are generated, this enzyme, in turn, activates prekallikrein and factor XI to form plasma kallikrein and factor XIa, respectively. Kallikrein and factor XIa then reciprocally activate factor XII. This reciprocal activation of factor XII, prekallikrein, and factor XI appears to accelerate the contact phase of blood coagulation. During activation, factor XII is cleaved at two specific sites in the molecule and becomes a serine protease. Recent studies suggest that surface binding of XII renders XII more susceptible to proteolytic cleavage by plasma kallikrein. Plasma prekallikrein and factor XI, however, are not absolute requirements for the activation of factor XII, since prolonged contact of prekallikrein-deficient plasma or factor XI-deficient plasma with surfaces lead to the activation of XII.

Plasma prekallikrein (Fletcher factor) has been known for a long time as a component of the plasma kinin-forming system. Its role in blood coagulation has recently become obvious through studies of congenital prekallikrein-deficient (Fletcher trait) plasma. Plasma prekallikrein is a single-chain polypeptide with an approximate molecular weight of 90,000. Its concentration in normal plasma is about 5 mg/dl. It is probably produced in the liver, since the titer of prekallikrein is greatly reduced in the plasma of patients with advanced hepatic cirrhosis. Plasma prekallikrein circulates in plasma as a complex with HMW kininogen. When blood comes into contact with a negatively charged surface, this complex is adsorbed onto the surface along with factor XII. The conversion of prekallikrein is brought about by activated factor XII. Factor XIIa activates prekallikrein by a proteolytic cleavage that changes the single chain to a two chain species composed of a heavy and a light chain linked by a disulfide bridge. The active site of kallikrein is associated with the light chain. Once activated, plasma kallikrein activates factor XII, as mentioned above. Kallikrein also releases a small peptide, bradykinin, from HMW kininogen. Bradykinin has many potent biological properties: it increases vascular permeability, induces pain, dilates small vessels, and contracts certain smooth muscles. It has been speculated, therefore, that bradykinin is one of the humoral mediators of acute inflammatory reactions.

The procoagulant activity of HMW kininogen has also become apparent recently through the studies of plasmas congenitally deficient in this protein. The kininogens are the precursors of biologically active peptide kinins such as bradykinin. Two groups of kininogens, of high and low molecular weight, are present in plasma. HMW kininogen is a plasma protein of approximately 120,000 molecular weight and consists of a single-chain polypeptide in which the bradykinin fragment is centrally located. Its plasma concentration is about 6 mg/dl. HMW kininogen has no known enzymatic functions and appears to be a cofactor in the contact activation of plasma. Both prekallikrein and factor XI exist in plasma as a complex with HMW kininogen. Binding of prekallikrein and factor XI to negatively charged surfaces is impaired in HMW kininogen-deficient plasma, suggesting that HMW kininogen may function as a carrier, bringing these proteins to the surface in juxtaposition to surface-bound factor XII. In this way, HMW kininogen augments the ability of factor XIIa to activate factor XI and prekallikrein and enhances the rate of activation of factor XII by kallikrein. At the same time, kallikrein releases bradykinin from HMW kininogen. Kinin-free HMW kininogen still appears to retain its procoagulant activity. LMW kininogen (50,000–60,000 molecular weight) has no known function in blood coagulation.

From the previous discussion, it is clear that factor XII, prekallikrein, and HMW kininogen participate in both blood coagulation and kinin release. Plasma kallikrein and activated factor XII (factor XIIa) also convert plasminogen to its active form, plasmin, and directly or indirectly activate the first component of complement (C1). These observations imply that blood coagulation, fibrinolysis, kinin formation, and complement activation are intimately interrelated via the contact phase.

Whereas the above-mentioned reactions represent the contact activation of plasma with foreign surfaces, enzymes present in cells are also known to be able to initiate the contact system. Both basophils and endothelial cells thus appear to contain enzymes that cleave and activate factor XII. The significance of the cellular activation of factor XII in vivo remains to be elucidated.

Factor XI is a plasma protein of approximately 160,000 molecular weight and is composed of two apparently identical polypeptide chains held together by a disulfide bond. Its concentration in normal plasma is about 0.5 mg/dl. As already noted, factor XI circulates in plasma as a complex with HMW kininogen. Factor XI is readily cleaved and activated by factor XIIa or trypsin. Cleavage occurs within an internal peptide bond in each chain, resulting in the formation of two heavy and two light chains. The active sites of activated factor XI (XIa) appear to be in each light chain. The function of factor XIa in blood coagulation is the activation of factor IX, the next factor in the line. Factor XIa also appears to activate plasminogen.

## The Activation of Factor IX (Christmas Factor).

Factor IX is one of the four vitamin K-dependent clotting factors. It is a glycoprotein (55,000 molecular weight) containing $\gamma$-carboxylglutamic acid residues, and it is functionally deficient in the plasma of patients with Christmas disease. The concentration in normal plasma is approximately 0.3mg/dl, and its half-life in the circulation is about 24 hours. Factor IX is a single-chain polypeptide and is converted to its activated form (factor IXa) by activated factor XI (factor XIa) in the presence of calcium ions. Factor XIa cleaves two peptide bonds, releasing a glycopeptide of 10,000 molecular weight from factor IX and converting it to a two-chain, activated form (factor IXa). Recent evidence suggests that factor IX is also activated by the factor VII–tissue factor–calcium complex that is formed via the extrinsic pathway.

Once activated, factor IXa converts factor X to its active form (factor Xa) in the presence of factor VIII, phospholipids, and calcium ions. The clotting factors form a multimolecular complex on the surface of the phospholipids, the $\gamma$-carboxylglutamic acid residues of factors IXa and X mediating their binding to the phospholipid. Under physiologic conditions, the platelets provide the phospholipids (PF 3) for this reaction. Factor VIII is a cofactor and appears to require modification by thrombin before it can function in the complex. The formation of the multimolecular complex accelerates the reaction several thousandfold by bringing factor X (substrate) and factor IXa (enzyme) into close approximation, increasing their chance of interaction. This process is very similar to the complex formation of factor Xa, prothrombin, factor V, phospholipid, and calcium ions in the activation of prothrombin.

### Factor VIII (AHF)

Factor VIII is an agent functionally deficient in the plasma of patients with classic hemophilia and von Willebrand's disease. It is present in normal plasma at an approximate concentration of 1 mg/dl, and its half-life in the circulation is about 12 hours. Factor VIII plays two distinct roles in hemostasis: procoagulant activity in the intrinsic pathway of blood coagulation and a role in primary hemostasis. Factor VIII is a huge plasma protein with a molecular weight in excess of one million that is a complex of two components.

One component of the factor VIII complex is associated with factor VIII procoagulant activity and is named *factor VIII:C*. This component is functionally decreased in the plasma of patients with classic hemophilia and von Willebrand's disease. The site of synthesis of factor VIII:C is not known. Its production is under the control of a gene on the X chromosome. Factor VIII:C is inactivated by human circulating anticoagulants against factor VIII that develop in multitransfused hemophilic patients or, rarely, in nonhemophilic individuals unrelated to transfusions. (see chapter 7) The structure of factor VIII:C is not known, since it has not yet been purified from human plasma. Recent studies suggest that the estimated molecular weight of factor VIII:C is approximately 280,000. The exact role of factor VIII:C in the activation of factor X has not yet been defined, but it seems likely that factor VIII:C acts as a regulatory protein, enhancing the rate of factor X activation in the same way that factor V accelerates the conversion of prothrombin. Initially, thrombin greatly enhances the ability of factor VIII:C to act as a cofactor and then inactivates it, thus providing both positive and negative feedback. Little is known of the molecular details of this reaction, but it appears to be associated with proteolytic modifications of the factor VIII:C structure.

The other component of the factor VIII complex is associated with primary hemostasis; it mediates adhesion of platelets to exposed subendothelial substances. This component is reduced in the plasma of patients with von Willebrand's disease but is normal in that of patients with classic hemophilia. It is identified by its ability to support agglutination of platelets by ristocetin (factor VIIIR:RC) and the retention of platelets by glass bead columns through which whole blood has been filtered. (see chapter 6) It is also recognized by heterologous antiserum against factor VIII (factor VIIIR:Ag) such as that produced in rabbits, but not by human circulating anticoagulants. Factor VIIIR:Ag comprises the majority of the protein mass of the factor VIII complex and is apparently synthesized by endothelial cells and megakaryocytes. The production of factor VIIIR:Ag is controlled by an autosomal gene. The structure of factor VIIIR:Ag has become apparent recently; it is composed of a population of multimers, and its molecular weight ranges from 850,000 to over 12 million. The capacity to induce platelet agglutination by ristocetin appears to be limited to the larger polymers.

Although factors VIII:C and VIIIR:Ag (or VIIIR:RC) have very distinct functions and biochemical and immunological properties, they seem to exist as a complex in plasma. The concentrations of these two components are closely correlated in normal plasma. How they form a complex is obscure, but it has been suggested that they may be linked by noncovalent bonds. The biological importance of complex formation is also uncertain, but the instability of factor VIII:C in the absence of factor VIIIR:Ag implies that complex formation may protect factor VIII:C from inactivation.

## Links between the Intrinsic and Extrinsic Pathways

In recent years, the distinction between the two independent pathways has become increasingly blurred as feedback mechanisms and interactions outside the classic schemes have been found. Activated factor XII (factor XIIa) can rapidly convert factor VII into a two-chain form that, upon combination with tissue factor, has increased activity as an activator of factor X. It seems that the activation of factor XII thus not only triggers the intrinsic pathway but also primes the extrinsic pathway. Similarly, activated factor X (factor Xa), whether generated via the intrinsic or the extrinsic pathway, also enhances factor VII activity. Large amounts of factor Xa, however, appears to inactivate factor VII and limit its own formation by the extrinsic pathway. Another link between the two pathways is the activation of factor IX by a factor VII–tissue factor–calcium complex. This implies that the intrinsic and extrinsic pathways converge at two levels, factor X and factor IX. The physiological significance of these newly discovered links remains to be clarified.

## ROLE OF FIBRINOLYSIS IN HEMOSTASIS

Fibrinolysis is the dissolution of fibrin clots. (see chapter 9) It may be considered as an essential host defense mechanism against the occlusion of blood vessels. Premature lysis of fibrin clots, however, may lead to rebleeding from the site of injury. Thus, fibrinolysis appears to play a role in hemostasis as well as in thrombosis.

Fibrinolysis is achieved, for the most part, by the digestion of fibrin by a potent plasma proteolytic enzyme, plasmin. Other proteases such as leukocytic enzymes may also be responsible for fibrinolysis under certain conditions. Plasmin is not present as such in normal circulating blood, but rather in the form of an inert precursor, plasminogen.

Figure 2-5 illustrates a simplified view of the human fibrinolytic system. Plasminogen is a plasma protein of 90,000 molecular weight composed of a single polypeptide chain. It is present in normal plasma at a concentration of approximately 20–40 mg/dl. Plasminogen is also present in lesser concentrations in all body fluids. Recent studies have shown that the liver is a site of the production of plasminogen.

Plasminogen is converted to plasmin by the action of specific enzymes called plasminogen activators. The activation of plasminogen involves a proteolytic cleavage of the single-chain zymogen and leads to the formation of plasmin, a two-chain polypeptide protease held together by a disulfide bond. Plasmin is a serine protease, and hydrolyzes susceptible arginine and lysine bonds in many proteins. Plasmin can digest fibrinogen, factor V, and factor VIII, as well as fibrin.

Plasminogen activators may be divided into two categories: intrinsic and extrinsic. Intrinsic activators are agents endogenous to blood and may convert plasminogen to plasmin when blood comes into contact with a foreign surface. Intrinsic activators include factor XII and other agents such as prekallikrein and factor XI (PTA). It should be pointed out that all of the intrinsic activators known to date are much weaker than the extrinsic activators in their ability to activate plasminogen. The significance of the intrinsic activators, however, lies in the fact that they are normal consituents of circulating blood. Extrinsic

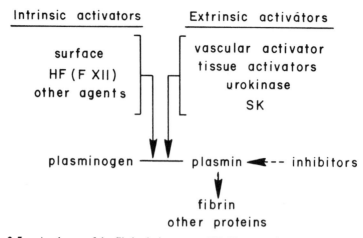

**Fig. 2-5.**    A scheme of the fibrinolytic system. HF: Hageman factor; SK: streptokinase.

activators are agents extrinsic to blood and are widely distributed in almost all body tissues including vascular endothelium. Plasminogen activator derived from endothelium has beeen speculated to play an important role in the activation of plasminogen because of its close proximity to blood. Urine also contains an activator called *urokinase* which is apparently produced by the kidney and excreted into urine. Urokinase is a serine protease of 53,000 molecular weight. Streptokinase (SK) is an activator derived from β-hemolytic streptococci. SK is not an enzyme, and it activates plasminogen by forming a complex with plasminogen. Both urokinase and SK, of course, are not present in normal circulating blood and do not appear to be involved in fibrinolysis in physiological states. They are used therapeutically in the treatment of thrombosis and embolism by inducing intense fibrinolysis.

When small amounts of plasmin are generated, they do not always lead to the digestion of fibrin or other proteins. This is because normal human plasma contains large amounts of inhibitors that quickly inactivate plasmin activity (see below). Among plasma inhibitors, $\alpha_2$-plasmin inhibitor ($\alpha_2$-antiplasmin, primary plasmin inhibitor) is probably the most important inhibitor in the regulation of in vivo fibrinolysis. $\alpha_2$-macroglobulin, antithrombin III, and C$\bar{\text{I}}$ INH (the inhibitor of the activated form of the first component of complement) are all able to inhibit plasmin activity when tested in vitro. Their physiological significance as plasmin inhibitors, however, appear to be minimal. $\alpha_2$-plasmin inhibitor is a fast-reacting potent inhibitor of plasmin; it inhibits plasmin instantaneously by forming a stable complex. It also inhibits adsorption of plasminogen to fibrin. The normal plasma concentration is approximately 5–7 mg/dl.

How the fibrinolytic system is activated and regulated in vivo is not fully understood. It is generally assumed that fibrinolysis is controlled by (1) release of plasminogen activator from vascular walls, (2) clearance of plasminogen activator by the liver, (3) activation of plasminogen, and (4) inhibition of the activation and action of plasmin. Circulating blood contains a small quantity of a labile plasminogen activator. The titer of this activator increases upon physical exercise or after local venous occlusion. This activator appears to be released from vascular endothelial cells. A number of vasoactive drugs such as epinephrine are also known to cause a transient rise in plasminogen activator activity by similar mechanisms.

When one considers the activation of plasminogen and inhibition of plasmin, it is important to distinguish the reactions in the fluid phase of plasma from those in the solid phase, that is, on the surface of fibrin. When free plasmin is generated in plasma, it can be readily inactivated by plasma inhibitors. Only when the amount of plasmin exceeds the amount of inhibitors available in plasma can the excess, uninhibited plasmin attack fibrinogen and other proteins. This is an unusual event. Recent evidence suggests that the activation of plasminogen in fibrin clots may be regulated as follows. When the vascular wall is injured, tissue factor and plasminogen activator are released. Tissue factor initiates the extrinsic pathway of thrombin formation, and thrombin then forms fibrin clots. Fibrin formation also occurs via the intrinsic pathway. Teleologically, it is interesting to note that local venous occulusion by clots may augment the release of plasminogen activator, whereas thrombin appears to inhibit its release. Both plasminogen and the vascular activator have the unique property of specifically binding to fibrin. This process seems to direct plasminogen and its activator to the fibrin surface. The formation of plasmin then takes place in situ, resulting in the dissolution of clots. $\alpha_2$-plasmin inhibitor is also incorporated into the clots by the action of factor XIIIa and may counteract the action of plasmin on fibrin.

The most direct evidence for the role of fibrinolysis in hemostasis comes from observations of human diseases. Several patients with a severe congenital deficiency of $\alpha_2$-plasmin inhibitor have now been found. All of them presented with a lifelong history of bleeding. It is likely that increased fibrinolysis due to the absence of potent plasmin inhibitors may have caused premature lysis of blood clots, leading to a bleeding tendency in these patients. A hemorrhagic tendency due to enhanced fibrinolysis is also seen as a side effect in some patients who receive urokinase or SK for the treatment of thromboembolism. The causes of the bleeding tendency in this case are several. Plasmin not only induces the dissolution of clots but also digests factor V, factor VIII, and fibrinogen. The proteolysis of fibrin and fibrinogen by plasmin generates a series of fragments of these proteins—fibrin/fibrinogen split products (FSP) or fibrin/fibrinogen degradation products (FDP)—that strongly inhibit both the action of thrombin on fibrinogen and platelet aggregation. Obviously, all of these changes would facilitate a bleeding tendency.

## CONTROL MECHANISMS IN HEMOSTASIS

When a blood vessel is injured, a platelet-fibrin plug forms at the site of injury, but does not usually extend into the lumen and occlude the blood vessel itself. As time passes, the platelet-fibrin plug is replaced by regenerating connective tissue. Growth of the platelet plugs and fibrin clots is thus closely regulated both temporally and topologically. Several mechanisms are known to control hemostasis.

### Blood Flow

The rapid movement of blood in the vessels may serve to wash away or dilute active coagulants generated locally at the site of injury. The importance of blood flow in preventing thrombosis is well illustrated by animal experiments. The intravenous injection of activated clotting factors into animals does not induce thrombus formation unless blood flow is stopped in a segment of vein during the period of "hypercoagulability." A combination of hypercoagulable states and venous stasis appears to be required for the formation of a thrombus.

### Hepatic Clearance of Activated factors

The liver seems to play a role in the removal of active coagulants or plasminogen activators from the circulation. Injection of active coagulants into the portal vein rather than into a systemic vein prevents the development of thrombi in the presence of venous stasis. It has also been shown in liver perfusion experiments that activated factor X (factor Xa) but not factor X is removed by passage through the liver. Furthermore, reticuloendothelial (RE) cells such as macrophages bind soluble fibrin but not fibrinogen. Recent studies also suggest the presence of specific binding sites for thrombin in vascular endothelial cells and peripheral blood monocytes. These observations suggest the importance of liver and RE cells in the clearance of activated factors and fibrin.

### Feedback Mechanisms in Blood Coagulation

A small event activating the clotting sequence may result in the generation of a significant amount of thrombin because of the amplification effect of the coagulation cascade. Both the intrinsic and extrinsic pathways of blood coagulation, however, appear to control their own activity by a series of feedback mechanisms such as the activation and inactivation of factors V and VIII by thrombin. These mechanisms were discussed earlier.

### Fibrinolysis

The fibrinolytic system is essential to dissolve and remove excess fibrin deposits to preserve vascular patency. Plasmin, a major fibrinolytic enzyme, also plays a role in inhibiting hemostasis. Plasmin can digest factors V and VIII, reducing their plasma concentrations. Fragments of fibrin and fibrinogen generated by plasmin (FDP, FSP) interfere with fibrin polymerization and platelet aggregation.

### Naturally Occurring Plasma Inhibitors

Human plasma contains many agents that inhibit the activity of activated clotting factors and fibrinolytic enzymes. Some well-characterized inhibitors include antithrombin III (heparin cofactor), $\alpha_2$-macroglobulin, $\alpha_1$-antitrypsin, $\alpha_2$-plasmin inhibitor ($\alpha_2$-antiplasmin), C$\overline{1}$ inactivator (C1 esterase inhibitor) and protein C (Table 2-2). It is interesting to note that the plasma concentrations of these inhibitors are much higher than those of the coagulation factors (Table 2-1) or plasminogen. In fact, these inhibitors comprise almost 20 percent of the globulin fraction of human plasma. It has been speculated that these inhibitors limit and localize thombosis, fibrinolysis, and inflammatory reactions. When studied in vitro, the spectra of these inhibitors are broad and, to some extent, overlapping. The clinical syndromes associated with inherited deficiencies of these inhibitors, however, are quite specific, suggesting that the physiological role of each inhibitor in vivo is distinct.

Antithrombin III (ATIII) is a plasma protein of 65,000 molecular weight that is composed of a single polypeptide chain. It inhibits thrombin by forming a stable 1:1 complex between an arginine residue of ATIII and the serine active site of thrombin. Its action is greatly accelerated by heparin, an acidic mucopolysaccharide present in mast cells. Heparin appears to bind to ATIII and to induce a conformational change in antithrombin that renders

**Table 2-2**
Naturally Occurring Plasma Inhibitors

| Inhibitors | Normal Plasma Concentration (mg/dl) | Hereditary Deficiency States |
|---|---|---|
| Antithrombin III (Heparin cofactor) | 18–30 | Thrombosis |
| $\alpha_2$-macroglobulin | 150–350 | ? |
| $\alpha_1$-antitrypsin | 200–400 | Pulmonary emphysema |
| $\alpha_2$-plasmin inhibitor ($\alpha_2$-antiplasmin) | 5–7 | Bleeding tendency |
| C$\bar{1}$ inactivator (C1 esterase inhibitor) | 15–35 | Hereditary angioneurotic edema (HANE) |
| Protein C | 0.4 | Thrombosis |

arginine at the reactive site more accessible to the active serine site of thrombin. ATIII is a major inhibitor of thrombin, but it also inhibits factors XIIa, XIa, Xa, IXa, plasma kallikrein, and plasmin. Its physiological importance is best shown by the occurrence of repeated episodes of thrombosis in patients with hereditary deficiencies of ATIII. This disorder becomes clinically apparent when ATIII levels are approximately half of those in normal persons.

$\alpha_2$-macroglobulin ($\alpha_2$M) is a large plasma protein (725,000 molecular weight) that appears to consist of several subunits. $\alpha_2$M inhibits thrombin, but it is less active than ATIII. Plasma kallikrein and plasmin are also inhibited by $\alpha_2$M. Heparin does not enhance this inhibition. The mode of the inhibition of thrombin by $\alpha_2$M is not precisely known, but it has been proposed that it occurs in 2 steps. First, thrombin splits a fragment of 85,000 molecular weight from $\alpha_2$M. Then the modified $\alpha_2$M undergoes a conformational change such that thrombin is trapped within the $\alpha_2$M molecule, preventing the escape or the interaction of thrombin with its substrates. Two families with inherited $\alpha_2$M deficiency have been recently described. Although plasma $\alpha_2$M levels in some members of the families were approximately 20–40 percent of the normal pooled plasma, these individuals appeared to be clinically asymptomatic.

$\alpha_1$-antitrypsin is a plasma protein of 50,000 molecular weight and inhibits factor XIa and plasmin. Whether it inactivates thrombin is debatable. Patients with a hereditary deficiency of $\alpha_1$-antitrypsin present with pulmonary emphysema or liver cirrhosis, but they do not have a thrombotic tendency.

$\alpha_2$-plasmin inhibitor ($\alpha_2$-antiplasmin) is a recently characterized, fast-reacting plasmin inhibitor. It inhibits plasmin instantaneously by forming a 1:1 complex, and it interferes with the binding of plasminogen to fibrin. The inherited deficiency of this inhibitor is associated with a severe hemorrhagic tendency.

C$\bar{1}$ inactivator (C1 esterase inhibitor) was initially identified as an inhibitor of C1 esterase in the complement system. Subsequently, it was found to inhibit plasmin, plasma kallikrein, and factors XIIa and XIa as well. The deficiency of this inhibitor, hereditary angioneurotic edema (HANE), however, is not accompanied by a thrombotic tendency.

Protein C is a newly identified vitamin K-dependent plasma protein. It is converted to its active serine protease form (activated protein C) by the action of thrombin. Activated protein C is a potent anticoagulant since it selectively inactivates factors V and VIII. A recent report claims that partial deficiency of protein C is associated with a thrombotic tendency.

## ROLE OF VITAMIN K

It has been long recognized that vitamin K (coagulation vitamin) is needed for the synthesis of 4 clotting factors (prothrombin and factors VII, IX, and X). How vitamin K functions in the production of these proteins, however, has only recently been clarified. Studies have revealed that these four clotting factors contain unique amino acid residues, γ-carboxylglutamic acids. As mentioned before, γ-carboxylglutamic acid residues are the sites of binding of calcium ions to these proteins and are required for their functions in blood coagulation. Formation of the vitamin K-dependent factors appears to occur in two steps. First, a polypeptide chain is produced on the ribosomes in the hepatocytes, a step that does not require the presence of the vitamin. Then a second carboxyl group is inserted into the gamma carbon of glutamic acid residues in the polypeptide chain. Carboxylation is carried out by a carboxylase enzyme. Vitamin K is an essential cofactor of this reaction. In this process, vitamin K is oxidized, but is conserved by a second enzyme, vitamin K reductase. The most commonly used oral anticoagulant, warfarin, is structurally similar to vitamin K and appears to inhibit vitamin K reductase competitively. In the presence of warfarin, therefore, vitamin K is depleted and γ-carboxylglutamic acid residues are not formed.

Recent studies have also demonstrated that, in addition to the four clotting factors, other proteins including protein C and protein S in plasma, and proteins of bone, lung, and kidney, contain calcium-binding γ-carboxylglutamic acid residues. The formation of these proteins also appears to be vitamin K dependent. The function of vitamin K thus is not restricted to the synthesis of four clotting factors, but rather is broader than was previously assumed.

## BIBLIOGRAPHY

1. Shattil SJ, Bennett JS: Platelets and their membranes in hemostasis: Physiology and pathophysiology. Ann Intern Med 94:108–118, 1981
2. Davie EW, Fujikawa K, Kurachi K, et al: The role of serine proteases in the blood coagulation cascade. Adv Enzymol Rel Areas Mol Biol 48:277–318, 1979
3. Jackson CM, Nemerson Y: Blood coagulation. Ann Rev Biochem 491:765–811, 1980
4. Cochrane CG, Griffin JH: Molecular assembly in the contact phase of the Hageman factor system. Am J Med 67:657–664, 1979
5. Saito H: The contact system in health and disease. Adv Intern Med 25:217–238, 1980
6. Hoyer H: The factor VIII complex: Structure and function. Blood 58:1–13, 1981
7. Mann KG, Taylor FB Jr (eds): The Regulation of Coagulation. New York, Elsevier North-Holland, 1980
8. Suttie JW: The metabolic role of vitamin K. Fed Proc 39:2730–2735, 1980

E. J. Walter Bowie
Charles A. Owen

# 3

# The Clinical and Laboratory Diagnosis of Hemorrhagic Disorders

Any patient with a bleeding disease, however mild, presents the clinician with a complex diagnostic problem. A careful history and clinical examination are essential in the evaluation of such a patient. This approach is of fundamental importance in a patient with a bleeding diathesis because the history is the only means of finding out whether or not a patient has a bleeding problem. The importance of the history cannot be overemphasized, but it is particularly important in patients with mild bleeding diseases in whom the results of screening tests of hemostasis may be normal. Results of laboratory tests alone can be misleading. Patients, for example, who have deficiencies of Hageman factor, prekallikrein, or high molecular weight kininogen may have abnormal partial thromboplastin times but are not bleeders. At the other end of the spectrum, the patient with a severe bleeding diathesis such as scurvy may have normal screening test results, and the only clue to a disorder is given by the history. Some clinicians substitute screening tests for a careful history, and as will be discussed later, this is an extremely hazardous practice.

## CLINICAL EVALUATION

### The History

Asking the patient if he is a bleeder is not usually very helpful, and sometimes the information produced may be misleading. Some patients may not admit to bleeding episodes that are significant. For example, a patient with von Willebrand's disease was unimpressed with his excessive bleeding from cuts because he was used to cutting himself, as he was a butcher. On careful evaluation, however, it was apparent that he bled more than normally. On the other hand, hypochondriacal patients may overemphasize the importance of insignificant bleeding. Furthermore, patients with mild bleeding diatheses may consider themselves to be normal, having never compared themselves with persons who have normal hemostasis. Such was true of the two daughters of the previously mentioned butcher; they did not consider their menstrual bleeding to be excessive, yet when they were first examined, their levels of hemoglobin were about 4 g/dl. It was subsequently proved that they had von Willebrand's disease. In other instances, bleeding may not be recognized for what it is; for example, hemarthroses in the hemophilic patient may be mistaken for some other type of joint involvement, such as rheumatic fever.

The physician, therefore, has to decide after careful questioning whether the patient has an abnormal hemostatic mechanism. Questioning should be specific and designed to ascertain if bleeding occurs in response to mild trauma. The most helpful historical technique is to compare the patient's response to challenges of the hemostatic mechanism with the response of a normal person to the same challenges. It is extremely helpful if the patient has had a major surgical procedure, because that experience is a more reliable test of the hemostatic mechanism than any laboratory test can provide. When dealing with a patient who has an acquired bleeding disease, it is important to make sure that the operation was performed after the disease was acquired.

If the patient has not undergone a major operation, information can be obtained about minor surgical procedures, such as circumcision, tonsillectomy, and dental extractions. It is important to get exact details of the bleeding after these procedures—in particular, exactly how long the bleeding persisted after the procedure was performed and whether blood transfusions were required.

To evaluate dental extractions, the history must include the number and type of teeth removed, whether sutures or packing had to be inserted, and whether the patient had to return to the dentist to control hemorrhaging. Dental extractions are a reliable measure of the hemostatic mechanism because the bleeding areas are associated with rigid bone and are not compressible. Presistent bleeding after removal of a small incisor is clearly more significant than excessive bleeding after removal of a large molar tooth. In fact, many people with a normal hemostatic mechanism may bleed excessively after molar tooth extractions, so this circumstance is not very helpful in deciding whether the patient has a bleeding problem. However, the absence of excessive bleeding after the extraction of molar teeth suggests that he has an effective hemostatic mechanism. The same comment can be made about tonsillectomy, which also may be a very bloody procedure in normal people because the tonsillar bed is extremely vascular. It is difficult, therefore, to interpret the significance of excessive bleeding at tonsillectomy, but if the bleeding has not been unusual, the implication is that the patient has a reasonably normal hemostatic mechanism. Tonsillectomy is also an example of the importance of taking an accurate history. Patients will often state that they bled excessively after the operation, when the bleeding actually occurred a week or 10 days after the procedure, at which time the operative slough separated.

The type of bleeding may also be of significance in making the diagnosis. Ecchymoses may be seen commonly in any type of bleeding diathesis and do not give a clue to the diagnosis. Petechiae, tiny pinpoint hemorrhages from the dermal capillary loops, are almost always diagnostic of platelet or vascular abnormality. In addition to the skin lesions, platelet abnormalities may cause superficial bleeding from the nose and gastrointestinal and genitourinary tracts. Deep bleeding into the subcutaneous tissues, muscles, retroperitoneal area, and abdominal viscera is seen most commonly in hereditary deficiencies of the coagulation factors, particularly classic hemophilia, but may also occur in scurvy. Spontaneous hemarthroses are limited almost entirely to patients with coagulation factor defects.

Epistaxis may occur with a number of bleeding diseases but is particularly associated with thrombocytopenia, hereditary hemorrhagic telangiectasia, and von Willebrand's disease. In von Willebrand's disease, it is not unusual to obtain a history of severe, recurrent epistaxis in childhood, which ameliorates about the time of puberty. Epistaxis may recur after menopause. It tends to occur in normal persons, particularly children, in the winter months, when the air is dry. If the nosebleeds are unilateral, a local lesion should be suspected. Gingival bleeding may result from gum disease but it is also seen with thrombocytopenia, uremia, scurvy, and the dysproteinemias. It is part of the pattern of the hyperviscosity syndrome. Hematuria occurs with thrombocytopenia, hemophilia, and oral anticoagulant therapy. Whatever the underlying hemostatic abnormality, however, the presence of hematuria should prompt a detailed investigation of the genitourinary tract to exclude the possibility of an underlying lesion such as a neoplasm. In any patient with unexplained hematuria, a factitial origin also must be considered. Patients with hemophilia may have recurrent episodes of hematuria, and it is usually not necessary to repeat the investigations in these patients.

Gastrointestinal bleeding may be associated with almost any type of hemorrhagic diathesis, particularly anticoagulant therapy, hereditary hemorrhagic telangiectasia, thrombocytopenia, von Willebrand's disease, pseudoxanthoma elasticum, and uremia. Paradoxically, essential thrombocythemia is commonly associated with gastrointestinal bleeding.[1] The diagnosis in these situations may present some difficulties initially because acute gastrointestinal hemorrhage increases the platelet count. The splenomegaly that is present in nearly all patients with essential thrombocythemia is an important clue to the diagnosis. Whatever the underlying hemorrhagic diathesis, patients with hemorrhage from the gastrointestinal tract should be completely investigated to determine if there is a local cause for their bleeding.

As pointed out, ecchymoses may be seen in almost any kind of hemorrhagic diathesis, and their significance is difficult to evaluate. Men rarely complain of bruising, and in our view, such a complaint by a man is an indication for an investigation of the hemostatic mechanism. Women, however, commonly complain of ease of bruising and frequently have one or two bruises. In these situations, inquiries should be made about whether the bruising is spontaneous or related to trauma and whether it occurs on the limbs, which are commonly exposed to minor trauma, or on the trunk, a more protected area. Information also should be obtained about the size and number of the bruises. It is often helpful to ask the patient, ''Do you usually have bruises, or do you usually have no bruises?'' In response to such a question, most patients who complain of ease of bruising will say that they usually have no bruises. It is difficult to be precise about the number of bruises, but if a woman consistently has more than half a dozen bruises, a hemostatic investigation is warranted. In general, bruises are not painful, and a complaint of painful bruises should raise the question of some form of psychogenic purpura.[2,3] If a bruise recurs at a site that is easily accessible to the fingers or mouth, a factitial origin should be suspected.

Menorrhagia may be the presenting symptom of thrombocytopenia or von Willebrand's disease as well as coagulation factor deficiencies. The evaluation of the amount of menstrual blood loss is difficult because most women have no way of knowing whether their periods are normal or excessive. The blood loss can be quantified historically by asking about the number of soaked pads (a soaked pad contains 50 ml or more of blood), the duration of bleeding, the use of superabsorbent and double pads, whether it is necessary to change at night, whether the patient soils herself, the presence of clots, and whether clots are passed with urination. Inquiries also should be made about the prescription of iron for anemia.

Questions should be asked of the parents: whether bleeding occurred with the eruption of the their child's deciduous teeth or with the separation of the umbilical cord; the latter is commonly seen in patients with factor XIII deficiency, afibrinogenemia, and factor VII deficiency. It is also helpful to ask the mother to compare the child's bruising and bleeding with those of siblings. One should always consider the possibility that one is dealing with a battered child, and the ecchymoses should be examined carefully for abrasions. Conversely, parents have been accused of maltreating their children when in fact the children had a bleeding disease.

The age at which hemorrhagic symptoms first appear may be helpful in deciding whether the bleeding is hereditary or acquired. When symptoms begin in infancy, an inherited type of bleeding diathesis is suggested, whereas most of the acquired hemorrhagic diseases occur later in life. These are broad generalizations, and there are exceptions. In the Ehlers-Danlos syndrome and hereditary hemorrhagic telangiectasia, for example, bleeding may not occur until later in life, although both are hereditary conditions. However, in idiopathic thrombocytopenic purpura, an acquired condition, the symptoms may start early in life and recur over a period of many years. In general, however, most of the bleeding disorders that develop later in life are acquired.

The history also should include details about exposure to toxic agents such as drugs and ionizing radiation. Numerous drugs have been associated with thrombocytopenia or vascular purpura; specific inquiry must be made in this regard, because a patient may not consider the pills he is taking as medications. The possibility that the patient may be taking an oral anticoagulant such as warfarin should always be considered. Occasionally, a patient is encountered who has a puzzling hemorrhagic diathesis and is found to be administering these drugs to himself or to have been given them without his knowledge. We have seen an occasional patient, for example, who has described his oral anticoagulant as "heart pills."

The family history may be helpful and, in some instances, characteristic. The best approach to taking a family history is to construct a pedigree chart and to inquire carefully about the evidence of bleeding in all of the relatives. Classic hemophilia, Christmas disease, and the Wiskott-Aldrich syndrome are transmitted as X-linked recessive traits, whereas factor XI deficiency and all other inherited bleeding diseases involve both sexes. The history of presumptive bleeding in relatives is of limited value unless there is medical documentation. Furthermore, the patient may be unaware of bleeding in relatives despite the fact that they have a significant bleeding diathesis. Four possibilities must be considered when both parents of a bleeder are asymptomatic:

1.  If the inheritance is X linked (for example, classic hemophilia or hemophilia A), the disease cannot occur in a father and his child unless the child's mother is a carrier.
2.  A genetic mutation may have occurred so that the disease has arisen de novo.
3.  The autosomal recessive diseases arise when both parents are asymptomatic heterozygotes. This is most common when relatives marry.
4.  The bleeding may be due to an acquired rather than an inherited abnormality.

Some patients administer oral anticoagulants to themselves,[4,5] and one should be aware of this in evaluating a long prothrombin time. Most of these patients are in one of the health professions, such as nursing, and many have histories of thrombosis. Most have deep emotional disturbances, and psychiatric advice should always be obtained.

## Physical Examination

The clinical evaluation of the patient is important to define the nature and extent of any current hemorrhage. It is also important, however, because many conditions are associated with unusual bleeding, so that, in the presence of one of these conditions, a hemostatic abnormality can be anticipated. A good example is liver disease, which may cause a complex hemostatic disorder, including decrease of the coagulation factors synthesized by the liver, thrombocytopenia, qualitative platelet abnormalities, dysfibrinogenemia, intravascular coagulation, and fibrinolysis. Significant abnormalities of platelet function may be associated with renal failure. Qualitative platelet abnormalities are found in association with many hematologic diseases, including the dysproteinemias, leukemias, and myeloproliferative diseases. Circulating anticoagulants may be associated with systemic lupus erythematosus, collagen diseases, malignancies, a number of other disorders, and certain drugs which induce a "lupuslike" syndrome.[6-9] This type of anticoagulant rarely results in abnormal bleeding.

If the patient has not been eating adequately and has recently received a broad-spectrum antibiotic, vitamin K deficiency should be considered. Vitamin K deficiency may occur preoperatively in a patient who has reduced his food intake because of abdominal discomfort from carcinoma of the colon and who preoperatively receives a drug that sterilizes the gut, removing the only remaining source of vitamin K. The deficiency may also occur postoperatively in patients who have not been eating well and who receive broad-spectrum antibiotics to treat a postoperative pneumonitis. Vitamin K deficiency also may occur in newborn infants because their gut is sterile, and there may be malabsorption of vitamin K in such conditions as sprue and biliary obstruction.

In many parts of the world, starvation is a way of life rather than a form of therapy, and in these countries, deficiency diseases may result in a bleeding tendency. An obvious example is kwashiorkor, which produces severe liver damage. Scurvy should always be considered in patients who are malnourished and whose diet does not contain adequate sources of vitamin C. Scurvy produces subperiosteal bleeding, gingival bleeding, and a characteristic type of perifollicular bleeding. Scurvy also may be seen in alcoholic persons, further complicating their hemorrhagic diathesis.

Many patients, particularly those with cancer, may have chronic compensated intravascular coagulation. The level of platelets and coagulation factors may be normal or even increased, but tests for fibrin complexes in the plasma are positive. These patients may be likely to develop acute decompensated intravascular coagulation, which can be triggered by the addition of another stimulus, such as a surgical operation.

## LABORATORY ASSESSMENT—GENERAL CONSIDERATIONS

After the history and physical examination, a clinical judgment can be made about whether or not the patient has a bleeding problem. The clinical evaluation allows patients to be divided into four main groups: (1) severe bleeding tendency, (2) minor bleeding tendency, (3) equivocal bleeding tendency, and (4) no bleeding tendency. At this point, the laboratory evaluation is begun, and, as will be shown, the type of bleeding may be of significant help in designing the program of hemostatic testing. Tests of hemostasis are then performed in order to assess the nature of the abnormality. There is a real diagnostic problem when bleeding is mild because these patients have histories that may be equivocal and the results of the usual screening tests of hemostasis may be normal. These patients require the most careful investigation in order to arrive at an accurate diagnosis. The patient who has a severe hemostatic defect usually presents no problem in either clinical recognition or laboratory diagnosis. Unfortunately, however, the patient with mild bleeding often receives an inadequate laboratory assessment. Patients with mild hemophilia, von Willebrand's disease, or qualitative platelet diseases may be overlooked, which may cause an unwelcome surprise when excessive bleeding occurs at surgery.

The situation is complicated because patients with mild bleeding tendencies may not have noted unusual bleeding, particularly if they have led sedentary lives. In the patient with mild hemophilia, for example, the diagnosis may be made only because excessive bleeding was noted at operation often in the later years of life. If the level of the factor VIII coagulant activity (antihemophilic factor) in such a patient were less than 25 or 30 U/dl, there would be an abnormality of the activated partial thromboplastin time so that if this test were performed routinely, the abnormality would be recognized preoperatively.

Currently, no simple, reliable screening test of hemostasis exists, and there is no completely satisfactory way of evaluating patients preoperatively. A careful history is essential, and a number of screening tests are useful.

In interpreting hemostatic tests, one should recognize that they are difficult to perform accurately. Quality control must be meticulous and must start at the time of venipuncture. A careful venipuncture is essential, because the release of tissue thromboplastin causes activation of the clotting mechanism and invalidates the result. Although some tests can be performed on frozen specimens of plasma, extensive hemostatic evaluation requires the presence of the patient. Assays of antihemophilic factor (factor VIII) and proaccelerin (factor V) on frozen specimens are particularly hazardous unless special precautions are taken. When tests of hemostasis are performed, patients are the best containers for their blood samples.

Hemostatic tests can be divided into two broad groups: screening tests and specific tests, such as coagulation factor assays and tests of platelet function.

## SCREENING TESTS OF HEMOSTASIS

Patients are often routinely referred for hemostatic evaluation before undergoing a surgical operation. Some clinicians perform preoperative tests of hemostasis in all patients, and others perform them only if the history is suggestive of a hemostatic disorder or if the patient's primary disease is associated with such a disorder. Each of these approaches has deficiencies, and neither provides a perfect approach to preoperative evaluation. The danger of using routine screening tests is that they may be substituted for a meticulous history, and the physician, unaware of their limitations, may rely on them. The most important clue to the presence of a minor bleeding tendency is the history, and even if the results of screening are normal, the history of unusual bleeding requires a thorough investigation of the mechanism of hemostasis.

Bleeding diseases may involve an abnormality of the blood vessel, the platelet, or the coagulation mechanism. If a bleeding diathesis is inherited, usually only one of these three areas is involved (with the exception of von Willebrand's disease), whereas in acquired bleeding diseases, there may be several hemostatic defects. In designing screening procedures, therefore, one must include tests of vascular, platelet, coagulation and fibrinolytic functions so that the whole hemostatic mechanism can be tested.

### Platelet Count

Thrombocytopenia has many causes. The thrombocytopenias are the most frequent cause of bleeding, so that measuring the level of circulating platelets is an extremely important screening test. All methods used for obtaining the platelet count have fairly wide standard deviations and may give occasional spurious results, so that the results must be confirmed by inspection of a blood smear. The electronic particle-counting machines may have a "gate" that excludes large cells. Large platelets may not be counted with this type of equipment, and an erroneously low platelet count will be reported. There is no difficulty in deciding from a blood smear whether the concentration of platelets is above or below normal, and it is also possible to observe other hematologic abnormalities and the morphologic characteristics of the platelets. If the blood smear is taken directly from the stab wound (that is, without the use of anticoagulants), the platelets will tend to form clumps. The platelets in Glanzmann's thrombasthenia, however, appear as single entities, and clumps are rarely found. The appearance of the platelets of Glanzmann's thrombasthenia is mimicked when normal blood is anticoagulated with ethylenediaminetetraacetic acid (EDTA).

In general, abnormal bleeding will not be encountered if the platelet count is higher than 100,000/$\mu$l, providing the platelets are normal. Actually, bleeding rarely becomes troublesome unless the platelet count is less than 50,000/$\mu$l. In certain congenital and acquired conditions, the thrombocytopenia may be associated with decreased platelet function. Such a situation may be suspected if the bleeding time seems to be unusually prolonged in relation to the platelet count and if the history of bleeding is out of proportion to the level of circulating platelets. In most qualitative platelet diseases, however, the level of circulating platelets is about normal and the bleeding is entirely due to abnormally functioning platelets. In conditions of increased peripheral platelet destruction, such as idiopathic thrombocytopenic purpura, the young platelets appear to have increased hemostatic competence, which is reflected in a bleeding time that is unusually short for the level of circulating platelets.

In certain myeloproliferative diseases, particularly essential thrombocythemia, the platelet count may be extremely high, and although thrombosis may be likely, bleeding is, paradoxically, a more usual complication. The platelets in these patients may show gross morphologic and functional abnormalities, which are presumably related to the hemostatic defect.

## The Bleeding Time

The bleeding time is defined by O'Brien[10] as the time between the infliction of a small, standard cut and the moment when the bleeding stops. This may be abrupt or taper off insensibly. Although the definition is admirably simple, the bleeding time has many variables. It is the most difficult test of hemostasis to standardize. If, however, it is carefully standarized, the test will give reproducible results, and it affords most important information in the evaluation of a patient with a bleeding tendency.

The bleeding time measures the interaction of the platelet with the blood vessel wall and the subsequent formation of the hemostatic plug. The bleeding time thus measures the early stages of hemostasis. A long bleeding time occurs when the level of circulating platelets is decreased, the platelets are abnormal in function, or the platelets cannot interact with the vessel wall. The bleeding time may be prolonged when there is a decrease or abnormality in certain plasma factors, such as von Willebrand factor, fibrinogen, or factor V, or abnormalities in the walls of the small blood vessels. Occasionsally, the bleeding time is prolonged for unexplained reasons. This condition was previously called *pseudohemophilia*.

There are numerous methods for performing the bleeding test. All are basically modifications of two techniques: the Duke technique,[11] in which a puncture or incision is made in the earlobe, and the Ivy technique,[12] in which a puncture or incision is made in the forearm while the capillaries are under increased constant pressure from an inflated blood pressure cuff on the upper arm. Earlier descriptions of the bleeding time were given by both Hayem and Milian.[13,14] Because Milian described the test as a coagulation test, it was overlooked in the bleeding time literature. Ratnoff[15] described a technique in which an incision is made in the ball of the finger rather than the ear, because this allows the bleeding to be more easily controlled. The ambient temperature is controlled in some methods by immersing the incised area in saline. In many other methods, saline immersion also has been used to quantitate the amount of blood loss.[16] Quantitation also has been obtained by the use of a flow cube that is placed over the wound and allows the amount of blood lost to be continuously recorded.[17,18]

The test is affected by a number of variables,[19,20] including the depth of the skin puncture, the length of the incision, the site of the incision, the direction of the incision, the capillary venous pressure, the skin temperature, and certain medications the patient may have ingested. The end point may be difficult to see because colorless liquid may still ooze from the wound after the escape of red blood cells has ceased. Because of the compliance of the skin, the most difficult variable to control is the depth of the incision. Unless the test is meticulously performed, the results obtained by using any method can be misleading.

One advantage of the Ivy method is that the forearm allows several bleeding tests to be performed and the skin in this area is less variable in thickness from one patient to another. The incision should be 1–2 mm deep so as to enter the subpapillary venous plexus. The Ivy method has been modified in many ways, and various automated devices have been developed to make the incision. The most useful way of performing the test is to use a template; the standardized template bleeding time introduced by Mielke and colleagues[21] has gained wide acceptance. Indeed, as Harker and Slichter have shown, the test is so reproducible that in thrombocytopenia due to impaired platelet production, the bleeding time has an inverse linear relationship to the platelet count.[22,23] An automated device (Simplate) made by General Diagnostics (Morris Plains, NJ) is commercially available for performing the bleeding time test.[24] This method requires two 5-mm-long by 2-mm-deep incisions and is extremely reproducible.

Template methods may produce keloid scars in a few patients. These can be minimized by apposing the sides of the wound with an adhesive dressing. In our own laboratory, we have continued to use a spring-loaded device. This does not result in scarring, and, although the results have a wider standard deviation than those produced by the template method, they are adequate for clinical purposes.[25] A template producing a 3-mm incision has been described by Hirsh et al.[26]

One of the most frequent causes of prolongation of the bleeding time is the ingestion of drugs, particularly aspirin; in evaluating the significance of prolonged bleeding time, a careful history of drug ingestion is essential.

In patients with mild von Willebrand's disease, the Ivy bleeding time may be prolonged when the Duke bleeding time is normal.[27,28] The Ivy bleeding time may therefore, be a more sensitive screening test in these situations, but the Duke test may give a more accurate reflection of treatment.

An intermediate syndrome of platelet dysfunction has been described[29] in which patients have an exaggerated response of the bleeding time to ingestion of aspirin as a result of the abnormality of platelet function. It has been suggested that these patients may bleed excessively at operation and that the response of the bleeding time to aspirin should be an integral part of the assessment of platelet function. It might be recalled that long ago Quick described this as the aspirin tolerance test.[30]

## The Partial Thromboplastin Time

Much information can be obtained from inspection of the citrated plasma used to perform the partial thromboplastin time test. Hemolysis, hyperlipemia, or bilirubinemia may be noted. Blue-green discoloration may be seen in the plasma of oral contraceptive users because of the high level of ceruloplasmin. If the plasma is centrifuged at a controlled rate to produce platelet-rich plasma, then the opalescence will indicate whether the platelet concentration is adequate or decreased.

The partial thromboplastin time measures the intrinsic coagulation activity of plasma. A partial thromboplastin such as cephalin or Inosithin (soya phosphatide) has an activity equivalent to that of platelet factor 3. These partial thromboplastins are added to the citrated plasma, and the clotting time is measured at 37°C after the addition of calcium.[25,31] As in all clotting tests, collection of the blood must be meticulous to minimize the activation of the contact system. The variable of contact activation is eliminated in a variant of the partial thrombloplastin time by producing maximal activation by the addition of kaolin, Celite, powdered glass, or ellagic acid before the partial thromboplastin is added to the plasma (activated partial thromboplastin time, APTT).[32]

Other tests that measure the intrinsic clotting mechanism are the whole-blood coagulation time and the plasma clot time (also called the plasma recalcification time). The whole-blood clot time is extremely insensitive, and the results will be normal if the levels of factor VIII coagulant activity, for example, are above 5 U/dl. All clotting factors except calcium and fibrinogen are said to be present in average normal plasma at a titer of 100 U/dl. We no longer perform this test and do not consider it to be a useful screening device. The whole-blood coagulation time, however, may be useful in Third World countries where lack of equipment and supplies precludes performance of the more complex procedures. It is also used by many to regulate heparin therapy.

The plasma clot time[33] has about the same sensitivity as the partial thromboplastin time, but it has fallen into disuse in most laboratories because of the difficulty of standardizing the platelet concentration. We perform it routinely, in addition to the partial thromboplastin time, and have found that in certain situations one of the times will be more prolonged than the other. For example, the plasma clot time may be prolonged by the "lupus" anticoagulant to a far greater extent than the partial thromboplastin time, and when the anticoagulant activity is mild, the partial thromboplastin time may be normal. Conversely, in patients who are taking oral anticoagulants, the partial thromboplastin time seems to be much more sensitive than the plasma clot time to the coagulation defects.

The partial thromboplastin time will be prolonged if there is decreased coagulation factor activity or if a circulating anticoagulant is present. Mixing the patient's plasma with normal plasma and retesting allows the two mechanisms to be distinguished. If mixing with an equal volume of normal plasma does not correct the abnormal clotting time, a circulating anticoagulant is present. If a smaller volume of normal plasma corrects the clotting time, an inhibitor probably is not present. Generally, 0.1 volume of normal plasma should correct the prolonged clotting time of 0.9 volume of the patient's plasma halfway toward the norm. Such a rule has exceptions, because a mild anticoagulant may be overcome by a small volume of plasma.

If the correction pattern indicates that the prolonged partial thromboplastin time is due to a coagulation factor deficiency, mixing tests are then performed with artificially depleted plasmas. Plasma, for example, can be depleted of factor V and factor VIII activities by aging because in human plasma these activities are labile. Often, however, factor VIII coagulant activity is difficult to remove completely. The vitamin K-dependent factors

deplete  $\overline{V}$ + $\overline{VIII}$  by aging
deplete  $\overline{II}$, $\overline{VII}$, $\overline{IX}$, $\overline{X}$ by adsorption.

II, VII, IX, and X can be removed by adsorption. Recently, we have been using a factor V-deficient plasma that has been produced artificially by affinity-adsorption, using a monoclonal antibody to factor V.[34] The plasma is an excellent reagent and is completely deficient in factor V. As more monoclonal antibodies to coagulation factors are developed, other plasmas that are artificially depleted of a specific coagulation factor can be developed.

The final identification of the coagulation factor deficiency is made by mixing the patient's plasma with plasma from patients in whom specific coagulation factors are deficient. The principle on which all coagulation mixing tests is based is that plasmas with different coagulation factor deficiencies will correct each other when mixed; if no correction occurs, it is assumed that the plasmas share the same deficiency. Coagulation factor assays are merely sophisticated mixing tests; they will be discussed later.

It is useful to perform both a partial thromboplastin time and an activated partial thromboplastin time as part of the screening procedure because this affords a simple way of examining the contact activation phase of the coagulation mechanism. An abnormality affecting the contact activation factors is suggested if the partial thromboplastin time does not become significantly shorter upon activation.

The sensitivity of the particular type of partial thromboplastin time that is being used should be known. In our laboratory, the result becomes abnormal when factor VIII coagulant activity decreases below 25 U/dl. This means that mild hemophilia in a patient with factor VIII levels above this value will not be detected by this test. Other modifications of the test are far less sensitive, and this knowledge is important in evaluating the significance of a normal test result.

## The Prothrombin Time

The prothrombin time is a measure of clotting initiated by the extrinsic coagulation system. Although important interactions occur between the intrinsic and extrinsic coagulation systems, the differentiation, although probably artificial, is helpful from a practical point of view in understanding the clinical significance of the screening coagulation tests.

The test is performed by adding a "complete" thromboplastin—the equivalent of tissue thromboplastin—to citrated blood and performing a coagulation time after the addition of calcium. Like the partial thromboplastin time, the prothrombin time is affected by deficiencies of factors V and X, prothrombin, and fibrinogen. Unlike the partial thromboplastin time, the prothrombin time is sensitive to deficiencies of factor VII. It bypasses the early stage of the intrinsic coagulation mechanism, however, and is normal in deficiencies of factors VIII, IX, XI, and XII, prekallikrein, and high molecular weight kininogen. The test was originally described by Quick et al.[35] and was called the *prothrombin time* because at that time factors V, VII, and X were unknown, and it was believed that the test reflected the concentration of prothrombin. In fact, it is much more sensitive to deficiencies of factors V, VII, and X.

The prothrombin time, like the partial thromboplastin time, may be prolonged because of the deficiency of a coagulation factor or the presence of a circulating anticoagulant. In exactly the same way as with a partial thromboplastin time, mixing tests will help to distinguish these two mechanisms. The use of artificially depleted plasmas and plasmas from patients with known coagulation factor deficiencies will allow the identification of the deficient coagulation activities.

As with the partial thromboplastin time, it is important to know the sensitivity of the prothrombin time. The situation is complicated because the sensitivity to coagulation factor deficiencies and inhibitors depends on the type of thromboplastin used. Each thromboplastin has a different sensitivity, and at present, there is no standardized method used in the United States. In some European countries and Australia, attempts have been made to set up national standards, and a number of committees have tried to bring some order into the international situation.

Our own thromboplastin is made from an aqueous extract of rabbit brain using Quick's original method, which is similar to that of the British—a method developed by Poller et al. with human brain.[36] The normal range for this method (as with Poller's method) is 17–19 seconds, longer than that of commercially produced acetone-extracted thromboplastin.

## The Thrombin Time

It is desirable, but not essential, to perform the thrombin time test as part of the screening procedures. The test consists of adding a solution of thrombin to anticoagulated plasma and performing a clotting time.[37] The thrombin time is prolonged when the levels of plasma fibrinogen are low, as well as in the presence of heparin, fibrinolytic split products, or abnormal fibrinogen. Occasionally, patients with abnormal fibrinogens have prolonged thrombin times but normal or only minimally prolonged partial thromboplastin times and prothrombin times. This means that, unless the thrombin time is performed, a certain proportion of patients with abnormal fibrinogens will not be detected. Like all other screening tests, the thrombin time is not perfect; in rare cases, patients have been described who have dysfibrinogenemia and normal or even short thrombin times.[38]

Another useful application of the thrombin time test is for the detection of heparin in patients who bleed after cardiac bypass surgery. If the concentration of thrombin added to the test plasma is adjusted to give a clotting time of more than 20 seconds with normal plasma, the test becomes extremely sensitive to small quantities of heparin. Large quantities of circulating heparin also will prolong the activated partial thromboplastin time and the prothrombin time. If, after cardiac bypass, the patient has a slightly prolonged thrombin time and a normal prothrombin time and partial thromboplastin time, one can conclude that the amount of circulating heparin is small and unlikely to be the cause of bleeding. The presence of heparin can be confirmed by removing it by adsorption with barium sulfate or by an ion-exchange cellulose (triethylaminoethyl) and by neutralization with protamine sulfate or platelet factor 4.

If the thrombin time is prolonged, a Reptilase or ancrod (Arvin) time should also be measured. Reptilase derived from the venom of the pit viper *Bothrops atrox* and ancrod, from *Ancistrodon Rhodostoma* venom, clot fibrinogen by splitting off fibrinopeptide A from the molecule and leaving fibrinopeptide B attached. The test is useful in differentiating the cause of a long thrombin time[39] because the Reptilase time is normal in the presence of heparin but prolonged in the presence of abnormal fibrinogens and fibrinolytic products.

## The Factor XIII (Fibrin-Stabilizing Factor) Test

All the screening tests enumerated so far are insensitive to deficiencies of factor XIII. Factor XIII is a transglutaminase that is activated by thrombin in the presence of calcium ions and causes covalent cross-linking of the fibrin clot. After the action of factor XIII, the clots are no longer soluble in $5 M$ urea or 1 percent monochloroacetic acid. Clot solubility in these reagents, therefore, can be used as a screening test for factor XIII deficiency,[40] al-

**Table 3-1**
Classification of Hemostatic Abnormalities Into Four Groups

| Deficiency | Prolonged Partial Thromboplastin Time | Prolonged Prothrombin Time | |
|---|---|---|---|
| High molecular weight kininogen | + | 0 | |
| Prekallikrein | + | 0 | |
| Factor XII | + | 0 | |
| Factor XI | + | 0 | Group 1 |
| Factor IX | + | 0 | |
| Factor VIII | + | 0 | |
| Factor VII | 0 | + | Group 2 |
| Factor V | + | + | |
| Factor X | + | + | |
| Prothrombin | + | + | Group 3 |
| Fibrinogen | + | + | Group 4 |
| Factor XIII | 0 | 0 | |

though the method is insensitive and detects only very severe deficiencies (2U/dl or less). There is some evidence, however, that only a small amount of factor XIII (above 2 U/dl) is required for normal hemostasis.

## Differential Diagnosis

Considerable discrimination of the inherited and acquired hemostatic disorders is possible by the use of three screening tests: the partial thromboplastin time and its activated variant, the prothrombin time, and the thrombin time (Tables 3-1 and 3-2).

Patients with the pattern shown in group 1 have abnormal activities of factors in the first stage of coagulation mechanism—namely, factors VIII, IX, XI, and XII, prekallikrein, and high molecular weight kininogen. The Passovoy factor also appears to be involved in this part of the coagulation mechanism. This large number of potential abnormalities can be divided into two groups on the basis of clinical findings. Three deficiencies (factor XII, prekallikrein, and high molecular weight kininogen) are not associated with bleeding, and three (factors XI, IX, and VIII) are. The first four factors, and possibly Passovoy factor, form the contact activation system. An abnormality in the contact activation factors can be suspected if the partial thromboplastin time does not shorten on the addition of an activator used in performing the activated partial thromboplastin time test (Table 3-3).

**Table 3-2**
Evaluation of Hemostatic Abnormalities with Three Screening Tests

| Group | Prothrombin Time | Partial Thromboplastin Time | Thrombin Time |
|---|---|---|---|
| Intrinsic factor abnormality | Normal | Abnormal | Normal |
| Extrinsic factor abnormality | Abnormal | Normal | Normal |
| Final common pathway abnormality or multiple defects | Abnormal | Abnormal | Usually normal |
| Fibrinogen abnormality | Normal* | Normal* | Abnormal |

*Unless the deficiency of fibrinogen or its inhibition is severe.

**Table 3-3**

Group I Patients with Prolonged Partial Thromboplastin Time

| Deficiency | Patient a Bleeder | Activated Partial Thromboplastin Time vs. Partial Thromboplastin Time* | Bleeding Time | Corrected by: | |
|---|---|---|---|---|---|
| | | | | Aged Normal Plasma | Adsorbed Normal Plasma |
| Factor VIII (classic hemophilia, | Yes | S | Normal | No | Yes |
| von Willebrand's disease) | | | Long | No | Yes |
| Factor IX | Usually | S | Normal | Yes | No |
| Factor XI | Yes | L | Normal | | |
| Factor XII | No | L | Normal | | |
| Prekallikrein | No | L | Normal | | |
| High molecular weight kininogen | No | L | Normal | | |

*S, activated partial thromboplastin time shorter than the partial thromboplastin time; L, same as the partial thromboplastin time.

The remainder of the patients with the group 1 pattern of abnormality have abnormal bleeding of the type outlined in the section on clinical evaluation. Patients with classic hemophilia (one type of functional deficiency of factor VIII) and Christmas disease (functional deficiency of factor IX) have an X-linked mode of inheritance, in contrast to patients with factor XI deficiency. In all of these patients, clues to the diagnosis can be given by specific mixing tests with artificial reagents, such as aged and adsorbed plasmas, but the final diagnosis depends on mixing the patient's plasma with the plasma from a subject with a known coagulation factor deficiency.

The group 2 pattern consists of a prolonged prothrombin time and a normal partial thromboplastin time and thrombin time. The only coagulation abnormality that causes this pattern of test results is factor VII deficiency, which is an extremely rare congenital disorder. Factor VII has the shortest in vivo half-life of all the coagulation proteins (3–5 hours), and so in vitamin K deficiency the concentration of factor VII is reduced before decreases are seen in the other vitamin K-dependent coagulation factors. In the early stages of vitamin K deficiency or oral anticoagulant therapy, therefore, an isolated deficiency of factor VII may occur as an acquired phenomenon and produce the group 2 pattern of coagulation tests.

The group 3 pattern consists of a prolonged prothrombin time and partial thromboplastin time and a normal or abnormal thrombin time. Patients have (1) inherited functional deficiencies (fibrinogen, prothrombin, factor V or X) or (2) acquired functional deficiencies, such as vitamin K deficiency (reduced prothrombin and factors VII, IX, and X), acute intravascular coagulation-fibrinolysis syndrome (reduced factors V and VIII, thrombocytopenia, increased FSP), or liver disease (reduced vitamin K-dependent factors and factor V, increased factor VIII). If fibrinogen is deficient or abnormal, the thrombin time is prolonged.

Deficiencies of proteins in the final common clotting pathway (namely, fibrinogen, prothrombin, and factors V and X) may cause this pattern of test results. Although most congenital deficiencies are single, occasionally combined deficiencies occur, particularly those of factors V and VIII,[41] and this would cause this same pattern of abnormalities in the screening tests. Other double deficiencies have been reported, and there have been extremely rare instances of deficiency in several or even all of the vitamin K-dependent coagulation factors.[42,43]

Much more commonly, prolongation of the partial thromboplastin time and prothrombin time is caused by acquired abnormalities (particularly vitamin K deficiency), oral anticoagulant therapy, liver disease, intravascular coagulation and fibrinolysis, or circulating anticoagulants.

In deficiencies of the vitamin K-dependent coagulation factors (due to oral anticoagulant therapy, antibiotic therapy, obstructive jaundice, or malabsorption), the stable cothromboplastic factors (factors VII and X) are decreased, whereas factor V is normal. In addition, specific assays for factor IX and prothrombin show decreases of these factors as well. However, in the acute intravascular coagulation–fibrinolysis syndrome, factors VII and X may be normal or only moderately decreased, whereas factors V and VIII are regularly decreased.[44,45] Simple mixing tests can give helpful information for determining which factors are depleted. In the acute intravascular coagulation–fibrinolysis syndrome, often called disseminated intravascular coagulation (DIC), there is also a decreased number of platelets and evidence of secondary fibrinolysis, based on an elevation of fibrinogen-related antigens. In significant liver disease, factor V is depleted in addition to the vitamin K-dependent coagulation factors, and eventually there is depletion of fibrinogen. Here again, simple mixing tests can give much information that is useful in the differential diagnosis. In many patients with liver disease, an abnormal fibrinogen is present, leading to pronounced prolongation of the thrombin time, and the activity levels in the factor VIII complex may be elevated.

Patients who have factor VII or X deficiency have a prolongation of the prothrombin time that is corrected by aged plasma but not by adsorbed plasma. The Russell's viper venom time helps in differentiating the abnormality.[46,47] The venom of the Russell's viper can activate factor X without the presence of factor VII. The clotting time with this test is therefore prolonged in factor X deficiency but normal in factor VII deficiency. Russell's viper venom also requires factor V and platelet factor 3, so the test time is prolonged in factor V deficiency; the test has been used as an assay for platelet factor 3. The situation regarding factor X is not as simple as was once believed because some patients have been described with factor X deficiency and normal Russell's viper venom times.[48,49]

The most frequent cause of a prolonged prothrombin time is oral anticoagulant therapy. Numerous patients are now taking long-term anticoagulants. Oral anticoagulant therapy thus should be the first possibility that is considered in evaluating a patient with a long prothrombin time.

The group 4 pattern consists of a prolonged thrombin time and a normal or abnormal prothrombin time and partial thromboplastin time. Patients may have hypofibrinogenemia, dysfibrinogenemia (inherited or acquired), or coagulation inhibitors (heparin, FSP).

If plasma fibrinogen is completely lacking, a truly rare afibrinogenemic state, there is no end point with any clotting test. In moderate hypofibrinogenemic states, the thrombin time tends to be more prolonged than the prothrombin time and partial thromboplastin time. Hypofibrinogenemia may be inherited, but more commonly it is secondary to decompensated intravascular coagulation or severe liver disease. In dysfibrinogenemia, the thrombin time may be prolonged and there may be little effect on the partial thromboplastin time or the prothrombin time. Dysfibrinogenemia may be an inherited abnormality but is commonly seen in association with liver disease. Lastly, inhibitors of the coagulation mechanism, such as FSP or heparin, may cause this pattern of abnormalities. We have seen patients with multiple myeloma who have prolonged thrombin times, and we have recently found

DIC → ↓ II̅, V̅, √III
      ↑ PTT
      ↑ reptilase t.
      ↑ thrombine t.

a heparin-like circulating anticoagulant in one of these patients.[50] The anticoagulant is probably related to heparan.

## SPECIFIC COAGULATION FACTOR ASSAYS

### Factor I (Fibrinogen)

The most reliable method for measuring fibrinogen is a quantitative technique that measures thrombin-coagulable protein.[51] The clotted fibrin is collected on glass beads or an applicator stick. The method requires meticulous attention to detail, particularly during washing, so that all serum proteins are removed without washing away the fibrin. The amount of fibrin in the sample is then measured. In our laboratory this is done colorimetrically with a biuret reagent.[52,53] A number of indirect methods for measuring fibrinogen depend on the clotting times, turbidity, and sedimentation rate of polymer beads.[54]

### Factor II (Prothrombin)

Prothrombin is measured by a 2-stage technique.[55,56] The anticoagulated plasma is defibrinated by the addition of a weak solution of thrombin. Tissue thromboplastin and calcium are then added so that the prothrombin begins to convert to thrombin. The amount of thrombin formed at various intervals is measured by adding the incubation mixture to a standard solution of fibrinogen. It is assumed that the maximal amount of thrombin generated reflects the concentration of prothrombin in the original plasma. If the plasma comes from a patient lacking factor V, VII, or X, the missing factor must be supplied to the assay mixture.

A two-stage method using Taipan snake venom also has been described.[57] This snake venom converts prothrombin directly to thrombin in the absence of any other known clotting factor. The first stage consists of generating thrombin by mixing the plasma with the Taipan snake venom in the presence of phospholipid and calcium chloride. The second stage is similar to that of the conventional test.

### Assays for Factors V, VII, and X

The unknown plasma is mixed with plasma that is congenitally deficient in factor V, VII, or X.[58] The prothrombin time test is performed, and the degree of correction of the clotting time is compared with that shown by normal plasma. In our laboratory, we continue to use the tilt-tube method in performing assays. Many commercial machines are useful for the clinical assessment of the prothrombin time and partial thromboplastin time, but when the clotting times are long, we have not found them to be reproducible enough to allow the performance of accurate assays.

Recently, we have started to use a substrate for factor V assays, which is artificially depleted of factor V by affinity chromatography using a hybridoma antibody.[34]

### Assays for Factors VIII, IX, XI, and XII

The substrate plasma is obtained from patients congenitally deficient in one of these factors.[58] The patient's plasma is mixed with the substrate plasma, and an activated partial thromboplastin time test is performed. The degree of correction of the clotting time is compared with that of normal plasma.

In Britain, a second method for measuring factor VIII activity is popular—the 2-stage-assay based on the thromboplastin generation test. In the first stage, an incubation mixture is prepared containing factor V, serum (supplies factors IX, X, XI, and XII), and a substitute for platelet factor 3. Factor VIII is provided by adding normal plasma, and calcium is also added. Various dilutions of the normal plasma containing factor VIII are used, the incubation mixture is transferred to tubes containing normal plasma, and the clotting time is recorded. The clotting time of the second stage is plotted against the concentrations of factor VIII in the normal plasma dilution; from this graph, the concentration of the factor in an unknown can be interpolated. It is stated that the two-stage technique is not affected by small traces of thrombin and thus is not likely to give the erroneously high results produced in a one-stage assay. Lupuslike inhibitors may inhibit the assay system in a one-stage assay, but because the plasma in the 2-stage method is more dilute, the activity of the inhibitors is less likely to affect the latter assay. It is also stated that the two-stage method is more precise than the one-stage method.[59,60] The disadvantage of the two-stage assay is that the reagents are difficult to prepare, and there are problems in standardization.

We have found no difference between the one- and two-stage methods. The reason may be that our one-stage assay differs from conventional assays in that we use a large amount of substrate (nine parts of substrate to one part of test plasma).

## Standardization of the Assay for Factor VIII:C

Because the level of factor VIII in the general population varies widely, a pool of plasma from many donors is necessary for a reference standard. The value of 1.0 U/ml is assigned to the pool. The concentrations of factor VIII among donors range from about 0.5 to about 2.0 U/ml. Because of the wide variation in the normal population, at least 20–30 donors should be used to form the standard pool, which must be prepared under highly standarized conditions and frozen at $-70°C$ or lower. The provision of such a large pool of donors is an obvious problem for laboratories that are not primarily engaged in coagulation work, and it would be helpful to have a commercially available reference standard. An international factor VIII reference preparation is now available at the National Institute for Biological Standards and Control in London. Recent observations, however, have shown that in these purified preparations the two-stage assay detects about 20 percent more activity than the one-stage assay. The two assays give comparable results when plasma samples are tested.[60,61]

## Tests for Factor VIII–Willebrand Factor

Factor VIII is a complex molecule, and there is compelling evidence that the factor VIII coagulant activity and the Willebrand factor activity are represented by two separate molecules that are associated but not covalently bound in vivo. The factor VIII coagulant molecule participates in the coagulation mechanism, and the Willebrand factor molecule is involved in platelet–blood vessel interaction. Various nomenclatures have been used for identifying the many factor VIII-related activities, and the following symbols will be used in this section: *factor VIII:C* refers to the factor VIII coagulant activity measured by the one-stage or two-stage coagulation assays, and *factor VIII-related antigen (VIIIR:AG)* refers to the antigenic activity related to factor VIII detected by a rabbit or goat antibody to purified Willebrand factor[62] as measured by Laurell's electroimmunossay.[63]

*Factor VIII-related Willebrand factor (VIIIR:WF)*, a term synonymous with *factor VIII–ristocetin–Willebrand factor* and *factor VIII–ristocetin cofactor,* refers to the normal plasma activity that allows ristocetin to induce platelet agglutination; this plasma activity is decreased or missing in the plasma in von Willebrand's disease. It is measured by the degree of correction of agglutination of washed human platelets.

## Assay for Factor VIII-Related Antigen

One of the most important developments in our knowledge of hemophilia and von Willebrand's disease is the observation that heterologous antisera to purified preparations of the factor VIII complex give immunoprecipitin reactions with normal plasma and hemophilic plasma but not with the plasma from patients who have severe von Willebrand's disease. The usual method for measuring factor VIIIR:AG uses the Laurell technique of immunolectrophoresis (Fig. 3-1).[64] An antibody to factor VIIIR:AG is dissolved in an agarose gel. Plasma is placed in a well in the gel, and the factor VIIIR:AG is electrophoresed toward the anode. The antigen–antibody reaction forms a precipitin line that has the appearance of a rocket ascending from the well.[65] The concentration of antigen is directly proportional to the area of the rocket, but conventionally only the height of the rocket is measured. Radioimmunosasays, immunoradiometric assays, and enzyme-linked assays also have been developed for the measurement of factor VIIIR:AG.

## Assay for Ristocetin–Willebrand Factor

Ristocetin is an antibiotic that was withdrawn from the commercial market because it produced thrombocytopenia. Howard and Firkin[66] observed that ristocetin induced platelet agglutination in normal platelet-rich plasma but not in the platelet-rich plasma of a patient with von Willebrand's disease. The addition of normal plasma to the patient's plasma produced platelet agglutination in von Willebrand's disease. The degree of agglutination in such a mixture is dependent on the amount of normal plasma added. This allowed the development of a functional assay for ristocetin–Willebrand factor or ristocetin cofactor using fresh human platelets that had been washed or gel-filtered to remove all the Willebrand factor.[67,68] To obviate the necessity to use fresh platelets, an assay has been developed in which platelets fixed with paraformaldehyde or formalin are substituted. Fixed platelets are stable for several weeks and give the same results as fresh-washed platelets.[69]

Another assay uses macroscopic platelet aggregation as the end point. Ristocetin is added to a platelet suspension, and the time required to produce the platelet aggregation (''snowstorm'') effect is measured.[70] The length of time is inversely proportional to the concentration of Willebrand factor. Fixed platelets can also be used in this way.[71]

## Factor XIII

The screening test for factor XIII has already been discussed (page 53).

The enzyme can be measured by a semiquantitative method in which fibrinogen, free of factor XIII, is added to various dilutions of normal and patients' plasma. Clotting is produced by the addition of thrombin, after which monochloroacetic acid is added. The greatest dilution of plasma at which the clot remains insoluble is recorded, and the value is compared with the control sample.[72]

Quantitative assays depend on factor XIII's transamidase properties, for example the incorporation of monodansylcadaverine into casein.[73]

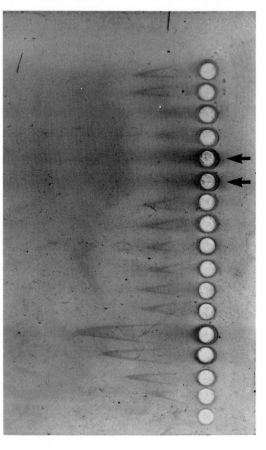

**Fig. 3-1.** Immunoelectrophoresis of factor VIII-related antigen by the Laurell technique. The first five wells are dilutions of the standard plasma from which the standard curve is constructed. The remaining wells contain samples of patients' plasmas (in duplicate). No "rockets" are seen above the wells (marked by arrows) that contain plasma from a patient with severe von Willebrand's disease.

## Special Tests of Platelet Function

Clinical platelet function tests measure platelet adhesion and aggregation, the release reaction, and coagulant activity. Like all tests of hemostasis, they must be meticulously performed. Unfortunately, they are usually available only in specialized laboratories.

Platelet disorders are one area of hemostasis in which physical signs may be helpful because petechiae are almost always diagnostic of a capillary or platelet abnormality. We have already discussed the bleeding time, which is the only test that measures directly the role of platelets in hemostasis. All of the other platelet function tests that will now be discussed assess the role of platelets in vitro, and there is not always a good correlation between an abnormal test result and clinical bleeding. Most of the platelet function tests are complicated, and they are affected by so many variables that it is important to standardize them carefully. Platelet function is affected by many drugs. If possible, patients should be tested only when they have stopped taking medications for at least 2 weeks.

## Platelet Aggregation

Platelet aggregation is the adherence of platelets to each other. Platelet-rich plasma is placed in the cuvette of a spectrophotometer and stirred with a magnetic stirrer.[74] After the addition of a solution of an aggregating agent (with the exception of epinephrine), the shape of the platelet changes from disc to sphere, and pseudopods are formed. The change in shape decreases light transmission; this decrease is followed by an increase in light transmission as platelet aggregates are formed. The platelets may disaggregate when the concentration of the aggregating agent is low, but at higher concentrations of most agents, a second phase of aggregation occurs, after which the platelets remain clumped.[75]

Usually, in the laboratory, the platelet-aggregating agents used are adenosine diphosphate (ADP), epinephrine, collagen, and arachidonic acid. Thrombin may also be used. ADP and epinephrine are primary aggregating agents and have specific receptors on the cell membrane. After the addition of these agents, thromboxane $A_2$ is formed and ADP is released from the platelet, resulting in the second phase of aggregation.[76–78] After the addition of collagen to platelet-rich plasma, a lag phase occurs, probably related to polymerization of the collagen. The platelets then aggregate, again after the formation of thromboxane $A_2$ and the release of ADP.[79] With collagen, therefore, only a single phase of aggregation occurs. Sodium arachidonate causes aggregation by its conversion to thromboxane $A_2$.

Platelet aggregation is affected by many variables, including the anticoagulant used, pH, time of storage,[80] rate of stirring and shape and size of the stir bar,[81] concentration of the platelets, and size and shape of the cuvette. Platelet aggregation is also affected by many drugs—most commonly aspirin, because it is widely used. Aspirin prevents the formation of thromboxane $A_2$ by inhibiting the cyclooxygenase of the platelet membrane. Use of arachidonate, therefore, is a useful screening test for aspirin ingestion.

Platelet aggregation tests are essential in the diagnosis of qualitative platelet disease.[25,82,83] In Glanzmann's thrombasthenia, there is no primary or secondary aggregation with any of the usual aggregating agents. Although they do not aggregate, the platelets do adhere to collagen and undergo a normal release reaction; they also agglutinate on the addition of ristocetin. In storage or release defects, there is no second wave of aggregation with ADP and epinephrine and disaggregation is often seen. Aggregation with collagen is decreased. The Bernard-Soulier syndrome is diagnosed by the presence of large platelets that are readily recognizable on the blood smear; aggregation with ADP, epinephrine, collagen, and arachidonate is normal. There is, however, no agglutination of

Bernard-Soulier platelets on the addition of ristocetin, because the platelets appear to lack receptors for Willebrand factor.

In the myeloproliferative diseases and other acquired qualitative platelet disorders, various platelet aggregation abnormalities have been described.[25,84-86]

If platelet aggregation is abnormal, the test should be repeated at least once because of the foibles of the test.

## Tests of Platelet Adhesion and Adhesion Aggregation

A number of tests measure platelet adhesion alone in the adherence of platelets to nonplatelet surfaces. These tests include immersion of glass slides and coverslips in blood or platelet-rich plasma,[87-90] adhesion of platelets to red cells,[91] and the use of rotating glass tubes[92-94] or glass rods[95] that have been coated with collagen or other proteins. The aggregometer also may be adapted to measure mainly platelet adhesion.[96-99] Adhesion-aggregation can be measured by the in vivo method of Borchgrevink,[84,100-103] an in vitro method using glass wool braid,[102] the Wright rotating glass bulb technique,[103-105] and the passage of blood through columns filled with small glass beads.[106-110]

With the exception of the glass bead column techniques, few of these methods have become popular in clinical laboratories. The methods using glass bead columns have been difficult to standardize, but they can give reproducible results and clinically useful information if the variables are taken into account. These variables include the presence or absence of red cells, temperature, the anticoagulant, the contact time of the blood with the glass beads, "disturbance" of the blood, and the type of plastic used to construct the columns.[111,112] It seems likely that the glass bead column test measures the primary phase of hemostasis, and it has been suggested that it provides a sensitive in vitro bleeding time.[113,114]

The results of the glass bead column tests are expressed as a percentage of platelets retained in the columns. Because it measures both adhesion and aggregation of platelets, the test is usually called a *platelet retention test*. It is not diagnostic of any specific disease; its main applications have been in von Willebrand's disease, and qualitative platelet diseases, and in testing drugs proposed as antithrombotic agents.[115-117] Although the platelet retention test was originally important in the diagnosis of von Willebrand's disease, it has now been superseded by more specific tests, including the measurement of factor VIII-related antigen and ristocetin cofactor.

The test remains useful in von Willebrand's disease when the diagnosis has been obscured by transfusions, pregnancy, and the use of birth control pills. In these conditions, the level of factor VIII coagulant activity, factor VIII-related antigen, and ristocetin cofactor may approach normal, but platelet retention remains abnormal. The test is also a useful screen for platelet function. It may be particularly valuable in laboratories that do not specialize in testing platelet function.

## Measurements of the Storage Pool and Release Reaction of Platelets

A number of substances are stored in the platelet organelles. During the release reaction, they are secreted by the platelet. The dense granules contain serotonin, calcium, ADP, adenosine triphosphate (ATP), pyrophosphate, and possibly antiplasmin. The $\alpha$-granules contain various proteins, including platelet factor 4, $\beta$-thromboglobulin, platelet-derived growth factor, fibrinogen, factor V, Willebrand factor, fibronectin, and albumin, as well as a number of other agents such as permeability factor, chemotactic factor, and bactericidal factor. The lysosomes contain acid hydrolases and cathepsins, and there are peroxisomes that contain catalase, as they do in other cells. The granules may be heterogeneous and store different proteins.

The contents of the dense granules and α-granules are released by all of the aggregating agents, but the lysosomes secrete their contents only in response to thrombin or to high concentrations of collagen.[118] In the condition known as *storage pool disease,* the contents of the platelet granules are decreased. In another type of qualitative disease, the granular contents are normal but secretion is abnormal. In both of these conditions, the aggregation patterns are identical, but they can be differentiated by measuring the storage pools of ADP, ATP, and serotonin. The nucleotide storage pool in the granules contains relatively more ADP than does the metabolic pool; thus, in storage pool disease, in which the granule nucleotides are decreased, there is relatively less ADP than in normal platelets, and the ATP:ADP ratio is high. In this way, storage pool defects can be differentiated from abnormalities of secretion. All of the serotonin in the plasma is contained in the dense granules of the platelets, and in storage pool disease affecting the dense granules, the uptake of serotonin is decreased. Radioactive serotonin can be used to measure the release reaction.

## Tests for Platelet Factor 3

Platelet factor 3 is a mixture of phospholipoproteins in the platelet membrane which furnishes the phospholipids needed for the clotting mechanisms. The phospholipids in the platelet membrane are made available during activation of the platelet and serve as a surface on which activation of the clotting factors occurs. The activity of platelet factor 3 increases during aggregation induced by ADP, epinephrine, serotonin, and collagen, and it probably is made available by a change in the platelet membrane.

The activity can be measured by a number of clotting tests, including the kaolin-activated plasma clot test, the clotting time using Russell's viper venom, the thromboplastin generation test, and the prothrombin consumption test. We have found the prothrombin consumption test to be the most reproducible way of gauging platelet factor 3 activity.[119] This test measures the residual coagulation activity in serum after clotting has occurred. In one tube, freshly drawn blood is allowed to clot spontaneously. In a second tube, a substitute for platelet factor 3, such as Inosithin, is added to the freshly drawn blood. If the prothrombin consumption abnormality in the first tube is due to a platelet factor 3 deficiency, the abnormality will be corrected in the second tube. In any condition in which platelet aggregation is abnormal, platelet factor 3 availability is decreased. There are occasional reports of an isolated deficiency of platelet factor 3, although this is a rare finding.[120–122] There is also a report of a patient with decreased platelet coagulant activity due to a diminished number of factor V binding sites, resulting in impaired factor Xa binding to the platelet membrane.[123,124]

## Miscellaneous Tests of Platelet Function

A number of other tests of platelet function have not found wide acceptance because they have been superseded by other tests or are of little clinical value. Capillary fragility is measured by increasing capillary pressures using local suction or the application of a sphygmomanometer cuff. There have been problems in standardizing the test, and its significance is not clearly understood. Clot retraction is widely used as a screening test for platelet function but gives little useful information. Clot retraction is abnormal in thrombocytopenia and thrombasthenia; both of these conditions can be more accurately diagnosed by other tests. The test should still be done in Glanzmann's thrombasthenia because this was the diagnostic criterion used by Glanzmann in his original paper.

The platelet contains specific proteins that are secreted during the release reaction, including β-thromboglobulin and platelet factor 4. An increase in the levels of these proteins in the circulating blood may be useful in diagnosing thrombotic states, and the levels are elevated in intravascular coagulation. Meticulous techniques must be used to prevent release of these proteins during the collection and preparation of the blood sample. In other bleeding disorders, however, measurement of these proteins is of no diagnostic help.

Finally, it must be emphasized that the clinical significance of abnormal platelet function tests should be interpreted in light of their limitations.

## SPECIAL PROBLEMS IN DIAGNOSIS

### Circulating Anticoagulants

In the preceding sections, much has been said about circulating anticoagulants. Although they will be dealt with in detail in a subsequent chapter, we will discuss them briefly here in relation to clotting tests. In systemic lupus erythematosus, circulating anticoagulants have frequently been recognized and generally regarded as interfering with the conversion of prothrombin to thrombin.[6-9] They may inhibit the phospholipid component of the prothrombin activator. It is of interest that, as previously pointed out, bleeding is unusual in these patients, and some of them may actually develop thrombosis. Hemorrhagic symptoms are usually associated with low platelet counts and occasionally with decreased prothrombin. The anticoagulant usually inhibits the partial thromboplastin time and, as noted previously, has a more pronounced effect on the plasma clot time. Sometimes the later stage of clotting is affected, with prolongation of the prothrombin time and occasionally of the thrombin time. Prolongation of the thrombin time, of course, must occur by some mechanism other than the inhibition of the prothrombin activators.

The other types of circulating inhibitors are antibodies that inhibit specific coagulation factors. The usual coagulation factor involved is factor VIII. The antibodies are found in patients with classic hemophilia, as well as in patients who do not have this disease.[7,9,125] They will be fully discussed in Chapter 7. The clotting tests in patients with factor VIII inhibitors show prolongation of the partial thromboplastin time. In contrast to patients with the lupus type of inhibitor, there is a gradual inhibition of the affected coagulation factor when the patient's plasma is mixed with normal plasma. Antibodies to factor VIII coagulant activity combine slowly with the factor and may take 30–60 minutes or even longer to exert their maximal effect. With the lupus anticoagulant, the inhibition is immediate. Another difference is that patients with factor VIII inhibitors usually have significant hemorrhagic symptoms.

Inhibitors to other coagulation factors, including factors V, IX, and XIII, have been described. In addition, several inhibitors have been described involving factor XI, as well as combinations of factors XI and XII and fibrinogen.[7,9]

### Hemophilia and von Willebrand's Disease

There is no difficulty in diagnosing severe classic hemophilia. The problem in diagnosis arises in recognizing mild classic hemophilia and in differentiating mild hemophilia from von Willebrand's disease. As pointed out in the discussion of the partial thromboplas-

**Table 3-4**

Characteristics of the Classic Types of Hemophilia (Factor VIII: C
Deficiency) and von Willebrand's Disease

| Characteristic | Classic Hemophilia | von Willebrand's Disease |
|---|---|---|
| Inheritance | X-linked | Autosomal |
| Partial thromboplastin time | Prolonged | Prolonged |
| Prothrombin time | Normal | Normal |
| Platelet count | Normal | Normal |
| Bleeding time | Normal | Prolonged |
| Factor VIII:C | Low | Low |
| Factor VIIIR:AG | Normal | Low |
| von Willebrand factor | Normal | Low |

tin time, clotting tests vary greatly in their sensitivity to factor VIII coagulant activity. The whole-blood coagulation time will become normal if the factor VIII coagulant activity is 5 percent of normal or higher, and the activated partial thromboplastin time will not become normal until the level is above 20–30 percent. The exact level depends on the type of test performed; some types are less sensitive than others. In any case, a certain proportion of patients with mild hemophilia will be missed, even with a sensitive test, and the history is the only way of recognizing these patients before operation.

Some problems occur in differentiating classic hemophilia from von Willebrand's disease. As in classic hemophilia, there is no difficulty in diagnosing severe von Willebrand's disease. In addition to having reduced factor VIII coagulant activity, which is present in both diseases, the patient who has von Willebrand's disease will have a long bleeding time and reduced platelet retention; the results of both of these tests are normal in hemophilia. The factor VIII-related antigen and the von Willebrand factor are reduced or absent in von Willebrand's disease but are normal in hemophilia. These activities may be completely absent in some forms of von Willebrand's disease, because the factor VIII-related antigen is not synthesized. In other forms of the disease, an abnormal VIIIR:AG molecule may be produced and the results of 1 or more of the diagnostic tests may be normal. These conditions are usually known as variant forms of von Willebrand's disease, and the diagnosis depends on identifying the molecular abnormality in the Willebrand factor.[126–128]

A comparison of the classic form of von Willebrand's disease with classic hemophilia is shown in Table 3-4. One or another of the abnormalities in von Willebrand's disease has been reported to be normal in the variant forms of the disease. In the milder forms, the bleeding time and the factor VIII coagulant level are usually normal. In the usual type of variant, the Willebrand factor measured by ristocetin agglutination is reduced out of proportion to the factor VIII-related antigen, and in these patients, factor VIII-related antigen may be normal or somewhat reduced. These findings clearly suggest an abnormal molecule. The Willebrand factor is a series of polymers,[129] and in some variant forms of the disease there is a preponderance of the less active, low molecular weight polymers. In an interesting and unusual variant, the spread of molecular weight is normal but the distribution of the polymers is abnormal. Such patients may actually show increased ristocetin agglutination of their platelets.[126] Lastly, there is a form of the disease in which the Willebrand factor is reduced in the plasma but is present in normal amounts in the platelets and endothelial cells.[130] In this last group of patients, the bleeding seems milder than in patients who lack Willebrand factor in the plasma, platelets, and endothelial cells.

The molecular abnormalities in von Willebrand's disease can be most readily diagnosed in the clinical laboratory by crossed immunoelectrophoresis. The introduction of immunologic methods has established the fact that many of the coagulation abnormalities are due to biologically inactive coagulation proteins.

## FUTURE DEVELOPMENTS

The problem with most tests of coagulation is that they depend on the timing of clot formation—an event that is the final stage of a sequence of enzyme reactions, It would be desirable to have more precise, specific tests that are easy to perform. The initial results from work with chromogenic substrates and monoclonal antibodies suggest that such procedures may be developed in the future.

Elucidation of the primary structure of many coagulant proteins has allowed the identification of proteolytic activation cleavage sites and the synthesis of peptides mimicking the amino acid sequence adjacent to the sites. The peptide is then linked to a dye, producing a colorless compound that develops a color after enzymatic cleavage. The rate of color development can be measured in a spectrophotometer and is proportional to the concentration of the enzyme.

Chromogenic substrates have been developed for thrombin, factor Xa, plasmin, plasma prekallikrein, Hageman factor, and plasma thromboplastin antecedent. These substrates, except for that of plasminogen, are nonspecific and can be used to assay antithrombin III, antiplasmin, and heparin. The assays so far available have not been very useful in the diagnosis of hemorrhagic diatheses. However, additional chromogenic substrates probably will be developed which are specific for the assay of various coagulation factors. We have assayed all of the coagulation factors (except fibrinogen and fibrin-stabilizing factor) by using a thrombin-sensitive chromogenic substrate.[131,132] The technique still requires the use of plasma deficient in a specific coagulation factor, and the chromogenic substrate is used to simplify the reading of the endpoint.

Monoclonal antibodies form another line of investigation which shows promise of being useful in the clinical coagulation laboratory. However, many of the so-called coagulation factor deficiencies are deficiencies of activity rather than absence of the protein; in many of these conditions, an abnormal protein molecule is produced which lacks clotting activity. Polyclonal antibodies will detect these abnormal molecules but cannot distinguish them from normal molecules; thus, these antibodies give no information about the function of the molecule. A clotting assay is still necessary. However, monoclonal antibodies eventually will probably be produced which are specific for the physiologic coagulation factor and will not recognize abnormal forms of the protein. Such a monoclonal antibody would allow the development of a practical immunologic assay that would reflect physiologic function and would obviate the need for any further clotting assays.

## REFERENCES

1.  Silverstein MN: Primary or hemorrhagic thrombocythemia. Arch Intern Med 122:18–22, 1968
2.  Agle DP, Ratnoff OD, Wasman M: Studies in autoerythrocyte sensitization: The induction of purpuric lesions by hypnotic suggestion. Psychosom Med 29:491–503, 1967
3.  Ratnoff OD, Agle DP: Psychogenic purpura: A re-evaluation of the syndrome of autoerythrocyte sensitization. Medicine (Balt) 47:475–500, 1968

4. Agle DP, Ratnoff OD, Spring GK: The anticoagulant malingerer: Psychiatric studies of three patients. Ann Intern Med 73:67–72,1970

5. Bowie EJW, Todd M, Thompson JH Jr, et al: Anticoagulant malingerers (the ''Dicumarol-eaters''). Am J Med 39:855–864, 1965

6. Bowie EJW, Thompson JH Jr, Pascuzzi CA, et al: Thrombosis in systemic lupus erythematosus despite circulating anticoagulants. J Lab Clin Med 62:416–430, 1963

7. Feinstein DI, Rapaport SI: Acquired inhibitors of blood coagulation. Prog Thromb Hemost 1:75–95, 1972

8. Margolius A Jr, Jackson DP, Ratnoff OD: Circulating anticoagulants: A study of 40 cases and a review of the literature. Medicine (Balt) 40:145–202, 1961

9. Shapiro SS, Hultin M: Acquired inhibitors to the blood coagulation factors. Semin Thromb Haemostas 1:336–385, 1975

10. O'Brien JR: The bleeding time in normal and abnormal subjects. J Clin Pathol 4:272–285, 1951

11. Duke WW: The relation of blood platelets to hemorrhagic disease: Description of a method for determining the bleeding time and coagulation time and report of three cases of hemorrhagic disease relieved by transfusion. JAMA 55:1185–1192, 1910

12. Ivy AC, Shapiro PF, Melnick P: The bleeding tendency in jaundice. Surg Gynecol Obstet 60:781–784, 1935

13. Milian MG: Influence de la peau sur la coagulabilité du sang. C R Soc Biol 53:576–578, 1901

14. Milian MG: Technique pour l'étude clinique de la coagulation du sang. Bull Mem Soc Med Hop Paris (s 3) 18:777–783, 1901.

15. Ratnoff OD: Bleeding Syndromes: A Clinical Manual. Springfield, Ill, Charles C Thomas, 1960

16. Adelson E, Crosby WH: A new method to measure bleeding time: The ''immersion'' method. Acta Haematol (Basel) 18:281–289, 1957

17. Sutor AH, Bowie EJW, Thompson JH Jr, et al: Bleeding from standardized skin punctures: Automated technic for recording time, intensity, and pattern of bleeding. Am J Clin Pathol 55:541–550, 1971

18. Sutor AH, Bowie EJW, Owen CA Jr: Effect of temperature on hemostasis: A cold-tolerance test. Blut 22:27–34, 1971

19. Bowie EJW, Owen CA Jr: The bleeding time. Prog Hemost Thromb 2:249–271, 1974

20. Bowie EJW, Owen CA Jr: Standardization of the bleeding time. Scand J Haematol Suppl. 37:87–94, 1980

21. Mielke CH Jr, Kaneshiro MM, Maher IA, et al: The standardized normal Ivy bleeding time and its prolongation by aspirin. Blood 34:204–215, 1969

22. Day HJ: Laboratory tests in platelet function, Schmidt RM (ed): CRC Handbook of Clinical Laboratory Science, vol. 1. Boca Raton, Fla CRC Press, 1979, pp 329–349

23. Harker LA, Slichter SJ: The bleeding time as a screening test for evaluation of platelet function. N Engl J Med 287:155–159, 1972

24. Kumar R, Ansell J, Deykin D: Clinical trial of a new bleeding time device, in Day HJ, Holmsen H, Zucker MB (eds): Platelet Function Testing. US Dept of Health, Education and Welfare Publication (NIH) 78–1087, 1978, pp 21–22

25. Owen CA Jr, Bowie EJW, Thompson JH Jr: The Diagnosis of Bleeding Disorders (ed 2). Boston, Little, Brown, 1975

26. Hirsh J. Blajchman M, Kaegi A: The bleeding time, in Day JH, Holmsen H, Zucker MB (eds): Platelet Function Testing. US Dept of Health, Education and Welfare publication (NIH) 78–1087, 1978, pp 1–12

27. Bowie EJW, Didisheim P, Thompson JH Jr, et al: Von Willebrand's disease: A critical review. Hematol Rev 1:1–50, 1968

28. Larrieu MJ, Caen JP, Meyer DO, et al: Congenital bleeding disorders with long bleeding

time and normal platelet count. II. Von Willebrand's disease (report of thirty-seven patients). Am J Med 45:354–372, 1968

29.  Czapek EE, Deykin D, Salzman E, et al: Intermediate syndrome of platelet dysfunction. Blood 52:103–113, 1978

30.  Quick AJ: Salicylates and bleeding: The aspirin tolerance test. Am J Med Sci 252:265–269, 1966

31.  Langdell RD, Wagner RH, Brinkhous KM: Effect of antihemophilic factor on one-stage clotting tests: A presumptive test for hemophilia and a simple one-stage antihemophilic factor assay procedure. J Lab Clin Med 41:637–647, 1953

32.  Proctor RR, Rapaport SI: The partial thromboplastin time with kaolin: A simple screening test for first stage plasma clotting factor deficiencies. Am J Clin Pathol 36:212–219, 1961

33.  Owen CA Jr, Mann FD, Hurn MM, et al: Evaluation of disorders of blood coagulation in the clinical laboratory. Am J Clin Pathol 25:1417–1426, 1955

34.  Katzmann JA, Nesheim ME, Hibbard LS, et al: Isolation of functional human coagulation Factor V by using a hybridoma antibody. Proc Natl Acad Sci USA 78:162–166, 1981

35.  Quick AJ, Stanley-Brown M, Bancroft FW: A study of the coagulation defect in hemophilia and in jaundice. Am J Med Sci 190:501–511, 1935

36.  Poller L: The British system of anticoagulant control. Thromb Diath Haemorrh 33:157–162, 1975

37.  Jim RTS: A study of the plasma thrombin time. J Lab Clin Med 50:45–60, 1957

38.  Egeberg O: Inherited fibrinogen abnormality causing thrombophilia. Thromb Diath Haemorrh 17:176–187, 1967

39.  Funk C, Gmür J, Herold R, et al: Reptilase-R—a new reagent in blood coagulation. Br J Haematol 21:43–52, 1971

40.  Duckert F, Jung E, Shmerling DH: A hitherto undescribed congenital haemorrhagic diathesis probably due to fibrin stabilizing factor deficiency. Thromb Diath Haemorrh 5:179–186, 1960

41.  Sibinga CTS, Gökemeyer JDM, ten Cate LP, et al: Combined deficiency of factor V and factor VIII: Report of a family and genetic analysis. Br J Haematol 23:467–481, 1972

42.  Biggs R: Some observations on the blood of patients with 'Factor-VII' deficiency. Br J Haematol 2:412–420, 1956

43.  Newcomb T, Matter M. Conroy L, et al: Congenital hemorrhagic diathesis of the prothrombin complex. Am J Med 20:798–805, 1956

44.  Owen CA Jr, Bowie EJW: Chronic intravascular coagulation and fibrinolysis (ICF) syndromes (DIC). Semin Thromb Hemostas 3:268–290, 1977

45.  Sharp AA: Diagnosis and management of disseminated intravascular coagulation. Br Med Bull 33:265–272, 1977

46.  Macfarlane RG: The coagulant action of Russell's viper venom: The use of antivenom in defining its reaction with a serum factor. Br J Haematol 7:496–511, 1961

47.  Prentice CRM, Ratnoff OD: The action of Russell's viper venom on Factor V and the prothrombin-converting principle. Br J Haematol 16:291–302, 1969

48.  Denson KWE, Lurie A, De Cataldo F, et al: The Factor-X defect: Recognition of abnormal forms of factor X. Br J Haematol 18:317–327, 1970

49.  Girolami A, Molaro G, Lazzarin M, et al: A 'new' congenital haemorrhagic condition due to the presence of an abnormal factor X (Factor X, Friuli): Study of a large kindred. Br J Haematol 19:179–192, 1970

50.  Khoory MS, Nesheim ME, Bowie EJW, et al: Circulating heparan sulfate proteoglycan anticoagulant from a patient with a plasma cell disorder. J Clin Invest 65:666–674, 1980

51.  Ratnoff OD, Menzie C: A new method for the determination of fibrinogen in small samples of plasma. J Lab Clin Med 37:316–320, 1951

52.  Mann FD, Shonyo ES, Mann FC: Effect of removal of the liver on blood coagulation. Am J Physiol 164:111–116, 1951

53.  Morrison PR: Preparation and properties of serum and plasma proteins. XV. Some factors

influencing the quantitative determination of fibrinogen. J Am Chem Soc 69:2723–2731, 1947

54. Exner T, Koppel JL: Fibrinogen–fibrin conversion as determined by polymer bead sedimentation technique. Experientia 28:1421–1423, 1972

55. Owen CA Jr, Hurn MM, Mann FD: Dextran as a substitute for acacia in assay of plasma prothrombin. Am J Clin Pathol 25:1279–1282, 1955

56. Warner ED, Brinkhous KM, Smith HP: A quantitative study on blood clotting: Prothrombin fluctuations under experimental conditions. Am J Physiol 114:667–675, 1936

57. Denson KWE, Borrett R, Biggs R: The specific assay of prothrombin using the Taipan snake venom. Br J Haematol 21:219–226, 1971

58. Bowie EJW, Thompson JH Jr, Didisheim P, et al: Mayo Clinic Laboratory Manual of Hemostasis. Philadelphia, WB Saunders, 1971

59. Bangham DR, Biggs R, Brozović M, et al: A biological standard for measurement of blood coagulation Factor VIII activity. Bull WHO 45:337–351, 1971

60. Kirkwood TBL, Rizza CR, Snape TJ, et al: Identification of sources of inter-laboratory variation in factor VIII assay. Br J Haematol 37:559–568, 1977

61. Kirkwood TBL, Barrowcliffe TW: Discrepancy between one-stage and two-stage assays of factor VIII coagulant activity. Br J Haematol 39:147, 1978 (abstract)

62. Olson JD, Brockway WJ, Fass DN, et al: Purification of porcine and human ristocetin–Willebrand factor. J Lab Clin Med 89:1278–1294, 1977

63. Nilsson IM, Blombäck B, Blombäck M. et al: Kvinnlig hämofili och dess behandling med humant antihämofiliglobulin. Nord Med 56:1654–1656, 1956

64. Laurell C-B: Quantitative estimation of proteins by electrophoresis in agarose gel containing antibodies. Anal Biochem 15:45–52, 1966

65. Zimmerman TS, Ratnoff OD, Powell AE: Immunologic differentiation of classic hemophilia (factor VIII deficiency) and von Willebrand's disease: With observations on combined deficiencies of antihemophilic factor and proaccelerin (factor V) and on an acquired circulating anticoagulant against antihemophilic factor. J Clin Invest 50:244–254, 1971

66. Howard MA, Firkin BG: Ristocetin—a new tool in the investigation of platelet aggregation. Thromb Diath Haemorrh 26:362–369, 1971

67. Olson JD, Brockway WJ, Fass DN, et al: Evaluation of ristocetin–Willebrand factor assay and ristocetin-induced platelet aggregation. Am J Clin Pathol 63:210–218, 1975

68. Weiss HJ, Hoyer LW, Rickles FR, et al: Quantitative assay of a plasma factor deficient in von Willebrand's disease that is necessary for platelet aggregation: Relationship to factor VIII procoagulant activity and antigen content. J Clin Invest 52:2708–2716, 1973

69. Macfarlane DE, Stibbe J. Kirby EP, et al: A method for assaying von Willebrand factor (ristocetin cofactor), letter to the editor. Thromb Diath Haemorrh 34:306–308, 1975

70. Griggs TR, Cooper HA, Webster WP, et al: Plasma aggregating factor (bovine) for human platelets: A marker for study of antihemophilic and von Willebrand factors. Proc Natl Acad Sci USA 70:2814–2828, 1973

71. Allain JP, Cooper HA, Wagner RH, et al: Platelets fixed with paraformaldehyde: A new reagent for assay of von Willebrand factor and platelet aggregating factor. J Lab Clin Med 85:318–328, 1975

72. Bohn H: Isolierung und Charakterisierung des fibrinstabilisierenden Faktors aus menschlichen Thrombozyten. Thromb Diath Haemorrh 23:455–468, 1970

73. Lorand L, Urayama T, de Kiewiet JWC, et al: Diagnostic and genetic studies on fibrin-stabilizing factor with a new assay based on amine incorporation. J Clin Invest 48:1054–1064, 1969

74. Born GVR: Aggregation of blood platelets by adenosine diphosphate and its reversal. Nature 194:927–929, 1962

75. Packham MA, Kinlough-Rathbone RL, Reimers H-J, et al: Mechanisms of platelet aggregation independent of adenosine diphosphate, in Silver MJ, Smith JB, Kocsis JJ (eds): Prostaglandins in Hematology. New York, Spectrum Publications, 1977, pp 247–276

76. Hamberg M, Svensson J, Samuelsson B: Thromboxanes: A new group of biologically active compounds derived from prostaglandin endoperoxides. Proc Natl Acad Sci USA 72:2994–2998, 1975

77. Mustard JF, Perry DW, Kinlough-Rathbone RL, et al: Factors responsible for ADP-induced release reaction of human platelets. Am J Physiol 228:1757–1765, 1975

78. Smith JB, Ingerman C, Kocsis JJ, et al: Formation of an intermediate in prostaglandin biosynthesis and its association with the platelet release reaction. J Clin Invest 53:1468–1472, 1974

79. Smith JB, Ingerman CM, Silver MJ: Malondialdehyde formation as an indication of prosta-glandin production by human platelets. J Lab Clin Med 88:167–172, 1976

80. Praga Ca, Pogliani EM: Effect of temperature on ADP-induced platelet aggregation: Its sig-nificance in studying antiaggregating drugs. Thromb Diath Haemorrh 29:183–189, 1973

81. Coller BS, Gralnick HR: The effect of stir bar size and shape on quantitative platelet aggregation. Thromb Res 8:121–129, 1976

82. Packham MA, Kinlough-Rathbone RL, Mustard JF: Aggregation and agglutination, in Day HJ, Holmsen H, Zucker MB (eds): Platelet Function Testing. US Dept of Health, Education and Welfare Publication (NIH) 78-1087, 1978, pp 66–92

83. Weiss HJ: Platelet physiology and abnormalities of platelet function. N Engl J Med 293: 580–588, 1975

84. Didisheim P, Bunting D: Abnormal platelet function in myelofibrosis. Am J Clin Pathol 45:566–573, 1966

85. Neemeh JA, Bowie EJW, Thompson JH Jr, et al: Quantitation of platelet aggregation in mye-loproliferative disorders. Am J Clin Pathol 57:336–347, 1972

86. Spaet TH, Lejnieks I, Gaynor E, et al: Defective platelets in essential thrombocythemia. Arch Intern Med 124:135–141, 1969

87. Breddin K: Zur Messung der Thrombozytenadhäsivität. Thromb Diath Haemorrh 12:269–281, 1964

88. George JN: Direct assessment of platelet adhesion to glass: A study of the forces of interac-tion and effects of plasma and serum factors, platelet function, and modification of the glass surface. Blood 40:862–874, 1972

89. Mason RG, Gilkey JM: A simple test for quantitation of platelet adhesion to glass: Studies in bleeder and nonbleeder subjects. Thromb Diath Haemorrh 25:21–29, 1971

90. Zucker MB, Vroman L: Platelet adhesion induced by fibrinogen adsorbed onto glass. Proc Soc Exp Biol Med 131:318–320, 1969

91. Zbinden G, Tomlin S: Effect of heparin on platelet adhesiveness. Acta Haematol (Basel) 41:264–275, 1969

92. Cazenave J-P, Packham MA, Mustard JF: Adherence of platelets to a collagen-coated surface: Development of a quantitative method. J Lab Clin Med 82:978–990, 1973

93. Jenkins CSP, Packham MA, Guccione MA, et al: Modification of platelet adherence to pro-tein-coated surfaces. J Lab Clin Med 81:280–290, 1973

94. Packham MA, Evans G, Glynn MF, et al: The effect of plasma proteins on the interaction of platelets with glass surfaces. J Lab Clin Med 73:686–697, 1969

95. Cazenave J-P, Reimers H-J, Kinlough-Rathbone RL, et al: Effects of sodium periodate on platelet functions. Lab Invest 34:471–481, 1976

96. Hirsh J, McBride JA, Dacie JV: Thrombo-embolism and increased platelet adhesiveness in post-splenectomy thrombocytosis. Australas Ann Med 15:122–128, 1966

97. Hovig T, Jørgensen L, Packham MA, et al: Platelet adherence to fibrin and collagen. J Lab Clin Med 71:29–40, 1968

98. Mustard JF, Hegardt B, Rowsell HC, et al: Effect of adenosine nucleotides on platelet aggre-gation and clotting time. J Lab Clin Med 64:548–559, 1964

99. Spaet TH, Lejnieks I: A technique for estimation of platelet-collagen adhesion. Proc Soc Exp Biol Med 132:1038–1041, 1969

100. Borchgrevink CF: A method for measuring platelet adhesiveness in vivo. Acta Med Scand 168:157–164, 1960

101. Borchgrevink CF: Platelet adhesion in vivo in patients with bleeding disorders. Acta Med Scand 170:231–243, 1961

102. Moolten SE, Vroman L: The adhesiveness of blood platelets in thromboembolism and hemorrhagic disorders. I. Measurement of platelet adhesiveness by the glass-wool filter. Am J Clin Pathol 19:701–709, 1949

103. Wright HP: The adhesiveness of blood platelets in normal subjects with varying concentrations of anti-coagulants. J Pathol Bacteriol 53:255–262, 1941

104. Wright HP: Adhesiveness of blood-platelets in haemophilia. Lancet 1:306–307, 1946

105. Wright HP: The adhesiveness of blood platelets in rabbits treated with Dicoumarol. J Pathol Bacteriol 57:382–385, 1945

106. Bowie EJW, Owen CA Jr, Thompson JH Jr, et al: Platelet adhesiveness in von Willebrand's disease. Am J Clin Pathol 51:69–77, 1969

107. Hellem AJ: The adhesiveness of human blood platelets in vitro. 2. The present method for determination of platelet adhesiveness. Scand J Clin Lab Invest Suppl. 51:12–26, 1960

108. Hellem AJ: Platelet adhesiveness in von Willebrand's disease: A study with a new modification of the glass bead filter method. Scand J Haematol 7:374–382, 1970

109. Rossi EC, Green D: A study of platelet retention by glass bead columns ('platelet adhesiveness' in normal subjects). Br J Haematol 23:47–57, 1972

110. Salzman EW: Measurement of platelet adhesiveness: A simple in vitro technique demonstrating an abnormality in von Willebrand's disease. J Lab Clin Med 62:724–735, 1963

111. Bowie EJW, Owen CA Jr: Some factors influencing platelet retention in glass bead columns including the influence of plastics. Am J Clin Pathol 56:479–483, 1971

112. Coller BS, Zucker MB: Reversible decrease in platelet retention by glass bead columns (adhesiveness) induced by disturbing the blood. Proc Soc Exp Biol Med 136:769–771, 1971

113. Bowie EJW, Owen CA Jr: Unpublished data

114. Weiss HJ: Platelet function tests and their interpretation, editorial. J Lab Clin Med 87:909–912, 1976

115. Bowie EJW, Owen CA Jr: The value of measuring platelet ''adhesiveness'' in the diagnosis of bleeding diseases. Am J Clin Pathol 60:302–308, 1973

116. Caen JP, Castaldi PA, Leclerc JC, et al: Congenital bleeding disorders with long bleeding time and normal platelet count. I. Glanzmann's thrombasthenia (report of fifteen patients). Am J Med 41:4–70, 1966

117. Salzman EW, Neri LL: Adhesiveness of blood platelets in uremia. Thromb Diath Haemorrh 15:84–92, 1966

118. Holmsen H, Weiss HJ: Secretable storage pools in platelets. Ann Rev Med 30:119–134, 1979

119. Owen CA Jr, Thompson JH Jr: Soybean phosphatides in prothrombin-consumption and thromboplastin-generation tests: Their uses in recognizing ''thrombasthenic hemophilia.'' Am J Clin Pathol 33:197–208, 1960

120. Bowie EJW, Owen CA Jr: Clinical disorders related to blood platelets, in Johnson SA (ed): The Circulating Platelet. New York, Academic Press, 1971, pp 473–539

121. Sultan Y, Brouet JC, Devergie A: Isolated platelet factor 3 deficiency, letter to the editor. N Engl J Med 294:1121, 1976

122. Weiss HJ: Platelet aggregation, adhesion and adenosine diphosphate release in thrombopathia (platelet factor 3 deficiency): A comparison with Glanzmann's thrombasthenia and von Willebrand's disease. Am J Med 43:570–578, 1967

123. Miletich JP, Kane WH, Hofmann SL, et al: Deficiency of factor $X_a$-factor $V_a$ binding sites on the platelets of a patient with a bleeding disorder. Blood 54:1015–1022, 1979

124. Weiss HJ, Vicic WJ, Lages BA, et al: Isolated deficiency of platelet procoagulant activity. Am J Med 67:206–213, 1979

125.  Biggs R: Jaundice and antibodies directed against factors VIII and IX in patients treated for haemophilia or Christmas disease in the United Kingdom. Br J Haematol 26:313–329, 1974

126.  Ruggeri ZM, Pareti FI, Mannucci PN, et al: Heightened interaction between platelets and Factor VIII/von Willebrand factor in a new subtype of von Willebrand's disease. N Engl J Med 302:1047–1051, 1980

127.  Ruggeri ZM, Zimmerman TS: Variant von Willebrand's disease: Characterization of two sub-types by analysis of multimeric composition of factor VIII/von Willebrand factor in plasma and platelets. J Clin Invest 65:1318–1325, 1980

128.  Zimmerman TS, Voss R, Edgington TS: Carbohydrate of the Factor VIII/von Willebrand factor in von Willebrand's disease. J Clin Invest 64:1298–1302, 1979

129.  Fass DN, Knutson GJ, Bowie EJW: Porcine Willebrand factor: A population of multimers. J Lab Clin Med 91:307–320, 1978

130.  Italian Working Group: Spectrum of von Willebrand's disease: A study of 100 cases. Br J Haematol 35:101–112, 1977

131.  Duncan A, Bowie EJW, Owen CA Jr: Automated activated partial thromboplastin APT screen using a thrombin specific chromogenic substrate. Fed Proc 40:807, 1981 (abstract)

132.  Duncan A, Bowie EJW, Owen CA Jr: Automated coagulation factor assays using a thrombin specific thromogenic substrate. Thromb Haemost 46:313, 1981 (abstract)

Barry S. Coller

# 4

# Disorders of Platelets

Blood platelets and the coagulation mechanism act in concert to form a complex ho-
meostatic system designed to prevent and arrest hemorrhage. The interaction of platelets with the blood vessel wall (adhesion) and with other platelets (aggregation), along
with the facilitatory role of platelets in thrombin generation, are required for normal hemostasis since both quantitative and qualitative defects in these functions may result in
hemorrhage.

## NORMAL PLATELET FUNCTION

### Anatomy and Biochemistry

Platelets circulate as variably sized, disc-shaped, anucleate cell fragments of $3.6 \pm$
$0.7$ μm (mean $\pm$ SD) diameter, $0.9 \pm 0.3$ μm thickness, and $7.06 \pm 4.85$ fl volume.[1] On
Romanowsky-stained peripheral blood smears, the platelets are the smallest formed element and usually exhibit purplish granules. When studied by scanning electronmicroscopy,
their surface is found to be fuzzy and to contain indentations which are thought to represent the openings of an elaborate system of tubules which extends throughout the interior
of the platelet (the open canalicular system)[2] (Figure 4-1). With the resolution achieved
by transmission electron microscopy, the platelet can be subdivided into several different
regions, including, according to White et al.,[3] a peripheral zone (composed of the plasma
membrane, along with an exterior coat and submembrane area), a sol-gel zone, and an
organelle zone (Fig. 4-2 and 4-3).

#### Peripheral Zone

The external membrane mediates all of the platelet's interactions with its
environment and thus occupies a central role in platelet physiology. Like many other mammalian cell membranes, it is composed of a double layer (i.e., bilayer) of phospholipids in
which are embedded glycolipids, cholesterol, and proteins. Among the membrane phospholipids, those that are negatively charged, such as phosphatidylinositol, phosphatidylserine,

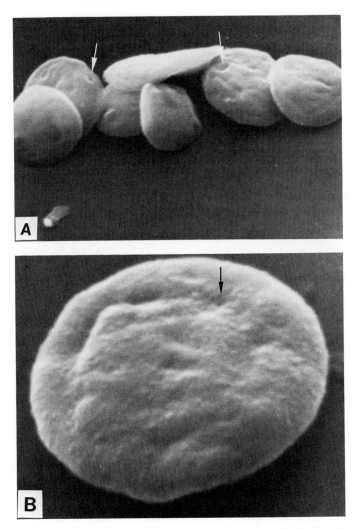

**Fig. 4-1.** Appearance of platelets viewed in the scanning electron microscope. The characteristic discoid form of the platelets is clearly apparent. Cell surfaces are quite smooth except for the identations (arrows), which are sites of communication between channels of the surface-connected canaliculi and the platelet membrane. From White JG, Gerrad JM[2] with permission of the American Association of Pathologists.

and phosphatidylethanolamine, are distributed primarily on the inner layer of the membrane, and thus are not exposed on the surface. Some controversial evidence suggests that these negatively charged phospholipids (which are very active in accelerating the clotting mechanism) move to the outer layer of the membrane when platelets are activated, thus accounting for the increased clot-promoting effect of activated platelets[4-6] (Figure 4-4). Platelet membrane phospholipids are particularly rich in arachidonic acid, the lipid precursor of the platelet-active prostaglandins and thromboxanes.[7]

The interior of the platelet membrane is viewed as a sea of lipid with a characteristic fluidity, a property reflecting the ease of motion of small molecular probes placed in that environment. Increasing the cholesterol content of the membrane tends to decrease the

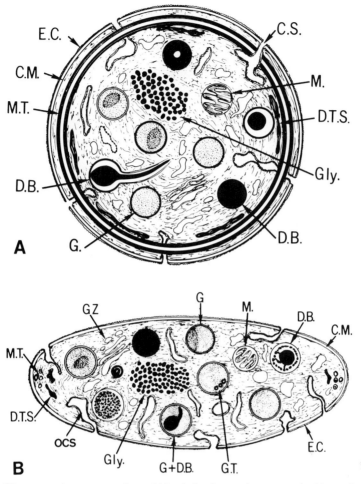

**Fig. 4-2.** Diagrammatic representations of blood platelets as they appear in thin sections by electron microscopy: a platelet cut in the equatorial plane (A) and a platelet in cross section (B). Components of the peripheral zone include the exterior coat (EC), trilaminar unit membrane (CM), and submembrane filament area which form the wall of the platelet and line the channels of the surface-connected open canalicular system (OCS). The matrix of the platelet is the sol-gel zone containing microfilaments, submembrane filaments (SMF), the circumferential band of microtubules (MT), and glycogen (Gly). Formed elements embedded in the sol-gel zone include mitochondria (M), granules (G), dense bodies (DB), and channels of the dense tubular system (DTS). Collectively, they constitute the organelle zone. A Golgi apparatus (GZ) is found in occasional platelets. From White JG, Gerrard JM[2] with permission of the American Association of Pathologists, p. 591.

overall fluidity,[8,9] and since cholesterol-rich platelets have been found by some (but not all) investigators to be especially sensitive to stimuli,[8] membrane fluidity may be an important factor in determining platelet responsiveness. In addition, there is some evidence that platelet activation alters lipid fluidity, but it is unclear as to whether this is a mechanism for transducing the activation message or a result of the activation.[9a,b] In other mammalian cells, it was recently found that sequential methylation of membrane phosphatidylethanolamine may be involved in transducing signals from the surface to the interior of the cell. Preliminary

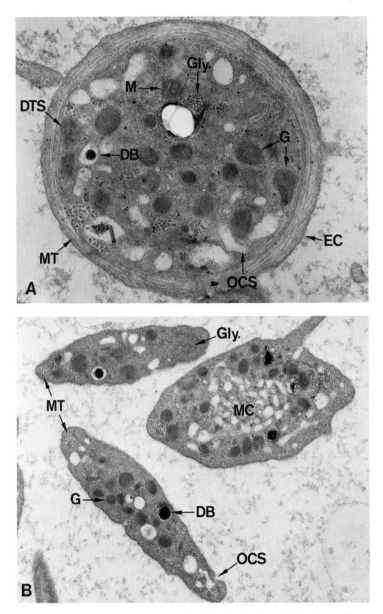

**Fig. 4-3.** Thin sections of glutaraldehyde–osmium-fixed, plastic-embedded normal human platelets. Most of the structures indicated diagrammatically in Figure 4-2 can be identified in these cells. The exterior coat is a relatively amorphous layer on the unit membrane. The submembrane region lies between the circumferential band of microtubules and the cell wall. In (A), the circumferential band of microtubules (MT) is sectioned in the equatorial plane and forms a complete circle. The cells in (B) are cut in cross section and reveal the bundle of microtubules at the polar ends of each cell. A membrane complex (MC) formed by interaction of the dense tubular (DTS) and surface-connected canalicular (OCS) systems is evident in one of the cells in (B). (A) X41,500; (B) X22,500. From White JG, Gerrard JM[2] with permission of the American Association of Pathologists.

## PLATELET LIPIDS

1. ~17 of dry weight, primarily in membranes.
2. Membranes 57 % protein, 35 % lipid, 8 % carbohydrate.
3. Membrane lipids : 75 % phospholipid, 20 % neutral lipid, 5 % glycolipid.
4. Phospholipids       a.) Uncharged and negatively charged.
                        b.) Rich in arachidonic acid.
5. Neutral lipids :    95 % cholesterol.
6. Cholesterol / Phospholipid = 0.5 on molar basis.

### PHOSPHOLIPID

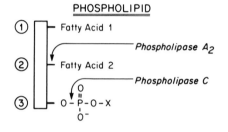

X = CHOLINE, SERINE, ETC.

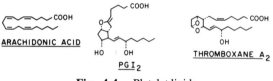

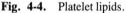

**Fig. 4-4.**   Platelet lipids.

evidence indicates that there is a basal level of phospholipid methylation in platelets, but that instead of increasing this activity, stimuli actually decrease it; it is unclear, however, whether this process is involved in stimulus translation.[10]

Extending out 150–200 Å from the phospholipid bilayer of the platelet membrane is an exterior fuzzy coat composed of several elements, including the carbohydrate-rich portions of the membrane-associated glycoproteins and glycolipids,[6,11–13] mucopolysaccharides, and plasma proteins which are adsorbed onto the platelet surface (Fig. 4-5). Platelets move in an electric field as if they have a considerable negative charge on their surface.[14] The major contributors to this negative charge are the sialic acid carboxyl groups associated with glycoproteins and glycolipids; a small number of amino groups contribute positive charges to the platelet's surface.[14] It is likely that the electrostatic repulsion between platelets that results from their negative surface charge plays an important role in preventing platelet aggregation since reducing the charge tends to increase platelet aggregation in several different systems.[15]

The platelet membrane proteins and glycoproteins have been studied intensively by the technique of detergent solubilization and subsequent electrophoretic separation in polyacrylamide gels according to size and isoelectric point. A variety of reagents have been employed to probe the chemical composition and location of these molecules.[16,17] At least 9 separate proteins have been identified, but only those which have been well characterized will be discussed.

Glycoprotein Ib(GPIb) consists of 2 disulfide-linked chains (alpha and beta of 143,000

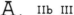

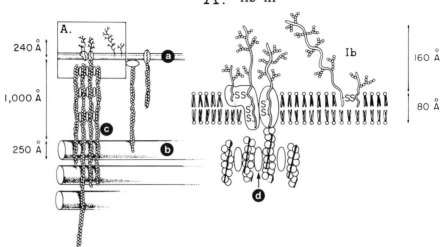

**Fig. 4-5.** The platelet membrane. A schematic depiction of the relationship between the external platelet membrane (a), the circumferential band of microtubules (b), microfilaments composed of actin polymers (c) and filamin (d in insert A), and the surface glycoproteins Ib, IIb, and III (shown in insert A). The actin polymers are shown attaching to the cytoplasmic portion of surface glycoproteins, and although there is preliminary evidence that glycoprotein III may subserve this function, attachment to other glycoproteins is shown to stress that the identity of proteins involved in microfibril attachment remains unknown. Although actin-containing microfibrils and tubulin-containing microtubules tend to copurify, the nature of the interaction between these structures is uncertain. The glycoproteins are schematically depicted, with their branching carbohydrate structures on the outside of the membrane and the appropriate location of their disulfide bonds in an adaptation of the structures proposed by Phillips DR,[17] with permission of Grune & Stratton.

and 22,000 molecular weight (Fig. 4-5). Chemical analysis indicates that it is very rich in carbohydrate in general and sialic acid in particular. Both protein chains stain for carbohydrate and are exposed on the outside of the membrane. GPIb is quite susceptible to proteolysis, and a fragment which is commonly split off during platelet membrane isolation has been given the name *glycocalicin*. The carbohydrate portion of GPIb appears to be similar to that of the major erythrocyte glycoprotein, glycophorin A, on which M and N blood groups are expressed.[18] Patients suffering from the rare Tn syndrome, in which there is an abnormality in the carbohydrate portion of glycophorin, seem to have a similar abnormality in GPIb.[19]

GPIb has been implicated in several different functional activities: (1) as a receptor for von Willebrand factor when platelets are stimulated with ristocetin;[17] (2) as a receptor for thrombin;[17] (3) as a receptor for drug-dependent antibodies;[20] and (4) as being in close proximity to the receptor for immune complexes.[21] Considerable evidence supports the role of GPIb as a von Willebrand factor receptor when platelets are stimulated with ristocetin: (1) congenital absence of GPIb in the Bernard-Soulier syndrome (see below) is associated with the inability to bind von Willebrand factor when platelets are stimulated with ristocetin; (2) selective proteolytic digestion of GPIb decreases ristocetin-induced von Willebrand factor binding; and (3) heterologous, homologous, and, most recently, monoclonal antibodies against GPIb selectively inhibit ristocetin-induced von Willebrand factor-dependent

**Table 4-1**
Phenotypic Frequency of Platelet
Antigens in the Dutch Population (%)

| Pl$^{A1}$ | (Zw$^a$) | 97.6 |
|---|---|---|
| Pl$^{A2}$ | (Zw$^b$) | 26.8 |
| Ko$^a$ | | 14.3 |
| Ko$^b$ | | 99.4 |
| Bak$^a$ | | 90.8 |

Adapted from van Leeuven EF, von dem
Borne AEGKr, von Riesz LE et al. Absence
of platelet specific alloantigens in Glanzmann's thrombasthenia. Blood 57:50, 1981.
With permission.

platelet agglutination.[17,17a,b] Studies with monoclonal antibodies also suggest that GPIb may exist in complex with a low molecular weight glycoprotein on the platelet's surface.[17b,c] Since the platelets of patients with the Tn syndrome, which lack the appropriate terminal carbohydrates of GPIb, appear to interact normally with von Willebrand factor, this region of the molecule is probably not involved in the binding function.

Glycoproteins IIb and III (GPIIb and GPIII) can be considered together since they seem to be associated with each other as a calcium-dependent complex in the membrane.[17,22] GPIIb is composed of 2 disulfide-linked subunits, a larger GPIIb$\alpha$ (molecular weight 132,000) and a smaller GPIIb$\beta$ (molecular weight 23,000) (Fig. 4-5). GPIII is a single-chain protein of molecular weight 114,000 whose carbohydrate moiety is also exposed on the platelet's surface. Available evidence suggests that both GPIIb and GPIII span the membrane. These proteins have been purified and found to have similar amino acid compositions[23,23a]. There is controversy as to whether proteolytic digests of the proteins show significant homology.[23,23a,b] The weight of evidence indicates that the GPIIb-III complex contains the determinants of the platelet receptor for fibrinogen since (1) patients with thrombasthenia who lack both of these proteins cannot bind fibrinogen;[24,25] (2) an alloantibody produced by a patient with thrombasthenia that reacted with the GPIIb–III complex inhibited fibrinogen binding to normal platelets;[26] (3) a monoclonal mouse hybridoma antibody that inhibited fibrinogen binding to platelets immunoprecipitated both GPIIb and III;[27] and (4) fibrinogen complexes with isolated GPIIb–III complex.[27a,27b] However, some conflicting evidence has also been reported.[28] Recent preliminary evidence indicates that the GPIIb–III complex may also function as a receptor for von Willebrand factor when platelets are activated by adenosine diphosphate (ADP) and thrombin, but not when stimulated with ristocetin.[28a–c] The GPIIb–III complex may also function as the backbone on which some of the platelet-specific antigens are expressed.[29,30] To date, 3 biallelic antigens [Pl$^A$(Zw), Ko, and Pl$^E$] and 1 monoallelic antigen (Bak$^a$) have been described on normal platelets; the frequencies of some of these antigens in the Dutch population are indicated in Table 4-1.[30] Platelets also contain recognition sites for drug-dependent and ethylenediaminotetraacetate (EDTA)-dependent antibodies as well as immune complexes. Patients with thrombasthenia lack or are severely deficient in the Pl$^{A1}$, Pl$^{A2}$, and Bak$^a$ antigens as well as the recognition site for EDTA-dependent antibodies. Recent biochemical evidence has, in fact, localized the Pl$^{A1}$ antigen specifically to GPIII.[31]

Glycoprotein V (GPV) is a single-chain protein with a molecular weight of 82,000 containing approximately 48 percent carbohydrate.[32] It probably has a peripheral, as opposed to a transmembrane, orientation in the membrane. Exposure of whole platelets or purified GPV to thrombin results in proteolytic cleavage of GPV; thus GPV cleavage may be involved in the stimulus-translation mechanism induced by thrombin.[33] Interestingly, recent evidence indicates that patients with Bernard-Soulier syndrome lack GPV and a low molecular weight glycoprotein in addition to GPIb.[34,34a]

### Sol-Gel Zone

One of the most striking features in platelet physiology is the platelet's ability to alter its shape dramatically and abruptly from a smooth disc to a spiny sphere with spikelike filopodia extending far out from its body. The maintenance of the resting disc shape and the explosive shape change are both thought to be controlled by what has been called the platelet's cytoskelton,[35-37] composed of (1) the contractile proteins actin and myosin (along with several associated proteins), and (2) the proteins involved in microtubule formation, namely tubulin and its associated proteins.

Actin is the most abundant of all the platelet proteins, representing approximately 20 percent of the total. Platelet actin is actually a mixture of 2 single-chain proteins (beta and gamma actin) of molecular weight 44,000[38,39] that are similar to, but not identical with, muscle actin. Actin can exist in a monomeric form (globular, or G actin) or undergo polymerization to a fibrous, filamentous form (F actin) (Fig. 4-6). One current hypothesis is that actin polymerization is responsible for the development of the filopodia that produce shape change. This concept is supported by data showing an increase in F actin when platelets are stimulated.[40] The equilibrium between G and F actin thus must be under a delicate control mechanism. Such control may be exercised by profilin, a small (16,000 molecular weight) basic protein found in platelets and other cells which forms a 1:1 complex with G actin (profil-actin) and thus prevents the G actin from undergoing polymerization.[40] When G actin does polymerize, the resulting F actin filaments are thought to incorporate a complex of troponin and tropomyosin, two proteins found in platelets which have been implicated in the control of actin–myosin interactions in skeletal muscle. Another platelet protein, filamin or actin-binding protein (260,000 molecular weight), also binds to F actin and has been implicated in organizing the actin filaments into bundles.[41] Filamin can be phosphorylated by a protein kinase which is controlled, at least in part, by the level of cyclic adenosine 5'-monophosphate (AMP), and it appears that the degree of phosphorylation of filamin determines its ability to interact with the actin filaments.[42] Additional control over the state of actin polymerization may be exercised by other proteins.[43,44] In order to generate a directed force, the actin filaments must be anchored into some structure in the platelet. A protein which serves this function in the Z discs of skeletal muscle, α-actinin, has been isolated from platelets; this protein may be located in the plasma and/or granule membranes of platelets and thus serve as an anchoring site for actin filaments. Several other anchoring proteins have been isolated from other cells, but their presence in platelets is still undetermined.

Platelet myosin (460,000 molecular weight) is composed of 6 polypeptide chains (2 each of molecular weight 200,000, 20,000, and 16,000), and although it is analogous to skeletal muscle myosin, it is immunologically distinct.[39] All 6 chains contribute to the dimeric head regions, which contain sites for both actin binding and the hydrolysis of ATP. The 20,000 molecular weight light chain of myosin can be phosphorylated by a specific myosin light chain kinase, and it is this phosphorylation which seems to determine the extent of actin–myosin adenosine triphosphatase (ATPase) activity, and thus contraction.[45] Control of the phosphorylation is quite complex, with the level of active myosin light chain kinase activity being controlled by the concentration of cytoplasmic

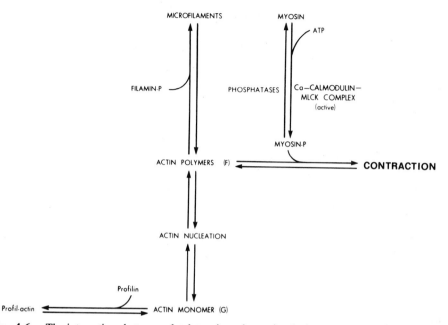

**Fig. 4-6.** The interactions between platelet actin and myosin. Actin monomers are in equilibrium with a complex composed of actin and the protein profilin (profil-actin). Under the appropriate conditions, actin monomers begin to polymerize into fibers. If these polymers interact with the phosphorylated form of the high molecular weight protein filamin, they apparently become microfilaments; they may be the structural support of the filopodia formed during the shape change reaction. Alternatively, the actin polymers can interact with the phosphorylated form of myosin, ultimately resulting in contraction. In order for platelet myosin to be phosphorylated (and thus able to produce contraction), a critical complex composed of calcium, the calcium regulatory protein calmodulin, and the phosphorylating enzyme, myosin light chain kinase, must be formed. An increase in the cytoplasmic level of calcium is thought to be needed for the complex to form. Phosphatases can reverse the phosphorylation of myosin and thus will decrease the amount of contraction.

$Ca^{2+}$ acting in concert with the protein calmodulin[45] (Fig. 4-6). Increases in cytoplasmic calcium result in activation of the kinase, phosphorylation of myosin, and increased contractile activity. An additional control mechanism exists since the kinase itself can be inhibited by increased intracellular cyclic AMP. Moreover, a phosphatase capable of dephosphorylating the myosin light chain also appears to play a role in the control of contraction. Since so much of the platelet's biochemistry is devoted to proteins involved in the contractile response in other cells, it is tempting to stress the similarity between platelets and muscle. However, as Cohen et al. pointed out,[35] the ratio of actin to myosin in platelets is much greater than in skeletal muscle (100:1 as against 6:1), and it is therefore not surprising that platelet actin appears to play a structural role in shape change (mediated by polymerization) that is probably independent of contraction. In addition, platelet myosin forms thinner and shorter filaments than skeletal muscle myosin, imposing serious limitations on the extent of contraction that can be achieved.

The platelet has a circumferential band of microtubules made up of molecular weight 110,000 subunits composed of 2 major proteins of 55,000 molecular weight ($\alpha$- and $\beta$-tubulin) in association with several high molecular weight proteins.[46] Interestingly, although the initial ultrastructural appearance suggested that the microtubules were closed, ringlike

**Table 4-2**
Platelet Granule Contents

| α-*Granules* | *Dense Bodies* |
|---|---|
| Platelet-specific proteins (low molecular weight) | ADP |
| PF4 | ATP |
| Low-affinity PF4 | |
| β-Thromboglobulin | Calcium |
| Platelet basic protein | Serotonin |
| Mitogenic factors | Pyrophosphate |
| High molecular weight glycoproteins | |
| Fibrinogen | *Lysosomal Enzymes* |
| Von Willebrand factor | Acid phosphatase |
| Fibronectin | β-*N*-Acetylglucosaminidase |
| Thrombospondin | |
| Factor V | β-Galactosidase |
| Albumin | β-Glycerophosphatase |
| | Aryl sulfatase |
| *Granular Proteins of* | |
| *Uncertain Location* | |
| Cathepsins | |
| Endoglucosidase | |
| Cyclic-3′,5′-phosphodiesterase | |
| Collagenase | |
| Vascular permeability factors | |
| Proelastase and elastase | |
| $\alpha_1$-Protease Inhibitor | |
| $\alpha_2$-Macroglobulin | |
| Antiplasmin | |
| Bactericidal protein | |

structures, studies using new lysing agents and microscopic techniques indicate that there may be only a single microtubule which winds around the platelet several times before terminating in 2 free ends.[47]

### Organelle Zone

The platelet contains a large number of granules that have been subdivided into α-granules, dense bodies (by virtue of their electronmicroscopic appearance), and lysosomes. The α-granules are the most numerous and contain a large number of proteins that can be released from platelets when they are stimulated (Table 4-2). Platelet factor 4 (PF4)[48,49] is composed of a single chain of 70 amino acids (7780 molecular weight); when released from the platelet, however, it is complexed with a proteoglycan carrier, giving it a high molecular weight. Low-affinity PF4 and β-thromboglobulin are immunologically similar, low molecular weight proteins, with the only structural difference being that low-affinity PF4 has four additional amino acids on the N-terminal portion of the molecule; several proteases can convert low-affinity PF4 into β-thromboglobulin. Platelet basic protein also reacts with antibodies prepared against β-thromboglobulin, but since it has a different iso-electric point, it must differ from the latter. All four of these proteins (PF4, low-affinity PF4, β-thromboglobulin, and platelet basic protein) can neutralize heparin's anticoagulant effect, but PF4 is considerably more potent than the others. Although the physiologic role of the antiheparin activity of these proteins is uncertain, the observation that there is a reservoir of PF4 adherent to the mucopolysaccharides which coat endothelial cells that is rapidly brought into the circulation when heparin is administered intravenously may account for the need to inject a bolus of heparin at the initiation of anticoagulation therapy. Recent studies have shown that PF4 is chemotactic for human polymorphonuclear leuko-cytes and monocytes at concentrations that may well be achieved at sites of vessel injury.[49a] Low-affinity PF4 and platelet basic protein have been shown to be mitogenic in some cell culture systems. Since only very low levels of β-thromboglobulin and PF4 normally circu-late in plasma, elevations of these levels have been interpreted as reflecting in vivo plate-let activation.

The platelet α-granule also contains at least one, and more likely several, cationic growth factors which have mitogenic activity for several different cell lines, including smooth muscle cells, fibroblasts, and glial cells.[48] These factors are released from plate-lets when they adhere to the subendothelium of damaged blood vessels. Although these factors may well function in normal repair processes, most studies have concentrated on their role in pathological processes. They have thus been implicated in the initiation of atherosclerosis by stimulating smooth muscle cells in the media of blood vessels to both proliferate and invade the intima.[50,50a] Since the platelet-derived growth factor(s) is mito-genic for fibroblasts,[51] it has been suggested that it might also play a role in the develop-ment of fibroblastic proliferation in other tissues, as for example, in myelofibrosis. Purified platelet-derived growth factors of 28,000 and 31,000 molecular weight which differ in carbohydrate content have been reported; the larger form has been shown to be chemotac-tic for neutrophils and monocytes.[51a] A very exciting recent observation is that the amino acid sequences of two forms of the platelet derived growth factor show extensive homology with a portion of a well characterized oncogene associated with simian sarcoma virus.[51b,c]

The α-granules also contain several high molecular weight glycoproteins. Fibrinogen and von Willebrand factor are discussed elsewhere, but it is interesting to point out that under the appropriate circumstances, the platelet can bind these proteins to its surface. Considerable controversy persists regarding the site of synthesis of platelet fibrinogen and von Willebrand factor and whether they are identical to those proteins which circulate in plasma. Fibronectin is a 2-chain glycoprotein of 450,000 molecular weight which is pres-ent both in the circulation and in association with cell surfaces, and appears to play an important role in the adhesion of a variety of cell types to different surfaces.[48] Although fibronectin may facilitate platelet spreading on collagen, it does not appear to be re-quired for platelet adhesion or aggregation.[52] Thrombospondin (thrombin-sensitive protein) is a glycoprotein of 450,000 molecular weight composed of 3 chains of 150,000 molecu-lar weight held together by disulfide bonds.[48] It can bind to the platelet surface after activation-induced released from the α-granules,[53] but its physiologic role has not been identified. Intraplatelet factor V is also probably localized in α-granules, and its activation and release appear to play an important role in the generation of thrombin on the platelet surface (see below).[48]

The platelet contains a significant number of lysosomes, membrane-bound organ-elles that are rich in hydrolytic enzymes. They are distinct from α-granules and are not readily detected by electron microscopy. A series of other proteins have been found in the "granular" fractions of platelets without specific localization to the granule type. Several of these proteins may play a role in the inflammatory response by altering vascular permeability, digesting the constituents of connective tissue or inhibiting certain proteases.

Dense bodies contain high concentrations of ADP, adenosine triphosphate (ATP), pyrophosphate, serotonin, and $Ca^{2+}$ along with small amounts of histamine, catecholamines, and $Mg^{2+}$.[54,55] In contrast to their relative concentrations in the platelet cytoplasm, the concentration of ADP in the dense granule is greater than that of ATP. Dense-body serotonin metabolism has been extensively studied in the platelet since it has some similarities to that in the granules of neurons.[54] Current evidence suggests that (1) megakaryocytes contain little serotonin; (2) after their release into the circulation, platelets take up serotonin from the plasma by active transport across the plasma membrane, with subsequent trapping in the dense bodies, perhaps by virtue of the reduced pH in the dense bodies; and (3) platelets contain monamine oxidase, an enzyme involved in serotonin metabolism, in their mitochondria, and there are conflicting data on whether this enzymatic activity is decreased in the platelets of patients with mental disorders.[54]

Other organelles found in platelets include (1) a calcium-sequestering membranous system analogous to the sarcoplasmic reticulum in muscle cells called the *dense tubular system*,[3] (2) several small mitochondria,[3] and (3) a Golgi apparatus (in occasional platelets).[2]

### *Biochemistry*[37,55-57]

With very low levels of ribonucleic acid (RNA) and without a nucleus to direct the synthesis of more RNA, the central biochemical feature of the platelet is its minimal ability to synthesize protein. Loss of enzymatic activity, as for example with the irreversible aspirin-induced inhibition of the enzyme cyclooxygenase, thus cannot be compensated for by synthesis of new protein.

*Energy metabolism.* Platelets contain the enzymes for glycolysis, oxidative phosphorylation, and fatty acid oxidation. A hexose monophosphate shunt is operative which, in turn, is linked to the reduction of glutathione. The platelet is also capable of synthesizing glycogen from glucose, and electron microscopy reveals that glycogen particles are quite prominent in some platelets.

*Lipids.* Platelets have the requisite enzymes to synthesize fatty acids and phospholipids. Two different enzymatic mechanisms for stimulation-induced release of arachidonic acid from phospholipids have been demonstrated (phospholipase $A_2$ and the combination of phospholipase C and diglyceride lipase), but the relative contributions of these 2 systems are still in dispute.[58] The released arachidonic acid can, in turn, be acted upon by 2 different enzymes[7] (Fig. 4-7): (1) lipoxygenase, in which case peroxy- and hydroxy–fatty acid products are generated, and (2) cyclooxygenase, which converts the arachidonic acid into a cyclic structure ($PGG_2$) that is first acted upon by a peroxidase (to become $PGH_2$) and can then enter one of several pathways leading to (a) thromboxane $A_2$, a labile but very potent aggregating agent, and its stable but inactive breakdown product, thromboxane $B_2$, (b) prostaglandins $E_2$, $F_{2\alpha}$ and $D_2$ (the last a labile, potent inhibitor of platelet aggregation), or (c) malondialdehyde and hydroxyheptadecatrienoic acid. Unlike endothelial cells, platelets lack the enzyme prostacyclin synthetase that converts the cyclic endoperoxide intermediates into $PGI_2$ (prostacyclin), a labile but very potent inhibitor of platelet aggregation. Another product of the action of phospholipase C on phosphatidylinositol, diacylglycerol, has been invoked as an important agent in platelet activation. There is con-

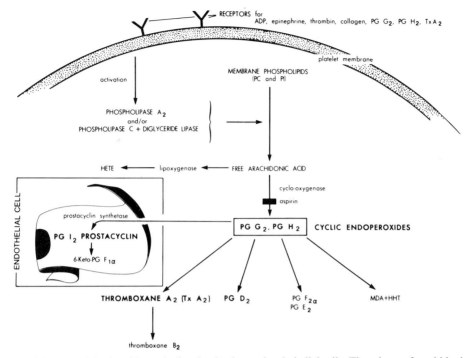

**Fig. 4-7.**   Arachdonic acid metabolism in platelets and endothelial cells. The release of arachidonic acid from membrane phospholipids occurs in response to platelet activation by a variety of agonists. Phospholipase $A_2$ and/or the combination of phospholipase C and diglyceride lipase are thought to be the enzymes involved in arachidonic acid release, but the relative contributions made by these 2 mechanisms are still uncertain. After release, the free arachidonic acid may be acted upon by either lipoxygenase or cyclooxygenase. The latter results in the production of the short-lived cyclic endoperoxides ($PGG_2$ and $PGH_2$), which are probably aggregating agents in their own right. These can be converted into a variety of products, the most important of which is thromboxane $A_2$, a very potent but short-lived aggregating and release-inducing agent. $PGD_2$ is an inhibitor of platelet aggregation and is also short-lived; its physiologic role is uncertain. Endothelial cells, in addition to having the enzymes to release arachidonic acid and convert it to cyclic endoperoxides, also have the enzyme needed to convert the cyclic endoperoxides into $PGI_2$ (prostacyclin synthetase), a very potent but short-lived inhibitor of platelet function. Platelets cannot make $PGI_2$, but may provide the cyclic endoperoxide intermediates to the endothelial cells under certain circumstances. Aspirin blocks prostaglandin synthesis by irreversibly inhibiting the enzyme cyclooxygenase.

siderable evidence that this lipid is involved in the phosphorylation of a 40,000 molecular weight protein whose appearance correlates with the induction of the release reaction when platelets are stimulated with thrombin or collagen.[58a] Recently, a unique phospholipid derivative (originally termed *platelet-activating factor*) identified as acetyl glyceryl ether phosphorylcholine (AGEPC) has been found to be an extremely potent aggregating agent.[59] Human basophils, and perhaps macrophages and neutrophils, have been shown to synthesize and/or release this compound when stimulated. Moreover, under some circumstances platelets themselves appear to be capable of making AGEPC. However, there is conflicting evidence as to whether platelets can synthesize significant amounts of AGEPC when stimulated with any of the agents that are thought to be of physiologic importance, and thus its role in platelet function in vivo remains in doubt.[59,60]

*Adenine nucleotides.* There are essentially 2 separate pools of adenine nucleotides in platelets: one in the cytoplasm (metabolic pool) and the other in the dense granules (storage pool). There is very little interchange between these two pools. The adenine nucleotides in the metabolic pool apparently cannot be synthesized de novo, but if platelets are supplied with exogenous adenine, adenosine, or hypoxanthine, they can take up these precursors and convert them into ADP and ATP; only hypoxanthine is normally present in plasma in significant concentrations. The storage pool of adenine nucleotides cannot be replenished after platelets release them from their dense granules in the course of the release reaction. Approximately 40 percent of the platelet's ATP and 50 percent of its ADP is present in the storage pool, and the ATP/ADP ratio is much lower in the storage pool than in the metabolic pool (approximately 0.7 compared to approximately 10.0). ATP hydrolysis is thought to be required for the conversion of G actin to F actin, and the ADP that results from the reaction apparently becomes associated with the F actin. Thus, a significant fraction of the cytoplasmic pool of adenine nucleotides is always associated with these cytoskeletal elements and is therefore unavailable for other metabolic processes.[55]

## Physiology

From a phenomenologic standpoint, platelets can be observed to undergo a stereotypic response when a blood vessel is injured (Fig.4-8): (1) within seconds platelets adhere to the site of injury; (2) shortly thereafter, platelets begin to aggregate, attaching themselves first to the platelets adhering to the vessel wall and then to platelets which lie on top of the adherent platelets; (3) platelets involved in both adhesion and aggregation are observed to degranulate, with the adherent platelets most notably affected and with the platelets that have aggregated farthest from the vessel wall least affected; (4) in time, the platelets pack together more tightly and fibrin strands are laid down, enmeshing the platelets in their network.[61] It is most convenient to consider platelet physiology in a manner which parallels these morphologic observations, with separate discussions of adhesion, aggregation, release of granule contents, and facilitation of coagulation. A discussion of the platelet response in its entirety, with emphasis on the controls which limit this response to loci where it is required, will then follow.

### Adhesion

One of the platelet's most dramatic properties is its ability to adhere rapidly to many different types of surfaces. Although a unitary mechanism for this phenomenon may have been anticipated, studies of the cofactor requirements for platelet adhesion to different surfaces indicate that a heterogeneous group of mechanisms operate. Adherence to glass requires the presence of an intact platelet receptor for fibrinogen[57] as well as exogenous fibrinogen and calcium. Adherence to collagen, on the other hand, requires neither fibrinogen nor calcium.[62] Many studies have shown that platelets will adhere to collagen only when the latter is organized into its insoluble fibrillar form. In fact, even though there are several types of collagen, differing in their polypeptide chain compositions, they appear to be equipotent with regard to their interaction with platelets when tested in their fibrillar forms.[62] The nature of the binding sites on the collagen molecule and on the platelet that are responsible for the adhesion remain obscure, but recent preliminary evidence points to the importance of a unique nonapeptide in type III collagen[63] and a platelet membrane receptor for collagen.[63a] The site to which platelets normally adhere, the subendothelium, is a complex structure that contains both collagenous and noncollagenous elements.

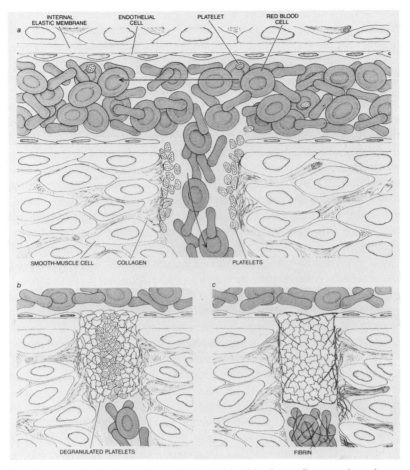

INTERNAL
ELASTIC MEMBRANE        ENDOTHELIAL        PLATELET        RED BLOOD
                           CELL                              CELL

SMOOTH-MUSCLE CELL        COLLAGEN                        PLATELETS

DEGRANULATED PLATELETS                              FIBRIN

**Fig. 4-8.**   The role of platelets in hemostasis. As blood begins to flow out through a cut in the vessel wall, platelets adhere to collagen in the wall (a). The platelets are thereby stimulated to secrete the contents of their granules, including ADP, and other passing platelets adhere to the first layer, building up a loose plug in the wound channel (b). Changes in the platelets and contact of blood with damaged cells convert the plasma protein prothrombin into the enzyme thrombin. The thrombin, in turn, converts fibrinogen into fibrin strands, which reinforce the platelet plug; it also causes platelets to pack together more closely (c). From Zucker MB[61] with permission of Scientific American, Inc., p. 96.

Baumgartner and his colleagues devised an adhesion technique to approximate more closely this in vivo situation;[61] a rabbit's aorta is deendothelialized in vivo with the aid of a balloon catheter, after which the aorta is removed and everted segments of it are mounted in a flow chamber through which blood is pumped at a predetermined rate corresponding to a certain shear rate (see below). After a period of time, the segment is fixed and the extent of platelet adhesion is determined microscopically. At high shear rates, the requirements for platelet adhesion in this system differ from those of both collagen and glass since exogenous von Willebrand factor, the platelet receptor for von Willebrand factor, and calcium are all necessary, whereas fibrinogen plays little or no role. At lower shear rates, the requirements more closely approximate those associated with collagen adhesion.[63] Recently, non-collagenous microfibrils have been purified from human placenta, and since they require exogenous von Willebrand factor to induce platelet aggregation, it has been suggested that they are the von Willebrand factor-dependent subendothelial element to which platelets adhere in the Baumgartner technique.[64,64a]

### Aggregation

The invention of the aggregometer[65,66] permitted the simple quantitative assessment of platelet aggregation with reasonable precision and accuracy when proper attention was given to technical considerations,[67] and thus resulted in a dramatic increase in studies of this phenomenon. Although each of the agonists commonly used to stimulate platelet aggregation in the clinical evaluation of platelet function has unique aspects with regard to mechanism of activation and pattern of aggregation, the responses to these stimuli appear to be composed of a mixture of the 5 fundamental platelet reactions indicated in Figure 4-9.

Shape change is an energy-requiring reaction characterized by the rapid extension of long, spikelike filopodia from the platelet associated with a change in the body of the platelet from its normal disc shape to a more spherical shape.[61] As previously indicated, actin polymerization is thought to be the major process responsible for this change.[39] Since shape change results in an extremely rapid and dramatic increase in platelet surface area, it is likely that the extensive internal membrane in the platelet's open canalicular system becomes part of the external membrane when the filopodia form. Even though several agonists induce shape change before inducing aggregation, shape change is clearly not an absolute requirement for aggregation since, for example, epinephrine can induce aggregation without producing any shape change. Although the precise physiologic role of shape change is thus unclear, 2 hypotheses can be considered: (1) the increase in surface area will permit a greater area for potential contact; (2) since electrostatic repulsion between two particles is directly related to both the radius of curvature of the particles and their surface charge densities,[68] the extension of long, thin filopodial spikes results in a dramatic decrease in the radius of curvature at the tips and thus reduces the electrostatic forces tending to keep platelets apart. The mechanism that triggers the development of filopodia remains unknown, but suggestions have included changes in divalent cation concentration, cytosolic pH, or exposure of nucleation sites on the cytosolic surface of the plasma membrane;[39,39a] all of these stimuli are presumed to initiate actin polymerization.

Some agonists have the capacity either to permit or to increase the binding of fibrinogen to the platelet surface,[24,25] and current evidence indicates that if a sufficient number of fibrinogen molecules bind to the platelet and the suspension is stirred, aggregation will occur. It is unclear how the binding of fibrinogen results in aggregation, but since fibrinogen is a very large (340,000 molecular weight) dimeric molecule, it is possible that single fibrinogen molecules could act as molecular bridges, attaching to identical binding sites on two platelets simultaneously, and thus ultimately leading to lattice formation. The localization of the platelet binding sites on fibrinogen to the carboxy-termini of the gamma chains, which are located at both ends of the molecule, is in accord with this hypothesis.[68a] Other aggregating agents appear to expose receptors for von Willebrand factor,[69,69a,b] and the binding of this protein also results in aggregation or, more precisely, agglutination (see the section on von Willebrand's disease below) if the suspension is stirred. As indicated above, it appears that von Willebrand factor can bind to different sites on the platelet membrane depending upon the agonist employed.[28a–c] The von Willebrand factor is not, in fact, a single molecular species, but rather a series of very high molecular weight (1-20 $\times$ 10$^6$) molecules composed of variable numbers of a single subunit.[69] It thus shares with fibrino-

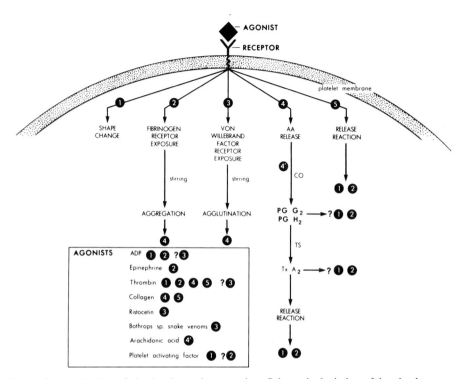

**Fig. 4-9.** Activation of platelets by various agonists. Schematic depiction of the platelet response to different agonists. After binding to a specific receptor, a signal is generated which results in 1 or more of the 5 responses shown. Pathway 1 results in platelet shape change, with the extension of long, thin filopodia and the assumption of a more spherical form for the main body of the platelet. There is no evidence that shape change itself leads to any other response. Several agonists result in the exposure of fibrinogen receptors on the platelets' surface. If the platelets are stirred and fibrinogen is available, aggregation will occur; this appears adequate for the initiation of pathway 4. Some agonists make von Willebrand factor receptors available, and if von Willebrand factor is present and the system is stirred, agglutination will occur. This is also sufficient to activate pathway 4. As just indicated, a variety of agents will ultimately result in release of arachidonic acid (pathway 4), which, in turn, will be converted into the potent aggregating agents $PGG_2$, $PGH_2$, and $TxA_2$. Moreover, the generation of these intermediates will cause release of ADP from the dense granules. The cyclic endoperoxides, $TxA_2$, and ADP can all result in additional aggregation by stimulating pathways 1 and 2. The addition of exogenous arachidonic acid (pathway 4) obviates the need to release this lipid from membrane phospholipids, but still requires cyclooxygenase (CO) and thromboxane synthetase (TS) activity. In pathway 5, the release reaction is stimulated by a mechanism that does not require intact arachidonic acid metabolism. The box on the lower left categorizes the agonists commonly used in assessing a patient's platelet function according to their ability to initiate the different pathways.

gen both a large molecular radius (due to its high molecular weight) and multiple valency (due to its composition of identical subunits), and therefore it too could function as a bridging molecule (see the section on von Willebrand's disease below).

Essentially all of the aggregating agents can stimulate the platelet to release arachidonic acid, although they vary in potency and in the requirement that the suspensions be stirred for aggregation to occur. Once arachidonic acid is released, it undergoes a series of reactions resulting in the generation of thromboxane $A_2$, which, in turn, is instrumental in inducing the release of granule contents. Since the strong aggregating agent ADP is one of the agents released, the system has a potent positive feedback loop. Moreover, the cyclic endoperoxides, $PGG_2$ and $PGH_2$, as well as thromboxane $A_2$, probably also induce shape change and aggregation, thus adding positive feedback loops of their own. Two aggregating agents, thrombin and collagen, in addition to stimulating arachidonic acid release and metabolism, are able to induce the platelet release reaction by a pathway independent of thromboxane $A_2$ production. It has been proposed that platelet production of the potent lipid stimulator of aggregation AGEPC (platelet-activating factor) may be responsible for this pathway of release, but currently available evidence on this point is conflicting.[59,60] In fact, thrombin is used clinically to subdivide patients who may have similar aggregation responses into (1) those who have abnormalities in arachidonic acid release or metabolism (who will have normal release of ADP), and (2) those who lack adequate stores of ADP in their dense granules (and thus will have abnormal release of ADP). Similarly, exogenous arachidonic acid, which can enter the platelet and be directly converted to its derivatives, can be used as an aggregating agent to differentiate patients with defective release of arachidonic acid from those with abnormalities in the subsequent metabolism of this fatty acid.

Several points require emphasis: (1) Agents that directly expose either fibrinogen or von Willebrand factor receptors produce aggregation even when thromboxane $A_2$ production and the release reaction cannot take place; this is appropriately termed *primary aggregation*. Conversely, the second waves of aggregation induced by the appropriate concentrations of ADP, epinephrine, thrombin, and ristocetin do require an intact release reaction and/or arachidonic acid metabolism and thus are properly termed *secondary aggregation*. A semantic problem arises with collagen-induced aggregation since aggregation occurs in a single wave, but only after platelets have adhered to the collagen and undergone arachidonic acid metabolism and the release reaction. Thus, despite the fact that this agent induces but a single wave, physiologically it is more akin to secondary aggregation in being dependent on arachidonic acid metabolism and the release reaction. (2) There is significant variation in the nature of the aggregates formed with different agonists, indicating the importance of factors that are still very poorly understood; for example, high concentrations of ristocetin can induce virtually all of the platelets to enter into a single aggregate, whereas no concentration of epinephrine or ADP will accomplish this. (3) Platelet aggregation in vitro is performed on citrated, platelet-rich plasma in which the concentration of ionized calcium is very low, and thus some of the observed responses (in particular, the ease with which the release reaction is induced) may be artifactual. Thus the relative roles of released ADP and the proaggregatory arachidonic acid metabolites in enhancing platelet aggregation in vivo remain uncertain. The complexity of the interrelationships involved in aggregation can be appreciated by considering the pathways outlined in Figure 4-9; for example, epinephrine can induce fibrinogen receptor exposure, resulting in both platelet aggregation (if the suspension is stirred) and release of arachidonic acid; the latter, in turn, results in the production of $PGG_2$, $PGH_2$, and thromboxane $A_2$ (all of which may be able to induce shape change and fibrinogen receptor exposure), as well as the release of ADP, which also can induce shape change, fibrinogen receptor exposure, von Willebrand factor receptor exposure, etc.

### Release Reaction

Extensive studies of the interaction of agonists with the platelet surface have been performed in an attempt to define the presumed receptors to which these agonists bind and the mechanism(s) that results in the platelet's response.[70] Unfortunately, serious methodologic and interpretative problems have plagued these studies. In particular, the difficulties involved in distinguishing a binding site from a true receptor (i.e., a site involved in producing a physiologic effect) have been especially hard to overcome. In brief (1) it appears that ADP may bind to at lease 2 different functional sites, one involved in inhibition of adenyl cyclase and another involved in shape change. Whether other sites exist for fibrinogen and von Willebrand factor receptor exposure is not known. (2) The platelet apparently contains primarily, if not exclusively, adrenergic receptors of the alpha$_2$ type, and it is to these that epinephrine presumably binds. The status of beta-adrenergic receptors on the platelet remains quite controversial.[71,72] (3) Thrombin binds to several different platelet proteins but apparently hydrolyzes only GPV. Since thrombin's proteolytic activity is required for it to initiate aggregation, it is possible that GPV proteolysis is involved in the stimulus-translation mechanism,[70] but this hypothesis has already been challenged.[72a] (4) Ristocetin appears to have a low-affinity interaction with the platelet surface that relies primarily on electrostatic forces (see the section on von Willebrand disease below).

Considerable evidence has accumulated in support of the hypothesis that the platelet release reaction is ultimately induced, regardless of the initial stimulus, by an increase in platelet cytosolic calcium.[39a,73,74] The increased calcium may initiate release by activating the contractile mechanism, as noted above, and/or by promoting the fusion of the granule membranes with the plasma membranes in the open canalicular system or at the cell surface. Although the platelet appears to have several separate pools of calcium (dense body, mitochondrial, membrane-associated, etc), current speculation is that the dense tubular system is the main source of the calcium that initiates the release reaction. One attractive although still preliminary, hypothesis is that thromboxane A$_2$ may act as an ionophore (a molecule which can transport ions across membranes) and thus transport calcium from the dense tubular system into the cytoplasm.[73]

In contrast to the proaggregatory effects of increased cytosolic calcium, increases in platelet cAMP are associated with inhibition of platelet function.[74] Intraplatelet cAMP is controlled by (1) the enzyme adenylate cyclase, which converts ATP into cAMP; this enzyme is stimulated by PGI$_2$ (prostacyclin), PGE$_1$ and PGD$_2$ and is probably inhibited by epinephrine and ADP; and (2) the cAMP-catabolizing enzyme phosphodiesterase, which is inhibited by xanthines such as theophylline (Fig. 4-10). Current evidence indicates that cAMP activates protein kinases which, in turn, alter cellular function by phosphorylating proteins. Several mechanisms may be involved in cAMP's inhibitory effect on the release reaction: (1) increased sequestration of calcium by the dense tubular system; (2) decreased arachidonic acid release from phospholipids; and (3) inhibition of myosin light chain kinase. Although considerable attention has been directed at cAMP's inhibition of the release reaction, it should be appreciated that increased cAMP also inhibits platelet adhesion and the primary wave of aggregation induced by ADP, epinephrine, thrombin, and ristocetin.[75] cAMP must therefore have an inhibitory mechanism(s) independent of its inhibition of the release reaction. Recently, cAMP was shown to alter the platelet membrane, perhaps through an effect on the cytoskeleton; this may account for the inhibition noted above.[75]

### Platelets and Coagulation

There is incontrovertible evidence that coagulation proceeds more rapidly when platelets are present in plasma than when they are not,[4,59,76] but considerable controversy exists concerning the mechanism(s) involved. This activity, operationally defined as platelet factor 3 (PF 3), appears to require that platelets be "activated" by one of several stimuli. A series of early observations pointed to the platelet membrane phospholipids or perhaps phospholipoproteins as the source of PF 3: (1) phospholipid mixtures from widely

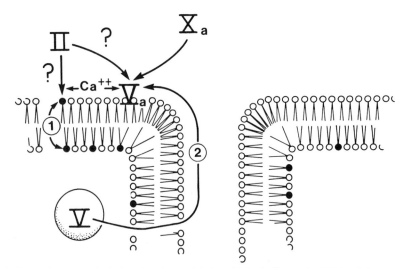

**Fig. 4-10.** PF 3. Hypothetical molecular models by which platelets make PF 3 activity (acceleration of prothrombin to thrombin conversion) available upon stimulation. In model 1, activation of the platelet results in a flip-flop motion of the negatively charged phospholipids from the inner leaflet of the bilayer to the outer leaflet. This produces a negative charge on the exterior surface of the lipid bilayer and may furnish (in the presence of calcium) a binding site for prothrombin (and perhaps other vitamin K-dependent factors). In model 2, factor V contained in the platelet's $\alpha$-granules is both released and activated (Va) when platelets are stimulated. The platelet membrane has specific receptor sites for the binding of Va. The bound factor Va (in the presence of calcium) then acts as a receptor for factor Xa. The factor Xa–Va–Ca$^{2+}$ complex then interacts with prothrombin (either by binding it directly or by lateral diffusion after the latter attaches as in model 1) to convert it to thrombin.

varying sources could substitute, at least in part, for platelets in accelerating coagulation; (2) unlike many other platelet factors that are released from the platelet with stimulation, PF 3 appears to stay with the platelet itself and become "available" on its surface; (3) the vitamin K-dependent proteins have been shown to bind to phospholipids (in the presence of calcium). Moreover, since negative phospholipids are the most potent substitutes for platelets,[77] the asymmetric distribution of phospholipids in the platelet membrane, with the negatively charged ones localized almost exclusively in the inner leaflet, would result in the shielding of PF 3 in resting platelets.[5,6] With platelet activation, these phospholipids may become available to the plasma factors either as a result of a generalized disruption of the membrane during aggregation ("lysis") or as a more specific alteration in which they move from the inner to the outer leaflet of the bilayer (Fig. 4-10). Although it is true that the potency of agonists in making PF 3 available parallels their ability to induce the release reaction, these two effects can be dissociated; thus, PF 3 availability is not simply a result of the release reaction.

Whereas there is general agreement that the platelet's phospholipids play a crucial role in the development of PF 3 activity, the observation that platelet membranes are more active than any combination of phospholipids[4] has led to the view that the platelet must play a more specific role than just making phospholipids available. Although unique phospholipoproteins may be responsible, in part, for this increased specificity, recent studies on the conversion of prothrombin to thrombin have identified another mechanism whereby platelets can accelerate coagulation, namely the presence of a high-affinity platelet membrane receptor for an activated form of factor V (proaccelerin).[78] If calcium ions are available, this membrane-bound, activated factor V can act as a receptor for factor Xa (activated Stuart factor) and speed the conversion of prothrombin (which may bind either to the factor V–Xa complex directly or perhaps to the platelet phospholipids) to thrombin.[79] The role of platelet activation in this system is unclear, but since activated factor V binds equally well to native or stimulated platelets, it is likely that it has more to do with the activation of the factor V in the platelet's α-granules than with changes in the platelet's factor V binding sites.[78,80] In fact, a platelet protease capable of activating factor V has recently been identified.[80a] The importance of platelet-associated factor V is supported by observations that platelet transfusions are often effective in treating patients with factor V deficiency and that prothrombin consumption is decreased when platelet-rich plasma from a patient with a deficiency in α-granule contents (presumably including factor V) is allowed to clot.[76] Thus, even if one accepts a recent suggestion to narrow the definition of PF 3 to "that activity . . . which represents the contribution of platelets to the interaction of factor Xa, factor V and calcium in the activation of prothrombin,"[81] both a phospholipid effect and this receptor effect are probably making contributions to the measured PF 3.

Although the role of platelets in prothrombin conversion has been the most intensively studied reaction, there is evidence that a similar platelet mechanism is involved in activation of factor X by factor IXa in the presence of activated factor VIII, platelets, and calcium.[81a] The platelet's role in this reaction has been termed *intrinsic factor-Xa forming activity*.[81] Specific receptor sites have not, however, been defined as yet.

Additional coagulation-accelerating effects of platelets have been proposed, including (1) ADP-induced factor XII activation (contact product-forming activity), (2) collagen-induced factor XIa-like activity and, (3) protection of bound Xa (and possibly XIa) from inactivation by plasma inhibitors.[81] The collagen-induced coagulant activity has been used to explain the variability of clinical bleeding symptoms in patients with thrombasthenia and hemophilia; the lack of bleeding symptoms in patients with factor XII, prekallikrein, or high molecular weight kininogen deficiencies; and the variability in thrombotic tendency in patients with a variety of disorders. There is, however, considerable controversy concerning the existence of contact product-forming activity and the quantitative contribution that activation of platelet-associated factor XI could make in normal hemostasis.[82,83] The precise physiologic significance of these activities thus remains to be determined.

Regardless of the precise mechanisms involved, morphologic studies make it clear that fibrin strands are laid down in intimate association with platelets and that the latter become enmeshed in the fibrin network. When clotting occurs in an undisturbed test tube containing platelet-rich plasma, the initial manifestation is a conversion of the fluid to a gellike state in which no fluid will be detectable even if the tube is turned upside down. If the tube does not contain platelets, it retains this property, but if platelets are present, the clot will be seen to retract with time until it takes up only a very small fraction of the total volume. This process of clot retraction probably involves a complex interaction of the platelet membrane with the fibrin strands (since it is abnormal in thrombasthenia), along with an intact platelet actinomyosin contractile mechanism.[35] Despite extensive investigation, the details of this phenomenon are still only poorly understood and its physiologic role in hemostasis remains uncertain.

### Control of Platelet Function

As indicated above, the ability of an activated platelet to produce proaggregatory arachidonic acid metabolites such as the cyclic endoperoxides and thromboxane $A_2$, and to release the potent aggregating agent ADP from its dense granules, constitutes a positive feedback mechanism that has the virtue of amplifying the initial response. It should be appreciated, however, that unopposed positive feedback systems are inherently unstable since, for example, one would predict that even a trivial stimulus would lead to an ever-increasing response until all the platelets in the body were aggregated. It is thus obvious that well-coordinated control mechanisms must exist to limit the response. Although it is possible to suggest several potential mechanisms, in truth very little is known about the physiologic contribution, if any, made by each of them.

Blood flow is probably the single most important factor establishing the limits of the platelet's contribution to in vivo hemostasis. It will determine the number of platelets passing a given point in the blood vessel in a given time, the length of time a platelet will have either to adhere to the vessel wall or to aggregate with another platelet before being carried downstream, and the force with which a given platelet will collide with the vessel wall or another platelet. In addition, blood flow will determine the shear rate acting on platelets that do adhere to the vessel wall.[84,85] An intuitive idea of the latter can be obtained if it is remembered that when fluids move through rigid tubes (i.e., under laminar flow), (1) the central cylinder of fluid moves fastest; (2) each succeeding concentric cylinder extending out from the center moves more slowly; (3) the cylinder of fluid at the vessel wall is essentially stationary; (4) a velocity gradient profile can be established by plotting the velocity as a function of the distance from the wall; and (5) the slope of the velocity gradient at the wall is the wall shear rate. In addition to its direct shearing effect, the presence of this velocity gradient is responsible for the phenomenon of axial streaming wherein the particles in a dilute suspension of fluid subjected to laminar flow move to the center of the stream and do not approach the wall. Were axial streaming the only factor controlling platelets' behavior in the circulation, they would not be able to function effectively in hemostasis since they would only rarely interact with the sites of injury. The presence of erythrocytes counteracts the tendency of platelets to stay in the axial stream by (1) selectively occupying the axial stream themselves, and thus enriching the blood near the wall with the remaining platelet-rich plasma, and (2) constantly colliding with each other and with platelets, thus insuring that some platelets will be forcefully directed at the vessel wall. Since shear rate is a function of velocity of flow and blood vessel diameter, it differs greatly in different parts of the normal circulation, complicating the analysis of platelet–vessel wall interactions. Moreover, where inhomogeneities exist in the circulation, as for example at branch points and stenoses, flow disturbance and vortex formation introduce even greater complexity. The importance of understanding these rheologic factors is underscored by the data discussed above indicating that the cofactor requirements for platelet adhesion to the subendothelium depend on the shear rate employed[63].

Perhaps even more remarkable than the platelet's ability to adhere to virtually all surfaces is the platelet's unique lack of adhesion to the blood vessel wall when the latter is covered with normal endothelial cells. Originally, this property was assigned to the highly negatively charged proteoglycans that coat the luminal surface of endothelial cells and thus help to establish a force of electrostatic repulsion between the endothelium and the negatively charged platelets.[86] The subsequent discovery that endothelial cells, unlike platelets, have the enzymes needed to synthesize prostacyclin ($PGI_2$), the most potent inhibitor of platelet adhesion and aggregation known, shifted the emphasis to a more active role of the endothelial cell in its nonthrombogenicity.[87] Although local levels of $PGI_2$ may be quite important, recent evidence casts doubts on whether the circulating level of $PGI_2$ under basal conditions is sufficiently high to inhibit platelet function, and so the issue remains undecided.[88] Additionally, the endothelium may play an important role in limiting the platelet response after it has been initiated by (1) taking up ADP released from platelets and converting it into adenosine, a potent platelet inhibitor;[89] (2) binding and removing thrombin;[90] and (3) increasing $PGI_2$ production or release upon exposure to thrombin.[90] Finally, there is evidence that endothelial cells can actually "steal" the proaggregatory cyclic endoperoxides that are produced by platelets in the course of their stimulation and convert them into the powerful platelet inhibitor, $PGI_2$.[91]

The poorly understood phenomenon termed the *refractory state*, in which platelets exposed to low concentrations of some agonists for a period of time respond poorly or not at all to a subsequent challenge with those same agonists,[59] may also help to limit the platelets' response; one can imagine that platelets at the periphery of a developing platelet aggregate are exposed to subaggregating levels of the agonists and thus may be inhibited from entering into the aggregate.

### Platelet Production and Kinetics[92,93]

Platelets are produced from the fragmentation of the cytoplasm of megakaryocytes. The latter are large, bone marrow-derived cells that are descendants of a multipotential cell which can form erythroid, myeloid, or megakaryocytic precursors. A stem cell committed exclusively to megakaryocyte production also probably exists. The megakaryocyte is unique among bone marrow cells in its ability to reproduce its deoxyribonucleic acid (DNA) without undergoing cell division (endomitosis). Current evidence supports a model in which a blastlike diploid precursor (conventionally referred to as being 2 N with regard to DNA content) undergoes endomitosis until its ploidy is anywhere from 4 to 64 N; approximately 70 percent are 16 N and the vast majority of the remaining 30 percent are 32 or 8 N. After DNA synthesis is complete, the megakaryoblast undergoes a maturation process during which proteins are synthesized, granules are formed, and an elaborate system of membranes (demarcation membranes) is developed. During the same time, the volume of cytoplasm increases and the nucleus takes on a multilobular appearance. The mature megakaryocyte has a granular cytoplasm and extensive demarcation membranes. At this point, pseudopodia are formed and find their way into the bone marrow sinusoids by passing between adventitial cells and through the cytoplasm of endothelial cells. Most commonly, these megakaryocyte pseudopodia then undergo fragmentation with release of platelets into the circulation, although an alternative mechanism in which whole megakaryocytes are first released into the circulation and then fragment after being trapped in the pulmonary circulation is probably also operative. It has been estimated that a single 16 N megakaryocyte gives rise to 1000 platelets. The entire maturation sequence has been estimated to take 4–5 days.

There is considerable circumstantial evidence that a thrombopoietic hormone(s), "thrombopoietin," exists, although both purification and characterization of it are still quite rudimentary. Plasma levels of this hormone(s) are thought to increase when the platelet count decreases and to decrease when the platelet count increases. It is interesting to speculate on the nature of the sensor that stimulates the production or release of thrombopoietin. It is quite unlikely that bleeding is involved in the sensing mechanism since the platelet count is normally maintained at approximately ten times the count needed to prevent spontaneous bleeding. Recent evidence suggests that there may, in fact, be 2 thrombopoietic hormones, one of which increases the number of stem cells committed to the megakaryocyte line and another that is involved in the maturation of the megakaryocytes. The former hormone may be controlled by the bone marrow megakaryocyte mass, whereas the latter probably varies inversely with the total platelet mass in the body, perhaps because platelets catabolize it.[94]

The thrombopoietic hormone(s) has several effects on megakaryocytes, including (1) an increase in their size; (2) an increase in their ploidy; (3) an increase in their numbers; and (4) perhaps a decrease in their maturation time. Under optimal conditions of thrombopoietic stress, it has been estimated that platelet production can increase eightfold, although somewhat lower estimates have also been reported. The platelets produced under such circumstances are larger than normal, but it is unclear whether this means that in the unstressed state young platelets are larger than old platelets.

When radiolabeled platelets are injected intravenously and a blood sample is taken soon thereafter, only approximately two-thirds of the injected platelets will be recovered in the circulation. Since the recovery is approximately 90 percent in asplenic patients, it has been concluded that at any given time, approximately one-third of the total platelet mass is sequestered in the spleen. When the spleen is enlarged, the recovery decreases and may be as low as 20 percent in the presence of severe splenomegaly. Platelet survival studies using $^{51}$Cr indicate that platelets normally survive for approximately 10 days. Under basal conditions, the kinetic data are most consistent with a selective removal of the oldest platelets (senescence), but when a pathologic process results in platelet consumption, the removal process becomes more random, affecting both young and old platelets alike. Both isotopic and nonisotopic methods of determining platelet life span are available for clinical use, although, from a practical standpoint, they are rarely required in deciding whether increased platelet destruction or decreased platelet production is the major pathogenetic mechanism in producing thrombocytopenia. These techniques have had their greatest benefit in documenting small reductions in platelet survival in patients with normal or near-normal platelet counts in a variety of disorders; they are also useful in assessing the effects of drug therapy in normalizing survival in these disorders.[95]

## PLATELET DISORDERS

### Quantitative Disorders

### THROMBOCYTOPENIA

Since most studies of normal individuals have found 150,000 platelets/$\mu$l to be the lower limit of normal, individuals with platelet counts lower than this are defined as having thrombocytopenia. Because there are many causes of thromboyctopenia, it is important to develop an orderly and systematic approach to the evaluation of this condition. Table 4-3 is organized according to the steps one might actually take in investigating a patient, while still retaining as much of a pathophysiologic categorization as is practicable.

#### Spurious Thrombocytopenia or Pseudothrombocytopenia

It is imperative that all abnormally low platelet counts obtained by electronic particle counters be confirmed by visual inspection of the peripheral smear. This will avoid unnecessary evaluation or, as has been reported,[96] inappropriate therapy of those patients with low instrument counts who actually have normal numbers of circulating platelets (*spurious thrombocytopenia* or *pseudothrombocytopenia*). The simplest approximation for evaluating platelet sufficiency on a peripheral smear is that each platelet identified in a 1000X oil-immersion objective field containing a monolayer of erythrocytes represents 20,000 platelets/$\mu$l whole blood.[97] When a discrepancy between the machine count and visual estimate is found, a count should be obtained by the reference technique, the manual hemocytometer method using a phase-contrast microscope.

The blood smears of patients with spurious thrombocytopenia may show one of the following three findings, each of which has several different etiologies: platelet aggregates, giant platelets, or "platelet satellism."

### Platelet Aggregates

Electronic particle counters count particles by detecting an abrupt change in electrical resistance when, as the particle passes through a small orifice, it displaces some of the electrolyte solution contained in the orifice. Since the change in resistance is proportional to the volume of the particle, platelets can be selectively counted by setting the instrument to count only those particles having volumes within a specific range, thus excluding white and red blood cells. Depending on the system, appropriate calculations are made to correct for dilution, the changes introduced by sample preparation, and the volume range of platelets actually counted. The final count is expressed as platelets per unit of whole blood. With the Coulter S + instrument, the whole blood is simply diluted and then counted. Thus, if platelet aggregates are present, not only will fewer particles be counted because the platelets are not single (an aggregate being counted as only a single particle), but also many of the aggregates will be excluded from the count because their volume is greater than the upper setting for platelets. A spuriously elevated erythrocyte and/or white blood cell count may result. Similar problems occur with instruments that rely on light scattering to detect platelets. With the Coulter ZBI instrument, the red blood cells are first sedimented by gravity and then the supernatant platelet-rich plasma is counted. When aggregates are present, they are more likely to sediment with the red blood cells instead of remaining in the supernatant as single platelets do, thus decreasing the instrument count. Moreover, even if some of the aggregates remain in the supernatant, they may not be counted as platelets for the reasons outlined above.

When reviewing a blood smear for the possibility of platelet clumps, it is important that the side edges of the smear away from the end on which the drop of blood was applied be carefully examined since large platelet aggregates tend to be pushed to the side by the smearing process. Improper blood collection and the presence of platelet agglutinins are the two major causes for the development of platelet aggregates after the blood leaves the patient's blood vessels. Problems related to both the method of anticoagulation and the technique of blood sampling may result in aggregate formation. When agglutinins are present, their effects are limited to the in vitro setting either as a result of their dependence on low temperature (cold agglutinin) or because of their requirement for anticoagulant (EDTA-dependent agglutinin).

*Collection into inadequate or improper anticoagulant.*   Blood for all cell counts, and especially for platelet counts, should be anticoagulated with EDTA, a very powerful chelator of the divalent cations ($Ca^{2+}$, $Mg^{2+}$) required for platelet aggregation induced by several stimuli. Counts performed with electronic particle counters are almost always lower in blood in which the anticoagulant is heparin rather than EDTA, due to the development of small aggregates in vitro.

**Table 4-3**
Thrombocytopenia

Thrombocytopenia branches into:

**True thrombocytopenia**

- Review of peripheral smear
  - **Platelet Size**
    - **Markedly increased**
      - May-Hegglin anomaly
      - Bernard-Soulier syndrome
      - Montreal platelet syndrome
      - Mediterranean macrothrombocytosis
      - Macrothrombocytes; hereditary deafness and nephritis
      - α-Storage pool disease
    - **Markedly decreased**
      - Wiskott-Aldrich syndrome
    - **Normal, somewhat increased, or decreased**
      - **Bone marrow megakaryocytes**
        - **Decreased**
          - A. Decreased stem cells
            - 1. Hypoplastic marrow
              - a. Aplastic anemia
                - 1) Idiopathic
                  - a) Constitutional (Fanconi's anemia)
                  - b) Acquired
        - **Normal or increased**
          - A. Increased removal
            - 1. Immunologic
              - a. Autoimmune or immune complex
                - 1) ITP—acute, chronic, neonatal
                - 2) Disease associated
                - 3) Drug related
                - 4) Sepsis associated

**Spurious thrombocytopenia**

1. Platelet clumps
   - a. Inadequate anticoagulation
   - b. Agglutinins
     - 1) Cold
     - 2) EDTA-dependent
2. Giant platelets
3. Platelet-leukocyte satellism

2) Secondary
    a) Drugs (chloramphenicol)
    b) Chemicals (benzene, etc.)
    c) Infections (hepatitis, miliary tuberculosis, etc.)
    d) Metabolic (pregnancy)
    e) Immunologic
    f) Paroxysmal nocturnal hemoglobinuria
  b. Chemotherapy
  c. Radiation therapy
2. Hyperplastic marrow (myelophthisic)
  a. Leukemias (acute and chronic)
  b. Lymphomas and myeloma
  c. Metastatic carcinoma
  d. Myelofibrosis
  e. Osteopetrosis
  f. Histiocytosis
  g. Gaucher's disease, etc.
3. Normocellular marrow
  a. Cyclic thrombocytopenia
  b. Congenital amegakaryocytosis
  c. Acute alcoholism
  d. Thiazides
  e. Thrombocytopenia with decreased megakaryocytes

  b. Alloimmune
    1) Isoimmune neonatal purpura
    2) Posttransfusion purpura
2. Increased utilization
  a. In association with increased fibrinogen consumption
    1) Disseminated intravascular coagulation
    2) Giant hemangioma
    3) Certain snake venoms
  b. Without increased fibrinogen consumption
    1) Thrombotic thrombocytopenic purpura
    2) Hemolytic-uremic syndrome
    3) "Thrombopoietin" deficiency
    4) Artificial or pathological surfaces
    5) Certain snake venoms
    6) Virus associated
    7) Allergy associated
B. Ineffective thrombopoiesis
  1. Megaloblastosis
  2. Paroxysmal nocturnal hemoglobinuria
  3. Erythroleukemia
  4. Hereditary thrombocytopenia
C. Increased pooling
  1. Hypersplenism
  2. Hypothermia

*Traumatic venipuncture.*    Blood samples drawn for platelet counts must be obtained with the utmost care and immediately anticoagulated since trauma or prolonged venipuncture can lead to the introduction of tissue factor into the specimen, with activation of the extrinsic pathway of coagulation and the generation of thrombin, a potent platelet-aggregating agent. This problem occurs most commonly when specimens are obtained by a fingerstick because the time for collection may be prolonged and the procedure, by its very nature, results in tissue damage. In addition, since the blood smear obtained with a fingerstick is taken directly from the drop of blood on the finger, it may not accurately reflect the blood sample actually used for the platelet count, since the latter will have entered the capillary tube a variable number of seconds before or after the blood for the smear was obtained. Thus, in the author's opinion, platelet counts should not be performed on fingerstick specimens unless the technician's technique is verified by periodically comparing counts obtained by venipuncture and fingerstick.

*Platelet agglutinins*

**Cold agglutinins.**[98]    Immunoglobulin G (IgG) and immunoglobulin M(IgM) agglutinins have been described in patients with systemic disorders such as metastatic carcinoma and in patients with serum protein abnormalities (i.e., cryoproteins and high gamma globulin levels). These agglutinins react with platelets only at temperatures below 34°C and thus usually have no effect on in vivo platelet function. The reaction is independent of the type and amount of anticoagulant used for specimen collection. In the presence of cold agglutinins the platelet count usually drops following blood collection for a period of 30 minutes to 2 hours. Unlike cold-induced red blood cell agglutination, platelet agglutination is not reversible upon rewarming, probably because platelets undergo irreversible alterations subsequent to their agglutination.

**EDTA-dependent platelet agglutinins.**[96,99,99a]    Aggregate formation usually occurs at 37°C as well as at lower temperatures, but only in the presence of EDTA. Moreover, there is heterogeneity in the mechanism by which EDTA permits the agglutinin to work: in some cases it appears to act by reducing the ionized calcium concentration, whereas in others a specific EDTA–membrane interaction is more likely. An association of this disorder with rheumatoid arthritis probably exists.

**Giant platelets.**    If giant platelets make up a large percentage of the total platelet number, a major underestimation by the electronic platelet count may occur since these megathrombocytes will (1) tend to sediment with the red blood cells if this step is employed (Coulter ZBI but not S + or automated optical systems) and (2) tend to be excluded by the upper sizing threshold of the particle counter. There are several rare hereditary congenital disorders associated with giant platelets (see below), and a considerable number of acquired disorders in which a significant subpopulation of giant platelets may be found (idiopathic thrombocytopenic purpura, myeloproliferative disorders, megaloblastic anemias). To give an example, a patient of the author's with the May-Hegglin anomaly (see below) has such large platelets that approximately 25 percent of them are as large as red blood cells. On one occasion, the platelet count on a single sample of her blood was 6,000/μl when measured by the Couler S + and 40,000/μl when measured by phase-contrast microscopy.

**Platelet satellism.**[100]    This is an uncommon in vitro hematologic finding about which little is understood. It is characterized by the presence of rosettes consisting of neutrophilic leukocytes (as well as rare band forms, monocytes, or eosinophils) surrounded by attached

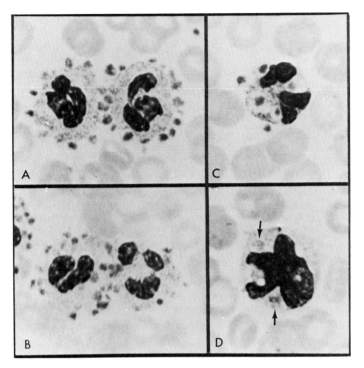

**Fig. 4-11.** Platelet satellism. (A) Platelet satellism. (B) Platelet satellism with early phagocytosis. (C) Platelet phagocytosis by a segmented neutrophil. (D) Platelet phagocytosis by a monocyte (arrows). Peripheral blood smear. Wright's stain, X2150. From Ravel R, Bassart JA, Platelet satellitosis and phagocytosis by leukocytes. Lab Med 5:41, 1974, with permission of JB Lippincott Co.

platelets (Fig.4-11). In most studies, this finding has been confined to blood anticoagulated with EDTA, but in two cases it also occurred in fingerstick blood. Phagocytosis of the platelets by neutrophils has also been observed. Forty-four cases have been reported since 1963 in patients ranging in age from 14 to 85 years, with a male:female ratio of 2.3:1. No specific symptoms, diseases, or medications have been consistently associated with this phenomenon. The in vitro rosetting of platelets around neutrophils seems to occur best at room temperature and appears to require the presence of EDTA rather than simply the low calcium concentration produced by the EDTA. The EDTA-dependent rosetting factor in plasma has been ascribed to a variety of plasma constituents, including gamma globulins, cryofibrinogen, fibronectin, and platelet-derived proteins. It should be noted that in a few cases the patient was thought to be truly thrombocytopenic; thus, one should be certain that one is not dealing with "pseudo-pseudothrombocytopenia." A platelet count performed by phase-contrast microscopy on blood anticoagulated with another anticoagulant (e.g., citrate) should suffice for this purpose.

If review of the blood smear confirms the presence of thrombocytopenia, the next logical step in the evaluation is a gross determination of the size of the platelets on the peripheral smear. As indicated in Table 4-3, there are several disorders in which the platelets are remarkably large (usually 4–6 times the volume of normal platelets, with a significant fraction as large as erythrocytes) and at least 1 disorder (Wiskott-Aldrich syndrome) in which they are quite obviously small. In addition, there is a considerable body of data correlating more subtle increases in platelet size with both thrombopoietic stress and bone

marrow megakaryocyte mass; this information may be of assistance in distinguishing decreased production of platelets from increased destruction as the pathogenetic mechanism
of thrombyocytopenia.[101,103] There are, however, a series of artifactual changes in platelet size resulting from a complex relationship between the anticoagulant, the temperature,
and the length of time after venipuncture that must be controlled if reliable information is
to be obtained about these more modest changes.[101-103] Particle counters can give a more
objective and statistically reliable determination of platelet volume than casual smear
observation, but they are equally subject to the artifactual changes noted above. Recent
evidence indicates that an increase in platelet volume by such counters may precede and
predict the recovery from thrombocytopenia in patients treated with chemotherapy.[103a]

*Thrombocytopenia associated with abnormal platelet size.*

**May-Hegglin anomaly.**   This disorder is characterized by the presence of giant platelets
and Döhle bodylike inclusions in granulocytes [104,106] (Fig. 4-12). Fewer than 100 cases
had been reported by 1980, with an autosomal dominant inheritance consistently found in
the families in which the inheritance could be evaluated. The anomaly is usually associated with mild to moderate thrombocytopenia, but both normal platelet counts and severe
thrombocytopenia have been reported, even within a single family. The presence of a hemorrhagic diathesis is also quite variable; approximately one-half of the patients will be
asymptomatic, whereas those who are affected usually have mild to moderate purpura,
epistaxis, menorrhagia, and gingival bleeding. More severe bleeding, however, may occur following dental extractions, surgery, or trauma. Overall, the bleeding tendency does
seem to correlate with the platelet count, but a few discrepancies have been reported.

Results of platelet function studies have also been variable. The bleeding time is almost always normal when the platelet count is above $75,000/\mu l$ and may even be normal at
counts under $50,000/\mu l$. This increased hemostatic effectiveness per platelet may result
from the large size of the platelets. Interestingly, it has been pointed out that the increase
in platelet size often compensates for the decrease in number, thus resulting in an essentially normal platelet mass; this observation may have implications for the feedback mechanisms involved in platelet production. Platelet aggregation studies with ADP, collagen,
and ristocetin have been interpreted as similar to those of control samples diluted to the
same count. Both normal and abnormal results have been reported with clot retraction;
normal, low, or high PF3 activity has been reported. Biochemically, other than increased
amounts of normal platelet constituents, no specific abnormalities have been found. The
finding of increased platelet$_\beta$-thromboglobulin levels suggests that the contents of the
$\alpha$-granules are increased proportionately to the increase in volume. [107] In one study, the
total platelet sialic acid was increased when expressed on a per platelet basis, but after
adjusting for differences in volume and surface area, the sialic acid content was normal;
this was in accord with the observed normal values for platelet electrophoretic mobility.[108]
The surface glycoproteins of May-Hegglin platelets are normal when analyzed by several
techniques.[108] In some patients, electron microscopy has revealed an abnormally tortuous
membrane complex along with unusually large granules and evidence of granule fusion,
whereas in others the electron microscopic anatomy has been reported to be normal.

The pathophysiology of the thrombocytopenia remains obscure. Patients have normal numbers of megakaryocytes, and the weight of evidence indicates that platelet survival is normal. No convincing evidence of ineffective thrombopoiesis has been presented.

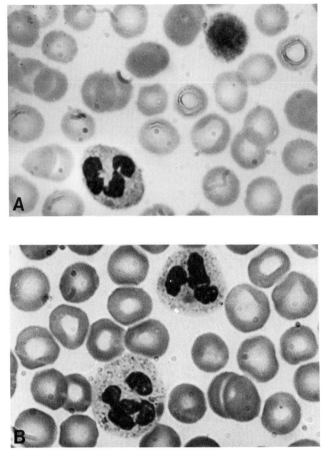

**Fig. 4-12.** May-Hegglin anomaly. (A) Giant platelet and neutrophil leukocyte from peripheral blood showing 1 inclusion body (X1000). (B) Neutrophil leukocytes from peripheral blood showing inclusion bodies. From Cabrera JR, Fontau G, Lorente F, et al[109] with permission of Blackwell Scientific Publications.

Thus, current thinking is that the total mass of platelets entering and leaving the circulation each day is normal in this disorder, but that an abnormality in megakaryocyte fragmentation results in the release of abnormally sized platelets. The Döhle bodylike inclusions are found in neutrophils, basophils, eosinophils, and monocytes, but there is controversy as to whether or not they are present in lymphocytes. Histochemical studies indicate that the inclusions contain RNA. The fraction of neutrophils containing inclusions varies widely, with reports ranging from 15 to 90 percent. Despite their similarity under light microscopy to the Döhle bodies found in infections, ultrastructural differences between May-Hegglin inclusions and Döhle bodies have been reported. Although increased susceptibility to infections has never been reported in the May-Hegglin anomaly, a defect in neutrophil mobility has recently been described.[109]

Therapeutically, patients with this disorder should be warned against the use of platelet-inhibiting medications and should carry identification indicating their increased risk of hemorrhage. Serious hemorrhage that cannot be conrolled with local measures should be treated with platelet transfusions. The role of splenectomy, if any, is unclear.

**Bernard-Soulier syndrome.**   This disorder is also characterized by dramatically large platelets. Since the qualitative defect in platelet function is usually more serious than the thrombocytopenia, this disorder will be discussed below with the qualitative disorders.

**Hereditary macrothrombocytopenia, deafness, and renal disease.**   This syndrome has been identified in only 3 families.[110–111]. This disorder appears to be inherited as an X chromosome-linked or autosomal dominant trait. Epistaxis beginning in childhood is common, and although bleeding from other sites is usually not severe, death due to subarachnoid hemorrhage has been reported. The hearing defect is of the sensorineural type, with frequent progression to deafness by mid-teens. The major manifestation of the renal disease is proteinuria beginning in childhood, and although it is usually not progressive, an illness indistinguishable from acute glomerulonephritis with progression to uremia has been reported. Interestingly, the familial association of deafness and renal disease in the absence of macrothrombocytopenia is a well-established syndrome. The thrombocytopenia in this syndrome is usually moderate, and normal or increased numbers of megakaryocytes are found in the bone marrow. The platelets are quite large on smear. Platelet function in two of the three families was reported to be abnormal with prolonged bleeding times, defective PF3 availabiltiy and abnormal aggregation responses to ADP, collagen, and epinephrine. In marked contrast, the patients in the third family were reported to have better bleeding times than would have been expected on the basis of their platelet counts, increased PF3 availability, and normal aggregation responses. Ultrastructural morphology was reported to be abnormal in the first two families and normal in the third, but the interpretation of the findings in the first two families has been challenged.[1] Therapeutically, other than avoiding antiplatelet medications and supplying the patients with appropriate identification, there is little to be done. Steroids and splenectomy do not seem to increase the platelet count. If serious hemorrhage occurs, platelet transfusions can be used with good effect since the platelet survival time is probably normal.

**The Montreal platelet syndrome.**   This is a poorly understood disorder, inherited in a dominant manner, and characterized by moderate to severe thrombocytopenia, prolonged bleeding times, spontaneous platelet aggregation, and normal clot retraction and PF3 availability.[112] It has been claimed that the greatly enlarged size of platelets found on peripheral smear is an artifact related to an abnormality in shape change since, when platelets are fixed while still in platelet-rich plasma, they are normal in size.

**Mediterranean macrothrombocytopenia.**   This disorder of moderate thrombocytopenia and large platelets is of uncertain inheritance and appears to be clinically benign.[113]

**Alpha-Storage pool disease (the "gray platelet" syndrome).**   This disorder is characterized by thrombocytopenia with a subpopulation of very large platelets. The biochemical and functional platelet abnormalities in this disease are significant, and thus this entity will be discussed below with the qualitative platelet disorders.

**Miscellaneous disorders of large platelets.**   A series of isolated reports of large platelets in association with thrombocytopenia and variable clinical manifestations exists in the literature.[114,155] The role of steroids and/or splenectomy in managing such patients is not clear.

**Wiskott-Aldrich syndrome.**    This disorder is characterized by small platelets, thrombocytopenia, recurrent infections, and eczema.[116,117] It is inherited as an X chromosome-linked trait and is associated with a wide variety of immunologic disturbances that are thought to account for both the infectious complications and the high frequency of lymphoreticular malignancies. The hemorrhagic manifestations resulting from the thrombocytopenia may be severe and are a common cause of death. The bleeding time is usually more prolonged than one would expect on the basis of the platelet count. This has been ascribed, at least in part, to the small size of the platelets. There is considerable controversy concerning the pathogenesis of both the small platelets and the thrombocytopenia. Autologous platelet survival has been reported to be anywhere from markedly to only minimally shortened, whereas there is general agreement that homologous platelet survival is essentially normal. Since the bone marrow megakaryocyte mass is normal or increased, the variation in autologous platelet survival data leads to two differing conclusions regarding the mechanism of thrombocytopenia, namely, (1) an intrinsic platelet defect resulting in premature removal or (2) ineffective thrombopoiesis. The recently described ability to cure the disorder by bone marrow transplantation does not help to distinguish between these two hypotheses. An autoimmune component may be superimposed on the underlying defect on occasion, and this may account for some of the reported variability. The majority of patients will have dramatic increases in their platelet counts and improvement in hemorrhagic manifestations with splenectomy. In the past, this procedure was considered to be contraindicated because of the very high likelihood of developing severe infections, but the use of pneumococcal vaccine and prophylactic antibiotics has prevented this complication to a large extent. It has also been reported that splenectomy results in a significant increase in platelet size, indicating that the platelets do not leave the bone marrow abnormally small. There is considerable controversy as to whether patients with this disorder have abnormal platelet function. Early studies of aggregation indicated significant abnormalities, but more recent studies performed with the near-normal counts achieved after splenectomy have been normal. Similar controversy surrounds the evaluation of platelet ultrastructure in this disorder, with some studies finding normal morphology and others reporting marked abnormalities in granules and mitochondria. Therapeutically, if bone marrow transplantation is not feasible and hemorrhage is a significant problem, splenectomy with preoperative vaccination against pneumococci and perhaps meningococci, and careful maintenance of prophylactic antibiotic treatment postoperatively should be considered. During acute hemorrhagic episodes, platelet transfusions can be administered.

The platelets of carriers of Wiskott-Aldrich syndrome have been reported to be particularly sensitive to the effects of 2-deoxy-D-glucose, an inhibitor of glycolysis, and a "stress" test based on the inhibition of epinephrine-induced aggregation produced by this agent has been proposed for carrier detection.[118] Incomplete forms of Wiskott-Aldrich syndrome characterized by X chromosome-linked inheritance of thrombocytopenia and small platelets, but without the severe immunologic abnormalities, have been reported. As might be expected, these patients tolerate splenectomy better than those with the complete form of the disease.[119]

## BONE MARROW EXAMINATION

The next step in the orderly evaluation of patients with thrombocytopenia is an examination of the bone marrow to assess specifically the adequacy of the megakaryocytes and the presence of any abnormalities. Although aspirate smears are usually quite adequate for the purpose of estimating megakaryocyte numbers, clot sections prepared from the aspirates are somewhat more reliable since a large number of spicules can be evaluated with less architectural disruption. If there is any possibility that an infiltrative process is present, a bone marrow biopsy should be performed in addition to the aspirate since it will permit the most reliable assessment of architectural disruption. A touch preparation made from a biopsy gives cytologic detail similar to that of an aspirate smear, and when an aspirate cannot be obtained (''dry tap''), it may permit a rapid assessment of the number of megakaryocytes.

## Thrombocytopenia Associated with Decreased Megakaryocytes

If the number of megakaryocytes is markedly decreased or absent, it is reasonable to conclude that the thrombocytopenia results from decreased platelet production due to an abnormality in number and/or differentiation of the stem cells. The absence of megakaryocytes may, in turn, be associated with a hypocellular, normocellular, or hypercellular bone marrow.

If the bone marrow demonstrates diffuse hypoplasia or aplasia, the thrombocytopenia is due to one of the diseases making up the broad category of disorders known as aplastic anemia; a recent classification of this group of diseases is given in Table 4-3.[120,121] A full description of each of these disorders is beyond the scope of this chapter, but a few comments can be made.

**Fanconi's anemia.**    This is a rare familial disorder characterized by pancytopenia, bone marrow hypoplasia, and various malformations, including brown skin pigmentation, hypoplasia of the kidney and spleen, absent or hypoplastic thumbs or radii, microcephaly, and mental and sexual retardation. The disease usually becomes manifest in the first decade of life, and although it often responds to therapy with androgens and corticosteroids, there is gradual deterioration with death due to infection, hemorrhage, or evolution into acute leukemia. It is interesting to note that the platelet count usually is the last hematologic parameter to respond to therapy. Chromosomal abnormalities and the extraordinary ease with which these patients' fibroblasts are transformed by viruses suggest a generalized defect in genetic information.

**Idiopathic, chemical- and drug-associated aplastic anemia.**    These forms of the disease have similarly grave prognoses. Although early studies of androgen therapy were quite encouraging, and follow-up studies do indicate that a fraction of patients who respond to androgens may have a relatively good long-term prognosis,[122] one can identify a group with severe disease (granulocytes less than $0.5 \times 10^9$/liter, platelet counts less than $20 \times 10^9$/liter, and reticulocyte counts less than $20 \times 10^9$/liter) whose median survival will be less than 6 months and whose 2-year mortality will be 80 percent. Patients in whom aplastic anemia follows hepatitis (usually non-A, non-B) also have a very grave prognosis, with a 1-year mortality rate as high as 90 percent. Bone marrow transplantation, despite its cost, morbidity, and mortality, appears to be the treatment of choice for those with a poor prognosis if a suitable donor is available, since a 40–60 percent 1–2-year disease-free survival can be achieved. Results with transplantation appear to be better with young patients and those who have not received transfusions. Although it may be very difficult to withhold all blood products from these patients, it seems prudent to avoid giving blood products obtained from the anticipated donor or other family members. The ability of transplantation to cure this form of the disorder has been taken as strong evidence that the defect is in the stem cell(s) and not in the bone marrow milieu. In contrast, there is at least inferential evidence that the bone marrow milieu may be the major factor responsible for aplastic anemia in pregnancy, since there have been several documented cases in which spontaneous remission followed either induced or natural termination of the pregnancy.[123] Moreover, recurrence of aplasia with subsequent pregnancies has also been reported. Considerable attention has recently been given to autoimmune etiologies of aplastic anemia, another possible milieu defect, but current evidence indicates that only a small minority of patients fit into this category.[120] The role of cytotoxic drugs and antilymphocyte globulin thus remains controversial.[120] *Paroxysmal nocturnal hemoglobinuria,* considered by most investigators to be a stem cell defect, may also present as aplastic anemia.

Both chemotherapy and radiation therapy can produce thrombocytopenia by myelosuppression. Unlike the idiosyncratic response in drug-associated aplastic anemia, these effects are dose related and predictable. Each group of chemotherapeutic agents has different characteristics with regard to the extent and duration of myelosuppression; these are summarized in Table 4-4.[124] It should be cautioned, however, that these drugs are most commonly given in combination, complicating one's ability to predict the severity and duration of thrombocytopenia. As a rule, phase-specific agents (e.g., methotrexate) produce the most rapid suppression and recovery, cycle-nonspecific agents (e.g., nitrosoureas) produce the most delayed and prolonged suppression, and cell cycle (but not phase-specific) agents (e.g., cyclophosphamide) are intermediate with regard to both the onset and the duration of suppression. A notable exception to this rule is the occasional patient who suffers severe, prolonged myelosuppression after busulfan therapy. Vinca alkaloids do not, as a rule, produce thrombocytopenia, and under certain conditions they actually increase the platelet count (see below).

When an infiltrating disease that replaces bone marrow elements produces thrombocytopenia, bone marrow examination will reveal a hyperplastic bone marrow, but with few or no megakaryocytes.[102,115] Although it is easy to conceive of this process as a mechanical "crowding out" of the normal elements, this is likely an oversimplification. Humoral inhibitors of hematopoiesis may be elaborated by these malignant cells, and in some of the leukemias the decrease in megakaryocytes may be related to the stem cell abnormality. This latter possibility is especially likely in patients with myelodysplastic syndromes ("preleukemia," "smouldering leukemia") in which extensive replacement of the marrow is not seen (and megakaryocytes may be present), and yet thrombocytopenia may be severe. Extensive replacement of the marrow by nonhematologic cells of any kind is usually associated with the presence of nucleated red blood cells and immature white blood cells in the peripheral blood, making these findings a very strong indication for bone marrow examination.

A heterogeneous group of disorders is characterized by thrombocytopenia in conjunction with decreased or absent megakaryocytes and an otherwise normocellular bone marrow.

**Cyclic thrombocytopenia.** This rare disorder is characterized by a predictable 20–40-day cycle of thrombocytopenia followed by normal platelet counts.[115] Whereas there have been reports of minor variations in the platelet count during the menstrual cycle (with the nadir usually before the onset of menses), and since many of the affected individuals are young women, an association with hormonal changes has been suggested. However, the thrombocytopenic cycle does not always follow the menstrual cycle, and the disease has been reported in both men and postmenopausal women. Clinically, the thrombocytopenia can be severe enough to cause spontaneous bleeding. The cause of the thrombocytopenia is thought to be a cyclical decrease in production since platelet survival is normal and the number of bone marrow megakaryocytes follows a cycle similar to that of the peripheral blood platelets. No benefit has been obtained from oophorectomy, splenectomy, or corticosteroid therapy.

**Table 4-4**
Myelosuppression Toxicity Chart

| Drug Class | Classification of Degree of Myelosuppression* | Median Time to Nadir | Median Time to Recovery | Characteristics of Myelosuppression | Blood Elements Primarily Affected | Organ System of Dose-Limiting Toxicity |
|---|---|---|---|---|---|---|
| **Alkylating agents** | | | | | | |
| Mechlorethamine (HN$_2$) | | 7–15 | 28 | Intermediate, nadir, and recovery | Pancytopenia RBC† WBC″ Platelets | BM‡ |
| Mephalan (Alkeran) | I | 10–12 | 42–50 | | | |
| Busulfan (Myleran) | | 11–30 | 24–54 | Uncharacteristically prolonged and delayed nadir and recovery | | |
| Chlorambucil (Leukeran) | | 14–28 | 28–42 | | | |
| Cyclophosphamide (Cytoxan) | II | 8–14 | 18–25 | | (Primarily WBC) | (Rarely bladder) |
| **Nitrosoureas** | | | | | | |
| Carmustine (BCNU) | I | 26–30 | 35–49 | Delayed onset and prolonged recovery (cumulative toxicity) | Leukopenia and thrombocytopenia (clinically severe anemia after 6 months of continuous therapy) | BM |
| Lomustine (CCNU) | | 40–50 | 60 | | | |
| Semustine (meCCNU) | | 28–63 | 82–89 | | | |
| **Antimetabolites** | | | | | | |
| Cytarabine (ARA-C) | I | 12–14 | 22–24 | (Intermediate) | Primarily thrombocytopenia and leukopenia | BM |
| Fluorouracil (5-FU) | | 7–14 | 16–24 | | | |
| Methotrexate (MTX) | II | 7–14 | 14–21 | Relatively short onset (nadir) and recovery | | |
| Mercaptopurine (GMP) | | 7–14 | 14–21 | | | |
| Hydroxyurea (Hydrea) | II | 18–30 | 21–35 | (Intermediate-long) | Leukopenia, thrombocytopenia | Gastrointestinal and BM |
| 5-Azacytidine | | | | | | |

| | | | | | | |
|---|---|---|---|---|---|---|
| Podophyllotoxins | | | | | | |
| VM-26 | I | 3–14 | 28 | Relatively short onset, nadir, and recovery | Leukopenia | BM |
| Etoposide (VP-16) | I | 16 | 20–22 | | Leukopenia, thrombocytopenia | |
| Steroids¶ | | | | | | |
| Androgens¶ | | — | — | None | None | Excessive endocrine changes |
| Estrogens¶ | | — | — | | | |
| Corticosteroids¶ (prednisone)¶ | IV | — | — | | | |
| Vinca Alkaloids | | | | | | |
| Vincristine (VCR)¶ | III | 4–5 | 7 | Rapid | — | Central and peripheral nervous systems |
| Velban (Vlb) | I | 5–9 | 14–21 | Relatively rapid | Leukopenia | BM |
| Antibiotics | | | | | | |
| Bleomycin¶ | III | — | — | — | None | Pulmonary |
| Mitomycin | II | 28–42 | 42–56 | Delayed, prolonged | Pancytopenia | Renal |
| Chromomycin A$_2$ | III | — | — | Probably intermediate | Leukopenia and thrombocytopenia (esp.) | Renal, hepatic |
| Mithramycin | III | 14 | 21–28 | Intermediate | Thrombocytopenia (esp.) | Hepatic |
| Anthracyclines | | | | | | |
| Rubidazone | II | 5–20 | — | Intermediate | Thrombocytopenia, leukopenia | Cardiac |
| Actinomycin | II | 14–21 | 22–25 | Intermediate | Thrombocytopenia, leukopenia | Gastrointestinal |
| Doxorubicin (Adriamycin) | II | 10–14 | 21–24 | Intermediate | Leukopenia | Cardiac |

*(continued)*

Table 4-4 (continued)

| Drug Class | Classification of Degree of Myelosuppression* | Median Time to Nadir | Median Time to Recovery | Characteristics of Myelosuppression | Blood Elements Primarily Affected | Organ System of Dose-Limiting Toxicity |
|---|---|---|---|---|---|---|
| Others |  |  |  |  |  |  |
| Procarbazine** | II | 25–36 | 36–50 | Intermediate | Leukopenia and thrombocytopenia (both) | BM |
| Dacarbazine (DTIC) | II | 21–28 | 28–35 |  |  | Gastrointestinal |
| Asparaginase¶ | III–IV | — | — |  | Leukopenia, thrombocytopenia | Immunologic, hepatic |
| Cisplatin | III | 14 | 21 | Intermediate | Pancytopenia | Renal |
| Razoxane (ICRF-159) | I | 11–16 | 19–24 | Intermediate | Leukopenia, thrombocytopenia | BM |

From Dorr RT, Fritz WL: Cancer Chemotherapy Handbook. New York, Elsevier/North-Holland, 1980 p. 104–106. With permission.

*I, primarily myelosuppressive; II, myelosuppressive but with other serious (dose-limiting) toxicities; III, myelosuppression not dose-limiting, toxicity of usual schedules; IV, myelosuppression rarely if ever present.

†Red blood cells.

‡Bone marrow.

″White blood cells.

¶Usually nonmyelosuppressive.

**Based on a 14-day course.

**Congenital amegakaryocytosis (thrombocytopenia with absent radii, TAR syndrome).**
This autosomal recessive disorder is characterized by thrombocytopenic hemorrhage beginning almost immediately after birth, an isolated decrease or absence of bone marrow megakaryocytes, and structural abnormalities of the skeleton, kidneys, and heart, the most consistent of which is an absence of radii in the arms.[102,115,125,126] Platelet survival is not significantly shortened. In addition to the thrombocytopenia, there may be a platelet function defect of the storage-pool deficiency type (see below). Clinically, this often a severe disorder, with more than one-third of the patients in one series dying in infancy. For those surviving infancy, the prognosis is considerably better, with hemorrhagic symptoms improving despite persistent thrombocytopenia. Although platelet transfusions are of clear short-term benefit, the results with splenectomy and corticosteroid therapy have been variable. It has recently been suggested that the tendency toward gastrointestinal hemorrhage in this syndrome is exacerbated in many cases by the presence of an allergy to cow's milk and that withdrawal of cow's milk results in clinical improvement, perhaps by decreasing the level of circulating immune complexes that can interfere with platelet function.[126]

**Alcohol-induced thrombocytopenia.**   This syndrome occurs in some chronic alcoholics during an acute period of excessive drinking and is characterized by the presence of isolated, sometimes severe, thrombocytopenia. When the patients are withdrawn from alcohol and placed on a normal diet, there is usually a rapid increase in the platelet count over the course of 1–2 weeks, culminating in the platelet count's "overshooting" to abnormally high levels prior to returning to normal values.[115] Bone marrow megakaryocytes tend to reflect the peripheral platelet counts, with marked decreases initially and supranormal levels with recovery and overshoot. When thrombocytopenia is present at a time when the bone marrow megakaryocytes are not severely depressed, ineffective thrombopoiesis may contribute to the thrombocytopenia. It is presumed that in certain susceptible individuals alcohol is toxic to the megakaryocytes, but the speed with which thrombocytopenia was documented to recur after reinstitution of alcohol in at least one study (4–6 hours) raises the possibility of a direct effect on circulating platelets.

**Thiazide diuretics and diethylstilbestrol-associated thrombocytopenia.[115]**   There is circumstantial evidence that these two drugs may produce thrombocytopenia by affecting the megakaryocytes since some reports have documented decreased megakaryocytes in the bone marrow, and the length of time for onset and recovery appear to follow the appropriate kinetics. It is especially intersting to note the reports of thrombocytopenia in a few newborns delivered of mothers who had ingested thiazide diuretics near delivery; bone marrow examination in these children usually showed reduced or absent megakaryocytes.

**The syndrome of thrombocytopenia with decreased megakaryocytes.**   Recently, a syndrome of thrombocytopenia with an isolated decrease in bone marrow megakaryocytes was described in 7 patients.[127] Platelet survival and size were normal. Of this group, two patients became aplastic, 1 developed "preleukemia," and the remaining 4 continued to have low platelet counts but were clinically stable. The authors concluded that this entity is more common than has heretofore been appreciated.

## Platelet Transfusion Therapy

Since the disorders enumerated above in the category of thrombocytopenia with reduced megakaryocytes are those most likely to require platelet transfusion therapy, a brief discussion of the principles and practice of this therapy will follow.[128–130] Platelets are harvested from normal donors either by a 2-step differential centrifugation process wherein approximately 85 percent of the platelets from 1 unit (approximately 500 ml) of a whole blood donation are concentrated into a small volume of plasma, or by the newer techniques in which centrifugation takes place in a spinning bowl, the platelets are collected from the stream of blood, and the remaining plasma and erythrocytes are returned to the donor. With the latter technique, one can collect 4–6 times as many platelets from a single donor as compared with the centrifugation of a single unit. Once collected, the platelet concentrates from single-unit blood donations can routinely be kept for up to three days at room temperature and still produce good clinical results. With the improved maintenance of pH attained with newer plastic containers, it appears that a five day shelf life can be attained.[131]

Based on the fact that the splenic pool contains 35 percent of the platelet mass and the known kinetics of autologous platelets, one would predict that a single unit (containing $5{-}10 \times 10^{10}$ platelets) should raise the platelet count of a 70-kg recipient by approximately $10,000/\mu$l immediately after transfusion

$$\left[ \frac{(7.5 \times 10^{10} \text{ platelets}) \, (0.65 \text{ recovery in circulation})}{(70 \text{ kg}) \, (72 \text{ ml blood volume/kg body weight})} \right]$$

and that one-half of these platelets should still be circulating after 4 days. However, these results are rarely achieved in clinical practice due to a combination of factors, including splenomegaly (primarily affecting recovery), fever, infection, diffuse intravascular coagulation, or bleeding (all primarily affecting survival) that are often present in patients requiring platelet transfusions. Both the recovery and survival of homologous platelets are thus reduced in these patients, even under relatively favorable conditions (in one study, mean recovery was 56 percent instead of 65 percent, and mean survival was 5.2 days instead of 9.6 days).[129] As a result, increments of greater than 5000 platelets/$\mu$l per unit of platelet concentrate infused are considered acceptable, and transfusions are usually required at least twice each week. From a practical standpoint, obtaining platelet counts 1 hour after the transfusion and 12–24 hours thereafter will permit determination of both recovery and survival in the patient so that subsequent needs can be estimated.

The single most important problem in the management of patients requiring long-term platelet support is the development of alloantibodies that make the patient refractory to additional platelet transfusions. The length of time and the number of units transfused before this happens are quite variable, but in aplastic anemia it can be expected to occur anywhere from 2 weeks to 6 months, with an average of 6 weeks. Patients with leukemia tend to become refractory more slowly, presumably as a result of the immunosuppression produced by the leukemia itself. In addition, since the length of time during which leukemic patients are thrombocytopenic is usually much shorter than that of patients with aplastic anemia, this problem is less frequent. There is abundant evidence that HLA-matched sibling platelets survive better than random-donor platelets in patients who become alloimmunized. Moreover, HLA-matched platelets from unrelated donors and platelets that are selectively "mismatched" for relatively nonimmunogenic HLA determinants may be quite effective.[132] This last observation is especially important since it indicates that one can probably select 10 appropriately matched or acceptably mismatched random donors for any new patient if one has a pool of HLA-typed donors of just a few thousand; this can be compared with the need for a pool of approximately 50,000 HLA-typed donors if perfect HLA matching were required. Given the remarkable success of HLA matching in extending the usefulness of platelet transfusion support, one might be tempted to use HLA-matched platelets exclusively. Several facts indicate that this approach is undesirable: (1) the expense and inconvenience are much greater in obtaining matched platelets than random donor platelets; (2) patients will usually respond well to random donor platelets and, even when they do become refractory, will probably respond well to matched platelets; (3) patients can eventually become sensitized even to matched platelets; and (4) if transplantation is considered, it is probably unwise to expose the patient to minor antigens found on the cells of family members for fear of sensitization.

The most controversial aspect of platelet transfusion therapy deals with whether platelets should be given prophylactically or only when bleeding is present. In acute leukemia or other malignancies treated with large doses of myelosuppressive drugs, most clinicians will give prophylactic transfusions to maintain the platelet count above 20,000/$\mu$l, since this is approximately the level below which serious spontaneous hemorrhage is thought to occur. This approach has been criticized recently for the following reasons: (1) the 20,000 platelets/$\mu$l criterion is based on incomplete data, and other evidence seems to support a count of 5000–10,000/$\mu$l as the cutoff for the spontaneous development of severe hemorrhage;[129] (2) other factors, such as the presence of infection, fever, diffuse intravascular coagulation, fibrinolysis, the underlying disease itself (e.g., blast crisis with leukostasis), and drugs (in particular, the semisynthetic penicillins that interfere with platelet function) are probably more important in determining the risk of hemorrhage than the platelet count alone; (3) clinical trials in which platelets were withheld until significant bleeding supervened did not result in excessive mortality or obvious morbidity and yet achieved a 50 percent reduction in the number of units of platelets transfused; and (4) patients on prophylactic regimens may become refractory to transfusions and fail to have their bleeding controlled later in their course. A crucial concern facing one who might opt to withhold platelets until bleeding occurs is the speed and certainty with which one can expect to obtain platelets. Until additional data become available, the author's preference is to continue using prophylactic transfusions during ablative chemotherapy when platelet concentrates are readily available, especially if the clinical setting puts the patient at high risk of bleeding. The author believes that withholding transfusions until clinical hemorrhage is apparent is the appropriate strategy for patients with aplastic anemia, especially if transplantation is contemplated, unless there is reason to believe that support may be needed only for a short period of time, as with the aplastic anemia of pregnancy.[123]

## Thrombocytopenia Associated with Normal or Increased Megakaryocytes

When the bone marrow of a thrombocytopenic patient contains a normal or increased number of megakaryocytes, it can be concluded that there is either an increased removal of platelets from the circulation or ineffective thrombopoiesis (that is, megakaryocytes do not mature and/or release platelets properly). Two major mechanisms of increased removal are recognized: (1) immunologic, in which platelets coated with immunoglobulins are prematurely removed by phagocytic cells of the reticuloendothelial system, and (2) increased utilization, in which the platelets either (a) adhere to and aggregate on abnormal or artificial surfaces or (b) undergo activation as a result of excessive thrombin generation or the presence of other agonists.

Immunologic causes for premature removal include (1) autoimmune or immune-complex disorders (which are not easily separated at present), and (2) alloimmune disorders. The major diseases in each category are indicated in Table 4-3.

**Acute idiopathic thrombocytopenic purpura (ITP).**[126,133-135]   This is primarily a disease of early childhood, affecting both sexes equally, and characterized by the abrupt onset of dependent and oral mucosal petechiae, ecchymoses, and, if severe, frank hemorrhage, in association with marked thrombocytopenia (usually less than 20,000 platelets/μl). The majority of patients will give a history of a viral infection several weeks before the onset of symptoms, most commonly a nondescript upper respiratory tract infection, but with the childhood exanthematous viral infections, infectious mononucleosis, mumps, and vaccination also reported. Perhaps as a result of this association, the disorder follows a seasonal pattern, with a peak in the winter and spring months. Clinical manifestations can be severe, and although mortality from central nervous system bleeding is quite uncommon (approximately 1 percent), hematuria and gastrointestinal hemorrhage are found in about 5–10 percent of cases.

The bone marrow virtually always contains increased numbers of large megakaryocytes whose morphology is characterized by a lack of both cytoplasmic granularity and platelet budding. These changes are thought to be nonspecific reflections of the increased platelet turnover found in this and related disorders, although they may be the result of antiplatelet antibodies that also react with megakaryocytes (see below). In addition to the thrombocytopenia, anemia due to blood loss, mild eosinophilia, and atypical lymphocytosis may be observed. The platelets may appear large on smear, but this has not been an invariable feature. The vast majority of patients will have an increased number of IgG molecules detectable on their platelets, using any one of the several tests currently available,[135a] and the extent of this increase will vary inversely with the platelet count. In contrast, fewer patients will have a positive test when their serum is incubated with normal platelets and the amount of platelet-associated IgG is quantified; moreover the results of this test do not correlate well with the platelet count. Although rarely needed for diagnosis, platelet survival studies show a dramatic decrease in survival, along with the frequent finding of platelet sequestration in the spleen.

The major considerations in the differential diagnosis of this disorder include the hemolytic-uremic syndrome, leukemia, drug-induced thrombocytopenia, sepsis, and hereditary thrombocytopenia. All but the last diagnosis should be easily differentiated on the basis of the clinical presentation, routine laboratory studies, and a bone marrow examination; hereditary thrombocytopenia may be more difficult to differentiate since it is characterized by thrombocytopenia and normal megakaryocytes.[102] Platelet counts on family members and a platelet survival study (short in ITP, normal in hereditary thrombocytopenia) may be required to distinguish between these disorders. One's index of suspicion of hereditary thrombocytopenia should be raised in those patients who do not remit spontaneously and who fail to respond to conventional therapy.

The pathophysiology of acute ITP is still uncertain. It is well established that (1) platelets have receptors for a site(s) on the Fc fragment of IgG molecules that is exposed when the latter enter into immune complexes, and (2) there is a close relationship between viral infections and the onset of this disease. The most commonly accepted hypothesis therefore is that children with this disorder make antibodies against a viral product that then results in the formation of an immune complex that attaches to platelets and results in premature platelet removal. In fact, circulating immune complexes have been detected in patients with acute ITP, but it is far from clear whether these are the cause or the result of the disorder since platelet-derived antigens could complex with antiplatelet antibodies. Alternatively, some investigators believe that platelets may play an important role in clearing immune complexes from the circulation; thus, thrombocytopenia of any cause may result in increases in circulating immune complexes.[136] It must be emphasized that none

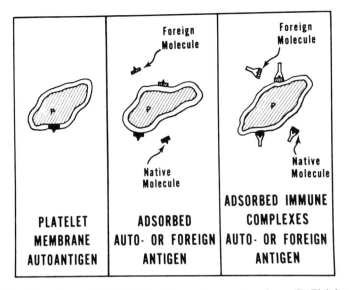

**Fig. 4-13.** Possible antigens in ITP. (A) Platelet membrane autoantigen. (B) Tightly adherent humoral molecule, either native or foreign. (C) Adsorbed immune complexes formed from a circulating native or foreign molecule and an antibody against this molecule. From McMillan R, The pathogenesis of immune thrombocytopenia. CRC Crit Rev Clin Lab Sci 8:303, 1977, p. 326. With permission.

of the currently employed assays for platelet-associated IgG or antiplatelet antibodies differentiate between immune complexes or antibodies directed against intrinsic or adsorbed platelet antigens (Fig. 4-13). Other pathophysiologic features of ITP will be discussed below in the section on chronic ITP.

The prognosis of acute ITP is excellent, with about 55 percent of patients achieving normal platelet counts within 4 weeks and about 85 percent recovering within 4 months. The high spontaneous remission rate has made it very difficult to assess the efficacy of different therapies, and some authorities believe that no therapy is required.[126,133,137] There is general agreement that the risk of serious hemorrhage is greatest during the first two weeks and that activity should be severely restricted during that time. The efficacy of corticosteroid therapy is unclear, with variable results reported as to the time required to achieve recovery. It has been suggested that corticosteroid therapy may even prolong the period of thrombocytopenia.[126,133-135,137] Regardless of their effect on the platelet count, some authorities recommend the use of corticosteroids to improve what has been called "capillary integrity" since it has been observed that hemorrhagic manifestations and the bleeding time often decrease before the platelet count increases in patients treated with these agents. A theoretical basis for such an effect comes from the evidence that corticosteroids inhibit $PGI_2$ synthesis by the endothelium by preventing the release of arachidonic acid from phospholipids.[138] This would result in less inhibition of platelet function and less vasodilatation, thus favoring improved hemostasis.[138] Given the minimal risk of short-term corticosteroid therapy, the author thinks that it is reasonable to initiate therapy in patients with significant hemorrhagic manifestations of acute ITP at a dose of about 2 mg/kg body weight/day (but not to exceed 80–100 mg/day) for several weeks, although one could justify withholding all therapy by reference to some reports in the literature. A detailed analysis of the pros and cons of corticosteroid therapy has recently been published.[126] With so many patients likely to have spontaneous remissions, rapid withdrawal of cortico-

**Table 4-5**

Quantitation of Platelet-Associated IgG (PAIgG) in Control Subjects and Patients with Acute and Chronic Immune Thrombocytopenic Purpura

| Assay | Controls | | Patients | | |
|---|---|---|---|---|---|
| | No. Studied | PAIgG* $\mu g/10^9$ platelets | No. Studied | PAIgG* $\mu g/10^9$ platelets | Positive Results(%) |
| Complement-lysis inhibition | | | | | |
| Dixon et al, 1975 | 16 | 300 ± 50 | 17 | 500 – 3400 | 100 |
| Hegde et al, 1977 | 17 | 4.5 (1.5–7.0) | 29 | 7–72 | 96 |
| Hauch and Rosse, 1977 | 21 | 4.1 ± 2.9 | 16 | 77.5 ± 24.1 | 88 |
| Kelton et al, 1979, 1980 | 30 | 4.7 ± 3.1 | 32 | 41.6 ± 32 | 91 |
| | 39 | 2.2 ± 0.1 | 37 | 20.0 ± 25 | 91 |
| Kernoff et al, 1980 | 48 | 1.8 – 14.8 | 17 | 21 – 213 | 100 |
| Fab-anti-Fab | | | | | |
| Luiken et al, 1977 | 70 | 1.2 ± 0.4 | 31 | 4.8 ± 3.8 | 94 |
| Radioactive Coombs' test | | | | | |
| Cines and Schreiber, 1979 | 20 | 2.4 ± 2.5 | 50 | 5 – 48 | 90 |
| Enzyme-linked anti-IgG | | | | | |
| Nel and Stevens, 1980 | 25 | 8.4 ± 3.5 | 9 | 100 – 405 | 78 |
| Leporrier et al, 1979 | 10 | 0.06 ± 0.02 | 11 | 0.2 – 1.7 | 100 |
| Staphylococcal Protein A | | | | | |
| Hymes et al, 1979 | 11 | 11.4 ± 7.4 | 35 | 150 ± 145 | 92 |
| Immunodiffusion | | | | | |
| Morse et al, 1981 | 20 | 3.8 ± 1.9 | 14 | 8.4 – 54.5 | 100 |

Adapted from McMillan R: Chronic idiopathic thrombocytopenic purpura. N Engl J Med 304:1135–1147, 1981. With permission.

*Data are reported as the mean ± S D or as the mean and range.

steroids is probably justified in those patients having a brisk response in order to avoid the more severe morbidity of long-term therapy in growing children. Recent studies suggest that high doses of the new preparations of gamma globulin that are suitable for intravenous administration may be efficacious in speeding recovery and avoiding splenectomy.[138a] Anecdotal evidence indicates that bleeding may be more severe in patients whose hemoglobin levels have dropped below 9 g/dl; hence, transfusion to maintain a higher level may be useful.[126] This interesting observation reinforces the importance of erythrocytes in facilitating the platelet's hemostatic function, perhaps on the basis of the rheologic factors discussed previously. Patients who develop evidence of life-threatening hemorrhage, in particular intracranial hemorrhage, should be treated immediately with platelet transfusions even if a significant increase in the circulating blood count is not achieved. In addition, some authorities recommend emergency splenectomy as the most rapid way of increasing the platelet count. One might also consider plasmapheresis in this setting, although there has not yet been a great deal of experience with this technique in acute ITP. Elective splenectomy should also be considered in patients who do not respond adequately to corticosteroids, who require toxic doses of corticosteroids for more than 6 months to maintain hemostasis, or who have purpura that is sufficiently severe to require curtailment of normal activities for more than one year.[126,133 135] Pneumococcal and perhaps meningococcal vaccines should probably be administered several weeks before elective splenectomies in all of these patients, and prolonged prophylactic antibiotic therapy should be considered postsplenectomy, especially in the younger age groups. It is important to emphasize that the platelet count alone should not be relied upon in deciding therapy since it is clear that some patients will be asymptomatic despite considerable thrombocytopenia.

**Chronic idiopathic thrombocytopenia purpura (ITP).** This disorder is characterized by the insidious onset of mucocutaneous hemorrhage—in particular, dependent and oral mucosal petechiae, spontaneous ecchymoses, epistaxis, and menorrhagia.[134,135,139] In the most severe cases, gastrointestinal, retinal, conjunctival, and central nervous system bleeding can occur. This disorder differs from acute ITP in 4 major ways: (1) it occurs primarily in adults aged 20–50 instead of children, (2) a history of an antecedent viral infection is very rare, (3) the female:male ratio is about 4:1 instead of 1:1, and (4) the disorder usually lasts for years, with thrombocytopenia persisting even during periods of clinical remission. An intermittent form of idiopathic thrombocytopenia is also recognized in which patients have discrete episodes of thrombocytopenia alternating with intervals of normal platelet counts and platelet survival; the episodes may be separated by many years.

The pathogenesis of chronic ITP has been the subject of intensive study ever since the pioneering observation by Harrington et al. that the plasma of patients with the disorder produced thrombocytopenia when infused into normal individuals.[139] Subsequent studies showed that platelets have increased amounts of IgG on their surface (Table 4-5) and that this results in a dramatic reduction in platelet survival (to as low as 20 minutes, with a mean of about 12 hours) as the antibody-coated platelets are prematurely and selectively removed by the phagocytic cells of the reticuloendothelial system. In those patients whose platelets have only small amounts of IgG on their surface, the major site of removal is likely to be the spleen since (1) the phagocytic cells in that organ recognize the Fc portion of the IgG molecule, (2) the circulation is slow, (3) the platelet pool is large, and (4) local (that is, intrasplenic) antibody production is high. The liver (which contains cells with receptors for IgM and the third component of the complement, C3) probably plays a more important role in platelet removal in patients who have surface-bound IgM in addition to IgG (estimated as 22 percent in one study), IgM only (about 5 percent), very high concentration of IgG, or C3 in addition to IgG.[139,140] The bone marrow may also contribute significantly to the removal process under the latter conditions.

Thrombokinetic studies indicate that the bone marrow can increase its effective production of platelets in response to decreased survival by up to 5–8 times normal, but with most chronic ITP patients having values between 2.5 and 5 times normal. Even though the antibodies in chronic ITP react with megakaryocytes as well as platelets, the weight of current evidence indicates that the bone marrow megakaryocyte mass increases in proportion to the increase in effective platelet production, indicating that ineffective thrombopoiesis probably does not make a significant contribution to the thrombocytopenia. Morphologic examination of the bone marrow reveals an increase in both the number and size of the megakaryocytes.

The platelet antigen(s) against which the antibodies are made in chronic ITP remains largely unknown. It is most likely that the antibodies are against a component(s) present on almost all normal platelets, in which case the disorder would be appropriately termed autoimmune. The possibility remains, however, that a foreign antigen(s) is tightly bound to the platelet, in which case the criteria for true autoimmunity would not be met. There is some preliminary evidence that the antibodies from different patients may be recognizing several different antigens, some of which are probably on the GPIIb–III complex.[141,141a,b] The limited amount of information available indicates that the immune response is usually polyclonal and that multiple IgG subclasses are present on the platelet surface. Several lines of evidence indicate that immune complexes are probably not responsible for this disorder, the most convincing of which are that (1) purified IgG alone is capable of reacting with platelets; (2) the responsible agent can cross the placenta; and (3) in the few cases tested thus far, F(ab)$_2$' fragments, devoid of the Fc portion of the IgG molecule, can bind to platelets.[135,139] The role, if any, for cell-mediated immunity in the pathogenesis of chronic ITP remains controversial. HLA typing has revealed equivocal results with the HLA-A, -B, and -C antigens. An increase in the HLA-D locus antigen, DRw2, has been reported; this is of special interest since this same antigen is said to be more common among patients with systemic lupus erythematosus[135] (see the section on disease-associated ITP below). Additional evidence supporting a link between chronic ITP and the collagen-vascular disorders systemic lupus erythematosus and rheumatoid arthritis is the high frequency of these disorders in the relatives of patients with chronic ITP.

The spleen plays a central role in the pathophysiology of chronic ITP since it is both a major source of antibody production and the major site of platelet removal. McMillan has proposed a scheme in which the spleen, by virtue of its role as the most important immunologic monitor of the intravascular space, may be the initial site of antibody production, with other lymphoid organs developing this capability only after memory cells leave the spleen to populate them.[139] If this is true, this model would furnish a justification for early splenectomy in an attempt to prevent the "metastasis" of the immune response to organs that cannot be surgically removed.

The diagnosis of chronic ITP is usually made quite easily when the typical clinical presentation is accompanied by thrombocytopenia (in the absence of other peripheral blood abnormalities) and increased numbers and size of bone marrow megakaryocytes. Platelets will usually appear somewhat large on smear. Abnormalities on physical examination are confined to those secondary to the thrombocytopenia; splenomegaly, in particular, occurs in no more than 3 percent of cases. It is vital that drug-induced thrombocytopenia be eliminated by the history and that consideration be given to the other disorders that may present with immune-induced thrombocytopenia, including systemic lupus erythematosus, lymphoma, sepsis, and the recently described acquired immunodeficiency syndrome.[135,139,141c] The diagnosis of immune-mediated thrombocytopenia can be confirmed by direct assay of platelet-associated IgG by any one of the many techniques available[139,141d] (Table 4-5). There is a reasonably good correlation between the amount of platelet-associated IgG and both platelet survival and platelet count; preliminary reports suggest that there may even be a correlation with response to therapy. Assays to detect antiplatelet antibodies in the patient's serum can also be performed. This test, however, is less sensitive, being positive in barely more than 50 percent of cases, and does not correlate well with the patient's clinical status. A recent hypothesis challenges the idea that all of the platelet-associated IgG is specifically directed at the platelet, raising the possibility that some may be nonspecifically associated with the platelet surface or with platelet fragments.[142,142a] Some techniques for measuring platelet-associated IgG, such as fluorescent anti-IgG antibody used in conjunction with a fluorescent cell analyzer, should be able to avoid interference from fragments. However, if "stress" platelets produced by means other than immunologic destruction do have increased levels of IgG, the interpretation of the specificity of these tests will require reassessment.

Perhaps the most important principle in the management of patients with chronic ITP is that the absolute platelet count cannot be relied upon as the sole criterion for determining whether treatment has succeeded or failed. Some patients will remain quite asymptomatic with counts considerably below 50,000/$\mu$l, whereas others may have bleeding manifestations at counts greater than 75,000/$\mu$l. There appear to be 2 separate factors, working in opposite directions, which may help to explain this paradox: (1) the increased functional capacity of large stress platelets and (2) the potential qualitative platelet abnormalities induced by the antiplatelet antibody. Early studies based on clinical observations and bleeding time tests indicated that both clinical hemostasis and the length of the bleeding time were much better in patients with chronic ITP than in patients whose platelet counts were reduced to the same extent as a result of decreased platelet production.[143] It was postulated that the large platelets produced as a result of the stress of thrombopoiesis in ITP, coupled with the skewing of the platelet population toward younger, more metabolically active platelets, resulted in this clinical benefit. In fact, the author believes that this observation remains accurate for the majority of patients. More recently, however, a storage pool disease-like syndrome has been reported in association with increased platelet-associated IgG by several investigators.[144] In addition, since in vitro studies indicate that the plasma of some patients with chronic ITP can inhibit normal platelet function, increasing concern about abnormal platelet function in these patients has been expressed. Finally, an abnormality in arachidonic acid metabolism has been reported in several patients with chronic ITP whose bleeding times were prolonged.[145] With the possibility that either hypo- or hyperfunctional platelets are present in patients with chronic ITP, it is vital that the individual patient's symptoms be carefully monitored. It may, however, be useful to perform a bleeding time when there is doubt. The author finds a normal bleeding time comforting after deciding, from clinical observations, that a count in the thrombocytopenic range is clinically acceptable and thus does not require an alteration in therapy.

If the patient presents with life-threatening hemorrhage, platelet transfusions should be administered and emergency splenectomy and/or plasmapheresis considered. In patients who are not in immediate jeopardy, prednisone at a dose of 1 mg/kg/day is considered the treatment of choice. One can expect improvement within the first week in most patients, and fully one-third will achieve normal counts. However, complete remissions (that is, normal counts while off corticosteroids) are unusual, probably occurring in considerably less than 25 percent of the patients.[135,139] Studies of thrombokinetics and platelet-associated IgG indicate that although corticosteroids initially act to decrease removal of platelets by the spleen, they may also interfere with the binding of antibody to the platelet surface and may eventually cause a decrease in antibody production (either directly or indirectly). In those patients who fail to respond to corticosteroids or who require toxic doses to maintain hemostasis, splenectomy is indicated. As noted previously, when practical pneumococcal and perhaps meningococcal vaccines should probably be adminsitered before splenectomy, and consideration should be given to the use of prophylactic antibiotics postsplenectomy. Between 50 and 80 percent of patients will have a significant postsplenectomy increase in platelet count, with a rapid increase in platelet survival and a similarly rapid decrease in platelet-associated IgG.[135,139] Although a good initial response to corticosteroids and documentation of abnormal sequestration of platelets in the spleen are said to correlate with a good response to splenectomy, there is currently no totally accurate test to predict the response. As a result, the author believes that patients should not be denied splenectomy on the basis of their response to corticosteroids or any of the scans or sequestration studies currently available. The overwhelming clinical experience is that patients tolerate splenectomy remarkably well despite severe thrombocytopenia. The platelet count in the immediate postoperative period is said to be a good indicator of the eventual response, with those having counts in excess of 500,000/μl having a favorable prognosis. Patients who either have an inadequate response to splenectomy or who relapse thereafter should be treated with corticosteroids again. If a response is obtained, it is desirable to attempt to control the patient's disease with alternate-day therapy in an attempt to minimize the complications of therapy. If the patient fails to respond to corticosteroids, the guidelines for choosing additional therapy become much more problematic. Some consideration can be given to the unlikely possibility that residual splenic tissue is still present, and a search for Howell-Jolly bodies in the peripheral smear should suffice to exclude it. The vinca alkaloids have been reported to be of benefit in some patients. Therapy is usually given as intravenous injections of vincristine (0.025 mg/kg, with an upper limit of 2 mg) or vinblastine (0.125 mg/kg, with an upper limit of 10 mg). Although relatively long-term responses have been reported, they are not common. Most patients will thus require frequent therapy (every 1–3 weeks), resulting in significant neurotoxicity with vincristine and the potential for leukopenia with vinblastine.[135,139] In an attempt to direct the alkaloid to the macrophage, vinblastine-loaded platelets have been infused intravenously. Although considerable success was reported in one series, subsequent series have reported a very low percentage of remissions.[146] Cyclophosphamide at a dose of 2–3 mg/kg/day or 300–600 mg/m² of body surface area every three weeks has been reported to induce remissions in 30–40 percent of refractory patients, but the maximum effect usually requires several months of therapy.[135,139] This drug may have serious side effects (including myelosuppression, hemorrhagic cystitis, and alopecia) as well as the potential to induce malignancies.

Azathioprine in daily doses of 1–3 mg/kg has been used with some success, but maximal responses are not achieved for several months and complete remissions are rare.[139] The combination of Cytoxan with vincristine and prednisone, as used in lymphoma protocols (cyclophosphamide 400 mg/m² orally on days 1–5; vincristine, 1 mg/m² intravenously on day 1; prednisone, 40 mg/m² orally on days 1–5; therapy to be repeated every 28 days for up to 6 cycles), has also achieved remissions in some patients, but its toxicity dictates that it be reserved for those cases refractory to all other measures.[139] Plasmapheresis may be considered in the control of acute hemorrhage or as a temporary measure to improve the platelet count when therapy has been initiated with one of the drugs which requires a longer period of time to act.[135,139] Other experimental therapies that have recently been reported include intravenous gamma globulin,[146a,b] colchicine,[146c] and danazol.[146d] It is too early to define each of their precise roles in the management of the disease.

As a final consideration, it is useful to consider the long-term fate of patients with chronic ITP who either fail with splenectomy or who relapse after the operation. A recent study identified 15 such patients.[147] In eight of them, hemostatically adequate platelet counts were eventually achieved either without additional therapy or, in those who did receive additional therapy, after subsequent withdrawal from all medication; the latter clinical remissions were all maintained for a minimum of three years. Of the 15 patients, 3 had complete responses to immunosuppressive therapy, 1 had a partial response and required continued therapy, and 3 were lost to followup. The authors emphasized the generally benign course of chronic ITP in those patients who undergo splenectomy, and thus cautioned against the indiscriminate use of toxic immunosuppressive therapy.

**Neonatal ITP.**    This is the disorder suffered by the fetuses and newborn children of mothers with chronic ITP as a result of the transplacental passage of antiplatelet IgG.[125,134,148] Clinically, the thrombocytopenia may be present at birth or may become apparent within several hours. Mucocutaneous hemorrhage predominates, and cephalohematomas have been reported. Intracranial hemorrhage, which probably occurs in less than 10 percent of cases, may be difficult to diagnose in the newborn and can result in permanent neurologic sequelae or death. Platelet counts should be monitored frequently during the first few days of life. If the count falls below 75,000/$\mu$l or if it is higher but dropping precipitously, corticosteroids (1–2 mg/kg/day of prednisone or an equivalent intravenous preparation) should be administered. The response is usually good, and the drug can be tapered quite rapidly if the count remains acceptable. Since no additional antibody enters the patient's circulation after delivery, recovery follows clearance of the IgG from the circulation, with the platelet counts rising to normal levels within 3–4 weeks postpartum in the majority of cases; occasionally, recovery may take considerably longer. If clinical hemorrhage is severe or if the count drops below 20,000–40,000/$\mu$l, platelet concentrates (2 units initially, repeated in 6–8 hours if necessary) are recommended by several authorities. If all else fails, exchange transfusion has a good theoretical justification and should probably be attempted.

There is considerable controversy concerning the use of corticosteroids and the optimal method of fetal delivery for pregnant patients with chronic ITP. In large part, this results from the difficulty of predicting whether the fetus of an affected mother will also be affected and, if so, to what extent. The maternal platelet count is not a good predictor of the newborn's count, especially if the mother has previously undergone splenectomy. A recent report suggests that the antiplatelet antibody level in maternal serum may be the best predictor of fetal platelet counts, but this hypothesis will require confirmation.[149] This uncertainty, and the fear of inducing head trauma during vaginal delivery, have led some authorities to suggest that cesarean section be performed on all pregnant women with chronic ITP who have previously undergone splenectomy, regardless of platelet count, and in those women with intact spleens who have counts below 100,000/$\mu$l.[139] Others have recommended vaginal delivery unless a specific obstetrical indication for cesarean section is present.[150] Recently, Karpatkin et al. reported that in all 12 of their cases, treating the mother for 10–14 days prior to delivery with 10–20 mg of prednisone resulted in newborns having platelet counts of more than 65,000/$\mu$l as compared with counts below 60,000/$\mu$l in 6 of 7 mothers not so treated. All of the treated mothers underwent routine vaginal deliveries, and there were not complications in the neonates. Hence, the authors concluded that if corticosteroid therapy is employed near term, there is no need to perform cesarean sections.[151] Others, however, have warned against using corticosteroids during pregnancy (although at higher doses and for longer durations), since there may be an increased risk of eclampsia, hypertension, and psychosis, along with the risk of adrenal suppression in the neonate.[139] Moreover, Cines et al. have reported that corticosteroid therapy may actually increase the fetus' risk of having severe thrombocytopenia by shifting the equilibrium from platelet-associated to serum antiplatelet antibody in the mother, thus facilitating its passage through the placenta to the fetus.[149] To avoid the uncertainty in predicting which fetuses will be thrombocytopenic, Scott et al. devised a technique wherein platelet counts are obtained from blood taken from the fetal scalp during labor after amniotomy is performed, and the results are used to decide whether to perform a cesarean section or a vaginal delivery.[150] They concluded that a count of 50,000/$\mu$l or above posed a sufficiently low risk to justify vaginal delivery. It should be noted, however, that labor must progress for a significant period of time before the head will be in position for the count to be performed; thus, some head trauma may occur.

**Disease-associated ITP.**    A disorder virtually indistinguishable from chronic ITP has been found in association with several other diseases, in particular systemic lupus erythematosus and various lymphoproliferative states.[134,135,139] It has been estimated that systemic lupus erythematosus may present as a chronic ITP-like illness in 10–15 percent of patients. The other manifestations of systemic lupus erythermatosus may require several years to appear. The high female predominance and the shared increase in the frequency of HLA-DRw2 also link the diseases.[135] Since as many as 25–30 percent of the patients presenting with a chronic ITP-like illness may actually have systemic lupus erythematosus, it is crucial that an investigation for the latter disorder be made in each patient. Other disorders associated with chronic ITP are Hodgkin's disease, non-Hodgkin's lymphoma, chronic lymphocytic leukemia, and sarcoidosis.[134] Links to thyrotoxicosis, tuberculosis, Hashimoto's thyroiditis, scleroderma, and carcinomatosis have also been reported, but are less definite.[134] The recent finding of an increased frequency of ITP in male homosexuals showing laboratory evidence of immunodeficiency suggests that ITP may be a manifestation of the acquired immunodeficiency syndrome.[141c] Current evidence implicates immune complexes rather than autoimmune antibodies in this disorder.[141c] Finally, the association of chronic ITP with a Coombs' positive autoimmune hemolytic anemia, occuring either simultaneously or sequentially, has been reported and serves to emphasize that the abnormality in immune regulation may be generalized; this combined disorder is referred to as *Evans' syndrome*.[134]

**Drug-related thrombocytopenias due to decreased platelet survival.**    In this heterogeneous group of disorders, there is a temporal association between drug ingestion and the onset of thrombocytopenia.[134] Bone marrow examination reveals increased numbers of megakaryocytes, and platelet survival is usually significantly decreased, indicating peripheral destruction as the major mechanism of thrombocytopenia. The appropriate therapy is, of course, drug withdrawal, and recovery is usually prompt and complete. In especially severe cases, corticosteroid therapy (1 mg/kg/day of prednisone) is appropriate in an attempt to speed recovery and improve capillary integrity. An immunologic basis for the disorder has been documented with some, but by no means all, of the drugs involved. Although this documentation is based in large part on analysis of platelet-associated IgG, it too has recently been challaenged on theoretical grounds as nonspecifically reflecting a decrease in mean platelet age.[142] Further complicating the analysis of the pathophysiology of these disorders is the convincing demonstration of an immunologically mediated case of drug-induced thrombocytopenia in which a metabolite of the drug acetaminophen, but not the drug itself, was the immunologically active agent.[152] Some of the more commonly used drugs that have been implicated in causing thrombocytopenia are discussed below, and a more comprehensive list is found in Table 4-6.

**Table 4-6**

Drugs Proved or Suspected to Induce Drug-Dependent,
Antibody-Mediated Immune Thrombocytopenia

| Drug | In Vitro Tests* | Rechallenge with Suspected Drug Resulting in Positive in Vivo Test* |
|---|---|---|
| Analgesics | | |
|   Acetylsalicylic acid | + | ∅ |
|   N-Acetyl-p-aminophenol sulfate | | |
|     (metabolite of acetaminophen) | + | ∅ |
|   Phenylbutazone | + | 0 |
| Antibiotics | | |
| *Antituberculous drugs* | | |
|   Isoniazid | ∅ | Unclear in vivo result, decreased platelets on 8th day after rechallenge |
|   Para-aminosalicylic acid (PAS) | ∅ | + |
|   Rifampicin | + | + |
|   Streptomycin | ∅ | + |
| *Penicillin group* | | |
|   Ampicillin | ∅ | ∅ |
|   Methicillin | + (Cross-reactivity to cloxacillin) | + |
|   Penicillin | ∅ | ∅ |
|   Phenoxymethyl penicillin | 0 | + |
|   Sodium cephalothin | + | + |
| *Other antibiotics* | | |
|   Lincomycin | ∅ | ∅ |
|   Novobiocin | + | + |
|   Oxytetracycline | ∅ | ∅ |
|   Pentamidine | − | ∅ |
|   Ristocetin | + (Nonimmune platelet aggregation and fibrinogen precipitation) | + (Due to nonimmune mechanism) |
| *Sulfonamides* | | |
|   Sulfamethoxazole and trimethoprim | ∅ | ∅ |
|   Sulfisoxazole | + | ∅ |
|   Sulfathiazole, sulfadiazine | ∅ | + |
|   Sulfadimidine | ∅ | ∅ |
| *Other sulfonamide derivatives* | | |
|   Acetazolamide | − | ∅ |
|   Chlorpropamide | ∅ | ∅ |
|   Diazoxide | ∅ | − |
|   Furosemide | ∅ | ∅ |
|   Tolbutamide | ∅ | ∅ |

*(continued)*

Table 4-6 (continued)

| Drug | In Vitro Tests* | Rechallenge with Suspected Drug Resulting in Positive in Vivo Test* |
|---|---|---|
| Anticonvulsants, sedatives, and hypnotics | | |
|   Allylisopropylacetylurea (Sedormid) | + | + |
|   Barbiturates | + | + |
|   Carbamazepine | + | + |
|   Phenytoin (diphenylhydantoin) | + | ∅ |
|   Ethchlorvynol | + | + |
|   Meprobamate | + | ∅ |
|   Paramethadione | ∅ | ∅ |
|   Primidone | ∅ | ∅ |
|   Sodium valproate | − | ∅ |
| Cinchona Alkaloids | | |
|   Quinidine | + | + |
|   Quinine | + | + |
| Foods | | |
|   Beans | ∅ | + |
| Miscellaneous | | |
|   Alpha-methyldopa | + | + |
|   Antazoline | + | + |
|   Antilymphocyte serum | + | ●+ |
|   Bacille Calmette-Guérin (BCG) therapy | − | ●+ |
|   Chlordiazepoxide and clidinium bromide (Librax) | ∅ | ∅ |
|   Chlorpheniramine | + | ∅ |
|   Chlorothiazide | + | ∅ |
|   Digitoxin | + | + |
|   Gold salts | − | ●+ |
|   Hydrochlorothiazide | + | ∅ |
|   Heparin | + | + |
|   Iopanoic acid | + | + |
|   Levamisole | ∅ | + |
|   Penicillamine | ∅ | ∅ |
|   Propylthiouracil | ∅ | ∅ |
|   Spironolactone | + | ∅ |
|   Stibophen | + | + |
|   Vinylchloride | ∅ | ●+ |

Adapted from Stuart MJ, McKenna R: Diseases of coagulation: The platelet and vasculature, in Nathan DG, Oski FA (eds): Hematology of Infancy and Childhood, Philadelphia, WB Saunders, 1981, p. 1263–1264. With permission.

*Key to symbols: ∅ = not done; + = positive; − = negative; ● = short platelet survival, no rechallenge;

**Heparin and platelets.**    The interactions between heparin and platelets are complex and still only incompletely understood. Part of this complexity results from the heterogeneity of the heparin preparations currently available, which are purified extracts of either the intestines of swine (porcine gut) or the lungs of cows (beef lung). The extracted heparins are mixtures of polysaccharides that differ considerably in their antithrombin-binding capacity, anticoagulant potency, molecular weight, and ability to interact with platelets.[153] One indication of the crudeness of the currently used extraction techniques is that the anti-coagulant potency of commercial heparin is approximately 180 U/mg (early preparations were only 100 U/mg), whereas subfractions of heparin have been purified which contain several times this specific activity.[153] Thus, at least some of the effects of ''heparin'' may not be due to the anticoagulant molecules at all. It is not surprising, therefore, that there is so much confusion and that different studies using different sources and purities of heparin (not to mention differences between lot numbers) have come to different conclusions. With this background as a caution, the various effects which have been reported will be described.

*Heparin as an ''antiplatelet'' agent.*    Heparin, in combination with antithrombin III, is an extremely potent inhibitor of thrombin. Moreover, this complex also inhibits several other serine proteases in the coagulation cascade that contribute to the generation of thrombin. Since thrombin is one of the most potent platelet-aggregating agents, there is no doubt that heparin exerts a dramatic ''antiplatelet'' effect when thrombin is being generated. This is most clearly deomonstrated in diffuse intravascular coagulation when the excessive gener-ation of thrombin results in a decrease in platelet survival sufficient to cause thrombocy-topenia.[134] In the appropriate circumstances heparin therapy can reverse this process, with a concomitant increase in platelets. Similarly, the clot that forms in venous thrombosis has large amounts of thrombin adsorbed to it and platelets adhere tenaciously to the clot. When these clots embolize to the lung, the vasoactive products produced or released by platelets can exert their effects on the pulmonary vasculature. In the presence of heparin, fewer plate-lets are associated with the clots and, presumably as a result of this antiplatelet effect, at least some of the pulmonary changes are arrested or even reversed quite quickly.

*Heparin-induced thrombocytopenia.*[154–157]    This disorder may be mild or severe.

**Mild disorder.**    Reductions in the platelet counts of a considerable fraction of pa-tients being treated with heparin have been reported in several recent articles.[154,155] Most of these reductions have been modest, with the count rarely dropping much below 100,000/µl, a level at which serious spontaneous bleeding is quite unlikely. Very few patients give a history of prior exposure to heparin. There is suggestive evidence that heparin extracted from beef lung is more likely to produce thrombocytopenia than that extracted from por-cine gut (31 vs. 3.7 percent and 26 vs. 7 percent in 2 studies), but this difference has not been confirmed in other studies.[155,157] Although an immunologic mechanism has been proposed to account for this mild thrombocytopenia, to date the evidence is against this hypothesis. It is well established that commercial heparin preparations will produce slight but consistent platelet aggregation in platelet-rich plasma in vitro; this phenomenon is inde-pendent of the platelet release reaction, but does require a cryoprecipitable plasma cofactor.[153] Interestingly, of the heparin subfractions having low molecular weight, those with high affinity for antithrombin III (and thus high anticoagulant activity) were the least potent inducers of this reaction, perhaps because the antithrombin competes with the platelets for the heparin. If this direct platelet aggregation effect is, in fact, responsible for the ob-served thrombocytopenia, it offers the hope that preparations of heparin may be obtained that will be potent anticoagulants without producing thrombocytopenia. Another mechanism that has been proposed is based on the observation that heparin can also potentiate aggregation induced by other agents.[158] Here again, of the low molecular weight fractions, those with high antithrombin III affinity are least active. It has been suggested that this results from heparin's ability to inhibit the enzyme adenylate cyclase since the latter is responsible for the production of cAMP, a potent platelet aggregation inhibitor.[159] Current data, however, indicate that this inhibition is observed only in broken platelet preparations, not in intact platelets.[158] The proaggregatory effect of heparin thus remains an enigma.

Clinically, this mild thrombocytopenia usually is observed between the 2nd and 15th day following full-dose heparin administration.[154] Platelet counts return to normal rapidly after heparin is discontinued and may do so even if therapy is continued. It need not be considered an absolute contraindication to further heparin therapy since it rarely produces hemorrhage or thrombosis, and the decision regarding continuation should weigh the original indication for heparin, the availability of frequent platelet counts to monitor further reductions, and the integrity of the other parts of the patient's hemostatic mechanism.

**Severe disorder.**    This is a much rarer reaction that usually begins several days after heparin is administered and becomes most severe between the 7th and 14th day. Although heparin is poorly antigenic, an immunologic mechanism is suggested by the interval between the onset of thrombocytopenia and the beginning of therapy, the rapid increase in the platelet count following discontinuation of heparin, and the equally rapid decline in circulating platelets after readministration of heparin.[154] Heparin-dependent antiplatelet antibodies (IgG, IgM, and IgA-IgG) have been identified in most patients with severe thrombocytopenia and increased amounts of platelet-associated IgG and C3 have been found in the few cases studies with these techniques.[154,154a,156] The antibody appears to be directed against a platelet–heparin complex, but there may be some antibody–heparin interaction as well, with the possibility that these latter complexes may directly aggregate circulating platelets. Ironically, this in vivo aggregation can itself produce thrombosis, the disease process for which the heparin was probably initially administered. These thrombotic events can be clinically disastrous, with major arterial occlusions, myocardial infarctions, and recurrent venous thrombosis (with or without pulmonary emboli) being reported.[154,154a] Hemorrhagic manifestations have been less frequently reported. The seriousness of these reactions makes repeated challenge with heparin very dangerous. The use of minidose heparin does not protect against the development of this complication. There is little evidence to suggest that the source of heparin affects the frequency of this problem or that switching to heparin obtained from the other species offers any advantage. One interesting observation is that patients often complain of vague symptoms, including low back and abdominal pain, a day or two prior to a major thrombotic event; these symptoms may be related to blood vessel occlusion and ischemia.

## Drug-induced, antibody-mediated thrombocytopenia (Table 4-6).

*Gold-induced thrombocytopenia.*    This phenomenon occurs in 1–3 percent of patients treated with this drug for the control of rheumatoid arthritis.[160] An immunologic mechanism is thought to be operative since (1) patients usually have normal to increased numbers of megakaryocytes in their bone marrow, (2) platelet survival was decreased in at least one patient in whom it was studied, and (3) antiplatelet antibodies have been found in the serum of some, but not all, patients.[160] Clinically, the onset is usually abrupt and may occur at widely varying total dosages (between 75 and 3500 mg of gold sodium thiomalate in 1 study.)[160] Thrombocytopenia has followed the use of both gold sodium thiomalate and aurothioglucose, and it is uncertain whether there is a difference in the frequency of thrombocytopenia with the two preparations. In addition, no consistent pattern has been observed with regard to the presence of other complications of gold therapy, such as proteinuria, stomatitis, or dermatitis. An association between gold-induced thrombocytopenia and HLA-DR3 has been demonstrated, and it has been suggested that HLA typing may be useful in screening patients who might be considered for chrysotherapy. Clinically, the platelet count is not infrequently less than 5,000/$\mu$l, and fatal hemorrhage, although rare, has been reported. Drug withdrawal and corticosteroid therapy (60 mg of prednisone/day) results in complete and permanent resolution of the thrombocytopenia in most patients within 2–3 weeks; splenectomy, however, may be required in some of the more persistent and severe cases. Although dimercaprol has been used to speed the removal of gold from the body, a recent study did not find this drug beneficial in treating the thrombocytopenia.[160]

*Quinine- and quinidine-dependent thrombocytopenia.*    These have been the most intensively studied of all the drug-related thrombocytopenias.[134] Clinically, the disorder is characterized by the abrupt onset of purpura after taking either of the medications for a variable period of time (days to years), but with the last dose almost always within 1 day of the onset of symptoms. When quinine-induced thrombocytopenia is suspected, specific questioning for ingestion of quinine-containing beverages such as tonic water is necessary. Some patients will give a history of constitutional symptoms soon after ingesting the drug and prior to the development of the purpura. Although ecchymosis is the most common symptom, petechiae also occur; in the more severe cases, hemorrhage may occur in the gastrointestinal or urinary tracts, the buccal mucosa, or the central nervous system. Laboratory investigation usually reveals severe thrombocytopenia, with platelet counts often below 10,000/$\mu$l and not infrequently below 1000/$\mu$l. Bone marrow examination reveals normal or increased megakaryocytes. Platelet-associated IgG levels are almost always increased, [161] and the patient's serum usually has an antibody which will attach to platelets (and in some cases fix complement) in the presence of the appropriate drug.[134] By these techniques, cross-reactivity between quinine- and quinidine-dependent antibodies is uncommon.

Several different mechanisms have been proposed to explain the pathogenesis of this disorder. Originally it was proposed that the drug became bound to the platelet surface, and this complex stimulated antibody production such that upon renewed ingestion of the drug, the antibody would behave as an antiplatelet antibody and result in rapid removal of the platelets.[162] Subsequent data appeared to conflict with this hypothesis and fit the "innocent bystander" mechanism better. [162,162a] In this model (1) the drug binds to a large carrier molecule in the plasma, presumably a protein; (2) an antibody is made against the complex, but upon rechallenge, the antibody will also bind to the drug (hapten) alone; (3) the drug–antibody complex has a high affinity for a site on the platelet and thus binds tightly to the platelet surface; and (4) the increased amount of antibody on the platelet surface results in premature removal of the platelets. It has been suggested that the platelet glycoprotein GPIb may be the site to which the complex binds since (1) the antibody does not appear to interact with platelets from patients with the Bernard-Soulier syndrome (which lack GPIb) even when incubated in the presence of the drug;[20] (2) partially purified GPIb inhibits the interaction of these antibodies with platelets; and (3) a quinidine-dependent antibody selectively precipitated GPIb (and a low molecular weight glycoprotein) from solubilized platelets.[162b] Studies employing formaldehyde fixation and proteolytic digestion of the platelet surface, however, have cast doubt on the identity of GPIb as the binding site for aggregated IgG.[162c]

Therapeutically, withdrawal of the drug usually results in return of the platelet count to normal within a few days, although more prolonged recoveries have been noted. It is unclear whether corticosteroids hasten recovery, but it seems reasonable to use them for their effects on the blood vessel and their possible effects on the thrombocytopenia, at least for a short course. Platelet transfusions may be necessary in cases complicated by serious hemorrhage. The use of a rechallenging dose of the drug to establish the diagnosis should be reserved for those situations in which no substitute drug is available since severe thrombocytopenia may occur even with very low doses.

*Trimethoprim–sulfamethoxazole-induced thrombocytopenia.*   This drug combination has been implicated in inducing immune-mediated thrombocytopenia. In vitro studies suggest that antibodies are directed against the trimethoprim and not the sulfamethoxazole.[161] In addition, the drug's antimetabolite action may affect platelet production adversely.[126] Since this drug is being used increasingly in the prophylactic therapy of patients treated with chemotherapy and those who have aplastic anemia, the resulting thrombocytopenia may be particularly serious. Moreover, in patients who already require platelet transfusions, it may be difficult to distinguish thrombocytopenia induced by this drug from alloimmunization. It is probably reasonable to discontinue this drug, if possible, in any patient who suffers a distinct decrease in response to platelet transfusions.

**Isoimmune neonatal purpura.**   This disorder can occur when a mother who lacks a platelet-specific antigen carries a fetus who has inherited that antigen from the father. If the mother then makes IgG antibodies against that antigen, they can cross the placenta and attach to the fetus' platelets.[125,134,148] The condition has been estimated to occur in a symptomatic form in at least one out of 5000 births. The $Pl^{A1}$ antigen, which is present on the platelets of all but 2–3 percent of the normal population, has been incriminated in the vast majority of cases, but several other specificities, including $Pl^{E2}$ and the recently described $Bak^a$ antigen, have also been involved.[163,164] Although anti-HLA antibodies have been detected in some cases, recent evidence suggests that these are probably not causal.[164] Although the pathogenesis of this disorder resembles that of erythroblastosis fetalis, it differs strikingly from the latter in that it occurs in the first pregnancy in almost one-half of the cases.

Clinically, the affected newborns are usually the products of uncomplicated pregnancies and deliveries, and may show little or no evidence of hemorrhage at birth. Within several hours, however, the platelet count drops, often to very low levels, and clinical evidence of hemorrhage with petechiae and ecchymoses appears.[134,148] Serious bleeding is not uncommon, and the mortality has been estimated at 10–15 percent, with intracranial hemorrhage being the most common cause of death. The thrombocytopenia usually abates within 2 weeks, but has been known to persist for up to 2 months. Bone marrow examination usually shows normal numbers of megakaryocytes, but they may be absent in some cases, presumably resulting from an action of the antibody directly on the megakaryocytes.[148]

Therapy for the disorder consists of corticosteroids and, in severe cases, platelet transfusions. Since the mother's platelets lack the antigen to which the antibody is directed, her platelets can be expected to be compatible. This is especially important since, in the case of the $Pl^{A1}$ system, so few random donors will be $Pl^{A1}$ negative. Whereas the mother's plasma contains the antibody, it is desirable to wash her platelets free of her plasma and resuspend them in compatible plasma prior to infusion. If need be, the platelets can be administered as part of an exchange transfusion. If the mother is unable to serve as a donor, some benefit can be expected from random donor platelets, but these should be reserved for serious hemmorhage. Splenectomy is usually not needed and poses serious risks if performed in infancy. In mothers who have previously had a child with isoimmune neonatal purpura, it has been recommended that subsequent deliveries be by cesarean section so as to avoid the cranial trauma associated with vaginal delivery, and to permit the harvesting of platelets from the mother immediately prior to the procedure so that they can be available immediately after delivery. This approach seems quite reasonable, but it is hoped that sequential assays of antiplatelet antibodies in the mother's serum during pregnancy may be able to predict which fetuses are truly at risk. Corticosteroid therapy for the mother near term has also been recommended.[125] It is obviously important to differentiate isoimmune neonatal purpura from neonatal ITP for both therapeutic and prognostic purposes, and since the mother of a child with neonatal ITP may be asymptomatic and give no history of chronic ITP, it is important that platelet counts and, if available, assays for antiplatelet antibodies and Pl$^{A1}$ phenotyping be performed on the mother.

**Posttransfusion purpura.**    This is a poorly understood disorder in which patients suffer severe thrombocytopenia approximately 1 week after receiving a whole blood transfusion.[126,134] The majority of cases reported to date have occurred in the 2–3 percent of individuals who lack the Pl$^{A1}$ antigen on their platelets. Other platelet-specific antigens are thought to account for the remainder of the cases. There is a striking female predominance, and since almost all of the women have previously been pregnant, it is presumed that sensitization takes place sometime during or shortly after pregnancy as a result of fetal platelets (containing the Pl$^{A1}$ antigen inherited from the father) gaining access to the maternal circulation. Since the patient's platelets lack the Pl$^{A1}$ antigen, it is paradoxical that the anti-Pl$^{A1}$ antibody should result in a decrease in the patient's own platelet count. One hypothesis for which there is preliminary supportive evidence is that the Pl$^{A1}$ antigen can be passively transferred to the patient's platelets after elution from the transfused platelets.[164a] The rarity of this disorder about (about 40 cases) compared with the expected frequency (one of 50 transfused parous women if all Pl$^{A1}$ negative patients were truly at risk) emphasizes our lack of understanding of all the factors involved. A recent report suggests that individuals who are Pl$^{A1}$ negative are more likely to become alloimmunized if they are HLA-B8 positive than if they are HLA-B8 negative.[164b] This may explain why only some Pl$^{A1}$ negative patients develop post-transfusion purpura.

   Clinically, these patients usually present with profound thrombocytopenia (less than 10,000/µl) and significant mucocutaneous hemorrhage. The bone marrow contains increased numbers of megakaryocytes, and anti-Pl$^{A1}$ antibodies are usually detectable in the patient's serum. Therapeutically, stringent precautions to prevent even the slightest trauma should be instituted. Based on the limited evidence currently available corticosteroids should probably be employed.[164c,d] Platelet transfusions from random donors should be avoided since they are likely to prolong the process and, more importantly, serious transfusion reactions have been reported. Plasmapheresis has a good theoretical rationale and appears to have been quite successful in the few cases in which it has been tried, shortening the interval for recovery from the usual 10–48 days to just a few days. If plasmapheresis is not available, exchange transfusions may have a role.[134]

**Increased platelet utilization.**    There are many disorders in which platelet consumption is sufficiently increased to produce thrombocytopenia.[126,134] In several of these conditions, platelet consumption is matched by increases in fibrinogen consumption, and it is presumed that increased thrombin production is responsible for both effects.[130,134] Diseases in this category include diffuse intravascular coagulation (regardless of the initiating stimulus), envenoming by certain snakes, and giant hemangiomas. These disease processes are discussed elsewhere. In other diseases, platelet consumption is increased, whereas fibrinogen survival is not affected. These conditions are discussed below.

*Thrombotic thrombocytopenic purpura (Moschcowitz' syndrome).*    This is a rare (about $1/10^6$ population/year) disorder characterized in its most complete form by the pentad of thrombocytopenia, microangiopathic hemolytic anemia, fluctuating neurologic symptoms, renal impairment, and fever.[126,134,165,166] Although its etiology and pathogenesis remain unknown, empiric advances in therapy have resulted in a dramatic improvement in the prognosis.

Clinically, the disorder is most common in women in the childbearing years, but both sexes and both young and old persons have been affected. In a minority of cases, the disorder has been associated with a variety of other conditions, including several collagen-vascular disorders, pregnancy, and antecedent upper respiratory tract infections, but there is no convincing evidence that these associations are causal rather than coincidental. The onset of symptoms is usually quite rapid, if not fulminant, with transient neurologic dysfunction and hemorrhage (menorrhagia, purpura, etc.) being the presenting symptoms in approximately one-half of the cases, and with malaise, weakness, fatigue, and abdominal pain occurring in approximately one-quarter. Fever (rarely above 102°F), nausea, vomiting, headache, jaundice, and pallor are present in only a minority of patients at the time of diagnosis, but the vast majority of patients will show these symptoms at some time during the course of the illness. The neurologic abnormalities most frequently observed are changes in mental status, paresis, paresthesias, headache, aphasia, seizures, dysarthria, visual changes, and coma.

Laboratory evaluation invariably reveals thrombocytopenia, with a platelet count nadir below 10,000/µl in more than one-half of the cases. Hematocrit values are reduced in virtually all cases, falling to about 20 percent in most patients. Review of the peripheral smear will show obvious microangiopathic changes with fragmented cells, nucleated red blood cells, and increased polychromasia. The reticulocyte count is almost always elevated, and values above 20 percent are not uncommon. Hematuria and proteinuria occur in the majority of patients, and elevations in blood urea nitrogen are also quite common; increases in serum creatinine occur less often. Serum bilirubin and lactate dehydrogenase values are almost always elevated, with the latter sometimes reaching incredibly high values (approximately 10,000 IU has been reported.) The majority of patients will have a normal prothrombin time, which helps to differentiate this disorder from diffuse intravascular coagulation. The activated partial thromboplastin time is also usually normal, but some patients will have a modest elevation in fibrin(ogen) degradation products. The latter apparently is not a reflection of a dramatic increase in the catabolism of fibrinogen since fibrinogen survival has been found to be normal in the few cases in which it has been measured. Serologic studies for antinuclear antibodies have given variable results in different series, but positive results have been reported in as many as 50 percent of patients. Bone marrow examination reveals erythroid hyperplasia and normal or increased numbers of megakaryocytes.

The microscopic pathology of thrombotic thrombocytopenic purpura is quite distinctive, with occlusive hyaline thrombi composed primarily of platelets (but with a small amount of fibrin admixed) filling the lumens of arterioles and capillaries. There is usually no evidence of vasculitis. Although it may be difficult to differentiate these lesions from those of classic diffuse intravascular coagulation, fibrin is said to play a much larger role in the latter. The hyaline thrombi are found throughout the body, with the heart, brain, kidneys, pancreas, and adrenals most heavily involved. It is common practice to obtain a biopsy specimen to confirm the diagnosis of thrombotic thrombocytopenic purpura, but there is controversy regarding the best site to biopsy. The bone marrow reveals thrombi in approximately 50 percent of cases, whereas the positive yield from gingival biopsy is anywhere from one-third to two-thirds. Even though random skin and muscle biopsies do not have good yields, it has recently been suggested that biopsy of a petechial site is preferred over gingival biopsy since microthrombi in dermal capillaries are very frequently seen.

The pathophysiology of this disorder remains the subject of remarkable controversy, but there is general agreement that the hallmark of the disease is platelet aggregate formation in small blood vessels, either as a result of blood vessel wall damage or an increase in the propensity of platelets to aggregate. Numerous factors have been suggested to contribute to this process, including (1) direct endothelial cell injury by viruses, immune complexes, etc.; (2) decreased circulating $PGI_2$ activity secondary to endothelial cell injury, deficiency of a plasma component that either stimulates $PGI_2$ production or stabilizes its activity, or the presence of a plasma component that antagonizes $PGI_2$; (3) decreased plasminogen activator in the affected blood vessel walls; (4) the presence of a high molecular weight plasma factor that induces aggregation of normal or patient platelets; (5) a deficiency of a normal plasma factor that inhibits such a platelet-aggregating factor; and (6) the presence of unusually large von Willebrand factor multimers, which in combination with an unidentified polycation may initiate platelet agglutination.[165,166,166a] Although evidence in favor of each of the above mechanisms has been reported, it is unclear what contribution, if any, each actually makes to the pathogenesis of the disorder.

Therapy remains controversial, but there is near unanimity on one point: the introduction of therapy designed to remove the patient's plasma and/or to supply the patient with normal plasma has dramatically improved the prognosis. Thus, when reviewed in 1966, only 17 of 271 patients were found to have had prolonged survival, with almost two-thirds of the patients dying within 3 months of the onset of symptoms. This is in stark contrast to the 70–80 percent response rate currently found in patients treated with plasma infusion, exchange transfusion, or exchange plasmapheresis. Preliminary evidence indicates that vincristine may also be highly efficacious, but this will require confirmation.[167,167a] Less clear, however, is whether any of the above therapies is clearly superior to the others and which additional therapeutic modalities should be employed. Corticosteroid therapy has not been convincingly shown to be of benefit, but since it has been used almost universally, it is difficult to be certain that it is not useful when combined with other therapies. The effect of corticosteroids in decreasing $PGI_2$ synthesis by endothelial cells might, however, be considered harmful on theoretical grounds, as it would tend to increase platelet aggregate formation in the microcirculation.[138] There are conflicting data about the efficacy of antiplatelet agents; some studies have shown a beneficial effect, especially when a combination of agents such as aspirin, dipyridamole, and sulfinpyrazone are used together, whereas a recent report indicates that they are probably of marginal benefit at best, and may actually contribute to the severity of the hemorrhagic diathesis.[168] Although there was some initial enthusiasm for the use of heparin, most recent studies have found it to be either of no use or potentially damaging. The role of splenectomy remains most controversial. A significant number of reports have documented a response to splenectomy in patients with severe disease who were previously unresponsive to pharmacologic interventions. However, retrospective analysis has emphasized that many of these patients received whole blood or plasma during the course of the procedure or postoperatively. The beneficial effect thus may have been due to the transfusions rather than to removal of the spleen. An occasional patient, however, may have benefited from splenectomy even though no plasma was given, and thus the issue remains moot. The results with thrombolytic therapy have been very poor, and these agents are probably contraindicated. Although there may be a great temptation to give platelet transfusions to patients with this disease who are severely thrombocytopenic and have hemorrhage, several investigators have noticed significant deterioration after platelet transfusions presumably reflecting an exacerbation of the thrombotic lesions. On theoretical grounds, infusion of $PGI_2$ would appear to be rational therapy. Early reports of its use were not encouraging, but at least 1 patient who failed to respond to all conventional measures, including plasma infusion and exchange, appears to have had a dramatic response to $PGI_2$.[169] Immunosuppressive drugs in general have not been of significant benefit.

A tentative therapeutic plan reflecting the literature as of the middle of 1983 might be as follows: (1) Initial therapy should probably consist of infusion of 10–20 units of plasma as rapidly as the patient's cardiovascular status permits. Although the data are quite limited, the author believes that it is reasonable also to give intravenous vincristine (1.4 mg/m$^2$, with an upper limit of 2 mg) at the outset since the toxicity is likely to be minimal and a response could obviate the need for more elaborate, expensive, and potentially dangerous therapy. If a response to vincristine is obtained, additional weekly injections should be given until disease activity abates, and then for 1 or 2 additional weeks. Most investigators would probably also use high doses of corticosteroids, but the author believes that the literature would support withholding them for at least a short period of time to see if a response can be obtained without committing oneself to long-term therapy with high doses; if a response is not obtained, it is probably reasonable to administer them. If the major manifestations of the disease are thrombotic, a combination of oral antiplatelet agents (for example, 600 mg aspirin every 12 hours, 200 mg dipyridamole every 12 hours, and 200 mg sulfinpyrazone every 6 hours) might be given. If hemorrhage is prominent, one might consider withholding these agents. (2) Patients who respond to the above regimen should be treated with additional plasma and/or vincristine to maintain the response. It should be appreciated that some patients may require enormous amounts (about 500 units) of plasma to maintain a response. (3) Patients who fail to respond to plasma infusion and/or vincristine should probably be treated with plasma exchange or whole blood exchange, depending on the facilities available, on the assumption that they have a noxious substance in their circulation instead of, or in addition to, a plasma factor deficiency. In patients who have a severely compromised cardiovascular status or who present in extremis, one of these modalities should probably be employed first. (4) If the above therapy fails, the more experimental measures (splenectomy or $PGI_2$ infusion) should be attempted.

*Hemolytic-uremic syndrome.* This disorder shares many clinical similarities with thrombotic thrombocytopenic purpura in that it is characterized by fever, thrombocytopenia, microangiopathic hemolytic anemia, and renal dysfunction.[126,134,165,166] However, its occurrence primarily in children, the rarity of neurologic findings, and the more severe renal involvement (often associated with hypertension) all help to distinguish it from thrombotic thrombocytopenic purpura. A disease essentially indistinguishable from hemolytic-uremic syndrome also occurs in women in the postpartum period. Antecedent viral infections of the gastrointestinal or upper respiratory tract are common in patients with the hemolytic-uremic syndrome and have led to speculation regarding an immune complex etiology for the disorder, but direct evidence to support this hypothesis is still fragmentary.

The laboratory findings are similar to those in thrombotic thrombocytopenic purpura except for the severe azotemia. The pathologic vascular changes are also similar to those in thrombotic thrombocytopenic purpura, but usually these changes are confined to the afferent arterioles and glomerular capillaries of the kidney.

Management remains controversial, although there is general agreement that early and vigorous dialysis is very important. Corticosteroids are of questionable value, but are generally used nonetheless. Heparin is also of questionable value, but judicious doses (50 U/kg every 4–6 hours) in patients manifesting laboratory evidence of diffuse intravascular coagulation are probably justified. Judgments concerning the efficacy of fibrinolytic therapy and antiplatelet agents are difficult to make. As in thrombotic thrombocytopenic purpura, concern has been expressed that platelet transfusions might exacerbate the disorder. Plasma infusion, plasma exchange, and whole blood exchange have been advocated in this disorder because of their efficacy in thrombotic thrombocytopenic purpura, but there has been less experience with these modalities in this disease. $PGI_2$ infusion has been proposed, not only for its antiplatelet effect but also for its vasodilating effect, which may help control the severe hypertension which is sometimes encountered; few data are available at present to assess its efficacy.

*"Thrombopoietin" deficiency.*    This interesting disorder has been well documented in only a single patient who had isolated thrombocytopenia, apparently from birth.[102,115,126] Although the patient had bone marrow megakaryocytes, they were described as being morphologically immature. After failing to respond to corticosteroids she underwent splenectomy. Although the operation did not improve her condition, it was noted that transfusions of whole blood or plasma resulted in megakaryocyte maturation and a rise in her peripheral platelet count. The patient went on to have several remissions, but ultimately developed a series of problems including infections, neurologic dysfunction, hemolytic anemia, hypertension, and nephritis by age 13. Since plasma infusion has been shown to be of benefit in some patients with thrombotic thrombocytopenic purpura, it was suggested that this patient had a very unusual form of that disease, in which case the defect may not have been in platelet production. In support of this contention is a report of a similar patient with episodes of severe thrombocytopenia who had dramatic responses to plasma infusion on many occasions and who also manifested a microangiopathic hemolytic anemia that responded to plasma.[126] Interestingly, this patient also had an abnormality of her right radius. Both of these patients were recently found to have elevated levels of von Willebrand factor during remission, with the latter containing unusually large multimeric forms.[166a] Since the levels decreased during relapse and the largest forms disappeared, a causal relationship was suggested. These patients have thus been classified as having a chronic relapsing form of thrombotic thrombocytopenic purpura.[166a]

*Artificial surfaces and abnormal blood vessels.*    Platelet survival has been shown to be decreased in a wide variety of disorders associated with the introduction of artificial surfaces into the circulation or when a pathologic process has altered the normal blood vessel wall (Table 4-7).[95,130,134,170] This is a very heterogeneous group of conditions in which it is presumed that platelets interact with the artificial or abnormal surface and then are either immediately lost to the circulation by direct attachment or are released from the surface but altered sufficiently so that they are prematurely removed. In addition, even if

**Table 4-7**
Conditions Associated with
Decreased Platelet Survival
and/or Thrombocytopenia

Artificial surfaces

    Cardiopulmonary bypass
    Renal dialysis
    Prosthetic heart valves
    Prosthetic vascular grafts
    Charcoal hemoperfusion
    Plasmapheresis
    Intra-aortic balloon pumping devices

Pathological surfaces

    Acute
        Sickle cell crisis
        Vasculitis
        Renal rejection

    Chronic conditions
        Coronary artery disease
        Rheumatic heart disease
        Gout
        Homocystinemia
        Smoking

Adapted from Mustard JF, Packham MA, Kinlough-Rathbone RL: Platelet survival, in Day HJ et al. (eds): Platelet Function Testing. (NIH) 78–1087. Department of Health, Education and Welfare, 1978, p. 551. With permission.

the platelets are not removed, they may be functionally impaired.[171] The extent of the shortening of survival and the capacity of the bone marrow to respond will determine whether thrombocytopenia occurs. With artificial surfaces, the deposition of platelets and the resulting thrombus formation may be the single most important factor in determining the biocompatibility of a given device. Interventions such as albumin precoating to decrease the platelet reactivity of the artificial surface, or $PGI_2$ infusion to decrease the interaction of platelets with the surfaces may prove to be very useful in devices that are used for only a brief period of time.[171] In fact, it has been reported that hemodialysis can be performed without any heparinization if $PGI_2$ is infused.[170] The shortened platelet survival found in most of the chronic disorders is thought to result from the pathological changes in the vasculature and usually is not severe enough to result in thrombocytopenia. The acute disorders, however, may well be associated with thrombocytopenia. It should be pointed out, however, that these are complicated diseases in which abnormalities other than those present in the blood vessel wall, (e.g., immune complex formation) may contribute to the thrombocytopenia.

*Snake venoms.*    Thrombocytopenia is known to occur after bites from several different snakes.[172] Although some of these venoms result in thrombin generation and thus are akin to diffuse intravascular coagulation in both pathogenesis and appropriate therapy, other

**Table 4-8**
Acute Viral-Induced
Thrombocytopenia

Congenital infections
  Cytomegalovirus
  Rubella virus

Acquired infections
  Hemorrhagic fever viruses
  Herpes viruses
    Herpes simplex virus
    Cytomegalovirus
    Varicella-zoster virus
    Epstein-Barr virus
  Exanthematous diseases
    Rubella
    Rubeola
    Exanthema subitum
  Enterovirus
  Mumps virus
  Adenovirus
  Variola virus
  Hepatitis virus

Vaccine-induced thrombocytopenia
  Rubeola vaccine
  Rubella vaccine

Adapted from Chesney PJ, and Shahidi NT:
Acute viral-induced thrombocytopenia: a review of human disease, animal models, and
in vitro studies, in Lusher JM, Barnhart MI
(eds): Acquired Bleeding Disorders in Children, New York, Masson Publishing USA,
1981, p. 66. With permission.

venoms appear to activate platelets directly; in the latter case, heparin therapy may not
be appropriate.

**Acute viral-induced thrombocytopenia.**    This is a well-recognized syndrome in both
humans and animals.[126,173] It can occur with congenital rubella or cytomegalovirus infections, a variety of acquired infections, and after vaccination with live viruses (Table 4-8). Although there has been a considerable amount of investigation of the pathogenesis of these
disorders, the precise mechanism(s) involved remains unclear. Among the suggested factors are (1) decreased platelet production secondary to viral infection of megakaryocytes
or (2) decreased platelet survival secondary to (a) direct virus–platelet interaction resulting in aggregation, release, and/or lysis, (b) direct virus–platelet interaction resulting in
premature phagocytosis, (c) viral-induced initiation of diffuse intravascular coagulation,
(d) viral-induced endothelial damage resulting in increased platelet utilization, (e) viral
antigen-containing immune complexes leading to premature platelet removal by an innocent bystander mechanism, (f) viral-induced erythrocyte hemolysis resulting in the release of platelet-activating agents such as ADP, or (g) loss of surface sialic acid from
platelets by viruses that contain neuraminidase activity.[126,173,174] Clinically, the throm-

bocytopenia associated with congenital infections is most often manifested as petechiae and ecchymoses occurring soon after birth. Serious hemorrhage is rare and, interestingly, the thrombocytopenia usually resolves spontaneously after several weeks even when there is evidence that the infection is persistent. The vast majority of episodes of thrombocytopenia associated with acquired infections are mild, but occasionally serious hemorrhage occurs. In this case, corticosteroid therapy and, if necessary, splenectomy should be considered since many of these cases may, in fact, be due to the development of postinfectious acute ITP.

**Allergy-induced thrombocytopenia.**   This mild form of thrombocytopenia has been reported in response to injected or ingested allergens.[126,134] Although symptomatic thrombocytopenia is very rare, the recent identification of a remarkably potent platelet-activating factor (PAF) derived from human basophils (and perhaps monocytes, neutrophils, and platelets) has renewed interest in the role of platelets in immune reactions.[59] In fact, an antigen-specific increase in circulating levels of PF 4 has been reported in association with changes in forced expiratory volume in asthmatic patients challenged by the aerosol inhalation of inciting allergens.[175]

**Ineffective thrombopoiesis.**   By analogy to erythropoiesis, ineffective thrombopoiesis is said to occur when, despite a normal mass of megakaryocytes in the bone marrow, there is a failure to produce and/or deliver a normal number of platelets to the circulation. Documentation thus requires careful quantitative analysis of the total megakaryocyte mass, megakaryocyte transit time, and platelet turnover. Total megakaryocyte mass determination requires precise evaluation of both megakaryocyte number and volume; these, in turn, are usually derived from estimates of the total erythroid marrow (based on erythron iron turnover) and determination of the erythroid/megakaryocyte ratio based on tedious analysis of bone marrow histologic sections. There are currently no direct ways to measure megakaryocyte transit time in humans; indirect evidence suggests that it is 7–8 days, and it is assumed that this time does not vary greatly with disease. Platelet mass turnover can be calculated from measurements of platelet count, platelet survival, and mean platelet volume. Given the demanding nature of these studies, it is not surprising that only a few careful measurements have been made; thus, the quantitative analysis of this category of disease is still rudimentary.

   *Thrombocytopenia with megaloblastic disorders.*   Megaloblastic states are usually associated with thrombocytopenia, with a fairly good correlation between the degree of anemia and thrombocytopenia.[134] It is, however, unusual for the thrombocytopenia to be severe or for hemorrhage to be a major factor in the clinical expression of the disease. Ineffective thrombopoiesis has been found in these disorders, as judged by a decrease in effective platelet production despite a significant increase in megakaryocyte mass. Platelet survival may also be mildly to moderately shortened. An increase in megakaryocyte mass is not universal since, at least in some severe cases, megakaryocytes may be reduced or even absent. Mild thrombocytopenia is usually found in paroxysmal noctural hemoglobinuria, and whereas platelet survival and megakaryocyte mass are not abnormal in most patients, ineffective thrombopoiesis is probably the major mechanism responsible for the decreased platelet count.[134] Current evidence indicates that *paroxysmal noctural hemoglobinuria* results from a stem cell abnormality. This hypothesis is supported by the observation that platelet membranes seem to share the increased sensitivity to lysis by complement that characterizes the erythrocyte membranes in this disease.[134] Early in the course of *erythro-*

*leukemia* there may be thrombocytopenia despite normal or increased numbers of mega-karyocytes in the bone marrow; hence, ineffective thrombopoiesis has been suggested to explain these findings.[134] The *congenital thrombocytopenias* that are characterized by nor-mal platelet survival and bone marrow megakaryocyte mass, and that may be confused with ITP if platelet survival and family studies are not performed, are also thought to re-flect ineffective thrombopoiesis.[102] Finally, the possible role of ineffective thrombopoiesis in some cases of alcohol-induced thrombocytopenia was alluded to above.

**Thrombocytopenia due to splenomegaly.**    Splenomegaly resulting from any etiology is frequently associated with mild to moderate thrombocytopenia.[134] The traditional view is that the thrombocytopenia results from sequestration of platelets in the spleen since it can be shown that the recovery of radiolabeled platelets in the circulation approaches 90 per-cent in the asplenic state, is approximately 65 percent in the normosplenic state, and may be as little as 10–30 percent when the spleen is markedly enlarged.[130] Moreover, direct assessment of platelet mass in spleens removed at operation has shown this organ to con-tain several times the number of platelets that are present in the general circulation. It should be stressed that when splenic enlargement alone is present, despite the marked re-duction in platelet recovery, the survival of the platelets that are recovered in the circula-tion should be normal. Thus, if the total of the circulating and spleen-containing platelet mass is increased severalfold and, on average, 10 percent of this total is destroyed each day, the bone marrow must increase its production to a like extent or else thrombocytopenia will occur. The platelet count at which equilibrium is established will depend primarily on the sensor which controls thrombopoietin production and the capacity of the bone marrow to increase production. Since current evidence seems to point toward the total extramedullary platelet mass (probably including the intrasplenic component) rather than the circulating platelet count as the major determinant of the hormonal feedback mechanism, it is not surprising that thrombocytopenia is common. Clinically, when splenic enlargement is the sole cause of thrombocytopenia, the platelet count is rarely sufficiently low to make hem-orrhage a problem. In those few cases in which bleeding does occur, splenectomy should be considered.

**Thrombocytopenia due to hypothermia.[134]**    A reduction in body temperature may pro-duce thrombocytopenia. Since it is usually quickly reversed upon rewarming, it is believed that the platelets are only transiently sequestered, primarily but not exclusively in the liver and spleen. Hypothermia has, however, been implicated in contributing to the neurologic dysfunction found in some patients operated on during profound hypothermia. It is inter-esting to speculate as to whether this phenomenon is related to the exposure of fibrinogen receptors on platelets known to occur with chilling.[176a]

## Thrombocytosis

The upper limit of platelet counts for the normal population is 350,000–400,000/μl; thus, patients with values above these levels are said to have thrombocytosis.[102,176] Since increases in platelet survival have not been documented in any of the conditions associated with thrombocytosis, the increase in platelet count must result from increased production, an acute increase in the release of stored platelets, or a decreased volume of platelets outside of the effective circulation (as after splenectomy). In some of the condi-tions in which production is increased, the thrombocytosis appears to be in response to the presence of another condition (reactive thrombocytosis); thus, it is presumed that the excessive thrombopoiesis is under the control of some humoral mechanism. In other disorders there is no obvious inciting condition (autonomous thrombocytosis); thus, it is presumed that the excessive thrombopoiesis results primarily from an abnormality in the megakaryocyte line. The latter disorders usually have the highest platelet counts.

There is a tendency to establish diagnostic and therapeutic criteria on the basis of the platelet count in these disorders, but the author believes that this approach gives insufficient weight to the important relationship that exists between the platelet count and the hematocrit. It should be remembered that although platelet counts are reported as the number of platelets per unit of whole blood, in fact platelets are excluded from the fraction of the whole blood composed of erythrocytes. The concentration of platelets in the circulating plasma thus will depend on both the platelet count and the hematocrit. For example, if one patient has a hematocrit of 30 percent and another patient has a hematocrit of 65 percent, the plasma concentration of platelets will be twice as great in the second patient when both have the same platelet count per unit whole blood. Moreover, as mentioned previously, it is the motion of the erythrocytes in the microvasculature imparting the radially directed force to the platelets that results in their interaction with the blood vessel wall.[84] These interactions therefore increase as a function of hematocrit. Hence, although the precise clinical implications of these complex interactions are just beginning to be evaluated, they emphasize that reliance on the platelet count as the sole criterion for evaluating the risk of either thrombosis or hemorrhage in these patients is probably overly simplistic. Some empiric support for the importance of the platelet–erythrocyte interaction derives from the observation that thrombotic phenomena are somewhat more common in patients with polycythemia vera than in patients with essential thrombocythemia despite the fact that the platelet count is often considerably higher in the latter disease. Moreover, the frequency of thrombotic episodes in polycythemia vera was found to correlate better with the hematocrit than with the platelet count.[177] Other factors must be involved, however, since within the group of patients with polycythemia vera, no simple analysis of platelet count and/or hematocrit is convincingly predictive of thrombosis.[177]

As with thrombocytopenia, it is imperative that all reports of elevated platelet counts by particle counters be confirmed by a visual estimate from the peripheral blood smear since the results may be spurious. A variety of particles, including Howell-Jolly bodies, nucleated red blood cells, cytoplasmic fragments from leukemic cells, malarial parasites, and Pappenheimer bodies, as well as paraproteins or aggregated erythrocyte stroma secondary to erythrocyte antibodies, may be mistaken for platelets by automated platelet counters based on their size and/or refractive index. If thrombocytosis is confirmed, it is important to consider its potential impact on other laboratory studies since release of platelet constituents during in vitro coagulation may result in spuriously elevated serum levels of potassium, calcium, phosphorus, uric acid, lactic acid dehydrogenase, and acid phosphatase. Attempts should thus be made to measure these substances in plasma rather than in serum.

*Reactive thrombocytosis.*[176]    Thrombocytosis may accompany a large number of *acute and chronic inflammatory* disorders (Table 4-9). *Acute hemorrhage* is also commonly associated with thrombocytosis, and sequential platelet counts may even be used to assess whether therapeutic measures to stop the bleeding have been successful. A variety of *malignant disorders* have been reported to cause thrombocytosis, but only a minority of patients with these diseases manifest increased platelet counts. *Epinephrine* administration results in the development of transient thrombocytosis; since asplenic patients fail to show this response, release of platelets from the splenic pool is presumed to be the major mechanism. *Exercise* also results in a short-lived increase in the platelet count, but the

**Table 4-9**
Reactive Thrombocytosis

Acute inflammation of diverse etiologies
Chronic inflammation
    Rheumatoid arthritis
    Polyarteritis nodosa
    Wegener's granulomatosis
    Ulcerative colitis
    Regional enteritis
    Tuberculosis
    Hepatic cirrhosis
    Chronic pneumonia
    Osteomyelitis
    Gonorrheal arthritis
Acute hemorrhage
Malignant disease of diverse types
Epinephrine
Exercise
Vincristine
"Rebound"
    Withdrawal of myelosuppressive drugs
    Vitamin $B_{12}$ therapy
Hemolytic anemias
Iron deficiency
Idiopathic sideroblastic anemia
Postsplenectomy

Adapted from Williams WJ: Thrombocytosis, in
Williams WJ et al (eds): Hematology, (2nd ed)
New York, McGraw-Hill, 1977, p. 1364. With
permission.

mechanism differs from that associated with epinephrine injection since a similar increase occurs in asplenic patients. The vinca alkaloid *vincristine* has been shown to increase the platelet counts of thrombocytopenic and nonthrombocytopenic patients alike, but the mechanism involved remains controversial. Several disorders are characterized by a *rebound thrombocytosis* following thrombocytopenia, including acute alcoholism, withdrawal of myelosuppressive drugs, and the administration of therapy for vitamin $B_{12}$ deficiency. It is reasonable to propose that the elevated counts result from a delay in the suppression of platelet production in the face of extreme stimulation, but direct data to support this view are not currently available.

The relationship between the stimulation of erythropoiesis and thrombopoiesis remains poorly defined.[102,176] The weight of current evidence indicates that purified erythropoietin does not stimulate thrombopoiesis, but several clinical observations suggest that some more complex relationship may exist. Patients with a variety of *hemolytic anemias* thus have been reported to have elevated platelet counts. Moreover, *iron deficiency anemia* is one of the most common causes of thrombocytosis (although it should be noted that the association is not invariable, and rare cases of thrombocytopenia have also been reported). Thrombocytosis has also been associated with *idiopathic sideroblastic anemia,* and its presence in that disorder has been found to correlate with a very low frequency of transformation to acute leukemia.[178] Perhaps the strongest evidence of a relationship derives from the observation that chronic *postsplenectomy* thrombocytosis (i.e., lasting for 3 or more months postoperatively) is inversely related to the postsplenectomy hemoglobin level and directly related to the postsplenectomy reticulocyte count.[179]

*Postsplenectomy thrombocytosis.*    The thrombocytosis that commonly accompanies splenectomy in the immediate postoperative period often presents management problems because of the risk of thrombohemorrhagic phenomena. The thrombocytosis is usually noted within the first few days, with the peak platelet count occurring 1–3 weeks later. In the majority of patients, the platelet count will then decrease over a period ranging from weeks to months until it returns to the normal range. A recent review of 318 patients who were not treated with anticoagulation or systematic aspirin prophylaxis found peak platelet counts of 400,000–1,000,000/μl in 53 percent of the cases, whereas 23 percent had counts greater than 1,000,000/μl.[180] A total of 10 patients (3 percent) suffered thromboembolic episodes (nine of which were thrombophlebitis and/or pulmonary embolism) in the immediate post-operative period, and although there was a trend in favor of a higher incidence in patients with thrombocytosis, it was not statistically significant. Moreover, five of the ten patients had underlying disorders (malignancies or cirrhosis) known to predispose one to thrombosis. It thus appears that the risk of thrombosis in untreated patients demonstrating thrombocytosis in the immediate postsplenectomy period is not dramatically increased and that measures beyond those that might routinely be employed for the patient's age and the nature of the surgery (e.g., minidose heparin, sequential leg compression) are probably not justified. In patients who have underlying diseases that predispose them to thrombosis, one should proba-bly consider the use of antiplatelet agents (e.g., aspirin and dipyridamole) if thrombocytosis occurs. Patients who have persistently elevated platelet counts after splenectomy have been reported to have a high incidence of both fatal and nonfatal thromboembolic phenomena. In one frequently quoted study, 5 of 49 postsplenectomy patients developed these compli-cations (2 of which were fatal), and all of them were in the group of 15 who had persistent thrombocytosis.[179] The thrombotic events, however, occurred four months, one year, five years, nine years, and ten years postsplenectomy, and other patients with equally high counts had no complications. Thus, although there may well be an increased risk, it is very hard to predict whether and when a given patient may suffer such a complication. The use of prophylactic antiplatelet agents must, therefore, be individualized based on the platelet count, the hematocrit, the presence of underlying disorders, and other pertinent clinical considerations.

*Autonomous thrombocytosis.*    Elevated platelet counts are found in all four diseases included in the myeloproliferative disorders *(essential thrombocythemia, polycythemia vera, myeloid metaplasia,* and *chronic myelogenous leukemia).*[102] In some patients there may be a transition from one form to another although a transition from chronic myelogenous leukemia to any of the others is less common than transitions between the others. Studies of glucose-6-phosphate dehydrogenase isoenzymes in all 4 myeloproliferative disorders indicate that these are clonal diseases and that the megakaryocytes are part of the disor-dered clone.[102,181]

*Essential thrombocythemia* is characterized by elevated platelet counts (almost al-ways above 1,000,000/μl) and morphologic evidence of a dramatic increase in megakaryo-cyte mass.[102,182] The platelets are quite large when assessed on blood smear or by particle counter and often have a variety of morphologic abnormalities, including decreased granula-tion and a more spherical shape than normal. Electron microscopy of platelets has revealed decreased microtubules, hypertrophy of the membranes of the dense tubular and open canalicular systems, and abnormal persistence of small amounts of nuclear material. The white blood cell count is commonly elevated and has been reported to be above 30,000/$\mu$l in as many as 40 percent of cases. A slight shift to the left is not uncommon, but immature granulocytic cells are only rarely encountered. When hemorrhage does not result in anemia, most patients will have normal or slightly increased hematocrits and the erythrocyte morphology is usually unremarkable. The spleen is increased in size in the majority of patients, but splenic atrophy secondary to infarction has also been reported. Removal of the spleen may result in catastrophic exacerbation of essential thrombocythemia (and may unmask this disease if performed on patients with the other myeloproliferative disorders), and thus is to be avoided unless other considerations make it absolutely necessary. Bone marrow examination usually shows generalized hyperplasia with a dramatic increase in both the size and number of megakaryocytes, many of which demonstrate features of dyspoiesis; increased fibrosis is quite common, reinforcing the relationship between this disorder and myeloid metaplasia. A specific chromosal abnormality (21q-) has been reported.[182]

Clinically, both hemorrhage and thrombosis occur and the relative frequencies of these complications vary from series to series.[182a] The gastrointestinal tract is the most common site of hemorrhage, but hematuria and easy bruising also occur. Thrombosis can occur in either the arterial or venous circulations; leg and portal-mesenteric vein thrombosis and cerebral, coronary, and peripheral arterial diseases are most common. One particular manifestation of peripheral arterial disease that deserves mention is the purple and painful toe and/or finger syndrome that is thought to reflect digital ischemia. Antiplatelet agents usually produce a dramatic improvement in these cases.[183,184]

Several studies of platelet function have been undertaken in an attempt to define abnormalities that may help predict which patients will develop hemorrhagic and/or thrombotic complications.[102,185] The bleeding time is prolonged in only a small minority of patients, and there is no clear correlation between this test and the tendency for hemorrhage. Abnormalities in platelet aggregation have been found in the majority of patients, with the most consistent finding being a remarkable decrease in epinephrine-induced aggregation such that not even a primary wave is obtained.[186] This defect appears to be quite specific for the myeloproliferative disorders and may even be of diagnostic help when one is not certain whether a patient's thrombocytosis is reactive or autonomous. However, although abnormalities in epinephrine-induced aggregation have correlated with the presence of hemorrhagic (and/or thrombotic) complications in some series, other studies have not found such an association. A recent study found that the platelets from two patients with essential thrombocythemia that failed to aggregate in response to epinephrine had fewer than one-half the number of $\alpha$-adrenergic receptors found on either normal platelets or platelets from patients with essential thrombocythemia who did respond to epinephrine.[186] Platelets from some patients with this disorder fail to produce one of the end products of prostaglandin metabolism, and although it has been suggested that this abnormality may correlate with clinical evidence of hemorrhage,[187] additional studies will be required to confirm this association. Similarly, preliminary reports indicating a correlation between hemorrhage and decreased platelet coagulant activities will require confirmation.[188,189] A variety of other in vitro platelet abnormalities have been described in essential thrombocythemia, including a deficiency of the storage pool of adenine nucleotides, but none of these has been documented to correlate with hemorrhage.[190]

Attempts to define in vitro assays to predict thrombosis have also been made. Increased levels of circulating platelet aggregates and increases in platelet coagulant activities have been reported to be useful in predicting which patients will have thrombotic complications.[184,188] Spontaneous platelet aggregation was found to correlate with thrombotic episodes in one study but not in another.[183,184] A defect in response to the inhibitory prostaglandin, $PGD_2$, has been found in the platelets of patients with all 4 myeloprolifera-

**Table 4-10**

Regimens for Treatment of Thrombocytosis

---

Radioactive phosphorus, 2.7 mCi/m$^2$. Repeat every 3 months when platelet count is > 600,000/μl.

Busulfan, 4 mg daily, until platelet count is <600,000μl. Then adjust continuous maintenance dose to keep platelet count below this level.

Melphalan, 10 mg daily for 7 days. Begin maintenance dose at 2 mg daily and adjust to keep platelet count <600,000/μl.

---

Adapted from Murphy S: Disorders of platelet production, in Colman RW et al (eds): Thrombosis and Hemostasis, Basic Principles and Clinical Practice, Philadelphia, JB Lippincott, 1982, p. 271. With permission.

tive disorders, apparently as a result of a decrease in the number of platelet PGD$_2$ binding sites.[191] It has been proposed that the PGD$_2$ synthesized by platelets is a physiologic regulator of platelet function and that the thrombotic tendency in these patients may result from this decreased inhibitory response.[191] This hypothesis, although attractive, is weakened by the observation that the marked overproduction of PGD$_2$ (18–120-fold) found in systemic mastocytosis is not associated with a bleeding diathesis.[192] Moreover, there was only a poor correlation between the decreased response to PGD$_2$ and a history of thrombosis in the patients studied.[191] At present, therefore, in vitro studies offer little prognostic information, and the clinician must be extremely cautious in deciding on therapeutic interventions lest he exacerbate the patient's problems.

Therapy in symptomatic patients with essential thrombocythemia should be directed primarily at controlling the platelet count, whereas antiplatelet therapy should be judiciously employed for those with thrombotic phenomena. Abrupt reductions in the platelet count can be achieved with the cell-separating instruments available, but the cost and inconvenience dictate that this therapy be reserved for acutely symptomatic patients. Radioactive phosphorus and several chemotherapeutic agents have been employed to reduce the platelet count,[191a] and the regimens recommended by Murphy are listed in Table 4-10.[102] Virtually all patients will respond to any of these regimens and attain a platelet count below 600,000/μl within 1–5 months, with the majority responding within the first 3 months. Treatment of asymptomatic patients is less clear-cut, since some of them will remain free of complications for many years without therapy and since the risk of inducing leukemia with radioactive phosphorus and alkylating agents is well established. Under these circumstances, the decision to treat must rest on an analysis of the patient's age, underlying diseases, platelet count, and hematocrit.

In patients manifesting definite thrombotic complications—in particular, painful and/or blue toes or fingers secondary to digital ischemia—antiplatelet agents (aspirin and dipyidamole) should be instituted immediately and maintained until the platelet count is lowered by definitive therapy. In cases in which it is uncertain whether there is a thrombotic complication related to the elevated platelet count, the author performs a bleeding time; if it is normal, antiplatelet therapy is instituted. If it is abnormally prolonged, the strength of the data supporting the presence of a thrombotic disorder is reassessed before instituting therapy. There are few long-term studies in these patients, but at least one report indicates that if the platelet count is well maintained, the patient may have quite a good long-term prognosis with long, unmaintained remissions.[183]

The other myeloproliferative disorders are also associated with thrombocytosis. A comparison of the platelet counts and the frequency of complications compiled by Murphy are presented in Table 4-11.[102] *Polycythemia vera* is characterized by less strikingly elevated platelet counts but a higher frequency of thrombotic disorders. As mentioned above,

**Table 4-11**

Frequency of Thrombotic and Hemorrhagic Complications in the
Myeloproliferative Disorders

|  | PV* | ET* | AMM* | CML* |
|---|---|---|---|---|
| Frequency of complications† | | | | |
| Thrombotic | + + + + | + + + | + + | + |
| Hemorrhagic | + + + | + + + + | + + + | + |
| Incidence of Thrombocytosis (%) | | | | |
| >400,000/μl | 65 | 0 | 30 | 65 |
| >1,000,000/μl | 10 | 100‡ | 5 | 25 |

Adapted from Murphy S: Disorders of platelet production, in Colman RW, et al (eds): Thrombosis and Hemostasis,
Basic Principles and Clinical Practice, Philadelphia, JB Lippincott, 1982, p. 269. With permission.
*PV, polycythemia vera; ET, essential thrombocythemia; AMM, agnogenic myeloid metaplasia; CML, chronic
myelogenous leukemia.
† + + + +, very common; + + +, common; + +, uncommon; +, rare; 0, absent.
‡Most series have required that the platelet count be >1,000,000/μl for entry.

if one adjusts for the differences in hematocrit, the concentration of platelets in the plasma
space in this disorder may be the same as or greater than that in essential thrombocythemia.
This finding, in conjunction with the rheologic and viscosity changes in this disorder, may
furnish an adequate explanation for the high frequency of thrombosis. Platelet functional
abnormalities, in particular an absence of the primary wave of epinephrine-induced
aggregation, are found in a significant number of patients.[193] *Myeloid metaplasia* is characterized by even less strikingly elevated platelet counts but by a relativey higher frequency
of hemorrhagic manifestations. Studies of platelet function, including bleeding times and
platelet aggregation, have found the highest frequency of abnormalities in this disease.
These functional abnormalities may, therefore, be making a significant contribution to the
hemorrhagic tendency.[102] *Chronic granulocytic leukemia* tends to stand apart from the
other disorders in that the frequency of both hemorrhagic and thrombotic complications is
much lower despite considerable increases in the platelet count.[194] No acceptable explanation for this observation has been advanced.

## Qualitative Platelet Disorders[114,195-197]

When the patient's history suggests a disorder of hemostasis and the platelet count
and tests of coagulation are normal, a qualitative platelet disorder should be considered. It
should be emphasized that, with the exception of the mild abnormality induced by the
nearly ubiquitous use of aspirin, these disorders are much less common than the quantitative platelet disorders. Figure 4-14 is a flowsheet for the evaluation of these disorders
based upon an orderly sequence of laboratory studies, although an attempt has been made
to group the disorders according to their pathophysiology as much as possible.

### Isolated PF 3 Deficiency

The bleeding time performed according to the template modification of the Ivy technique is probably the most sensitive test of platelet plug formation. It is abnormal, though
to a variable extent, in all of the qualitative platelet disorders except for isolated deficiency of PF 3, a condition in which the defect is in the platelet's ability to accelerate the
generation of thrombin, not in platelet plug formation. Only five patients have been re-

## Qualitative Platelet Disorders

**Bleeding time**

- **Increased**
  - **Platelet retention**
    - **Markedly decreased**
      - **Platelet aggregation/agglutination**
        - **Abnormal primary wave**
          1. Fibrinogen dependent (ADP, etc.)
             a) Afibrinogenemia
             b) Thrombasthenia
          2. Von Willebrand factor dependent (ristocetin, etc.)
             a Von Willebrand's disease
             b Bernard-Soulier syndrome
          3. Drugs
             a Penicillin derivatives
             b Ticlopidine
          4. Hypergammaglobulinemia
    - **Decreased or normal**
      - **Platelet aggregation**
        - **Variably abnormal second wave**
          Uremia
        - **Normal**

- **Normal**
  - **Serum prothrombin time**
    - **Decreased**
      Isolated PF 3 abnormality
    - **Normal**
      1. Normal initial slope von Willebrand factor-dependent aggregation
      2. ADP and epinephrine aggregation: normal first wave, absent second wave

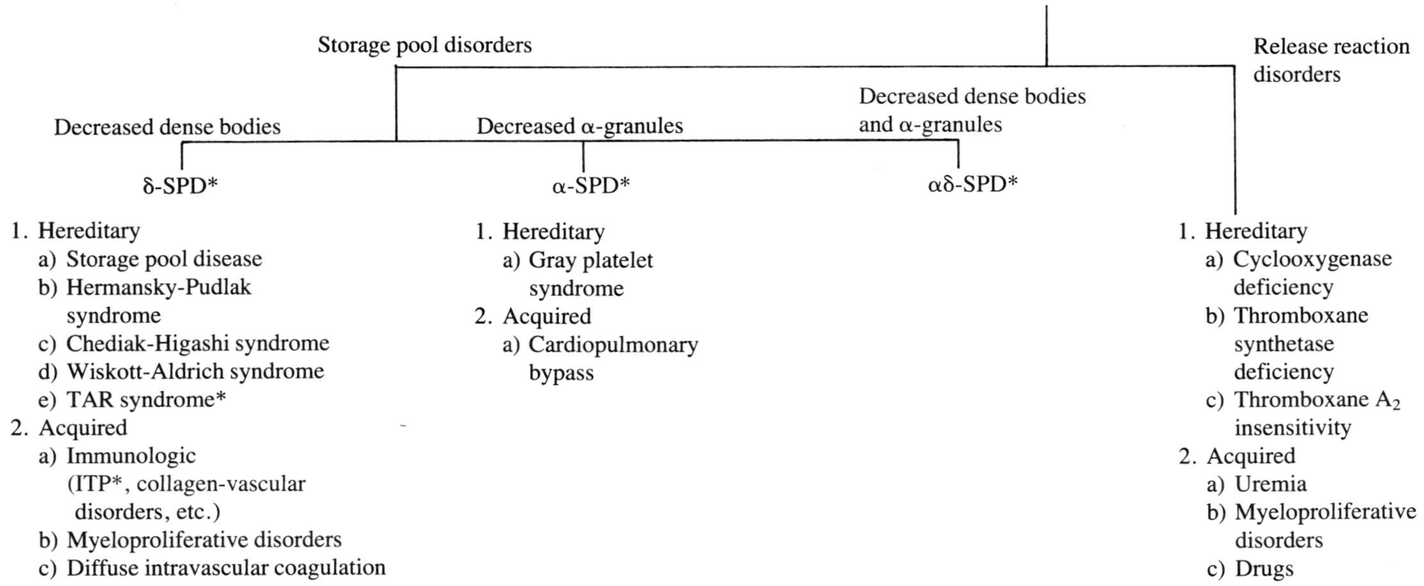

Storage pool disorders

Release reaction disorders

Decreased dense bodies
δ-SPD*

Decreased α-granules
α-SPD*

Decreased dense bodies and α-granules
αδ-SPD*

**Decreased dense bodies — δ-SPD***

1. Hereditary
   a) Storage pool disease
   b) Hermansky-Pudlak syndrome
   c) Chediak-Higashi syndrome
   d) Wiskott-Aldrich syndrome
   e) TAR syndrome*
2. Acquired
   a) Immunologic (ITP*, collagen-vascular disorders, etc.)
   b) Myeloproliferative disorders
   c) Diffuse intravascular coagulation

**Decreased α-granules — α-SPD***

1. Hereditary
   a) Gray platelet syndrome
2. Acquired
   a) Cardiopulmonary bypass

**Release reaction disorders**

1. Hereditary
   a) Cyclooxygenase deficiency
   b) Thromboxane synthetase deficiency
   c) Thromboxane A$_2$ insensitivity
2. Acquired
   a) Uremia
   b) Myeloproliferative disorders
   c) Drugs

**Fig. 4-14.** Qualitative platelet disorders.

*SPD, Storage pool disease; TAR, thrombocytopenia with absent radii; ITP, idiopathic thrombocytopenic purpura.

145

**Table 4-12**

Isolated PF 3 Deficiency

| | |
|---|---|
| Platelet count | Normal |
| Bleeding time | Normal |
| Platelet morphology | |
|   Light microscope | Normal |
|   Electron microscope | Normal |
| Platelet retention | Normal |
| Platelet interaction with subendothelium | |
|   Adhesion | Normal |
| Platelet aggregation | |
|   ADP | Normal |
|   Epinephrine | Normal |
|   Collagen | Normal |
|   Ristocetin | Normal |
| Platelet release of | |
|   ADP by | |
|     Thrombin | Normal |
|     Kaolin | Normal |
|   Serotonin by | |
|     Kaolin | Decreased |
|   $\beta$-$N$-Acetyl glucosaminidase by | |
|     Thrombin | Normal |
| Prothrombin consumption | Decreased |
| "PF-3" | |
|   Kaolin-induced by: | |
|     Recalcifiction time | Decreased |
|     Russell's viper time | Decreased |
|   Freezing and thawing induced by | |
|     Recalcification time | Decreased |
|     Russell's viper time | Decreased |

ported with this disorder, and in two it appeared to be secondary to other coexisting diseases (Ehlers-Danlos syndrome and Hashimoto's thyroiditis in one and chronic myelocytic leukemia in the other).[198-200] All three patients in whom the defect was present in an isolated fashion had significant but variable bleeding histories. One patient had had an uncomplicated appendectomy at age three, but she subsequently bled excessively after tooth extraction, tonsillectomy, parturition, and hysterectomy; she also suffered a spontaneous retroperitoneal hemorrhage. The second patient's symptoms began at age three and included multiple episodes of abrupt, severe hemorrhage in muscles in addition to a single posttraumatic hemarthrosis. The third patient had a lifelong history of epistaxis and suffered from severe postpartum hemorrhage, menorrhagia, and bleeding after tooth extraction. None of the patients had a family history of abnormal hemostasis. A patient with a similar history and laboratory findings, but with a markedly prolonged bleeding time, has also been reported, suggesting heterogeneity in the defects in this disorder.[201]

The laboratory data on these patients are shown in Table 4-12. The shortened serum prothrombin time, a reflection of decreased prothrombin consumption during the clotting of whole blood, is the most consistent abnormality. Since this assay is easy to perform, it is reasonable to use it as a screening test for this disorder. Specific assays of PF 3 are abnormal whether measured as that fraction which is made available by a variety of inducers (most commonly kaolin) or as the total amount of PF 3 (determined after freezing and thawing). Since prothrombin consumption and the inducible PF 3 activity will also be abnormal in many other disorders of platelet function, it is very important to assess both PF 3 and platelet aggregation.

Whereas it is now believed that assays of PF 3 reflect contributions from both the platelet phospholipids and the presence of activated factor V bound specifically to the platelet, so that a defect in one or the other of these systems could result in a decrease in measurable PF 3 activity. One patient has, in fact, been studied in detail and found to have normal quantities of platelet phospholipids, but a 75–80 percent decrease in the number of binding sites for activated factor V.[199,202] Therapeutically, platelet transfusions have been effective in both preventing and treating hemorrhage. Interestingly, one patient had a consistent response to prothrombin complex concentrates, suggesting the possibility that activated factors present in these products may have bypassed the need for PF 3.

### Disorders with Markedly Reduced Platelet Retention

The platelet retention test can distinguish a group of disorders in which the test is severely abnormal from another group in which it is either normal or only mildly abnormal. Many laboratories, however, do not use this assay because it lacks specificity and requires considerable technical competence in both preparing the columns and performing the test. Although it does not offer definitive information concerning the site of the defect, the author has found the retention test to be useful in several settings: (1) as probably the most sensitive test for mild von Willebrand's disease (see Chapter 6 below), (2) in helping to decide when a platelet function defect is present when other studies are equivocal, and (3) in helping to distinguish aspirin ingestion (which does not result in abnormal retention) from other release reaction defects and storage-pool diseases, which usually are associated with abnormal retention.

The disorders in which platelet retention is markedly decreased include (1) a decrease in plasma fibrinogen (afibrinogenemia) or a platelet defect resulting in an inability to bind fibrinogen (thrombasthenia), (2) a decrease in plasma von Willebrand factor activity (von Willebrand's disease) or a platelet defect resulting in an inability to bind von Willebrand factor (Bernard-Soulier syndrome), or (3) uremia, in which the defect is unknown. In addition, several drugs (penicillin derivatives and ticlopidine) can induce a similar abnormality.

*Afibrinogenemia.*[203,204]  In this rare disorder, there may be abnormalities in fibrinogen-dependent platelet function, including prolonged bleeding times; abnormal primary platelet aggregation induced by ADP, epinephrine, and thrombin; abnormal platelet retention; and abnormal spreading of platelets on glass. Clinical symptoms are quite variable but may be severe, with muscle and joint bleeding in addition to mucocutaneous bruising. Needless to say, it is impossible to differentiate clinical hemorrhage due to lack of clot formation from that due to defective platelet function. Therapy for bleeding episodes consists of fibrinogen replacement with cryoprecipitate, with hemostasis usually achieved at fibrinogen concentrations of 50–100 mg/dl.

*Glanzmann's thrombasthenia.*  This is a rare hemorrhagic disorder characterized by abnormal platelet function. The clinical manifestations of the 30 patients from 26 families reported in the English literature since the aggregometer became available for definitive diagnosis have recently been reviewed by George and Reimann;[205] similar findings were reported by Reichert et al. in the 42 patients with thrombasthenia they identified in the Iraqi-Jewish population in Israel.[205a] Mucocutaneous hemorrhage predominates, with epistaxis and easy bruising in addition to petechial, menorrhagic, gingival, gastrointestinal, post-tooth extraction, postpartum, and postoperative bleeding. Hemarthroses are rare but have been reported. Onset of symptoms can occur at birth, and most patients become symptomatic within the first year of life. Excerpts from the histories of a severely affected and a mildly affected patient reported by Caen et al.[206] are reproduced below.

[Severely affected.] Since [age 3] epistaxis has recurred at intervals not longer than three months. Following the loss of the first dentition there was bleeding from the gums, and hemorrhage occurred once from infected adenoids. Severe cutaneous bleeding has been occasioned by venipuncture and bleeding time determination. The patient has received transfusions fourteen times, variously with fresh whole blood, platelet rich plasma and platelet concentrates . . . p.7.

[Mildly affected.] Although this patient has a mild form of the disease, menorrhagia has complicated the history since the menarche at thirteen years. The first hemorrhagic manifestation was at the age of eight months when severe epistaxis persisted for three days. Except for occasional bruising and mild epistaxis lasting from two to three days and recurring three or four times each year, the patient was well; she received no treatment until the onset of menstruation at thirteen years of age which necessitated blood transfusion. Since that time, despite an attempt to control menstruation with estrogen therapy, menorrhagia has been sufficiently severe to require blood transfusion on three further occasions. p.7.

It is interesting to note that although menorrhagia is both a common and a severe symptom, spontaneous parturition has been reported to occur without incident in several patients, although profuse bleeding has been reported in at least one patient.[114] In contrast, spontaneous abortions appear to be more commonly associated with serious hemorrhage.

Genetics. All currently available data point to an autosomal recessive mode of inheritance since (1) the sexes appear to be affected equally; (2) consanguinity was present in 4 of the 26 families reviewed by George and Reiman[205] and in a higher percentage of the Iraqi-Jewish patients[205a], and (3) the parents of thrombasthenics are minimally symptomatic or asymptomatic. More recent analyses of platelet membrane glycoproteins in patients and family members also support an autosomal recessive inheritance pattern and permit the identification of heterozygotes.[207,208,208a]

Laboratory studies. The results of laboratory studies in patients with thrombasthenia are listed in Table 4-13. The diagnosis is made easily since the failure to obtain primary platelet aggregation with ADP or thrombin is virtually unique to this disorder. There is heterogeneity among patients with thrombasthenia, as manifested by significant variations in the extent of impairment of clot retraction, the reductions in GPIIb and GPIII, and the deficiencies in platelet fibrinogen. It has been reported that in a given patient there is a concordance in the above defects, thus allowing for easy division into those with absent (type I) or reduced (type II) levels,[26] but other studies have challenged this scheme.[209] Two unusual patients with thrombasthenia have been reported who have the characteristic clinical and laboratory abnormalities except that their platelets contain normal amounts of GPIIb and GPIII.[209a,209b] Qualitative defects in the glycoproteins affecting their ability to complex normally may be responsible for this form of the disease.[209b]

Pathophysiology. Although multiple enzymatic deficiencies, primarily affecting the platelet's reductive capacity, have been described in thrombasthenia,[196] it is the defects in membrane GPIIb and GPIII[210,211] that are believed to be responsible for the major manifestations of the disorder. The platelet surface antigen defects probably result from GPIIb and GPIII serving as precursor molecules on which these antigens are expressed.[29,30] Most importantly, the inability of thrombasthenic platelets to bind fibrinogen[24,25] suggests a unifying hypothesis to explain the failure of clot retraction and aggregation induced by all

**Table 4-13**

Thrombasthenia

| | |
|---|---|
| Platelet count | Normal |
| Bleeding time | Prolonged |
| Platelet morphology | |
|    Light microscope | Normal |
|    Electron microscope | Normal |
| Clot retraction | Decreased |
| Platelet retention | Decreased |
| Platelet spreading on glass | Decreased |
| Platelet interaction with subendothelium* | |
|    Adhesion | Normal |
|    Aggregation | Decreased |
| Electrophoretic mobility | Conflicting results |
| Platelet aggregation | |
|    ADP | Absent primary and second waves |
|    Epinephrine | Absent primary and second waves |
|    Collagen | Decreased |
|    Thrombin | Absent |
|    Ristocetin† | Cyclical |
| ADP and thrombin binding | Normal |
| Shape change | Normal |
| Platelet release | |
|    ADP, epinephrine | Decreased |
|    Thrombin, collagen | Normal |
| PF3 | Decreased |
| Prothrombin consumption | Variable results |
| Platelet fibrinogen | Decreased or absent |
| Platelet binding of fibrinogen | Decreased or absent |
| Glycoproteins | |
|    Ib | Normal or increased |
|    IIb | Decreased or absent |
|    III | Decreased or absent |
|    V | Normal |
| Platelet surface antigens | |
|    $Pl^{A1}$   ($Zw^a$) | Reduced or absent |
|    $Pl^{A2}$   ($Zw^b$) | Reduced or absent |
|       $Ko^a$ | ? |
|       $Ko^b$ | Normal |
|       $Pl^{E1}$ | ? |
|       $Pl^{E2}$ | ? |
|       $Bak^a$ | Absent |
|       EDTA-dependent antibody sites | Reduced or absent |

*See reference 216.
†See reference 217.

of the agonists that are known to expose the fibrinogen receptor (ADP, epinephrine, thrombin, collagen). It is tempting, therefore, to hypothesize that GPIIb and GPIII are, in fact, involved in fibrinogen binding. Strong preliminary data do support this view,[27,27a,27b] but some controversy persists.[28,212] The contribution, if any, to the hemorrhagic diathesis produced by the defect in binding von Willebrand factor when thrombastheric platelets are stimulated with thrombin[28a] remains to be defined.

The reduction or absence of platelet fibrinogen in thrombasthenia is an intriguing finding with important implications for the origin of this protein. Since platelet fibrinogen is localized to the α-granules, it is reasonable to suggest that megakaryocytes synthesize and transport it to the granules before megakaryocyte fragmentation and release of platelets into the circulation. Synthesis of fibrinogen by megakaryocytes, however, has not been demonstrated to date; moreover, it would suggest the seemingly unlikely possibility that thrombasthenics have a fibrinogen synthesis defect isolated to their megakaryocytes (their plasma fibrinogen levels are normal) in addition to the GPIIb and GPIII defects. Alternative hypotheses, in which GPIIb and GPIIIa are either involved in taking up fibrinogen from plasma or keeping the fibrinogen in α-granules, appear to have simplicity on their side but remain undocumented. The recent report of the presence of GPIIb and GPIII in the α-granule membranes of normal platelets[213] is consistent with these latter hypotheses. Considerable controversy persists, however, as to whether unstimulated platelets can bind fibrinogen and whether normal platelets have fibrinogen on their surface.[24,25]

It is also interesting to speculate on how a genetic alteration that presumably affects only a single site results in a marked reduction of 2 separate proteins. Among the alternatives, one might consider that (1) the genes for GPIIb and GPIII are adjacent to each other on the DNA and are transcribed as a single unit, (2) the defect is in an enzyme required for a posttranslational modification of both glycoproteins, or (3) one of the glycoproteins serves as a binding site for the other.

Treatment. With the exception of hormonal agents to control menses, the only available therapy is platelet transfusion.[214] Since nearly all patients may ultimately become refractory to platelet transfusions as a result of antibody development, it is reasonable to try to withhold transfusion unless clinical hemorrhage is significant. The use of HLA-matched platelets may be helpful. The most serious complication in these patients, however, is the development of an antibody against the antigens missing from thrombasthenic platelets since this antibody may actually interfere with the function of transfused platelets.[215] When dealing with such a patient and a severe hemorrhage, it would be reasonable to consider plasmapheresis in addition to platelet transfusions.

*Von Willebrand's disease.*   See Chapter 6.

*Bernard-Soulier syndrome.*   This rare hemorrhagic disorder is characterized by the combination of large platelets, mild thrombocytopenia, and a severe defect in von Willebrand factor-dependent platelet function. The clinical manifestations of the 16 patients from 13 families reported in the literature who meet the criteria for diagnosis have recently been reviewed by George and Reimann.[205] Mucocutaneous and posttraumatic bleeding predominate, with the onset usually in early infancy (often at circumcision). Hemorrhage is variable but often severe, as judged by the need for transfusion in many of the reported cases. A typical history from the report by Maldonado et al.[218] is presented:

The patient had bled profusely at circumcision when 2 months old, and at age 2 years he had a massive hematoma of the forehead after a blow to his head. Abnormal bruising and bleeding occurred at age 3½ from an injured toe and another head injury. At age 5, facial petechiae were noted after a severe bout of coughing. When he was 6 years old, a tooth was knocked loose and he had

**Table 4-14**

Bernard-Soulier Syndrome

| | |
|---|---|
| Platelet count | Decreased |
| Platelet survival | Decreased |
| Bleeding time | Prolonged |
| Platelet morphology | |
|    Light microscope | Large, increased granules |
|    Electron microscope | Nonspecific changes |
| Shape change | Decreased |
| Clot retraction | Decreased |
| Platelet retention | Decreased |
| Platelet interaction with subendothelium | |
|    Adhesion | Decreased |
|    Aggregation | Normal |
| Electrophoretic mobility | Decreased |
| Platelet aggregation | |
|    ADP | Normal or increased |
|    Epinephrine | Normal or increased |
|    Collagen | Normal |
|    Thrombin | Decreased |
|    Ristocetin | Absent |
|    Bovine von Willebrand factor | Absent |
| Prothrombin consumption | Decreased |
| PF3 | Decreased |
| Platelet von Willebrand factor | Normal |
| Platelet-binding of von Willebrand factor | Decreased |
| Glycoproteins | |
|    Ib | Decreased or absent |
|    IIb | Normal |
|    III | Normal |
|    V | Decreased or absent |
|    GP17 | Decreased or absent |

bled profusely. At age 9, his gums were lacerated accidentally by a dental drill and bleeding persisted for 3 weeks. About 1 year later, he fell and suffered multiple lacerations and bruises of the extremities. Infusion of platelet concentrates appeared to control the bleeding. Frequent epistaxis and easy bruising persisted. . . . p. 402.

The expected laboratory data are listed in Table 4-14. The marked decrease in platelet GPIb is probably responsible for many of the observed abnormalities: (1) Since GPIb is extremely rich in the negatively charged carbohydrate sialic acid, the surface charge of the platelets, and thus their electrophoretic mobility, is decreased. (2) Since a normal complement of surface sialic acid appears to be required for normal platelet survival, the survival of Bernard-Soulier platelets is significantly decreased. (3) The decrease in platelet survival is probably the major cause of thrombocytopenia. (4) There is considerable evidence that GPIb is the receptor for von Willebrand factor when platelets are stimulated with ristocetin and when platelets adhere to subendothelial structures, explaining the severe defect in von Willebrand factor-dependent platelet function (bleeding time, platelet retention, adhesion, ristocetin- and bovine von Willebrand factor-induced agglutination).[17,219] The defect(s) resulting in decreased thrombin-induced platelet aggregation is less clear. It may also be a result of the GPIb deficiency since thrombin binds to GPIb.[17] Alternatively or additionally, the deficiency in platelet GPV may be responsible for the thrombin-induced aggregation defect since this glycoprotein appears to be a substrate for the proteolytic action of thrombin.[34,70] The reason(s) why Bernard-Soulier platelets do not support the normal consumption of prothrombin during clotting remains unknown[221], but several defects in their facilitation of thrombin generation have been reported.[220]

Autosomal recessive inheritance has been proposed for the disorder based upon the high frequency of consanguinity in the reported cases and the absence of hemorrhagic symptoms in the parents.[205] Careful analysis, however, revealed that some of the parents of affected individuals did have abnormally large platelets and decreased amounts of GPIb, indicating that there is subtle expression of the defect in presumed heterozygotes. Despite these abnormalities, parents whose platelets contained a 50 percent decrease in GPIb had normal hemostasis.[222]

Platelet transfusion is the mainstay of therapy. The risk of sensitization makes it prudent to reserve transfusion for significant hemorrhage. Moreover, a patient who had received many transfusions developed an antibody that was apparently directed against GPIb and inhibited von Willebrand factor-dependent platelet function.[222a] Hormonal therapy to prevent menstruation is an important adjunctive measure since menorrhagia is often a problem. Neither splenectomy nor corticosteroid therapy has been of demonstrable benefit.

*Uremia.*[195,223,224]   Uremic patients are known to suffer from an increased risk of hemorrhage. The effect of renal failure upon hemostasis is discussed at length in Chapter 15. Defective platelet function is thought to be the major cause of bleeding since mucocutaneous sites are most commonly affected and since prolongation of the bleeding time and decreased platelet retention are the most consistent laboratory abnormalities. Additional but more variable abnormalities have been found in prothrombin consumption, PF 3 availability and total PF 3, and platelet aggregation induced by ADP, epinephrine, and collagen. Several metabolites known to accumulate in uremia have been proposed as platelet toxins (urea, guanidinosuccinic acid, phenol, phenolic acids, "middle molecules"), but the data remain inconclusive.[223–225] More recently several other causes for the defective platelet function have been proposed: (1) a qualitative abnormality in ristocetin cofactor activity (found in uremic patients in one study, but normal or increased values were found in several other studies),[226,227] (2) defective prostaglandin synthesis,[195,224] and (3) increased $PGI_2$ synthesis.[228,229]

Clinically, the introduction of dialysis has dramatically decreased the risk of serious bleeding in uremic patients, giving strong support to the contention that the defect is not intrinsic to the platelet. It has been pointed out, however, that avoidance of drugs that interfere with platelet function and careful attention to vitamin K therapy to avoid the superimposition of a coagulation defect may have also contributed to this improvement.[223,224] Available evidence suggests that peritoneal dialysis is more effective in reversing the platelet defect than hemodialysis, either as a result of the inefficiency in removing specific molecules by hemodialysis or damage inflicted on platelets by the dialysis membrane.[224] The bleeding time is the best predictor of the likelihood of excessive bleeding. Occasional patients will have serious hemorrhage despite dialysis. A recent report indicates that cryoprecipitate is effective in correcting both the bleeding time and the clinical hemorrhage in these patients;[230] the mechanism remains unclear. Similarly, the infusion of deamino-8-D-arginine vasopressin, an agent known to release von Willebrand factor from endothelial cells, into uremic patients also shortens the bleeding time.[230a] In bleeding patients who have even mild thrombocytopenia in conjunction with uremia, platelet transfusions may help to control the bleeding.

*Penicillin and its derivatives.*[224,231]   High doses of penicillin G, carbenicillin, and ticarcillin have been shown to produce a rather striking defect in platelet function that is associated with an increased risk of hemorrhage. There is a time lag between administration of the drug and the onset of platelet abnormalities, suggesting either that the active agent is a metabolite of the administered drug or that a prolonged exposure to the administered drug is necessary for the defect to develop. The abnormalities can be reproduced by the drugs in vitro, but the concentrations required are higher than those achieved in vivo. In addition to prolonging the bleeding time and decreasing platelet retention, the antibiotics appear to interfere with both fibrinogen- and von Willebrand factor-dependent platelet function as judged by a decrease in the primary waves of aggregation induced by ADP, epinephrine, collagen, ristocetin, and bovine von Willebrand factor. The platelet's adenine nucleotides and prostaglandin synthetic capacity are not affected. In vitro studies suggest that these antibiotics decrease the binding of ADP, epinephrine, and von Willebrand factor to the platelet, presumably on the basis of a nonspecific "coating" effect. Carbenicillin and ticarcillin are equipotent in producing platelet abnormalities, but ticarcillin is used in lower doses to treat infection, so that the latter is preferable for maintaining hemostasis. Recognition of the antiplatelet effect of these drugs is especially important when high doses are administered to immunocompromised hosts who may also be thrombocytopenic. Should hemorrhage occur, the drug should be discontinued if possible, but platelet transfusions will probably also be needed since the platelet defect tends to persist for more than a week after drug withdrawal.

*Ticlopidine.*[232]   This new antiplatelet agent prolongs the bleeding time and inhibits the primary wave of fibrinogen-dependent platelet aggregation when administered orally. It is currently undergoing trials as an antithrombotic agent.

*Hypergammaglobulinemia.*[233]   Although hypergammaglobulinemia is known to produce abnormalities in clot formation as a result of its effects on the conversion of fibrinogen to fibrin, it appears as if a bleeding diathesis due to abnormal platelet function is present in some patients with multiple myeloma. Prolongation of the bleeding time and decreased platelet retention, along with variable abnormalities in platelet aggregation, are the most characteristic findings. There is said to be a reasonably good correlation between the plasma concentration of the myeloma protein and the degree of platelet dysfunction. Patients with IgA myeloma may have a disproportionately high risk of having platelet abnormalities. When the immunoglobulin level is reduced to normal, the platelet function defects disappear. Protein coating of the platelet surface has been proposed to explain these phenomena and, in fact, it has recently been shown that there is an increase in firmly bound, platelet-associated IgG whenever the plasma level of IgG is increased, even in benign diseases such as systemic lupus erythematosus and rheumatoid arthritis.[233] This last observation has significant implications for the interpretation of increased levels of platelet-associated IgG as evidence in favor of an autoimmune platelet disorder in these hypergammaglobulinemic states.

### Second-Wave Aggregation Defects

The second wave of fibrinogen-dependent platelet aggregation requires an intact release reaction mechanism and a normal pool of platelet-active agents in the platelet granules, especially ADP in the dense granules. Defects in either of these processes thus result in abnormal platelet aggregation. Recent advances in the analysis of platelet function have permitted these disorders to be subdivided into those in which the primary defect is in the release reaction mechanism and those in which there is a storage granule defect. The latter can be further subdivided into those in which the dense bodies are primarily affected ($\delta$-storage pool disorder), those in which the $\alpha$-granules are primarily affected ($\alpha$-storage pool disorder), and those in which both types of granules are affected ($\alpha\delta$-storage pool disorder). Further subdivision of the abnormalities in second-wave aggregation can be made on the basis of whether the disorder is hereditary or acquired. It should be emphasized that despite the subcategorization of these disorders, there remains considerable heterogeneity within each group in both the clinical and laboratory expression of the diseases.

*Hereditary release reaction disorders.*[195,234,235] The full expression of the platelet release reaction appears to require (1) release of arachidonic acid from phospholipid followed by its conversion into thromboxane $A_2$, and (2) the action of thromboxane $A_2$ at some still unknown site, resulting in the release of calcium into the cytoplasm. As might be expected, there are multiple sites at which a defect can occur in this complex mechanism. Thus, although these disorders were originally described simply as "aspirin-like" defects, in some patients it has been possible to identify the locus of the abnormality more precisely.

**Cyclooxygenase deficiency.**[234,236–238] Cyclooxygenase is one of the enzymes required for the conversion of arachidonic acid to thromboxane $A_2$. Four unrelated patients with a deficiency of this enzyme have been reported. Clinically, they had mild lifelong bleeding disorders with mucocutaneous bleeding but little postpartum or postsurgical hemorrhage. The inheritance of the disorder is unclear, but it is interesting to note that all four cases occurred in women. The bleeding time is only slightly prolonged. Platelet retention in a glass bead column was abnormal in the two patients in whom it was tested. This finding may be useful in differentiating this disorder from the effect of aspirin ingestion since platelet retention is not affected by aspirin. Although ADP and epinephrine failed to produce the release reaction, thrombin did cause release since it can activate a mechanism independent of prostaglandin synthesis. The presence of normal thrombin-induced release is useful in distinguishing this disorder from the $\delta$-storage pool disorders in which thrombin does not result in secretion. This essentially normal platelet response to thrombin has been proposed as a possible explanation for the freedom from severe postoperative hemorrhage, since in the latter setting thrombin generation might be expected to be significant. As one would predict, these patients' platelets cannot make thromboxane $A_2$ when supplied with arachidonic acid, but they can make thromboxane $A_2$ if supplied with the cyclic endoperoxides $PGG_2$ and $PGH_2$. Since cyclooxygenase is also the first enzyme in the pathway for $PGI_2$ synthesis in endothelial cells, one would expect that a deficiency of this enzyme would also result in a decrease in $PGI_2$. This was confirmed in one patient whose endothelium was unable to produce normal amounts of $PGI_2$. Whereas primary hemostasis has been viewed as a balance between thromboxane $A_2$ production by platelets and $PGI_2$ synthesis by endothelial cells, it is interesting that a deficiency in both results in a mild bleeding diathesis without evidence of thrombosis. This seems to indicate that thromboxane plays a greater role than $PGI_2$ in determining the balance. Therapeutically, other than avoiding antiplatelet medication and using hormonal therapy to control menorrhagia, there is little to be done short of using platelet transfusions for serious episodes of hemorrhage, should they occur.

**Thromboxane synthetase deficiency.**[239,240]   Thromboxane synthetase is the enzyme that converts the cyclic endoperoxides into thromboxane $A_2$. Only two families with a deficiency of this enzyme have been reported; the clinical manifestations have ranged from mild to quite severe. The platelets of these patients do not form thromboxane $A_2$ as normal platelets do, even when supplied with cyclic endoperoxides. Interestingly, the platelets make increased amounts of the other prostaglandins (including the inhibitor, $PGD_2$), presumably because the block in thromboxane $A_2$ synthesis increases the availability of the endoperoxide precursors. Moreover, the plasma levels of $PGI_2$ appear to be increased, perhaps because the cyclic endoperoxides produced in the platelet gain access to the endothelium, where they are converted to $PGI_2$ (endothelial "steal"). Treatment is as noted above for the cyclooxygenase deficiency.

**Thromboxane $A_2$ insensitivity.**[241–243]   The site of action for thromboxane $A_2$ is unknown, but presumably it involves a receptor recognition step. It appears that two families and one isolated patient have an abnormality in the response of their platelets to thromboxane $A_2$. This insensitivity has been postulated to result from (1) an increase in platelet cAMP, [242] (2) an inability to mobilize calcium normally, [243] or (3) an abnormality in thromboxane $A_2$ receptors.[241] Clinically, this disorder results in a mild to moderate mucocutaneous hemorrhagic diathesis.

*Acquired release reaction disorders.*   A large number of drugs have been shown to inhibit the platelet release reaction, and a variable fraction of patients with uremia or myeloproliferative disorders have been shown to have similar defects.

**Drugs.**[126]

*Aspirin.*   Considering the number of individuals at risk, aspirin is by far the most important drug inhibitor of platelet function. Within minutes of ingesting a single 300-mg tablet, abnormalities in the release reaction and the second wave of aggregation induced by ADP and epinephrine are observed. Collagen-induced aggregation is decreased, but the defect can be overcome by increasing the concentration of collagen employed. Thrombin-induced aggregation and release is not significantly affected. The bleeding time is slightly but significantly prolonged. It has been shown that aspirin irreversibly inactivates the enzyme cyclooxygenase by acetylating one of its amino acids. As would be expected, therefore, arachidonic acid cannot induce platelet aggregation or release of aspirin-treated platelets, but the cyclic endoperoxides can. Since platelets have little or no capacity to synthesize protein, once the platelet's cyclooxygenase has been inactivated, the platelet will be without this enzymatic activity for the rest of its life. As a result, the defect produced by a single exposure to aspirin can usually be detected in vitro for 3–9 days, depending on the assay employed. It should also be appreciated that although the half-life of detectable salicylates may be relatively long, the acetyl group of aspirin is hydrolyzed quite rapidly in plasma; thus, the platelet population is at risk of becoming inhibited for only a brief period of time after aspirin ingestion. This observation permitted the development of a novel method for determining platelet survival based on the speed with which platelet cyclooxygenase activity returns to normal after aspirin ingestion. Since cyclooxygenase is also required for the production of $PGI_2$, aspirin also inhibits $PGI_2$ synthesis by endothelial cells. The effect of aspirin on $PGI_2$ synthesis is more short-lived than its effect on platelet synthesis of thromboxane $A_2$, however, because endothelial cells have an active protein synthetic mechanism and so can replace the inactivated enzyme. Moreover, there is some evidence to suggest that the endothelial cell cyclooxygenase is less sensitive to aspirin's effects than the platelet enzyme.

Clinically, since aspirin ingestion is so widespread, it is clear that the vast majority of users do not develop a significant hemorrhagic diathesis. On the other hand, the slight but significant prolongation of the bleeding time probably does indicate that a subtle defect is established even in normal individuals. Studies of blood loss in patients subjected to the hemostatic challenges of childbirth and open-heart surgery suggest that recent aspirin ingestors do, indeed, lose more blood. In addition, the neonates of mothers who have taken aspirin just prior to delivery appear to have a significantly increased risk of hemorrhage. Moreover, platelets from donors who have recently ingested aspirin are less effective hemostatically than those from donors who are aspirin free. Despite these observations, other than perhaps a slight increase in bruising and a slight increase in gastrointestinal blood loss, normal individuals who are not undergoing a major hemostatic challenge rarely show evidence of a significant hemorrhagic diathesis.

In striking contrast to the mild effect of aspirin on normal individuals is its exaggerated and often dramatic effect on individuals ingesting alcohol[243a] or with compromised hemostatic mechanisms. Hemophiliacs and patients with von Willebrand's disease develop markedly prolonged bleeding times after aspirin ingestion and appear to be at considerably increased risk of spontaneous hemorrhage. It has been suggested that patients with mild von Willebrand's disease, in whom the diagnosis is equivocal, be given an aspirin tolerance test wherein the bleeding time is performed before and after aspirin ingestion; a marked prolongation beyond what would be expected from normal individuals would be taken as a positive response. The author has not utilized this test, in part because it would require careful standardization of bleeding times in normal persons who have taken aspirin. The author prefers to rely on the platelet retention test in equivocal cases of von Willebrand's disease.

After all of the above considerations have been taken into account, there remains a small number of patients with minimal and variable abnormalities of in vitro platelet function who are essentially asymptomatic when free of aspirin but who have significant spontaneous bleeding when taking aspirin. This syndrome has been named the *intermediate syndrome* of platelet dysfunction, a term that merely serves to emphasize our lack of understanding of the pathophysiology of the disorder. It is obviously important to identify these patients since they can derive considerable benefit from simply avoiding aspirin.

*Nonsteroidal anti-inflammatory agents.* (indomethacin, phenylbutazone, naproxen, ibuprofen, etc.). Virtually all of these agents produce inhibition of the release reaction, although, unlike aspirin ingestion, the effect appears to last only as long as the drug remains in the circulation. Much less information is available about the clinical risks with the use of these drugs, but it is prudent to avoid them in patients who are at risk of excessive hemorrhage. When managing patients with inflammatory diseases who have either a coagulation or a platelet disorder (quantitative or qualitative), the appropriate course of action may be very difficult to decide. If the disorder is severe enough to warrant the use of corticosteroids, these can, of course, be used with impunity. If analgesia is the major indication for drug therapy, alternative choices include acetaminophen, choline salicylate, and narcotics or various congeners of narcotics (codeine, morphine, dextropropoxyphene, pentazocine, etc.). From a practical standpoint, the author has found it useful to be sure that patients have an adequate supply of the appropriate medication in their possession in

**Table 4-15**

Drugs That Inhibit Platelet Function (After Ingestion)*

Antibiotics (ampicillin, carbenicillin, cephalosporin, methicillin, penicillin G. ticarcillin)
Antihistamines (chlorpheniramine maleate, diphenhydramine)
Nonsteroidal anti-inflammatory agents (aspirin, naproxen, phenylbutazone, sulindac, sulfinpyrazone)
Chemotherapeutic agents (mithramycin)
Ethyl alcohol
Glyceryl guaiacolate
Heparin
Macromolecules (dextran)
Nitrofurantoin
Phenothiazines (chlorpromazine, promethazine)
Pseudoephedrine hydrochloride
Pyrimido-pyrimidine compounds (dipyridamole)
Tricyclic antidepressants (amitriptyline, desmethylipramine, imipramine, nortriptyline)
Triprolidine
Vinca alkaloids
Valproate sodium

From Stuart MJ, McKenna R: Diseases of coagulation: The platelet and vasculature, in Nathan DG, Oski FA (eds): Hematology of Infancy and Childhood, (2nd ed), Philadelphia, WB Saunders, 1981, p. 1306. With permission.
*Following administration, these drugs have been demonstrated to affect platelet function in vitro or in vivo, with or without concomitant abnormalities in the bleeding time.

order to avoid their taking the antiplatelet medications that are available at home when they may not have access to a pharmacy. It is also important that patients be told which over-the-counter medications contain aspirin or other proscribed drugs.

*Miscellaneous medications.*[126] A large variety of medications have been implicated in causing platelet function abnormalities. A majority of these studies were performed by adding the drugs to platelets in vitro, and it is difficult to extrapolate the findings to the in vivo risk of taking the medication. Even the drugs that have been shown to cause defects of in vitro platelet function do not uniformly lengthen the bleeding time when administered to individuals; the risk of using them thus remains unclear. Tables 4-15 and 4-16, taken from reference 126, summarize these data.

**Uremia and myeloproliferative disorders.**[187,223] Both of these conditions have been associated with defects in the release reaction. In uremia the defect is believed to be secondary to a toxic substance that accumulates when renal function deteriorates since dialysis readily reverses the defect. In contrast, the platelet defect in the myeloproliferative disorders is thought to reflect the fundamental abnormality in the megakaryocyte cell line.

**Storage pool disorders.** Both dense bodies and α-granules are considered to be storage sites since their contents are not in rapid equilibrium with the cytoplasm of the platelet. Moreover, if for any reason the platelet loses the contents of one or the other of these granule types, it appears to be unable to replenish the granule's contents. It is convenient to categorize these disorders according to both the predominant granule involved and whether the disorder is hereditary or acquired. It should, however, be stressed that various combi-

**Table 4-16**
Drugs That Inhibit Platelet Function (When Added to Platelets)*

---

Alpha-adrenergic blocking agents (dihydroergotamine, phentolamine)
Anesthetics, local (cocaine, nupercaine, procaine, xylocaine)
Anesthetics, general (cyclopropane diethyl ether, halothane, nitrous oxide, methoxyflurane)
Anti-inflammatory agents, nonsteroidal (flufenamic acid, ibufenac, ibuprofen, meclofenamic acid,
    mefenamic acid, phenoprofen, solufenum)
Atropine
Barbituric acid derivatives (sodium pentobarbital)
Beta-blocking agents (propranolol)
Chelating agents
Chemotherapeutic agents (azathioprine, carmustine, melphalan)
Chloroquine compounds
Clofibrate
Colchicine
Contrast agents used in diagnostic radiology
Dihomo-δ-linolenic acid
Furosemide
Halofenate
Methyl xanthines (aminophylline, caffeine, theophylline)
Mercurial diuretics (meralluride, mersalyl)
Onion extracts
Reserpine
Serotonin antagonists (cyproheptadine, metergoline)
Steroids (hydrocortisone, methyl prednisolone)
Vasodilators (papaverine, quazodine, suloctidil)
Vitamin C
Vitamin E

---

From Stuart MJ, McKenna R: Diseases of coagulation: The platelet and vasculature, in Nathan DG, Oski, Fa (eds): Hematology of Infancy and Childhood, (2nd ed), Philadelphia, WB Saunders, 1981, p. 1306. With permission.
*These drugs have been demonstrated to affect platelet function when added to platelets in the in vitro experimental situation. Following ingestion in humans, these agents may also cause abnormalities in in vitro platelet function tests. No data, however, are available concerning bleeding times or clinical evidence of bleeding following the administration of these drugs to humans.

nations of partial deficiencies also exist and that there is great heterogeneity within these categories. In fact, it has become clear that some of these patients also have defects in the arachidonic acid pathway and adhesion.[195,235]

δ **and** αδ **Storage pool disorders.**[195,235,244,245]   This group of diseases is characterized by a mild to moderate history of mucocutaneous, postpartum, and postoperative hemorrhage. As shown in Table 4-17, bleeding time and platelet retention results are variable. Platelet aggregation usually shows the classic pattern of absent second-wave aggregation with ADP and epinephrine. Confirmation of the diagnosis can be made by demonstrating (1) an absence or abnormalities of dense bodies by either electron microscopy or mepacrine staining, (2) decreases in serotonin, the storage pool of adenine nucleotides, and calcium by biochemical analysis, and (3) decreased release of serotonin and adenine nucleotides by thrombin. Platelet serotonin uptake demonstrates a characteristic abnormality in which there is a normal initial velocity of uptake, but with a distinct reduction in the total amount taken up and an increased fraction undergoing metabolism. This pattern is thought to reflect

**Table 4-17**
δ-Storage Pool Deficiency

| | |
|---|---|
| Platelet count | Normal |
| Bleeding time | Normal or slightly prolonged |
| Platelet morphology | |
|   Light microscope | Normal |
|   Electron microscope | Absent dense bodies |
| Platelet retention | Variably abnormal |
| Platelet interaction with subendothelium | |
|   Adhesion | Variably abnormal |
|   Aggregation | Abnormal |
| Platelet aggregation | |
|   ADP | Absent second wave |
|   Epinephrine | Absent second wave |
|   Arachidonic acid | Variable abnormal |
|   Collagen | Decreased |
|   Ristocetin | Normal initial slope |
| Serotonin uptake | Normal rate; decreased plateau |
| Platelet serotonin | Markedly decreased |
| Platelet ADP, ATP | Reduced storage pool; normal metabolic pool |
| Thrombin-releasable ATP and ADP | Decreased |
| Platelet β-thromboglobulin and PF 4 | Normal |
| Membrane glycoproteins | Normal |

normal transport of serotonin across the plasma membrane and an absence of the storage granules that sequester the serotonin and thus protect it from the enzymes which catabolize it. In the patients who also have deficiencies in their α-granules, low levels of β-thromboglobulin and PF 4, as well as other α-granule proteins, are found. The hereditary forms of this disorder include (1) *storage pool disease,* which appears to be inherited as an autosomal dominant trait and may be found in association with partial or severe α-granule deficiency and abnormalities in arachidonic acid metabolism; (2) *Hermansky-Pudlak syndrome,* an autosomal recessive disorder characterized by tyrosinase-positive oculocutaneous albinism, a lifelong bleeding disorder, and a ceroid-like pigment in macrophages; these patients have the most severe decrease in dense body contents and appear to have normal α-granules; (3) *Chediak-Higashi syndrome,* an autosomal recessive disease characterized by oculocutaneous albinism, recurrent pyogenic infections, abnormally large granules in granule-containing cells, and a hemorrhagic diathesis; (4) the *Wiskott-Aldrich syndrome,* discussed above; and (5) the *thrombocytopenia with absent radii syndrome* mentioned above.

Defects in the storage pool of adenine nucleotides have been reported in several acquired disorders,[195] including (1) *ITP* and other disorders (*collagen-vascular disorders,* lymphoproliferative disorders, etc.) in which antiplatelet antibodies are present; it is proposed that the antibodies induce release of dense body contents in vivo and thus result in dense body depletion; (2) *myeloproliferative disorders* in which the defective megakaryocytes produce platelets deficient in dense body contents; and (3) *disseminated intravascular coagulation* in which thrombin is presumed to induce in vivo release of dense body contents. Several *drugs* may induce a decrease in dense body serotonin, including reserpine, methysergide, tricyclic antidepressants, and phenothiazines, but they do not seem to induce a clinically significant hemostatic defect.

Treatment of these disorders consists of avoiding antiplatelet agents, hormonal control of menorrhagia, and platelet transfusions for severe episodes of hemorrhage. The role of splenectomy in Wiskott-Aldrich syndrome has already been discussed. A very interesting but poorly understood recent observation is that infusions of cryoprecipitate can decrease the bleeding time of patients with these disorders without affecting in vitro aggregation responses or the contents of the dense granules.[246] Cryoprecipitate rather than platelet transfusions has, therefore, been recommended in the preoperative therapy of these patients so as to avoid the risk of platelet immunization.

$\alpha$-Storage pool disorders.[195,247-249]   Isolated deficiency of the contents of $\alpha$-granules occurs as a hereditary disorder ($\alpha$-storage disease, gray platelet syndrome) and on an acquired basis in association with cardiopulmonary bypass.

The gray platelet syndrome has been reported in only four patients from three families. The patients had had bleeding symptoms from early infancy, with petechiae, easy bruising, and epistaxis being most common; postoperative and postpartum hemorrhage and hemarthroses have also been observed. There may be a tendency for the bleeding symptoms to decrease with age. One patient also suffered from oculoauriculovertebral dysplasia. Although the data are obviously limited, autosomal recessive inheritance seems most likely. The platelet count is variably decreased, but not severely; in 1 patient, corticosteroid therapy produced a temporary increase in platelet count, and splenectomy resulted in a permanent increase in platelet count to above 100,000/$\mu$l. The laboratory data found in this disorder are outlined in Table 4-18. The combination of a low platelet count and large, degranulated platelets (gray) on blood smear should raise one's suspicion; confirmation requires assessment of platelet $\beta$-thromboglobulin and PF 4 by commercially available radioimmunoassays. A rare patient with an EDTA-dependent platelet agglutinin may also have degranulated platelets on peripheral blood smear, but it should not be difficult to differentiate these disorders.

The pathophysiology of the gray platelet syndrome remains unclear. Since these patients have normal or increased levels of plasma $\beta$-thromboglobulin and PF 4, proteins that are thought to be made exclusively in megakaryocytes, it is presumed that these patients have a defect in packaging the $\alpha$-granule contents rather than in synthesizing them. The presence of fibrosis in the bone marrow of two patients has been ascribed to leakage of mitogenic factors out of the megakaryocytes and into the surrounding bone marrow as a result of this packaging disorder. The mild but consistent abnormalities in platelet aggregation by ADP, epinephrine, and thrombin and the more severe abnormality in collagen-induced aggregation indicate that there may be a role for $\alpha$-granule contents in these functions. The most likely $\alpha$-granule proteins to be involved in aggregation are thrombospondin (which binds to the platelet after release is induced and may serve a "lectinlike" function),[250] fibronectin, and fibrinogen. Similarly, the mild abnormality in agonist-induced release of serotonin in this disorder has raised the possibility of a role for $\alpha$-granule contents in this reaction.

$\alpha$-Granule depletion during cardiopulmonary bypass.[195]   The initiation of cardiopulmonary bypass is associated with prolongation of the bleeding time and release of $\alpha$-granule (but not dense body) contents ($\beta$-thromboglobulin and PF 4) into the circulation. Interestingly, despite persistence of the $\alpha$-granule defect, the bleeding time in these patients reverts to normal after bypass is completed, indicating that the $\alpha$-granule abnormality is not the exclusive cause of the prolonged bleeding time. An occasional patient, however, may have a persistently abnormal bleeding time, and as these patients appear to have excessive post-

**Table 4-18**

α-Storage Pool Deficiency (Gray Platelet Syndrome)

| | |
|---|---|
| Platelet count | Variably decreased |
| Bleeding time | Variably prolonged |
| Platelet morphology | |
|     Light microscope | Large, ungranulated ("gray") |
|     Electron microscope | Marked vacuolization, decreased α-granules |
| Megakaryocyte morphology | Decreased α-granules |
| Platelet interaction with subendothelium | |
|     Aggregation | Abnormal |
| Platelet aggregation | |
|     ADP | Decreased at limiting doses |
|     Epinephrine | Decreased at limiting doses |
|     Collagen | Decreased |
|     Thrombin | Decreased |
|     Ristocetin | Normal |
| Arachidonic acid metabolism | Normal |
| Serotonin uptake | Normal |
| Serotonin release | Decreased at limiting doses of agonists |
| Membrane glycoproteins | Normal |
| β-thromboglobulin and PF 4 | |
|     Plasma level | Increased |
|     Platelet content | Markedly decreased |
| Fibrinogen | |
|     Plasma level | Normal |
|     Platelet content | Markedly decreased |
| Platelet mitogenic activity | Markedly decreased |
| Thrombospondin | Markedly decreased |

operative bleeding, platelet transfusion therapy may be indicated. The use of $PGI_2$ during bypass in experimental animals has protected against both the loss of α-granule contents and the prolongation in bleeding time.

### Miscellaneous Disorders

*Bartter's syndrome.*[251]    Abnormalities in both the first and second waves of fibrinogen-dependent platelet aggregation have been reported in this disorder, which is otherwise characterized by juxtaglomerular cell hyperplasia, hyperreninism, severe hypokalemia, and excessive urinary excretion of prostaglandins. An increase in platelet cAMP has been demonstrated, and this abnormality is postulated to result from the presence of a stable prostaglandin-derived inhibitor in these patients' plasmas. Despite these in vitro abnormalities, the patients studied to date have had normal bleeding times and have not had excessive hemorrhage.

*Alcohol-induced platelet dysfunction.*[224]    Platelet dysfunction, independent of alcohol-induced thrombocytopenia, has been demonstrated in some individuals who have ingested large amounts of alcohol. Prolonged bleeding times, especially after aspirin ingestion,[243a] and abnormal second-wave aggregation are the most consistent abnormalities. Proposed mechanisms for these effects include (1) decreased cyclic endoperoxide synthesis, (2) membrane alterations secondary to changes in osmolality, (3) decreased adenine nucleotide levels, and (4) changes in platelet cAMP.

*Glycogen storage disease.*[195]   Patients with glucose-6-phosphatase deficiency and fructose-1,6-diphosphate deficiency have been reported to have a mild mucocutaneous bleeding disorder; prolonged bleeding times and abnormalities in second-wave platelet aggregation have been demonstrated. Since the platelets do not share the enzyme defect, and since the platelet defect would be corrected with glucose infusion, it has been concluded that the chronic hypoglycemia has compromised the metabolic pool of adenine nucleotides, resulting in a decrease in ATP sufficient to affect the release reaction.

*Acute leukemias and preleukemic states.*[195]   In addition to the quantitative defects in platelets in these disorders, qualitative abnormalities have been described. Defects in both the release reaction and the storage pool of adenine nucleotides have been suggested. An interesting report of a patient with preleukemia who had a bleeding diathesis despite a normal number of platelets proposed a defective form of thromboxane $A_2$ to account for the observed findings.

*Newborns.*[195]   A mild defect in platelet function in newborns has been reported, with the evidence pointing to a deficiency of metabolic ATP as the major cause. It is usually of no clinical consequence, but maternal aspirin ingestion can apparently exacerbate the disorder so as to make it clinically significant.

*Essential fatty acid deficiency.*[4]   Prolonged dietary deficiency of essential fatty acids results in a complex disorder in which hemorrhage is one manifestation. The platelet defect results from a deficiency of arachidonic acid and the attendant defects in prostaglandin synthesis. Although it is very rare now, prolonged hyperalimentation with fat-free solutions may produce this disorder.

*Other disorders.*[195,252]   Hypothyroidism, infectious mononucleosis, pernicious anemia, and cyanotic heart disease have all been associated with mild platelet function defects.

## REFERENCES

1.   Frojmovic MM, Panjwani R: Geometry of normal mammalian platelets by quantitative microscopic studies. Biophys J 16:1071–1089, 1976
2.   White JG, Gerrard JM: Ultrastructural features of abnormal blood platelets. A review. Am J Pathol 83:589–632, 1976
3.   White JG, Clawson CC, Gerrard JM: Platelet ultrastructure, in Bloom AL, Thomas DP (eds): Haemostasis and Thrombosis. Edinburgh, Churchill Livingstone, 1981, pp 22–49
4.   Marcus AJ: The role of lipids in blood coagulation, in Paoletti R, Kritchevsky D (eds): Advances in Lipid Research, vol. 4. New York, Academic Press, 1967, pp 1–37
5.   Zwaal RFA, Rosing J, Tans G, et al: Topological and kinetic aspects of phospholipids in blood coagulation, in Mann KG, Taylor FB Jr. (eds): The Regulation of Coagulation. New York, Elsevier North-Holland, 1980, pp 95–112
6.   Schick PK: The role of platelet membrane lipids in platelet hemostatic activities. Semin Hematol 16:221–233, 1979
7.   Marcus AJ: The role of lipids in platelet function: With particular reference to the arachidonic acid pathway. J Lipid Res 9:793–826, 1976
8.   Shattil SJ, Cooper RA: Role of membrane lipid composition, organization, and fluidity in human platelet function, in Spaet TH (ed): Progress in Hemostasis and Thrombosis, vol. 4. New York, Grune & Stratton, 1979, pp 59–86

9.  Shattil SJ, Bennett JS: Platelets and their membranes in hemostasis: Physiology and patho-physiology. Ann Intern Med 94:108–118, 1980

9a. Nathan I, Fleisher G, Livne A et al: Membrane microenvironmental changes during activation of human platelets by thrombin. J Biol Chem 254:9822–9828, 1979

9b. Hayward JA, Scandella CJ, Simon SR, et al: Thrombin activation decreases platelet membrane fluidity. Clin Res 30:503A, 1982 (abstract)

10. Shattil SJ, McDonough M, Burch JW: Inhibition of platelet phospholipid methylation during platelet secretion. Blood 57:537–544, 1981

11. Karpatkin S: Composition of platelets, in Williams WJ et al (eds): Hematology (2nd ed). New York, McGraw-Hill, 1977, pp 1176–1187

12. Marcus AJ, Ullman HL, Safier LB: Studies on human platelet gangliosides. J Clin Invest 51:2602–2612, 1972

13. Wang C-T, Schick PK: The effect of thrombin on the organization of human platelet membrane glycosphingolipids. The sphingosine composition of platelet glycolipids and ceramides. J Biol Chem 256:752–756, 1981

14. Seaman GVF: Electrochemical features of platelet interactions. Thromb Res 8(suppl 2):235–246, 1976

15. Greenberg J, Packham MA, Cazenave J-P, et al: Effects on platelet function of removal of platelet sialic acid by neuraminidase. Lab Invest 32:476–484, 1975

16. Nurden AT, Caen JP: The different glycoprotein abnormalities in thrombasthenic and Bernard-Soulier platelets. Semin Hematol 16:234–250, 1979

17. Phillips DR: An evaluation of membrane glycoproteins in platelet adhesion and aggregation, in Spaet TH, (ed): Progress in Hemostasis and Thrombosis. Vol. 5. New York, Grune & Stratton, 1980, pp 81–109

17a. Ruan C, Tobelem G, McMichael AJ, et al: Monoclonal antibody to human platelet glycoprotein I. II. Effects on human platelet function. Br J Haematol 49:511–519, 1981

17b. Coller BS, Peerschke EI, Scudder LE, et al: Studies with a murine monoclonal antibody that abolishes ristocetin-induced binding of von Willebrand factor to platelets: Additional evidence in support of GPIb as a platelet receptor for von Willebrand factor. Blood, 61: 99–110, 1983

17c. Berndt MC, Gregory C, Castaldi PA, et al: Purification of human platelet membrane glycoprotein IB complex using a monoclonal antibody. Thromb Haemostas 50:361, 1983 (abstract)

18. Anstee DJ: The blood group MNSs-active sialoglycoproteins. Semin Hematol 18:13–31, 1981

19. Cartron JP, Nurden AT, Blanchard, et al: The Tn receptors of human red cells and platelets. Rev Fr Trans Immunohematol 23:613–628, 1980

20. Kunicki TJ, Russell N, Nurden AT, et al: Further studies of the human platelet receptor for quinine- and quinidine-dependent antibodies. J Immunol 126:398–402, 1981

21. Moore A, Ross GD, Nachman RL: Interaction of platelet membrane receptors with von Willebrand factor, ristocetin and the Fc region of immunoglobulin G. J Clin Invest 62:1053–1060, 1978

22. Kunicki TJ, Pidard D, Rosa J-P, et al: The formation of $Ca^{++}$-dependent complexes of platelet membrane glycoproteins IIB and IIIa in solution as determined by crossed immuno-electrophoresis. Blood 58:268–278, 1981

23. Leung LLK, Kinoshita T, Nachman RL: Isolation, purification, and partial characterization of platelet membrane glycoproteins IIb and IIIa. J Biol Chem 256:1994–1997, 1981

23a. McEver RP, Baenzinger JU, and Majerus PN: Isolation and structural characterization of the polypeptide subunits of membrane glycoprotein IIb-IIIa from human platelets. Blood 59: 80–85, 1982

23b. Newman PJ, Kahn RA: Structural relationship of human platelet membrane glycoproteins IIb and IIIa. Submitted for publication.

24.  Bennett JS, Vilaire G: Exposure of platelet fibrinogen receptors by ADP and epinephrine. J Clin Invest 64:1393–1401, 1979

25.  Coller BS: Interaction of normal, thrombasthenic, and Bernard-Soulier platelets with immobolized fibrinogen: Defective platelet-fibrinogen interaction in thrombasthenia. Blood 55:169–178, 1980

26.  Lee H, Nurden AT, Thomaidis A, et al: Relationship between fibrinogen binding and the platelet glycoprotein deficiencies in Glanzmann's thrombasthenia Type I and Type II. Br J Haematol 48:47–57, 1981

27.  Coller BS: Preliminary characterization of hybridoma antibodies that inhibit fibrinogen–platelet interactions. Blood 58:191a, 1981 (abstract)

27a. Nachman RL, Leung LLK: Complex formation of platelet membrane glycoproteins IIb and IIIa with fibrinogen. J Clin Invest 69:263–269, 1982

27b. Gogstad GO, Brosstad F, Krutnes M-B, et al: Fibrinogen-binding properties of the human platelet glycoprotein IIb-IIIa complex: A study using crossed-radioimmunoelectrophoresis. Blood 60:663–671, 1983

28.  Kornecki E, Niewiarowski S, Morinelli TA, et al: Effects of chymotrypsin and adenosine diphosphate on the exposure of fibrinogen receptors on normal human and Glanzmann's thrombasthenic platelets. J Biol Chem 256:5696–5701, 1981

28a. Ruggeri ZM, Bader K, DeMarco L: Glanzmann's thrombasthenia: Deficient binding of von Willebrand factor to thrombin-stumulated platelets. Proc. Natl. Acad. Sci. USA 79:6038–6041, 1982

28b. Gralnick HR, Coller BS: Platelets stimulated with thrombin and ADP bind von Willebrand factor to different sites than platelets stimulated with ristocetin. Clin Res 31:482A, 1983 (abstract)

28c. Ruggeri ZM, De Marco L, Montgomery RR: Platelets have more than one receptor for von Willebrand factor. Clin Res 31:322A, 1983 (abstract)

29.  Kunicki TJ, Aster RH: Deletion of the platelet-specific alloantigen $Pl^{A1}$ from platelets in Glanzmann's thrombasthenia. J Clin Invest 61:1225–1231, 1978

30.  van Leeuwen EF, von dem Borne AEGKr, von Riesz LE, et al: Absence of platelet-specific alloantigens in Glanzmann's thrombasthenia. Blood 57:49–54, 1981

31.  Kunicki TJ, Aster RH: Isolation and immunologic characterization of the human platelet alloantigen, $Pl^{A1}$. Molec Immunol 16:353–360, 1979

32.  Berndt MC, Phillips DR: Purification and preliminary physicochemical characterization of human platelet membrane glycoprotein V. J Biol Chem 256:59–65, 1981

33.  Phillips DR, Agin PP: Platelet plasma membrane glycoproteins. Identification of a proteolytic substrate for thrombin. Biochem Biophys Res Commun 75:940–947, 1977

34.  Nurden AT, Dupuis D: The reduced aggregation response of Bernard-Soulier platelets to thrombin may be related to an abnormal glycoprotein V. Thromb Haemost 46:22, 1981 (abstract)

34a. Clemetson KJ, McGregor JL, James E, et al: Characterization of the platelet membrane glycoprotein abnormalities in Bernard-Soulier syndrome and comparison with normal by surface-labeling techniques and high-resolution two-dimensional gel electrophoresis. J Clin Invest 70:304–311, 1982

35.  Cohen I, Gerrard JM, Bergman RN, et al: The role of contractile filaments in platelet activation, in Peters H (ed): Protides of the Biological Fluids, Proceedings of the 26th Colloquium. Oxford, Pergamon Press, 1979, pp 555–556

36.  Crawford N: Platelet microfilaments and microtubules, in Gordon JL (ed): Platelets in Biology and Pathology. Amsterdam, Elsevier North-Holland, 1976, pp 121–157

37.  Holmsen H, Smith JB, Daniel JL, et al: Platelet biochemistry, in Schmidt RM (ed): CRC Handbook Series in Clinical Laboratory Science, sec I: Hematology, vol. I. Boca Raton, Fla, CRC Press, 1979, pp 273–312

38.  Harris HE, Weeds AG: Platelet actin: Sub-cellular distribution and association with profilin. FEBS Lett 90:84–88, 1978

39.  Harris H: Regulation of motile activity in platelets, in Gordon JL (ed): Platelets in Biology
     and Pathology, vol. 2. Amsterdam, Elsevier/North-Holland, 1981, pp 473–500

39a. Rink TJ: Calcium in platelet activation: Studies with a fluorescent indicator of cytoplasmic
     free $Ca^{2+}$. Thromb Haemostas 50:92, 1983 (abstract)

40.  Markey F, Lindberg U: Biochemical evidence for actin filament formation as a primary re-
     sponse in stimulation of platelets with thrombin: The possible role of the profilin:actin complex,
     in, Peters H (ed): Protides of the Biological Fluids, Proceedings of the 26th Colloquium. Oxford,
     Pergamon Press, 1979, pp 487–492

41.  Wallach D, Davies PJA, Pastan I: Purification of mammalian filamin. Similarity to high mo-
     lecular weight actin-binding protein in macrophages, platelets, fibroblasts, and other tissues.
     J Biol Chem 253:3328–3335, 1978

42.  Lucas RC, Rosenberg S, Shafiq S, et al: The isolation and characterization of a cytoskeleton
     and a contractile apparatus from human platelets, in Peters H (ed:) Protides of the Biological
     Fluids, Proceedings of the 26th Colloquium. Oxford, Pergamon Press, 1979, pp 465–470

43.  Grumet M, Lin S: A platelet inhibitor protein with cytochalasin-like activity against actin
     polymerization in vitro. Cell 21:439–444, 1980

44.  Lind SE, Yin HL, Stossel TP, et al: Human platelets contain gelsolin, a regulator of actin
     filament length. J Clin Invest 69:1384–1387, 1982

45.  Hathaway DR, Eaton CR, Adelstein RS: Regulation of human platelet myosin kinase by
     calcium-calmodulin and cyclic AMP, in Mann KG, Taylor FB Jr (eds): The Regulation of
     Coagulation. New York, Elsevier/North Holland, 1980, pp 271–276

46.  Castle AG, Crawford N: Platelet microtubule subunit proteins. Thromb Haemost 42:1630–1633,
     1979

47.  Nachmias VT, Sullender J, Fallon J, et al: Observations on the ''cytoskeleton'' of human
     platelets. Thromb Haemost 42:1661–1666, 1979

48.  Niewiarowski S: Platelet release reaction and secreted platelet proteins, in Bloom AL,
     Thomas DP (eds): Haemostasis and Thrombosis. Edinburgh, Churchill Livingstone, 1981,
     pp 73–83

49.  Kaplan KL: Platelet granule proteins: Localization and secretion, in Gordon JL (ed): Platelets
     in Biology and Pathology, vol. 2. Amsterdam, Elsevier/North-Holland, 1981, pp 77–90

49a. Deuel TF, Senior RM, Chang D, et al: Platelet factor 4 is chemotactic for neutrophils and
     monocytes. Proc Natl Acad Sci USA 78:4584–4587, 1981

50.  Ross R, Glomset JA: The pathogenesis of atherosclerosis. N Engl J Med 295:369–377, 420–
     425, 1976

50a. Goldberg ID, Stemerman MB, Handin RI: Vascular permeation of platelet factor 4 after endo-
     thelial injury. Science 209:611–612, 1980

51.  Castro-Malaspina H, Rabellino EM, Yen A, et al: Human megakaryocyte stimulation of pro-
     liferation of bone marrow fibroblasts. Blood 57:781–787, 1981

51a. Deuel TF, Senior RM, Huang JS, et al: Chemotaxis of monocytes and neutrophils to platelet-
     derived growth factor. J Clin Invest 69:1046–1049, 1982

51b. Waterfield MD, Scrace GT, Whittle N, et al: Platelet-derived growth factor is structurally re-
     lated to the putative transforming protein p $28^{sis}$ of simian sarcoma virus. Nature 304:35–39,
     1983

51c. Doolittle RJ, Hunkapiller MW, Hood LE, et al: Simian sarcoma virus *onc* gene, v-*sis*, is
     derived from the gene (or genes) encoding a platelet-derived growth factor. Science 221:275–
     277, 1983

52.  Hynes RO, Ali IU, Destree AT, et al: A large glycoprotein lost from the surfaces of trans-
     formed cells. Ann NY Acad Sci 312:317–342, 1978

53.  Phillips DR, Jennings LK, Prasanna HR: $Ca^{2+}$-mediated association of glycoprotein G
     (thrombin-sensitive protein, thrombospondin) with human platelets. J Biol Chem 24:11629–
     11632, 1980

54.  DaPrada M, Richards JG, Kettler R: Amine storage organelles in platelets, in Gordon JL (ed):

Platelets in Biology and Pathology, vol. 2. Amsterdam, Elsevier/North-Holland, 1981, pp 107–145

55.  Urgurbil K, Holmsen H: Nucleotide compartmentation: Radioisotopic and nuclear magnetic resonance studies, in Gordon JL (ed): Platelets in Biology and Pathology, vol. 2. Amsterdam, Elsevier/North-Holland, 1981, pp 147–177

56.  Karpatkin S: Metabolism of platelets, in Williams WJ et al (eds): Hematology (2nd ed). New York, McGraw-Hill, 1977, p 1187–1200

57.  Marcus AJ, Zucker MB: The Physiology of Blood Platelets. New York, Grune & Stratton, 1965

58.  Rittenhouse-Simmons S, Deykin D: Release and metabolism of arachidonate in human platelets, in Gordon JL (ed): Platelets in Biology and Pathology, vol. 2. Amsterdam, Elsevier/North-Holland, 1981, p 349–372

58a. Sano K, Takai Y, Yamanishi J, et al: A role of calcium-activated phospholipid-dependent protein kinase in human platelet activation. Comparison of thrombin and collagen actions. J Biol Chem 258:2010–2013, 1983

59.  Vargaftig BB, Chignard M, Benveniste J, et al: Background and present status of research on platelet-activating factor (PAF-acether). Ann NY Acad Sci 370:119–137, 1981

60.  Marcus AJ, Safier LB, Ullman HL, et al: Effects of acetyl glyceryl ether phosphorylcholine on human platelet function in vitro. Blood 58:1027–1031, 1981

61.  Zucker MB: The functioning of blood platelets. Sci Am 242(6):86–103, 1980

62.  Santoro SA, Cunningham LW: The interaction of platelets with collagen, in Gordon JL (ed): Platelets in Biology and Pathology, vol. 2. Amsterdam, Elsevier/North-Holland, 1981, pp 249–264

63.  Legrand YJ, Karniguiah A, Lefrancier P, et al: Interaction of platelets with a nonapeptide derived from type III collagen. Blood 58:198a, 1981 (abstract)

63a. Chiang TM, Kang AH: Isolation and purification of collagen α1(I) receptor from human platelet membrane. J Biol Chem 257:7581–7586, 1982

64.  Legrand YJ, Fauvel F, Gutman N, et al: Microfibrils (MF) platelet interaction: Requirement of von Willebrand factor. Thromb Res 19:737–739, 1980 (letter)

64a. Fauvel F, Grant ME, Legrand YJ, et al: Interaction of blood platelets with a microfibrillar extract from adult bovine aorta: Requirement for von Willebrand factor. Proc Natl Acad Sci USA 80:551–554, 1983

65.  Born GV, Cross MJ: The aggregation of blood platelets. J Physiol 168:178–195, 1963

66.  O'Brien JR: Platelet aggregation. II. Some results from a new method of study. J Clin Pathol 15:452–455, 1962

67.  Coller BS: Platelet aggregation by ADP, collagen and ristocetin: A critical review of methodology and analysis, in Schmidt RM (ed): CRC Handbook Series in Clinical Laboratory Sciences, sec. 1: Hematology, vol. I. Boca Raton, Fla, CRC Press, 1979, pp 381–396

68.  Pethica BA: The physical chemistry of cell adhesion. Exp Cell Res 8(suppl): 123–140, 1961

68a. Kloczewiak M, Timmons S, Hawiger J: Recognition site for the platelet receptor is present on the 15-residue carboxy-terminal fragment of the γ chain of human fibrinogen and is not involved in the fibrin polymerization reaction. Thromb Res 29:249–255, 1983

69.  McKee PA: Observations on structure–function relationships of human antihemophilic/von Willebrand factor protein. Ann NY Acad Sci 370:210–226, 1981

69a. Fujimoto T, Ohara S, Hawiger J: Thrombin-induced exposure and prostacyclin inhibition of the receptor for factor VIII/von Willebrand factor on human platelets. J Clin Invest 69:1212–1222, 1982

69b. Fujimoto T, Hawiger J: Adenosine diphosphate induces binding of von Willebrand factor to human platelets. Nature 297:154–156, 1982

70.  Berndt MC, Phillips DR: Platelet membrane proteins: Composition and receptor function, in, Gordon JL (ed): Platelets in Biology and Pathology, vol. 2. Amsterdam, Elsevier/North-Holland, 1981, pp 43–75

71. Scrutton MC, Wallis RB: Catecholamine receptors, in Gordon JL (ed): Platelets in Biology and Pathology, vol. 2. Amsterdam, Elsevier/North-Holland, 1981, pp 179–210

72. Owen Ne, Feinberg H, Le Breton GC: Epinephrine induces $Ca^{2+}$ uptake in human blood platelets. Am J Physiol 239:H483–488, 1980

72a. Detwiler T: Interactions of thrombin with platelets. Thromb Haemostas 50:326, 1983 (abstract)

73. Gerrard JM, Peterson DA, White JG: Calcium mobilization, in Gordon JL (ed): Platelets in Biology and Pathology, vol. 2. Amsterdam, Elsevier/North-Holland, 1981, pp 407–436

74. Feinstein MB, Rodan GA, Cutler LS: Cyclic AMP and calcium in platelet function, in Gordon JL (ed): Platelets in Biology and Pathology, vol. 2. Amsterdam, Elsevier/North-Holland, 1981, pp 437–472

75. Coller BS: Inhibition of von Willebrand factor-dependent platelet function by increased platelet cyclic AMP and its prevention by cytoskeleton-disrupting agents. Blood 57:846–855, 1981

76. White BN, Cox AC, Taylor FB: The procoagulant effect of platelets on conversion of prothrombin to thrombin in nonanticoagulated plasma. J Lab Clin Med 95:827–841, 1980

77. Bangham AD: A correlation between surface change and coagulant action of phospholipids. Nature 192:1197–1198, 1961

78. Tracy PB, Peterson JM, Nesheim ME, et al: Platelet interaction with bovine coagulation factor V and Va, in Mann KG, Taylor FB Jr (eds): The Regulation of Coagulation. New York, Elsevier/North-Holland, 1980, pp 237–243

79. Majerus PW, Miletich JP, Kane WH: The formation of thrombin on the platelet surface, in Mann KG, Taylor FB Jr (eds): The Regulation of Coagulation. New York, Elsevier/North-Holland, 1980, pp 215–222

80. Østerud B, Rapaport SI, Lavine KK: Factor V activity of platelets: Evidence for an activated factor V molecule and for a platelet activator. Blood 49:819–834, 1977

80a. Kane WH, Mruk JS, Majerus PW: Activation of coagulation factor V by a platelet protease. J Clin Invest 70:1092–1100, 1982

81. Walsh PN: Contributions of platelets to intrinsic coagulation, in Schmidt RM (ed): Handbook Series in Clinical Laboratory Sciences, sec. 1: Hematology, vol. 1. Boca Raton, Fla, CRC Press, 1979, pp 351–359

81a. Hultin MB: Role of human factor VIII in factor X activation. J Clin Invest 69:950–958, 1982

82. Schiffman S, Rimon A, Rapaport SI: Factor XI and platelets: Evidence that platelets contain only minimal factor XI activity and antigen. Br J Haematol 35:429–436, 1977

83. Vicic WJ, Ratnoff OD, Saito H, et al: Platelets and surface-mediated clotting activity. Br J Haematol 43:91–98, 1979

84. Dormandy JA: Haemorheology and thrombosis, in Bloom AL, Thomas DP (eds): Haemostasis and Thrombosis. Edinburgh, Churchill Livingstone, 1981, pp 610–625

85. Turitto VT, Muggli R, Baumgartner HR: Physical factors influencing platelet deposition on subendothelium: Importance of blood shear rate. Ann NY Acad Sci 283:284–292, 1977

86. Wight TN: Vessel proteoglycans and thrombogenesis, in Spaet TH (ed): Progress in Hemostasis and Thrombosis, vol. 5. New York, Grune & Stratton, 1980, pp 1–39

87. Moncada S, Vane JR: Arachidonic acid metabolites and the interactions between platelets and blood-vessels. N Engl J Med 300:1142–1147, 1979

88. Macintyre DE: Platelet prostaglandin receptors, in Gordon JL (ed): Platelets in Biology and Pathology, vol. 2. Amsterdam, Elsevier/North-Holland, 1981, pp 211–247

89. Crutchley DJ, Ryan US, Ryan JW: Effects of aspirin and dipyridamole on the degradation of adenosine diphosphate by cultured cells derived from bovine pulmonary artery. J Clin Invest 66:29–35, 1980

90. Lollar P, Owen WG: Active-site-dependent, thrombin-induced release of adenine nucleotides from cultured human endothelial cells. Ann NY Acad Sci 370:51–56, 1981

91. Marcus AJ, Weksler BB, Jaffe EA, et al: Synthesis of prostacyclin from platelet-derived endoperoxides by cultured human endothelial cells. J Clin Invest 66:979–986, 1980

92. Aster RH: Production, distribution, life-span and fate of platelets, in Williams WJ et al (eds): Hematology (2nd ed). New York, McGraw-Hill, 1977, pp 1210–1220

93. Penington DG: Formation of platelets, in Gordon JL (ed): Platelets in Biology and Pathology, vol. 2. Amsterdam, Elsevier/North-Holland, 1981, pp 19–41

94. Hoffman R, Mazur E, Bruno E, et al: Assay of an activity in the serum of patients with disorders of thrombopoiesis that stimulates formation of megakaryocytic colonies. N Engl J Med 305:533–538, 1981

95. Mustard JF, Packham MA, Kinlough-Rathbone RL: Platelet survival, in Day HJ et al (eds): Platelet Function Testing. Dept of Health, Education and Welfare publication (NIH) 78-1087, 1978, pp 545–560

96. Onder O, Weinstein A, Hoyer LW: Pseudothrombocytopenia caused by platelet agglutinins that are reactive in blood anticoagulated with chelating agents. Blood 56:177–182, 1980

97. Bell A, Neely CL: Smear platelet counts, South Med J 73:899–901, 1980

98. Watkins SP Jr, Shulman NR: Platelet cold agglutinins. Blood 36:153–158, 1970

99. Veenhoven WA, van der Schans GS, Huiges W, et al: Pseudothrombocytopenia due to agglutinins. Am J Clin Pathol 72:1005–1008, 1979

99a. Pegels JG, Bruynes ECE, Engelfreit CP, et al: Pseudothrombocytopenia: An immunologic study on platelet antibodies dependent on ethylene diamine tetra-acetate. Blood 59:157–161, 1982

100. McGregor DH, Davis JW, Liu PI, et al: Platelet satellism: Experimental studies. Lab Invest 42:343–355, 1980

101. Karpatkin S: Platelet sizing, in Schmidt RM (ed): CRC Handbook Series in Clinical Laboratory Science, sec 1: Hematology, vol. I. Boca Raton, Fla, CRC Press, 1979, pp 409–434

102. Murphy S: Disorders of platelet production, in Colman RW et al (eds): Thrombosis and Hemostasis, Basic Principles and Clinical Practice. Philadelphia, JB Lippincott, 1982, 259–273

103. Holme S, Simmonds M, Ballek R, et al: Comparative measurements of platelet size by Coulter counter, microscopy of blood smears, and light transmission studies. Relationship between platelet size and shape. J Lab Clin Med 97:610–622, 1981

103a. Eldor A, Avitzour M, Or R, et al: Prediction of haemorrhagic diathesis in thrombocytopenia by mean platelet volume. Br Med J 285:397–400, 1982

104. Oski FA, Naiman JL, Allen DM, et al: Leukocytic inclusions—Döhle bodies—associated with platelet abnormality (the May-Hegglin anomaly). Report of a family and review of the literature. Blood 20:657–667, 1962

105. Hamilton RW, Shaikh BS, Ottie JN, et al: Platelet function, ultrastructure and survival in the May-Hegglin anomaly. Am J Clin Pathol 74:663–668, 1980

106. Godwin HA, Ginsburg AD: May-Hegglin anomaly: A defect in megakaryocyte fragmentation? Br J Haematol 26:117–128, 1974

107. Fabris F, Casonato A, Randi ML, et al: Plasma and platelet beta-thromboglobulin levels in patients with May-Hegglin anomaly. Haemostasis 9:126–130, 1980

108. Coller BS, Zarrabi MH: Platelet membrane studies in the May-Hegglin anomaly. Blood 58:279–284, 1981

109. Cabrera JR, Fontau G, Lorente F, et al: Defective neutrophil mobility in the May-Hegglin anomaly. Br J Haematol 47:337–343, 1981

110. Eckstein JD, Filip DJ, Watts JC: Hereditary thrombocytopenia, deafness, and renal disease. Ann Intern Med 82:639–645, 1975

111. Epstein CJ, Sahad MA, Piel CF, et al: Hereditary macrothrombocytopathia, nephritis and deafness. Am J Med 52:299–310, 1972

112. Mitton JG, Frojmovic MM: Shape-changing agents produce abnormally large platelets in a hereditary "giant platelets syndrome." J Lab Clin Med 93:154–161, 1980

113. Von Behrens WE: Mediterranean macrothrombocytopenia. Blood 46:199–208, 1975

114. Lusher JM, Barnhart MI: Congenital disorders affecting platelets. Semin Thromb Hemost 4:123–186, 1977

115.  Aster RH: Thrombocytopenia due to diminished or defective platelet production, in Williams WJ et al (eds): Hematology (2nd ed). New York, McGraw-Hill, 1977, pp 1317–1325

116.  Lum LG, Tubergen DG, Corash L, et al: Splenectomy in the management of the thrombocytopenia of the Wiskott-Aldrich syndrome. N Engl J Med 302:892–896, 1980

117.  Ochs HD, Slichter SJ, Harker LA, et al: The Wiskott-Aldrich syndrome: Studies of lymphocytes, granulocytes, and platelets. Blood 55:243–252, 1980

118.  Nathan DG: Splenectomy in the Wiskott-Aldrich syndrome. N Engl J Med 302:916–917, 1980

119.  Zeigler Z, Murphy S, Gardner FH: Microscopic platelet size and morphology in various hematologic disorders. Blood 51:479–486, 1973

120.  Gale RP, Champlin RE, Feig SA, et al: Aplastic anemia: Biology and treatment. Ann Intern Med 95:477–494, 1981

121.  Erslev AJ: Aplastic anemia, in Williams WJ et al (eds): Hematology (2nd ed). New York, McGraw-Hill, 1977, pp 258–278

122.  Najean Y: Long-term follow-up in patients with aplastic anemia. A study of 137 androgen-treated patients surviving more than two years. Am J Med 71:543–551, 1981

123.  Goldstein I, Coller BS: Aplastic anemia in pregnancy. Ann Intern Med 82:537–539, 1975 (letter)

124.  Dorr RT, Fritz WL: Cancer Chemotherapy Handbook. New York, Elsevier/North-Holland, 1980, pp 104–106

125.  Buchanan GR; Hemorrhagic diseases, in Nathan DG, Oski FA (eds): Hematology of Infancy and Childhood (2nd ed). Philadelphia, WB Saunders, 1981, pp 119–143

126.  Stuart MJ, McKenna R: Diseases of coagulation: The platelet and vasculature, in Nathan DG, Oski FA (eds): Hematology of Infancy and Childhood (2nd ed), Philadelphia, WB Saunders, 1981, pp 1234–1338

127.  Stoll DB, Blum S, Pasquale D, et al: Thrombocytopenia with decreased megakaryocytes: Evaluation and prognosis. Ann Intern Med 94:170–175, 1981

128.  Gardner FH: Preservation and clinical use of platelets, in Williams WJ et al (eds): Hematology (2nd ed). New York, McGraw-Hill, 1977, pp 1553–1561

129.  Slichter SJ: Controversies in platelet transfusion therapy. Ann Rev Med 31:509–540, 1980

130.  Harker LA: The kinetics of platelet production and destruction in man. Clin Hematol 6:671–693, 1977

131.  Simon TL, Nelson EJ, Carmen R, et al: Extension of platelet concentrate storage, Transfusion 23:207–212, 1983

132.  Duquesnoy RJ, Filip DJ, Rodey GE, et al: Successful transfusion of platelets "mismatched" for HLA antigens to alloimmunized thrombocytopenic patients. Am J Hematol 2:219–226, 1977

133.  McClure PD: Idiopathic thrombocytopenic purpura in children, in Lusher JM, Barnhart MI (eds): Acquired Bleeding Disorders in Children. Platelet Abnormalities and laboratory Methods. New York, Masson Publishing USA, 1981, pp 83–91

134.  Aster RH: Thrombocytopenia due to enhanced platelet destruction, in Williams WJ et al (eds): Hematology (2nd ed). New York, McGraw-Hill, 1977, pp 1326–1360

135.  Karpatkin S: Autoimmune thrombocytopenic purpura. Blood 56:329–343, 1980

135a. Cheung N-K V, Hilgartner MW, Schulman I, et al: Platelet–associated immunoglobulin G in childhood idiopathic thrombocytopenic purpura. J Pediatrics 102:366–370, 1983

136.  Trent RJ, Clancy RL, Danis V, et al: Immune complexes in thrombocytopenic patients: Cause or effect? Br J Haematol 44:645–654, 1980

137.  Lusher JM, Emami A, Ravindranath Y, et al: Idiopathic thrombocytopenic purpura in children—the case for management without steroids. Prog Ped Hematol Oncol, In Press

138.  Blajchman MA, Senyl AF, Hirsh J, et al: Shortening of the bleeding time in rabbits by hydrocortisone caused by inhibition of prostacyclin generation by the vessel wall. J Clin Invest 63:1026–1035, 1979

138a. Salama A, Mueller-Eckhardt C, Kiefel V: Effect of intravenous immunoglobulin in immune thrombocytopenia. Competitive inhibition of reticuloendothelial system function by sequestration of autologous red blood cells? Lancet 2:193–195, 1983

139.   McMillan R: Chronic idiopathic thrombocytopenic purpura. N Engl J Med 304:1135–1147, 1981

140.   Von dem Borne AEGKr, Helmerhorst FM, van Leeuwen EF, et al: Autoimmune thrombocytopenia: Detection of platelet autoantibodies with the suspension immunofluorescence test. Br J Haematol 45:319–327, 1980

141.   McMillan R, Woods VL: Antibodies and antigens in chronic immune thrombocytopenic purpura. Thromb Haemostas 50:330, 1983 (abstract)

141a.  Woods VL Jr, Oh EH, Mason D, et al: Autoantibodies against the platelet glycoprotein IIb/IIIa complex in patients with idiopathic thrombocytopenic purpura. Blood 60(suppl 1):142a, 1982 (abstract)

141b.  Beardsley DJS, Spiegel JE, Jacobs MM, et al: Identification of antigen-bearing proteins: Localization of the target antigen in a subset of patients with idiopathic (or immune) thrombocytopenia purpura. Blood 60(suppl 1):184a, 1982 (abstract)

141c.  Morris L, Distenfeld A, Amorosi E, et al: Autoimmune thrombocytopenic purpura in homosexual men. Ann Intern Med 96:714–717, 1982

141d.  LoBuglio A, Court WS, Vinocur L, et al: Immune thrombocytopenic purpura: Use of $^{125}$I-labeled antihuman IgG monoclonal antibody to quantify platelet-bound IgG. N Engl J Med 309:459, 1983

142.   Shulman NR, Leissinger CA, Hotchkiss A: An in vivo model demonstrating that elevated platelet-associated IgG is a non-specific consequence of platelet destruction. Blood 60(suppl 1):191a, 1982 (abstract)

142a.  Murphy S: In search of a platelet Coombs test. N Engl J Med 309:490, 1983

143.   Harker LA, Slichter SJ: The bleeding time as a screening test for evaluation of platelet function. N Engl J Med 287:155–159, 1972

144.   Weiss HJ, Rosove MH, Lages BA, et al: Acquired storage pool deficiency with increased platelet-associated IgG. Report of five cases. Am J Med 69:711–717, 1980

145.   Stuart MJ, Kelton JG, Allen JB: Abnormal platelet function and arachidonate metabolism in chronic idiopathic thrombocytopenic purpura. Blood 58:326–329, 1981

146.   Kelton JG, McDonald JWD, Barr RM, et al: The reversible binding of vinblastine to platelets: Implications for therapy. Blood 57:431–436, 1981

146a.  Fehr J, Hofman NV, Kappeler U: Transient reversal of thrombocytopenia in idiopathic thrombocytopenia purpura by high-dose intravenous gammaglobulin. N Engl J Med 306:1254–1258, 1982

146b.  Bussel J, Kimberly R, Inman R, et al: Intravenous gammaglobulin treatment of chronic idiopathic thrombocytopenic purpura. Blood 62:480–486, 1983

146c.  Strother SV, Zuckerman KS, LoBuglio AF: Colchicine therapy of refractory immune thrombocytopenia. Blood 60(suppl 1):192a, 1982 (abstract)

146d.  Ahn YS, Harrington WJ, Simon SR, et al: Danazol for the treatment of idiopathic thrombocytopenic purpura. N Engl J Med 308:1396–1399, 1983

147.   Picozzi VJ, Roeske WR, Creger WP: Fate of therapy failures in adult idiopathic thrombocytopenic purpura. Am J Med 69:690–694, 1980

148.   Karpatkin M, Karpatkin S: Immune neonatal thrombocytopenia, in Lusher JM, Barnhart MI (eds): Acquired Bleeding Disorders in Children. Platelet Abnormalities and Laboratory Methods. New York, Masson Publishing USA, 1981, pp 93–105

149.   Cines DB, Dusak B, Tomaski A, et al: Immune thrombocytopenic purpura and pregnancy. N Engl J Med 306:826–831, 1982

150.   Scott JR, Cruikshank DP, Kochenour NK, et al: Fetal platelet counts in the obstetrical management of immunologic thrombocytopenic purpura. Am J Obstet Gynecol 136:495–499, 1980

151.   Karpatkin M, Porges RF, Karpatkin S: Platelet counts in infants of women with autoimmune thrombocytopenia: Effect of steroid administration to the mother. N Engl J Med 305:396–399, 1981

152. Eisner EV, Shahidi NT: Immune thrombocytopenia due to a drug metabolite. N Engl J Med 287:376–381, 1971

153. Salzman EW, Rosenberg RD, Smith MH, et al: Effect of heparin and heparin fractions on platelet aggregation. J Clin Invest 65:64–73, 1980

154. Carreras LO: Thrombosis and thrombocytopenia induced by heparin. Scand J Haematol Suppl 36:64–80, 1980

154a. Chong BH, Pitney WR, Castaldi PA: Heparin-induced thrombocytopenia: Association of thrombotic complications with heparin-dependent IgG antibody that induces thromboxane synthesis and platelet aggregation. Lancet 2:1246–1249, 1982

155. Bell WR, Royall RM: Heparin-associated thrombocytopenia: A comparison of three heparin preparations. N Engl J Med 303:902–907, 1980

156. Cines DB, Kaywin P, Bina M, et al: Heparin-associated thrombocytopenia. N Engl J Med 303:788–795, 1980

157. Kwaan HC, Kampmeier PA, Gomez HJ: Incidence of thrombocytopenia during therapy with bovine lung and porcine gut mucosal heparin preprations. Thromb Haemost 46:215, 1981 (abstract)

158. MacIntyre DE, Handin RI, Rosenberg RD, et al: Pro-aggregatory action of heparin reverses the effect of inhibitors of human platelet aggregation. Circulation 62(Suppl III):III–274, 1980 (abstract)

159. Reches A, Eldor A, Salomon Y: Heparin inhibits $PGE_1$—sensitive adenylate cyclase and antagonizes $PGE_1$ antiaggregating effect in human platelets. J Lab Clin Med 93:638–644, 1979

160. Coblyn JS, Weinblatt M, Holdswort D, et al: Gold-induced thrombocytopenia. A clinical and immunogenetic study of twenty-three patients. Ann Intern Med 95:178–181, 1981

161. Kelton JB, Meltzer D, Moore J, et al: Drug-induced thrombocytopenia is associated with increased binding of IgG to platelets both in vivo and in vitro. Blood 58:524–529, 1981

162. Shulman NR: Immunologic reactions to drugs. N Engl J Med 287:408–409, 1972

162a. Christie DJ, Aster RH: Drug–antibody–platelet interaction in quinine- and quinidine-induced thrombocytopenia. J Clin Invest 70:989–998, 1982

162b. Castaldi PA, Berndt MC, Koutts J, et al: Quinidine-induced thrombocytopenia and leukopenia: demonstration and characterisation of the quinidine-dependent antiplatelet and antileukocyte antibodies. Thrombos Haemostas 50:331, 1983 (abstract)

162c. Pfueller SL, Jenkins CSP, Lüscher EF: A comparative study of the effect of modification of the surface of human platelets on the receptors for aggregated immunoglobulins and for ristocetin-von Willebrand factor. Biochem Biophys Acta 465:614–626, 1977

163. Von dem Borne AEGKr, von Riesz E, Verheugt FWA, et al: Bak[a], a new platelet-specific antigen involved in neonatal alloimmune thrombocytopenia. Vox Sang 39:113–120, 1980

164. Von dem Borne AEGKr, van Leeuwen EF, von Riesz LE, et al: Neonatal alloiummune thrombocytopenia: Detection and characterization of the responsible antibodies by the platelet immunofluorescence test. Blood 57:649–656, 1981

164a. Kickler TS, Ness PM, Bell WR: Ability of PLA-1 negative platelets to acquire PLA-1 specificity from plasma obtained from stored blood: A proposed mechanism to explain the autologous destruction of platelets in posttransfusion thrombocytopenia. Blood 60(suppl 1):179a, 1982 (abstract)

164b. Reznikoff-Etievant MF, Dangu C, Lobet R: HLA-B8 antigen and $P1^{A1}$ alloimmunization. Tissue Antigens 18:66–68, 1981

164c. Shulman NR, Jordan JV Jr: Platelet immunology, in Colman RW, et al (eds): Thrombosis and Hemostasis, Basic Principles and Clinical Pratice. Philadelphia, JB Lippincott, 1982, pp 274–342

164d. Slichter SJ: Post-transfusion purpura. Response to steroids and association with red blood cell and lymphocytotoxic antibodies. Br J Haematol 50:599–605, 1982

165. Kwaan HC (ed): Management of thrombotic thrombocytopenic purpura. Semin Thromb Haemost 7:1–51, 1981

166.  Kwaan HC (ed): Thrombotic thrombocytopenic purpura, Part I. Semin Thromb Haemost 6:328–429, 1980

166a. Moake JL, Rudy CK, Troll JH, et al: Unusually large plasma factor VIII: von Willebrand factor multimers in chronic relapsing thrombotic thrombocytopenic purpura. N Engl J Med 307:1432–1435, 1982

167.  Gutterman L, Stevenson TD: Treatment of thrombotic thrombocytopenic purpura with vincristine. JAMA 247:1433–1436, 1982

167a. Gutterman LA, Meek LE, Stevenson TD: Treatment of thrombotic thrombocytopenic purpura (TTP) and hemolytic-uremic syndrome with vinca alkaloids. Blood 60(suppl 1):186a, 1982 (abstract)

168.  Rosove MH, Ho WG, Goldfinger D: Ineffectiveness of aspirin and dipyridamole in the treatment of thrombotic thrombocytopenic purpura. Ann Intern Med 96:27–33, 1982

169.  Fitzgerald GA, Maas RL, Stein R, et al: Intravenous prostacyclin in thrombotic thrombocytopenic purpura. Ann Intern Med 95:319–322, 1981

170.  Forbes CD: Thrombosis and artificial surfaces. Clin Haematol 10:653–668, 1981

171.  Malpass TW, Hanson SR, Savage B, et al: Prevention of acquired transient defect in platelet plug formation by infused prostacyclin. Blood 57:736–740, 1981

172.  Schmaier AH, Claypool W, Colman RW: Crotalocytin: Recognition and purification of a timber rattlesnake platelet aggregating protein. Blood 56:1013–1019, 1980

173.  Chesney PJ, Shahidi NT: Acute viral-induced thrombocytopenia: A review of human disease, animal models, and in vitro studies, in Lusher JM, Barnhart MI (eds): Acquired Bleeding Disorders in Children. Platelet Abnormalities and Laboratory Methods, New York, Masson Publishing USA, 1981, pp 65–81

174.  Scott S, Reimers H-J, Chernesky MA, et al: Effect of viruses on platelet aggregation and platelet survival in rabbits. Blood 52:47–55, 1978

175.  Knauer KA, Lichtenstein LM, Adkinson NJ Jr, et al: Platelet activation during antigen-induced airway reactions in asthmatic subjects. N Engl J Med 304:1404–1407, 1981

176.  Williams WJ: Thrombocytosis, in Williams WJ, et al (eds): Hematology (2nd ed). New York, McGraw-Hill, 1977, pp 1364–1367

176a. Peerschke EI, Zucker MB; Fibrinogen receptor exposure and aggregation of human blood platelets produced by ADP and chilling. Blood 57:663–670, 1981

177.  Glass JL, Wasserman LR: Primary polycythemia, in Williams WJ et al (eds): Hematology (2nd ed). New York, McGraw-Hill, 1977, pp 624–641

178.  Steeter RR, Presant CA, Reinhard E: Prognostic significance of thrombocytosis in idiopathic sideroblastic anemia. Blood 50:427–432, 1977

179.  Hirsh JA, Dacie JV: Persistent post-splenectomy thrombocytosis and thromboembolism: A consequence of continuing anaemia. Br J Haematol 12:44–53, 1966

180.  Boxer MA, Braun J, Ellman L: Thromboembolic risk of postsplenectomy thrombocytosis. Arch Surg 113:808–809, 1978

181.  Fialkow PJ, Fagnet GB, Jacobson RJ, et al: Evidence that essential thrombocythemia is a clonal disorder with origin in a multipotent stem cell. Blood 58:916–919, 1981

182.  Petit P, Van den Berghe H: A chromosomal abnormality (21q-) in primary thrombocytosis. Hum Genet 50:105–106, 1979

182a. Laszlo J, Iland H, Murphy S, et al: Essential thrombocythemia: Clinical and laboratory characteristics at presentation. Clin Res 31:535A, 1983 (abstract)

183.  Hussain S, Schwartz JM, Friedman SA, et al: Arterial thrombosis in essential thrombocythemia. Am Heart J 96:31–36, 1978

184.  Wu KK: Platelet hyperaggregability and thrombosis in patients with thrombocythemia. Ann Intern Med 88:7–11, 1978

185.  Weinfeld A, Branehög I, Kutti J: Platelets in the myeloproliferative syndrome. Clin Hematol 4:373–392, 1975

186.  Kaywin P, McDonough M, Insel PA, et al: Platelet function in essential thrombocythemia.

Decreased epinephrine responsiveness associated with a deficiency of platelet $\alpha$-adrenergic receptors. N Engl J Med 299:505–509, 1978

187. Keenan JP, Wharton J, Shepherd AJN, et al: Defective platelet lipid peroxidation in myeloproliferative disorders, a possible defect of prostaglandin synthesis. Br J Haematol 35:275–283, 1977

188. Walsh PN, Murphy S, Barry WE: The role of platelets in the pathogenesis of thrombosis and hemorrhage in patients with thrombocytosis. Thromb Haemost 38:1085–1096, 1977

189. Cortellazzo S, Colucci M, Barbui T, et al: Reduced platelet factor X-activating activity. A possible contribution to bleeding complications in polycythemia vera and essential thrombocythaemia. Haemostasis 10:37–50, 1981

190. Nishimura J, Okamoto S, Ibayashi H: Abnormalities of platelet adenine nucleotides in patients with myeloproliferative disorders. Thromb Haemost 41:787–795, 1979

191. Cooper B, Ahern D: Characterization of the platelet prostaglandin $D_2$ receptor. Loss of prostaglandin $D_2$ receptor in platelets of patients withh myeloproliferative disorders. J Clin Invest 64:586–590, 1979

191a. Murphy S, Rosenthhal DS, Weinfeld A, et al: Essential thrombocythemia: Response during first year of therapy with melphalan and radioactive phosphorous. A polycythemia vera study group report. Cancer Treat Rep. 66:1495–1500, 1982

192. Roberts LJ II, Sweetman BJ, Lewis RA, et al: Increased production of prostaglandin $D_2$ in patients with systemic mastocytosis. N Engl J Med 303:1400–1404, 1980

193. Berger S, Aledort LM, Gilbert HS, et al: Abnormalities of platelet function in patients with polycythemia vera. Cancer Res 33:2683–2687, 1973

194. Mason JE Jr, DeVita VT, Canellos GP: Thrombocytosis in chronic granulocytic leukemia: Incidence and clinical significance. Blood 44:483–487, 1974

195. Hardisty RM, Caen JP: Disorders of platelet function, in Bloom AL, Thomas DP (eds): Haemostasis and Thrombosis. Edinburgh, Churchill Livingstone, 1981, pp 301–320

196. Weiss HJ: Congenital qualitative platelet disorders, in Williams WJ et al (eds): Hematology (2nd ed). New York, McGraw-Hill, 1977, pp 1368–1377

197. Weiss HJ. Acquired qualitative platelet disorders, in Williams WJ et al (eds): Hematology (2nd ed). New York, McGraw-Hill, 1977, pp 1377–1384

198. Sultan Y, Brouet JC, Devergie A: Isolated platelet factor 3 deficiency. N Engl J Med 294:1121, 1976 (letter)

199. Weiss HJ, Vicic WJ, Lages BA, et al: Isolated deficiency of platelet procoagulant activity. Am J Med 67:206–213, 1979

200. Minkoff IM, Wu KK, Walasek J, et al: Bleeding disorder due to an isolated platelet factor 3 deficiency. Arch Intern Med 140:366–367, 1980

201. Girolami A, Brunetti A, Fioretti D, et al: Congenital thrombocytopathy (platelet factor 3 defect) with prolonged bleeding time but normal platelet adhesiveness and aggregation. Acta Haematol 50:116–123, 1973

202. Miletich JP, Kane WH, Hofman SL, et al: Deficiency of factor Xa-factor Va binding sites on the platelets of a patient with a bleeding disorder. Blood 54:1015–1022, 1979

203. Weiss HJ, Rogers J: Fibrinogen and platelets in the primary arrest of bleeding. Studies in two patients with congenital afibrinogenemia. N Engl J Med 285:369–374, 1971

204. Gralnick HR: Congenital disorders of fibrinogen, in Williams WJ et al (eds): Hematology (2nd ed). New York, McGraw-Hill, 1977, pp 1423–1431

205. George JN, Reimann TA: Inherited disorders of the platelet membrane: Glanzmann's thrombasthenia and Bernard-Soulier disease, in Colman RW et al (eds): Thrombosis and Hemostasis, Basic Principles and Clinical Practice. Philadelphia, JB Lippincott, 1982, pp 496–506

205a. Reichert N, Seligsohn U, Ramot B: Clinical and genetic aspects of Glanzmann's thrombasthenia in Israel. Thromb Diath Haemorrh 34:806–820, 1975

206. Caen JP, Castaldi PA, Leclerc JC, et al: Congenital bleeding disorders with long bleeding time and normal platelet count. I. Glanzmann's thrombasthenia (report of fifteen patients). Am J Med 41:4–26, 1966

207. McEver RP, Baenziger NL, Majerus PW: Isolation and quantitation of the platelet membrane glycoprotein deficient in thrombasthenia using a monoclonal hybridoma antibody. J Clin Invest 66:1311–1318, 1980

208. Kunicki TJ, Pidard D, Cazenave J-P, et al: Inheritance of the human platelet alloantigen, Pl$^{A1}$, in Type I Glanzmann's thrombasthenia. J Clin Invest 67:717–724, 1981

208a. Stormorken H, Gogstad GO, Solum NO, et al: Diagnosis of heterozygotes in Glanzmann's thrombasthenia. Thromb Haemostas 48:217–221, 1982

209. Holahan JR, White GC II: Heterogeneity of membrane surface proteins in Glanzmann's thrombasthenia. Blood 57:174–181, 1981

209a. Lightsey AL, Throma WJ, Plow EF, et al: Glanzmann's thrombasthenia in the absence of glycoprotein IIb and III deficiency. Blood 58(suppl 1):199a, 1981 (abstract)

209b. Nurden AT, Rosa J-P, Boizard B, et al: Evidence that GPIIb-IIIa complexes are required for ADP-induced platelet aggregation from studies on the platelets of a patient with a new type of Glanzmann's thrombasthenia. Thromb Haemostas 50:216, 1983 (abstract)

210. Nurden AT, Caen JP: An abnormal platelet glycoprotein pattern in three cases of Glanzmann's thrombasthenia. Br J Haematol 28:253–260, 1974

211. Phillips DR, Agin PP: Platelet membrane defects in Glanzmann's thrombasthenia. J Clin Invest 60:535–545, 1977

212. Clemetson KJ, Capitanio A, Pareti FI, et al: Additional platelet membrane glycoprotein abnormalities in Glanzmann's thrombasthenia: A comparison with normals by high resolution two-dimensional polyacrylamide gel electrophoresis. Thromb Res 18:797–806, 1980

213. Gogstad GO, Hagen I, Korsmo R, et al: Evidence for a separate localization of platelet glycoprotein IIb and IIIa in the $\alpha$-granule membrane. Thromb Haemost 46:109, 1981 (abstract)

214. Brown CH III, Weisberg RJ, Natelson EA, et al: Glanzmann's thrombasthenia: Assessment of the response to platelet transfusions. Transfusion 15:124–131, 1975

215. Degos L, Dautiguy A, Brouet JC, et al: A molecular defect in thrombasthenic platelets. J Clin Invest 56:236–240, 1975

216. Tschopp TB, Weiss HJ, Baumgartner HR: Interaction of thrombasthenic platelets with subendothelium: Normal adhesion, absent aggregation. Experimentia 31:113–116, 1975

217. Chediak J, Telfer MC, Vander Laan B, et al: Cycles of agglutination-disagglutination induced by ristocetin in thrombasthenic platelets. Br J Haematol 43:113–126, 1979

218. Maldonado JE, Gilchrist GS, Brigden LP, et al: Ultrastructure of platelets in Bernard-Soulier syndrome. Mayo Clin Proc 50:402–406, 1975

219. Coller BS: Preliminary characterization of platelet-derived hybridoma antibodies that inhibit ristocetin and bovine von Willebrand factor-induced platelet aggregation. Blood 58:191a, 1981 (abstract)

220. Walsh PN, Mills DCB, Pareti FI, et al: Hereditary giant platelet syndrome: Absence of collagen-induced coagulant activity and deficiency of factor XI binding to platelets. Br J Haematol 29:639–655, 1975

221. Bithell TC, Parekh SJ, Strong RR: Platelet-function studies in the Bernard-Soulier syndrome. Ann NY Acad Sci 201a:145–160, 1972

222. George JN, Reimann TA, Moake JL, et al: Bernard-Soulier disease: A study of four patients and their parents. Br J Haematol 48:459–467, 1981

222a. Degos L, Tobelem G, Lethielleaux P, et al: Molecular defect in platelets from patients with Bernard-Soulier syndrome. Blood 50:899–903, 1977

223. Rabiner SF: Uremic bleeding. In Spaet TH (ed), Prog Hemost Thromb Vol. I, New York: Grune & Stratton, 1972, pp 233–250

224. Malpass TW, Harker LA: Acquired disorders of platelet function. Semin Hematol 17:242–258, 1980

225. Gallice P, Fournier N, Crevat A, et al: In vitro inhibition of platelet aggregation by uremic middle molecules. Biomedicine (Paris) 33:185–188, 1980

226. Kazatchkine M, Sultan Y, Caen JP, et al: Bleeding in renal failure: A possible cause. Br Med J 2:612–615, 1976

227. Warrell RP Jr, Hultin MB, Coller BS: Increased factor VIII/von Willebrand factor antigen and von Willebrand factor activity in renal failure. Am J Med 66:226–228, 1979

228. Remuzzi G, Marchesi D, Cavenaghi AE, et al: Bleeding in renal failure: A possible role of vascular prostacyclin (PGI$_2$). Clin Nephrol 12:127–131, 1979

229. Defreyn G, Vergara Dauden M, Machin SJ, et al: A plasma factor in uremia which stimulates prostacyclin release from cultured endothelial cells. Thromb Res 19:695–699, 1980

230. Janson PA, Jubelirer SJ, Weinstein MJ, et al: Treatment of the bleeding tendency in uremia with cryoprecipitate. N Engl J Med 303:1318–1322, 1980

230a. Mannucci PM, Remuzzi G, Pusineri F et al: Deamino-8-D-arginine vasopressin shortens the bleeding time in uremia. N Eng J Med 308:8, 1983

231. Shattil SJ, Bennett JS, McDonough M, et al: Carbenicillin and penicillin G inhibit platelet function in vitro by impairing the interaction of agonists with the platelet surface. J Clin Invest 65:329–337, 1980

232. O'Brien JR, Etherington MD, Shuttleworth RD: Ticlopidine—an antiplatelet drug: Effects in human volunteers. Thromb Res 13:245–254, 1978

233. McGrath KM, Stuart JJ, Richard F II: Correlation between serum IgG, platelet membrane IgG and platelet function in hypergammaglobulinemic states. Br J Haematol 42:585–591, 1979

234. Wu KK: Bleeding disorders due to abnormalities in platelet prostaglandins, in Wu KK, Rossi EC (eds): Prostaglandins in Clinical Medicine. Chicago, Year Book, 1982, 81–92

235. Weiss HJ. Congenital disorders of platelet function. Semin Hematol 17:228–241, 1980

236. Malmsten C, Hamberg M, Svensson J, et al: Physiological role of an endoperoxide in human platelets: Hemostatic defect due to platelet cyclo-oxygenase deficiency. Proc Natl Acad Sci USA 72:1446–1450, 1975

237. Lagarde M, Byron PA, Vargaftig BB, et al: Impairment of platelet thrombaxane A$_2$ generation and of the platelet release reaction in two patients with congenital deficiency of platelet cyclo-oxygenase. Br J Haematol 38:251–266, 1978

238. Pareti FI, Mannucci PM, D'Angelo A, et al: Congenital deficiency of thromboxane and prostacyclin. Lancet 1:898–900, 1980

239. Mestel F, Oetiliker O, Beck E, et al: Severe bleeding associated with defective thromboxane synthetase. Lancet 1:157, 1980 (letter)

240. Machin SJ, Carreras LO, Chamone DAF, et al: Familial deficiency of thromboxane synthetase. Br J Haematol 47:629, 1981 (abstract)

241. Wu KK, Le Breton GC, Tai H-H, et al: Abnormal platelet response to thromboxane A$_2$. J Clin Invest 67:1801–1804, 1981

242. Samama M, Lecrubier C, Conard J, et al: Constitutional thrombocytopathy with subnormal response to thromboxane A$_2$. Br J Haematol 48:293–303, 1981

243. Lages B, Malmsten C, Weiss HJ, et al: Impaired platelet response to thromboxane-A$_2$ and defective calcium mobilization in a patient with a bleeding disorder. Blood 57:545–552, 1981

243a. Deykin D, Janson P, McMahon L. Ethanol potentiation of aspirin—induced prolongation of the bleeding time. N Eng J Med 306:852–854, 1982

244. Weiss HJ, Lages B: Platelet malondialdehyde production and aggregation responses induced by arachidonate, prostaglandin-G$_2$, collagen, and epinephrine in 12 patients with storage pool deficiency. Blood 58:27–33, 1981

245. Weiss HJ, Witte LD, Kaplan KL, et al: Heterogeneity in storage pool deficiency: Studies on granule-bound substances in 18 patients including variants deficient in α-granules, platelet factor 4,β-thromboglobulin, and platelet-derived growth factor. Blood 54:1296–1319, 1979

246. Gerritsen SW, Akkerman J-WN, Sixma JJ: Correction of the bleeding time in patients with storage pool deficiency by infusion of cryoprecipitate. Br J Haematol 40:153–160, 1978

247.  Gerrard JM, Phillips DR, Rao GHR, et al: Biochemical studies of two patients with the gray platelet syndrome. J Clin Invest 66:102–109, 1980

248.  Levy-Toledano S, Caen JP, Breton-Gorius J, et al: Gray platelet syndrome: α-Granule deficiency. J Lab Clin Med 98:831–848, 1981

249.  Raccuglia G: Gray platelet syndrome. A variety of qualitative platelet disorder. Am J Med 51:818–828, 1971

250.  Jaffe EA, Leung LLK, Nachman RL, et al: Thrombospondin is the endogenous lectin of human platelets. Blood 58(suppl 1):196a, 1981 (abstract)

251.  Stoff JS, Stemerman M, Steer M. A defect in platelet aggregation in Bartter's syndrome. Am J Med 68:171–180, 1980

252.  Qualitative disorders of platelet function, in Wintrobe MM, et al (eds): Clinical Hematology (8th ed). Philadelphia, Lea & Febiger, 1981, pp 1135–1157

Charles D. Forbes

# 5

# Clinical Aspects of the Hemophilias and Their Treatment

## CLASSIC HEMOPHILIA AND CHRISTMAS DISEASE

Classic hemophilia (hemophilia A) and Christmas disease (hemophilia B) are life-long hemorrhagic diseases, both inherited as X chromosome-linked disorders and thus limited almost exclusively to males. Both disorders are heterogeneous. The coagulant defect in classic hemophilia is the functional deficiency of antihemophilic factor (AHF, factor VIII), as measured in clotting assays. The plasma of affected patients, however, contains normal or elevated amounts of antigens related to factor VIII that can be detected by heterologous antiserum against this agent.[1] A minority of patients also have antigens that react with human antibodies against the coagulant properties of factor VIII.

In Christmas disease, the coagulant defect is the functional deficiency of factor IX (Christmas factor). Several varieties of Christmas disease have been described. In most patients, the coagulant deficiency of factor IX is paralleled by a deficiency of antigens recognized by antiserum against this agent, that is, the defect is cross-reacting material negative (CRM⁻). In others, disproportionately high titers of factor IX-like antigens can be detected, that is, the defect is CRM⁺. Such individuals synthesize one or another abnormal variant of factor IX.[2-5a] In this latter group of patients there is a subset, said to have hemophilia $B_m$, who have a long prothrombin time, but this is demonstrable only when the tissue thromboplastin used in this assay is of bovine origin.[6] Doubt has been expressed that all patients who have hemophilia $B_m$ are CRM⁺.[7]

The diagnosis of classic hemophilia or Christmas disease is suggested by the coincidence of an abnormally long activated partial thromboplastin time and a normal prothrombin time; the bleeding time is normal. The defect is then delineated by specific assays (Chapter 3). These tests allow a semi-quantitative estimation of the degree of the coagulant defect, which, in most instances, parallels the severity of the patient's symptoms. Classic hemophilia must also be distinguished from von Willebrand's disease (Chapter 6), in which a coagulant deficiency of factor VIII is coupled with a long bleeding time and impaired agglutination of platelets upon addition of ristocetin to platelet-rich plasma.

Additionally, in most patients with von Willebrand's disease, antigens detected by heterologous antiserum against factor VIII are depressed.

## Incidence and Distribution

Classic hemophilia and Christmas disease have been recorded in all human races and in many animal species. Variations in the incidence of disease may represent problems of assay, accelerated death rates due to lack of treatment, and true variations in genetic incidence. In the United Kingdom, about 1–2 persons per 10,000 population are affected with hemophilia, giving about 3,500 patients. A similar incidence has been estimated in the United States, with 20,000 patients,[8] and in continental Europe.[9] In Africa it is said to be uncommon in the Bantu,[10-14] which may represent, in part at least, excessive mortality associated with ritual circumcision as well as underdiagnosis.[11,12] The disorder does, however, seem to be significantly less common in American blacks.[15]

The incidence of Christmas disease is about one-sixth to one-tenth that of classic hemophilia.[16,17] Exceptions occur in certain instances, in which for geographical or religious reasons a high incidence has appeared in specific areas, such as the Tenna Valley in Switzerland,[18] certain African countries,[10,19] and the Amish communities in Ohio and Pennsylvania, in the United States.[20] Christmas disease is rare in Japan.[21]

The incidence of von Willebrand's disease varies widely according to the ability of centers to define it accurately. In addition, there are probably true geographical variations due to interbreeding in closed communities.[22] Heterozygotes for the disease are reported to be half as common as in classic hemophilia, but the incidence of homozygotes is about one per million of the United Kingdom population.[23]

The other genetic disorders of clotting are either rare or extremely rare. Their importance, however, lies in the role they have played in elucidation of the mechanisms of blood coagulation, hemostasis, and thrombosis.

## Clinical Presentation

The presentations of classic hemophilia and Christmas disease are identical and will be described in detail. Many of the other disorders show significant differences from hemophilia in the type and site of bleeding; these will be described later.

The time at which bleeding starts is determined by the clinical severity of the defect. The clinical severity usually correlates with the assayed level of factor VIII (AHF) or factor IX (Christmas factor), as measured in clotting assays. A severe defect is manifested by recurrent spontaneous bleeding and is associated with a factor level less than 0.01 U/ml (where the average normal standard is 1.0 U/ml or 100 percent). A moderate defect is one in which bleeding may occur spontaneously but often appears after trauma or surgery; the factor level ranges from 0.01 to 0.05 U/ml. A mild defect is associated with bleeding after trauma or surgery but not spontaneously; the factor level is 0.05–0.5 U/ml. Occasionally, patients are found in whom the clinical grade of defect does not match the assayed level of factor; for example, a patient with a factor level of less than 0.01 U/ml may never have had spontaneous bleeding.

Although the level of factor VIII in normal people increases with exercise, emotion, and epinephrine (adrenaline) infusion,[24-26] this is of little importance under physiological conditions in classic hemophilia. Many of the patients who have been observed carefully over many years go through "bleeding phases" in which they lurch from one bleeding crisis to another. There seems to be no good reason for this; undoubtedly in the past, some of these patients probably had developed factor VIII inhibitors and became unresponsive to infusions, and probably some had taken analgesics which compounded their hemostatic abnormality, but such phases of bleeding are still seen in patients who do not have either problem. Repeated assays of factor VIII show no variation which can account for this pattern. It has also been suggested that bleeding is seasonal, with most bleeds occurring in the winter.[27] This has been our experience with certain patients, but curiously, the stated peak of incidence of bleeding in winter does not coincide with the peak demand for blood products.

The level of factor VIII recorded in members of any one family remains remarkably constant, and the clinical severity is usually similar. The exception to this is an unusual variant in which the levels of factor VIII fluctuate (Heckathorn's disease).[28] This constancy of defect within a family is often an important factor to emphasize during genetic counseling, as it will often sway a patient toward or away from termination of a pregnancy.

Because platelet function is normal, primary hemostasis (and the bleeding time) are normal. Bleeding in hemophilia is more typically manifested by the formation of internal hematomas rather than by mucosal bleeding. Excess bleeding at birth is rare; the first manifestations usually occur when the baby starts to move around in his cot. However, bleeding will occur after surgery (e.g., circumcision) or intramuscular injections, and these should be avoided. The first signs the parents may notice are large skin bruises, often on the head and arms; these may be severe enough to raise accusations of a battered baby syndrome. Abnormal bleeding may then occur from or into any part of the body. The most common sites are joints, muscles, renal tract, gut, and mouth after dental extraction.

## Joint Disease

The clinical features of acute hemarthrosis in hemophilia were well described in early clinical case reports,[29] but it was not initially appreciated that the acutely swollen joint contained blood. This was first proposed by Dubois in 1838,[30] but the suggestion was met with great resistance until Reinert, in 1869,[31] described a patient with a bleeding tendency who developed an acute swelling of the shoulder joint which suppurated and liberated a great quantity of blood. This observation was confirmed when the knee joint of a hemophiliac was aspirated and a large volume of fluid blood escaped.[32]

The earliest postmortem examination of the chronic joint changes in hemophilia was that of Lemp,[33] who in 1857 described the pigmentation and hypertrophy of the synovium associated with dissolution of the articular cartilage. In 1892, Konig[34] published the first detailed account of the pathological changes in a large series of joints and correlated these changes with the number of acute bleeding episodes. The histology of both acute and chronic joint changes has now been well documented by a variety of authors,[35-37] and observations have also been made in hemophilic dogs with joint disease.[38,39]

### Acute Hemarthrosis

Joint disease is the single most important cause of morbidity in hemophilia. The incidence varies with the severity of the bleeding tendency, and up to 90 percent of severely affected patients may have had this complicaton.[40]

The joint most commonly affected is the knee, followed by the elbow, ankle, and wrist. Bleeding into other joints is less common, and bleeding into the hip is distinctly less frequent.[41] This is surprising, as weight bearing is one of the important factors responsible for the initiation of bleeding, but the hip may gain protection from trauma by the large muscle cuff of flexors and extensors. It seems that once a joint has been "targeted" by a series of bleeds, it is liable to recurrent bleeding, probably due to the chronic changes of hyperplasia and hyperemia of the synovium.[41a] Curiously, the hands are usually spared.

*Clinical features.*   Premonitory symptoms of bleeding are often found in patients before overt signs are present. These include a feeling of warmth or prickling. Administration of the appropriate plasma concentrate may abort the bleed at this stage. Pain is the most common feature of the acute joint bleed. This is probably due partly to an acute inflammatory response associated with kinin generation and partly to distention of the joint capsule by blood. Bleeding is associated with limitation of movement, and the joint is held in the position in which the volume of the joint space is maximal, usually in flexion.[42] The other signs are those of acute inflammation with tenderness to the touch, an easily detectable rise in temperature, and obvious distention of the capsule. The amount of distention varies greatly, and may be restricted in a patient with previous recurrent bleeding and fibrous adhesions.

*Investigation.*   Radiological examination is of little value except when trauma is involved and a fracture may be suspected. X-ray may also show the chronic degenerative changes of previous bleeds, but this is of little practical importance in the management of the acute event.

Thermography may be of value in determining the extent of inflammation, as the local temperature of the skin over the joint may be as much as 5°C higher than that of the normal joint.[43,44] Thermography is also a good test for objective assessment of therapeutic regimens. Surprisingly, thermography remains abnormal for several weeks after the joint has returned to clinical normality.

In addition, radionuclide scanning of the acute joint with $^{99m}$Tc-pertechnetate shows grossly abnormal uptake of the isotope.[45] Although visualization of the isotope in an inflamed joint reflects mainly increased vascularity of the synovial membrane and other joint tissues,[46,47] part of the localization of the radioactivity is due to binding of the technetium by the hypertrophied synovium.[48,49] These isotope scans also remain abnormal for several months following clinical resolution of the acute bleed, probably reflecting the presence of the hypertrophied, hyperemic synovium. It is probable that these changes are associated with the onset of chronic degenerative changes in cartilage and bone.

*Pathology.*   The etiology of the joint changes is poorly understood. Much of this knowledge is derived from pathological studies of hemophilic dog joints which are similarly affected.[36,38,39] It is probable that bleeding originates in the rich vascular bed of the synovial plexus and probably starts in one of the hypertrophied synovial villi that is trapped by the joint action. The expanding hematoma rapidly ruptures into the joint space, with production of the classic signs of acute inflammation. Within a few hours, an acute inflammatory exudate forms, with migration of polymorphonuclear leukocytes and an increase in synovial lining cells. Synovial hypertrophy occurs within a few days, and the frondlike villi are full of lymphocytes, histiocytes, and polymorphonuclear cells. Macroscopically, the joint surfaces are stained brown from hemosiderin; microscopically, this pigment may be seen in the pericytes. It has been suggested that the presence of iron stimulates the production of cathepsins, which lead to cartilage destruction.[50]

*Management.*   As hemarthrosis is an acutely painful condition, adequate amounts of potent analgesics are required, and it may be necessary to control the pain with morphine. Such treatment must not be continued for more than a few days because of the possibility of drug dependence. Adequate amounts of clotting factor concentrates are also necessary to stop further bleeding. In their own right, they seem to be effective in reducing pain and facilitating resorption of blood. Therapy should be aimed at raising the clotting factor level to at least 0.3 U/ml, which should be maintained for several days. The majority of minor and moderate bleeds will respond to these simple measures, and the patient can be rapidly mobilized in a few days. In addition, there is some evidence of benefit from the use of a short course of steroids (page 214). If immobilization is prolonged, active and passive exercises are required to ensure that no wasting of the muscle cuffs occurs. Exercise is best carried out immediately after infusion of concentrates.

There is little evidence that aspiration of blood in acute bleeding is of value. In a controlled trial, such a procedure was shown to have slight immediate benefit, but on assessment six weeks after the event, there was no evidence of benefit in the group with aspirated joints. Additionally, aspiration produces the risks of infection and hemorrhage from the needle track.

In a major acute bleed associated with severe pain and muscle spasm, admission to the hospital may be necessary and splinting is of value in providing protection from movement. This may be done using plaster of paris back slabs or a plastic equivalent. Analgesia, concentrates, and intensive physiotherapy are required. In addition, many patients find benefit from the use of ice packs or a commercial equivalent. Elevation of the limb may also improve comfort.

### Chronic Hemophilic Arthritis

The chronic degenerative lesions of the joints in hemophilia have been well described both microscopically and macroscopically.[34,36,37,51,52] Such chronic changes usually predominate in the large weight-bearing jonts and have the following incidence: knee, 68 percent; ankle, 56 percent; elbow, 53 percent; and hip, 16 percent. Smaller joints are rarely involved.[53] Such changes usually appear only with increasing age, and the severity is often directly related to the number of hemarthroses into the joint.

*Clinical features.*   Many affected joints are free of pain despite the presence of gross deformity. Loss of movement is an invariable feature, and many joints have fixed flexion contractures. The muscle cuffs around the joint may be severely atrophied despite attempts to avoid this with intensive physiotherapy. In addition, unbalanced actions of muscle groups may lead to severe deformity before apparent changes occur in the joint itself. For example, rotational and valgus deformities may occur in the knee as a result of wasting of the quadriceps muscles that oppose the more powerful hamstrings.

It is inevitable that, as the changes of osteoarthrosis appear, the symptoms change. There may be chronic pain which requires constant analgesia. Episodes of acute hemarthrosis may result in a much smaller volume of blood in the joint, but because of the contracted, fibrous capsule, they are acutely painful. Chronic effusions may present as a painless ''boggy'' swelling of the joint. About 20 percent of every group of hemophilic patients will require mobility aids such as crutches or sticks, and 8 percent will require a wheelchair.[51] With time and repeated bleeding, the progression is toward reduction in movement due to fibrous ankylosis and the development of pain due to osteoarthrosis.

*Pathology.* The gross appearance of the synovium resembles that of pigmented villonodular synovitis, with extensive areas of brown pigment in the synovium and in the articular cartilage. The cartilage loses its normal sheen and becomes irregularly pitted. Loose flakes of cartilage may be found in the joint cavity, and at the edges of the articular surface synovial membrane may replace cartilage. There is also a great variation in cartilage thickness; in some areas cartilage may be totally eroded, with exposure of the underlying bone. Bone cysts may form deep in the cartilage as a result of hemorrhage.

Microscopically, the synovium is greatly hypertrophied and heavily infiltrated with extensive deposits of iron, lymphocytes, and monocytes. There is also extensive fibrosis, and the superficial layers contain leashes of dilated blood vessels which are of venous origin. It is thought that these thin-walled veins form the site of repeated hemorrhage. In addition, the walls of these veins are a rich source of plasminogen activator, which may be one source of continuing bleeding.

*Radiology.* In the chronic hemophilic arthritic joint, radiological findings[51,54–56] are diverse and are characteristic of the disease. As a result of acute bleeding, which results in hyperemia, osteoporosis is invariable and soft tissue shadows due to synovial iron are seen.[57] Loss of cartilage results in loss of joint space, and as cartilage is replaced peripherally, the underlying bone is resorbed, with formation of subchondral cysts which are typical of hemophilic joint disease. With progression of the disease, eburnation of bone occurs and osteophytic outgrowth may be marked. Bony ankylosis is rare, and the limited movement of the joint is almost always due to soft tissue changes.

In some joints, notably the knee, resorption of bone may result from synovial hypertrophy, with production of an enlarged intercondylar fossa, and there may be differential overgrowth of one of the femoral condyles. Such valgus deformity may be associated with instability of the joint, with posterior subluxation of the tibia and lateral shift of the tibia on the femur.[36]

*Management.* The mainstay of management is conservative, with adequate analgesia to relieve pain, physiotherapy to maintain and improve mobility, corrective devices to restore flexion deformities, and lightweight splints to maintain the correction. Lastly, when all else has failed, reconstructive surgery may be required.

Such surgery must be undertaken in highly specialized orthopedic units in association with a hemophilia center.[58,59] Minor procedures include patellectomy for painful disease localized to the retropatellar region and synovectomy; gentle manipulation[51] or synoviorthesis[60,61] under anesthesia may overcome a flexion deformity with extreme muscle spasm.

It must be remembered that teen-age patients with hemophilic disease are also liable to the usual problems of other adolescents. In the knee joint, the diagnosis of a torn meniscus may be made by arthroscopy.[62] Such patients merit a standard meniscectomy.

In many older patients with painful fixed flexion contractions, the last approach is arthrodesis or arthroplasty.[63,64] An alternative to surgery in patients with synovial hypertrophy is the use of injections of radionuclides. Success has been claimed for this procedure, but the long-term effects need to be fully evaluated.[60] We currently favor a more conservative approach with synovectomy first, followed by joint replacement if this fails. The results of replacement of the knee joint to date are good in the short term, but the procedure is known to have a substantial failure rate in the long term in other types of arthritis,[65] and as yet no group has had enough long-term experience with hemophilia.[66,67] The main advantage of joint replacement is the immediate relief of chronic pain, and if simultaneous synovectomy is carried out, reduction of bleeding episodes is also found.[66,68] If such procedures fail, then arthrodesis may be of value. The usual indication is failure of conservative management, but it has a place in the correction of severe deformity and instability of a joint. The long-term results are good, with reasonable mobility and freedom from chronic pain.[58]

Orthopedic procedures are rarely required on the upper limb, as the joints there are usually less severely affected. The most common surgical operation is excision of the radial head for chronic pain and stiffness of the elbow joint.

## Muscle Bleeding and Hematoma

Bleeding into muscles has long been recognized as a frequent and disabling cause of morbidity in coagulation disorders. Usually this occurs after trauma, but it can also occur spontaneously or after emotional stress. Not until 1839 was it appreciated that these large swellings contained altered blood.[69] In the original patient, the swelling was opened surgically and the patient died from exsanguination.

In numerous studies, bleeding into muscles is recorded as being the third most common type of bleeding, occurring in as many as 75 percent of severely affected patients.[70,71]

In the upper limb, most hematomas are in the anterior surface in the flexor group of muscles, whereas in the lower limb, the soleus and gastrocnemius muscles are most commonly affected. The clinical features depend on the muscle involved, its size and fascial confines, and the severity of the coagulation defect. If the cause of hematoma is direct trauma, there may be superficial bruising followed by an expanding, painful lesion in the muscle. Often, however, there seems to be no particular precipitating cause; the patient simply presents with pain and swelling. On occasion, such a lesion may follow an intramuscular injection; this procedure must be prohibited.

Bleeding produces a tender, swollen lesion in the muscle which rapidly goes into protective spasm and causes flexion of the adjacent joint, with restriction of movement and severe pain.

Little work has been done on the pathology of such muscle hematomas, but it would seem that muscle necrosis occurs rapidly due to ischemia of the fibers as the expanding hematoma strips off the neurovascular bundles. Death of muscle is evidenced by the rise in the serum levels of enzymes associated with muscle function, that is, creatine kinase, lactic dehydrogenase, the aminotransferases, and aldolase. Levels of these enzymes may be used as a diagnostic aid.[72] As a result of bleeding, there is an acute inflammatory reaction, with infiltration of the muscle with polymorphonuclear leukocytes and later with phagocytic mononuclear cells. Healing takes place slowly, with replacement of the muscle fibers with collagen and no effective regeneration of muscle fibers.[73]

Large muscle hematomas may produce compression of adjacent nerves, blood vessels, and other structures. It is usually when such lesions become chronic that they assume major significance (see the section on pseudotumors). Muscle hematomas do not usually present a major diagnostic problem, as they are generally found in a peripheral location and are easily palpated. If, however, they occur within the abdomen, the diagnosis is more difficult. In this situation, the diagnosis may be made by serial estimation of muscle enzymes,[72] and the extent and position of hematomas may be determined by ultrasonography[74-76] or by computed tomography (CT). An ultrasonic technique will show that such lesions are poorly transonic, that is, they behave as cystic lesions and are of varying consistency. All hematomas contain reflecting speckles which probably represent isolated muscle bundles as well as nerves and blood vessels. In a large series of cases we have shown rapid resorption of the muscle hematoma, but the muscle volume was significantly reduced after the healing phase was complete.

The fate of the blood clot is unknown, but it is presumably digested by local tissue and white cell enzymes. Serial estimation of the levels of fibrin degradation products (FDP) shows no change in level.

An important site of hematoma formation is the iliopsoas muscle. This results in compression of the femoral nerve (see the section on peripheral nerve lesions). CT is of great value in establishing the diagnosis in this condition and following the patient's progress. Sublingual hematomas were once a common cause of death in young hemophiliacs, but they are now rarely a problem as they respond rapidly to concentrates. Spontaneous or traumatically induced bleeding into the retroperitoneal tissues may occur, and because of tracking of blood between tissue planes, a volume sufficient to produce severe hypotension may be lost. Diagnosis may be made by CT scanning or ultrasonography.

The treatment of all hematomas is conservative, with adequate analgesia and factor replacement. Relief of pain may also be achieved with an ice pack and a plaster of paris back slab to stop movement of the affected part. One should not attempt to aspirate these hematomas due to the likelihood of introducing infection and creating a chronic sinus.

## Pseudotumors (Hemophilic Blood Cysts)

The formation of pseudotumors in patients with bleeding disorders is rare; the incidence in several large series of patients with hemophilia ranges from 0.5 to 2.0 percent.[77-79] The most common anatomical sites are the thigh and pelvis, but a small number of cases have been reported in the calves, feet, arms, and hands. Bilateral pseudotumors have been recorded in only 3 patients; these involved the cuboid bones of the feet[80] and the pelvis.[74,81]

Pseudotumors are found in both classic hemophilia and Christmas disease[82] despite the suggestion that Christmas disease patients are more likely to have a less serious defect.[83] It is of great interest that a pseudotumor has also been reported in a patient with an exceptionally mild bleeding defect and an AHF titer of 23 percent.[84]

In several of the case reports, including the original, there has been some clinical doubt about the diagnosis, the suspicion being that the destructive lesion might be osteogenic sarcoma.[84-87] In many of the cases in which biopsy was undertaken, serious complications ensued, including death from infection introduced at the time of diagnostic aspiration or uncontrollable hemorrhage from the needle track.[82,84,87,88] Osteogenic sarcoma has, however, been described in a hemophilic patient[89] and should always enter into the differential diagnosis despite its rare occurrence.

### Pathology

The cause of the expanding lesion is not clear but, it almost certainly has its origin either in a deep muscle hematoma, which may be retained under pressure inside the muscle fascia and aponeurosis, or as bleeding between the bone and the periosteum, which is easily detached from the diaphysis of the long bones in the young. In both situations there may be no history of trauma or injury. The encapsulated collections of blood undergo further bleeding, with gradual increase in size, the production of pressure on surrounding structures[90]—in particular on nerves and blood vessels—and necrosis of surrounding bone. These cysts are often enormous in size and multilobulated. They contain a large mass of clot with a small amount of dark brown fluid. The wall of the pseudotumor is a tough membrane which probably represents the thickened fascia or periosteum. The wall tends to be very vascular and is heavily infiltrated with tissue macrophages stuffed with hemosiderin.[91]

### Clinical Presentation

The patient usually presents with a painless mass which has become larger over a period of months or years. The mass is usually firm and attached to deep structures such as muscle or bone. Pain may supervene if a pathological fracture of the adjacent bone occurs or if overlying nerves are involved. Occasionally, the overlying skin may be involved, with ulceration followed by infection of the cavity, septicemia, and death.

### Investigations

The diagnosis is confirmed by x-ray. The picture varies according to the site, size, and duration of the hematoma. Usually there is a large, soft tissue mass associated with destruction of adjacent bone, new bone formation in the elevated periosteum, and irregular calcification of the soft tissue mass.[92] Additional information may be obtained by ultrasonography and radionuclide scanning[74] and, in a pelvic lesion, by intravenous pyelography and barium enema.

Treatment should be aimed at prevention, and all deep hematomas should be treated vigorously with plasma factor concentrates. For the established pseudotumor, there are three avenues of treatment: immobilization and replacement therapy, radiotherapy, and extensive surgery. The choice will depend on the size and site of the lesion. There is some evidence that in younger children with open epiphyses where the lesions are small and peripheral, immobilization and replacement therapy can lead to permanent resolution without loss of function.[93–96] In large lesions of the femur and pelvis, radiotherapy has not been successful[97] but has been used to gain relief of pain.[98] In the small, peripheral pseudotumors of the hands and feet, however, radiotherapy (1500 rads) has resulted in total resolution of the lesion.[80,99]

Before the advent of adequate plasma concentrates, surgery carried a 75 percent mortality. With the appearance of better concentrates, more experience with surgical techniques, and newer antibiotics, the mortality from surgical intervention has fallen.[92] Surgery is probably less hazardous in patients with a peripheral lesion.[100] In addition, more accurate localization using ultrasonography, CT scanning, and radionuclide scanning has enabled the surgeon to plan ahead more accurately. It is essential that complete removal of the cyst wall be undertaken; this involves identification and dissection of neuromuscular bundles and bone grafting if indicated. Amputation may be required if restorative surgery is not feasible.

## Gastrointestinal Bleeding

### Upper Gastrointestinal Bleeding

In his review of 256 cases of hemophilia and related bleeding disorders, Grandidier[101] in 1855 found gastrointestinal hemorrhage to be a common cause of spontaneous bleeding; this has been confirmed in numerous recent clinical case series.[71,102] In addition, many individual case histories with gastrointestinal bleeding were recorded in the early literature, usually due to peptic ulcer and often associated with heroic attempts at surgery.[103,104] Often such attempts were doomed to failure because of deficient hemostasis, and uncontrolled gastrointestinal hemorrhage or its sequellae accounted for up to one-third of the deaths in this disease.[71,105,106] In a retrospective study of 80 adult hemophiliacs, it was found that 20 percent had suffered from gastrointestinal bleeding.[105] Most of these patients were shown to have duodenal ulceration, and one-half required either partial gastrectomy or pyloroplasty and vagotomy to control bleeding. With the advent of better concentrates infused in adequate amounts, the incidence of gastrointestinal bleeding has diminished.

The incidence of proven peptic ulceration, diagnosed either at endoscopy or on barium meal, in our patients[107] is 13 percent of the adult hemophilic population, an incidence significantly greater than that found in a comparable section of society. It is well established that such a population is under continuous stress,[108,109] and there is a proven association between stress and presentation with bleeding symptoms.[27,110,111]

About 50 percent of the patients surveyed have had no symptoms suggestive of alimentary disease before the first intestinal bleed.[107] In this group of previously symptom-free patients, there was a significantly greater number of severely affected hemophiliacs. The eupeptic and dyspeptic groups (at the time of first bleed) were identical with regard to age, blood group, age at which the first gastrointestinal bleed occurred, and ingestion of alcohol and salicylate. In patients with previous dyspeptic symptoms, 90 percent had evidence of duodenal ulcer by barium meal or endoscopy at the time of bleeding. Gastric ulcer seems to have been uncommon. On the other hand, 80 percent of patients who had been symptomless up to the time of intestinal bleeding had no evidence of an abnormality; it seems likely that in severely affected patients bleeding occurs when the mucosal injury is minimal, whereas in the dyspeptic group, in which the majority of patients are only moderately affected, the mucosal lesion must be more advanced before bleeding occurs.

Ingestion of aspirin and related anti-inflammatory drugs impairs platelet function and, in patients with coagulation defects, may produce severe alimentary hemorrhage.[112,113] All patients with coagulation defects should be warned against taking such drugs and provided with a list of proprietary drugs which contain aspirin.

The recurrence rate for alimentary bleeding is high, with two-thirds of patients having multiple episodes which eventually necessitate surgery. Mortality from gastrointestinal hemorrhage has changed considerably and now is a rare event compared to the 33 percent mortality recorded in 1961.[106] This dramatic reduction is almost totally due to the advent of plasma concentrates.

*Management.*    Patients with bleeding disorders who present with gastrointestinal bleeding should be managed the same way as patients with normal coagulation mechanisms after the hemostatic defect has been corrected with appropriate plasma concentrates. Such therapy may have to be given for 5–7 days until healing of the ulcer is complete.

Intravenous plasma, plasma expanders, or blood are necessary to correct hypotension and anemia if present. Emergency endoscopy should be carried out to define the lesion. If dyspeptic symptoms are present, oral administration of alkalis may be of value, and some physicians use a nasogastric tube to instill alkalis and milk. This may also be used to detect further bleeding. We routinely use an $H_2$-receptor blocker such as cimetidine, the first doses of which are given intravenously if peptic ulceration is present at endoscopy. Thereafter, oral medication is continued at 200 mg three times daily and 400 mg at night for 6 weeks. In addition, the patient may require oral iron for six weeks. After this time, the patient should again receive endoscopy; if the ulcer has healed, the cimetidine may be stopped. We do not yet have enough experience to predict how $H_2$ receptor blockers have affected the natural history of peptic ulcer in hemophilia, but the impression is that they are of considerable value and may also be given prophylactically.

### Intramural Hematoma of the Bowel

Bleeding into the wall of the bowel presents acutely with severe pain, often referred, and signs of intestinal obstruction. This may mimic a variety of surgical emergencies such as acute appendicitis, perforation of peptic ulcer, and acute cholecystitis; the diagnosis is difficult to make and often requires elimination of the other possibilities. It is, however, of major importance to avoid an unnecessary laparotomy; thus, it is worthwhile to give a large dose of the appropriate coagulation factor concentrate and await the response. No laboratory tests are diagnostic, but on occasion a barium meal and follow-through will determine the site of the narrowing; such a test should be done with great caution in the presence of signs of obstruction.

### Rectal Bleeding

As in any other patient, rectal bleeding requires investigation. The usual cause is hemorrhoids, but rectal carcinoma and anal fissure have been described in hemophilia. Treatment of hemorrhoids should be along conservative lines, and most patients will respond to such measures. If bleeding persists, operative treatment is necessary. We have had success with the technique of ''banding'': using a special tool, an elastic band is slipped over the base of the hemorrhoid, which is then sloughed off over the next day or so. Hemostatic cover is required during this period, and the usual nursing precautions must be taken.

## Intracranial Bleeding

Intracranial bleeding remains one of the most common causes of death in patients with bleeding disorders; the mortality rate is about 50 percent.[114] Subdural hematomas occur in hemophilic infants as a result of falls, but many episodes appear to be spontaneous, especially in severely affected patients. Often there are frank signs of neurological damage by the time the patient presents, and the diagnosis is not in doubt. A diagnostic problem, however, arises in the hemophilic patient who has received a blow to the head and who may have been unconscious but has no neurological signs. Because of the high mortality and morbidity in these patients, we treat such cases prophylactically with plasma concentrates for seven days to ensure adequate hemostasis.[115,116] In addition, all patients should have CT scanning to ensure early diagnosis of small intracerebral bleeds. We believe that by using this routine, we have significantly reduced the number of patients requiring neurosurgery—an impression also found in other clinics.[116]

It has been suggested that in hemophilic children there is a high incidence of abnormal electroencephalograms (EEGs), which may reflect previous subclinical intracerebral bleeding.[117] In a study of adult hemophiliacs in the west of Scotland, we have shown that the incidence of abnormal EEGs is similar to that of any other hospital group of patients.[118] This test is therefore of little routine value.

In the event that intracerebral bleeding is diagnosed, a massive infusion of concentrates should be given urgently to maintain a plasma factor level of 0.8–1.0 U/ml, and the patient should be investigated and treated by the neurosurgeon. Therapy must be continued until healing is complete; after craniotomy in a severely affected patient, this may require several weeks of intensive therapy.[119] At autopsy or surgery the site of bleeding is rarely found; presumably most bleeds start following trauma to small vessels. The site of bleeding may be either subdural, intracranial, or subarachnoid.[120-124] In over one-half of the patients there is no history of injury.

About 15 percent of intracerebral bleeds are associated with epileptiform seizures which may coincide with the acute event or occur months later as a result of fibrosis during the healing process. Many clinics advocate the use of anticonvulsive therapy as a prophylactic measure to protect the patient from further epileptiform fits, which may trigger a recurrence of the bleeding due to the dramatic rise in intracranial pressure which occurs during the tonic phase of a seizure. It is recommended that anticonvulsive therapy be withdrawn after several months if the EEG is normal.

### Bleeding into the Vertebral Canal

Bleeding into the vertebral canal is a rare complication of hemophilia and tends to present without any history of trauma. The signs are usually dramatic, with acute onset of pain in the neck or back and progressive onset of paralysis. The site of bleeding is rarely found but, in those patients coming to operation or autopsy, 75 percent of bleeds are extramedullary and only 25 percent are intramedullary.[116] Rarely, intramedullary bleeding is associated with a lesion of the spinal cord, for example, cavitation due to syringomyelia.[125,126]

Such patients require urgent plasma concentrate replacement, and myelography should be carried out once hemostasis is secured. If the hematoma is large, no cerebrospinal fluid may be obtained and cisternal puncture may be required to localize the lesion. About one-half of the patients described[127-129] have required operation, but in most cases surgery has had little effect and is associated with high mortality and morbidity. In one of our own patients who was shown to have a cervical extramedullary bleed with total quadriplegia, improvement was observed after he had been infused with massive amounts of concentrate prior to surgery. Subsequently, he made a gradual improvement and 5 years later he had no neurological signs.[130]

### Peripheral Nerve Lesions Due to Bleeding

The incidence of peripheral nerve lesions varies from about 5 to 15 percent of reported series of patients.[70,131] The diagnosis may be difficult to make in some patients due to associated muscular atrophy resulting from degenerative joint disease. The nerve is probably affected by compression from the expanding hematoma but may be involved as a result of ischemia.

The femoral nerve is the one most commonly affected (over 90 percent of cases), usually as a result of bleeding into the iliopsoas muscle. [131,132] Such patients present with acute pain in the lower abdomen and groin brought on by violent flexion-extension of the hip. The patient is found to be in extreme pain and lies with the hip flexed and externally rotated. Movement produces excruciating pain, and any movement is resisted. Nerve compression produces loss of knee jerk and loss of sensation over the area from the anterior thigh to below the knee. Powerful analgesics and plasma concentrates are urgently required. Immobilization of the leg with a plaster of paris back slab is of great comfort and allows the patient to sleep without inducing pain. Hemostasis must be continued until the patient has been fully mobilized, a process which requires graduated physiotherapy over several weeks to months.[133]

Rarely is the diagnosis in doubt. Occasionally, however, a right-sided lesion may be mistaken for acute appendicitis. In this case, the creatine kinase levels and other muscle enzyme assays will confirm intramuscular bleeding[72,134] and the lesion can be demonstrated by ultrasonography[74-76] and CT scanning.

## Renal Abnormalities in Bleeding Disorders

### *Hematuria*

Hematuria is a relatively common symptom in hemophilia and in various surveys was the presenting feature in up to 25 percent of cases.[70] It occurs most commonly in the 12–21 age group, and it is reported as having occurred in 60 percent of hemophilic boys.[102] It is rare to find hematuria before the age of 12 years,[135] but 90 percent of severely affected patients will have one or more episodes in their lifetime.[136] The majority of these episodes are not associated with trauma, are of short duration (2–3 days), and cease spontaneously. Because of this, they have always been felt to be benign and not intrinsically harmful to the renal tissues.[137] When qualitative studies are made of red cell excretion rates, however, there is a recorded incidence of 20 percent of subclinical hematuria.[138,139] The true incidence of hematuria, therefore, is far greater than that documented in the past.

The clinical course of untreated frank hematuria has been well documented, and even in the era preceding replacement therapy the condition was self-limited.[27] Anemia was produced occasionally, but death from exsanguination was rare. Usually there is no history of direct or indirect trauma, and there seems to be no association with recent sexual intercourse. Exceptionally, there may be a history of injury, and urgent investigation is required to ensure the integrity of the organs.[136,140,141]

It is generally believed that, with the advent of self-treatment and prophylaxis, the incidence of hematuria has significantly declined, as has the incidence of microscopic hematuria.

Paradoxically, in the untreated hemophilic patient with hematuria, clotting of the extravasated blood may occur in the urinary tract, with the production of clot colic or obstruction. This is probably a result of the presence of thromboplastins in the urine. Renal obstruction may then result from administration of plasma products[142,144] or fibrinolytic inhibitors (page 215).

### *Tests of Renal Function*

We believe that all hemophilic patients with hematuria merit investigation to eliminate other types of pathology such as renal stone,[145] malignant tumors,[140,146] traumatic rupture of the kidney or ureter,[140,141] or renal tuberculosis.

Intravenous pyelography is the technique of choice, as it will localize the side, site, and extent of an obstruction.[147,149] In our previous studies of a series of patients who had a history of hematuria but no recent bleeding, we found filling defects in the renal tract due to old clot in 38 percent of patients,[139] and in a follow-up series of patients self-treated or on prophylactic treatment, a similar incidence has been found. In addition, evidence of previous obstruction of the urinary tract with dilatation of the ureter, calices, or pelvis of the kidney was found in 10 percent of the sample.

Isotope renography using [131]I-hippuran may be used as a screening test, as it is sensitive, easily carried out, and can be repeated due to the low radiation dose involved. In our previous studies, screening by this technique showed an incidence of obstruction of 20 percent, and there was a good correlation with the pyelogram. Biochemical tests of renal function (urea, creatinine, and creatinine clearance) are also of value. Thirty percent of patients have been found to have abnormal renal function as measured by the most sensitive test, creatinine clearance.[139] Similar results have been published in other series.[145]

### Obstruction of the Renal Tract

The natural history of renal tract bleeding is very variable, and follow-up reports of renal obstruction are rare. It has been claimed that resolution of the clot occurs within two weeks.[148] However, there is now abundant evidence of long-standing unlysed clots undergoing calcification.[139,149] Surprisingly, such calcified clots, even when causing partial obstruction, do not seem to be a focus for secondary infection.

There is also evidence that in some patients with hematuria, bleeding has occurred within the renal substance and extended into the pelvis of the ureter.[149] This may cause distortion of the caliceal pattern and produce the picture of papillary necrosis by pressure or impairment of blood supply.[145]

In many of our patients with radiological evidence of obstruction, no cause was apparent. This has been confirmed in other studies,[145] and has been suggested to represent previous retroperitoneal bleeding with fibrosis and contraction. In our opinion, however, it represents slow lysis of a clot in the ureter or bladder.

Although there is a risk of producing unlysable clots in the renal tract with the use of fibrinolytic inhibitors such as epsilon-aminocaproic acid or cyclokapron, there has been little evidence of an increased incidence of renal abnormalities on the pyelogram or isotope renogram, or any significant differences in tests of renal function in a group of patients taking these drugs.[139]

A rare cause of obstruction of the renal tract is an expanding hemophilic pseudotumor of the pelvis. At least two such cases have been recorded.[74,149] In addition, four cases of nephromegaly have been reported, three of which were associated with pseudotumors of the pelvis, but with no radiological evidence of obstruction.[150] It has been suggested that the renal enlargement was due to multiple blood and plasma transfusions.

### Management of Hematuria

The patient should receive sufficient fluid to ensure a high fluid output, which will dilute the level of urokinase in the urine and flush away small clots. Hemostasis should be maintained during the period of clinical hematuria by infusion of the appropriate plasma concentrate. Blood transfusion is rarely required, but if hematuria is heavy and prolonged, a prophylactic course of iron is indicated. Adequate analgesia in combination with an antispasmodic drug should be given if colic is present (e.g., pethidine with atropine).

Routine use of fibrinolytic inhibitors is not recommended due to the theoretical risk of producing unlysable clots (page 215). However, in patients in whom bleeding continues despite adequate hemostasis or in patients with inhibitors, they may be used. We have one severely affected patient who refuses to take blood products because of his religion (Jehovah's Witness). This patient has been successfully treated on several occasions for heavy hematuria with tranexamic acid alone. In patients who do not respond to conventional treatment a trial of high-dose steroids should be given (see the section on steroid treatment). The rationale for this is not clear, but steroids act on capillary permeability, although they have little effect on either the level of AHF (factor VIII) or its duration of action.[151] In one study, however, treatment with prednisolone alone, in a dose of 2 mg/kg for 2 days followed by 1 mg/kg for 2 days, resulted in clearing of the urine.[152] These results have been confirmed, and it has been convincingly shown that although steroids alone may stop hematuria, when plasma concentrates and steroids are used in combination, treatment is 100 percent successful in a shorter period of time.[153]

### Other Renal Disorders

Renal disorders other than those due to hematuria occur. These include nephrotic syndrome, trauma, acute tubular necrosis, analgesic nephropathy, chronic pyelonephritis, renal stone, and renal neoplasia.

*Nephrotic syndrome.*  Cases of nephrotic syndrome and nephritis have been associated with hemophilia and its treatment.[138] In one case,[154] deposits of amyloid were found in the kidneys, and it was believed that this represented a response to long-standing incompatible plasma infusions; serological studies showed that the patient had a circulating anti-Gm(1) antibody. In this patient, treatment with selected Gm(−1) plasmas markedly reduced the number and severity of the reactions. Another case of nephrotic syndrome was associated with infusion of bovine factor VIII preparations to produce hemostasis for laparotomy.[155] Nephritis, which was reversible, has been induced by porcine factor VIII.[156] It is possible that the lesions were caused by the platelet-aggregating action of animal factor VIII.[157,158]

*Mismatched transfusion.*  In older patients with bleeding disorders, transfusion of whole blood was frequently necessary to combat the anemia associated with recurrent hemorrhage. As a consequence, many such patients (11 percent) had antibodies to the various blood groups, and reactions with acute hemolysis were not uncommon.[115] Acute tubular necrosis as a result seems to have been rare.[159]

*Analgesic nephropathy.*  Adequate control of pain in hemophilia (see the section on pain) remains a major problem and is often associated with abuse of anti-inflammatory and analgesic drugs. Phenacetin has no antiplatelet action but is known to have nephrotoxic activity. At least 1 such patient who ingested large amounts over a period of years was found to have hypertension, small shrunken kidneys, and sterile urine.[149]

*Pyelonephritis.*  Recurrent pyelonephritis seems to be uncommon in bleeding disorders despite the high incidence of complete or partial obstruction due to the presence of clots. In our study, none of the patients at the time of study had a positive urine culture. One patient, however, has died of chronic pyelonephritis associated with paraplegia from spinal cord hematoma; this has been recorded elsewhere.[145]

*Perirenal hematoma.*  This rare complication of bleeding disorders usually presents after trauma but may occur spontaneously. The usual presentation is acute abdominal and loin pain associated with abdominal swelling. Hematuria may or may not be found depending upon whether bleeding into the renal substance has also occurred. Retroperitoneal spread of the hematoma occurs rapidly and may mimic other abdominal catastrophies.[141] The diagnosis of retroperitoneal bleeding may be made by ultrasonic or CT scanning.

*Renal failure.*  Chronic renal failure is rare in bleeding disorders, but it presents a major management problem. As renal decompensation occurs, the platelet dysfunction of uremia becomes apparent, and correction of the clotting defect may not be possible with factor VIII concentrates. In addition, if chronic dialysis is required, it is technically more difficult, and the use of heparin to prevent platelet-fibrin deposition on the dialysis membranes may exacerbate the bleeding tendency.[160] Renal transplantation may be of value in selected patients.[160,161]

## Dental Bleeding

In bleeding disorders, dental extraction and other dental procedures have represented some of the most common hemostatic challenges to these patients. In the era before concentrates became available, they were frequent sources of morbidity and occasionally of death.

Local applications of styptics such as silver nitrate are of little value, and swabs soaked in thrombin have only a transient effect. Administration of plasma products to produce a hemostatic level of clotting factor is essential, as is immaculate dental technique, with care being taken to secure hemostasis from the gum at the time of surgery.

The keystone of dental care in hemophilia is prevention of problems, and a designated child dentist should routinely see all of these patients as part of a comprehensive care system. We encourage our parents to use fluoride tablets in order to supplement normal intake from the water supply to reduce tooth decay. Regular routine dental care starts with the appearance of the first tooth. Dental fillings can be carried out under local anesthesia, and nerve block can be safely done after a single dose of concentrate is given. We have also carried out fillings and extractions without concentrate cover under hypnosis, a procedure used elsewhere.[162]

After dental extraction, the fibrin which forms in the socket is exposed to the lytic action of plasminogen activator present in saliva. In clinical trials in which a placebo was given, bleeding from the socket occurred on the third postoperative day, suggesting that the fibrinolytic process slowly removes fibrin.[163] In the normal patient this is of little importance, but in the hemophilic patient inhibition of fibrinolysis by drugs may tilt the balance and ensure stability of the fibrin clot.

Routine extractions are carried out on an outpatient basis. The hemophiliac reports to the center for concentrate and a dose, calculated to raise his level to 0.5 U/ml, is given. He is started on tranexamic acid, 0.5 g three times a day, or epsilon-aminocaproic acid, 4 g every 4 hours for 10 days in adults and pro rata in children. An antibiotic is also routinely given to prevent infections in the socket, a factor that we believe potentiates hemorrhage. Rarely is a further dose of factor concentrate necessary. If major dental surgery is contemplated, the patient requires admission to the hospital and is treated as for other surgical procedures.

Various studies have been carried out using either epsilon-aminocaproic acid (EACA, Amicar, Epsikapron) or tranexamic acid (AMCA, Cyclokapron); some studies have been single-blind and other double-blind, with random allocation and placebo control.[163-167] Using a variety of objective criteria such as transfusion requirements, days spent in the hospital, fall of hemoglobin, and measurement of blood lost (with labeled red blood cells), there seems little doubt of the value of these inhibitors. They significantly reduce the need for factor VIII or factor IX concentrates and also reduce blood loss from the socket.[163,165] Such therapy has now been incorporated into our standard regimen for dental extraction in hemophilia.

## Inheritance

*Classic hemophilia* is transmitted as an X-linked recessive disorder and always affects males who are hemizygous. As a result, all of the sons of a hemophilic male are normal but all of his daughters are obligatory carriers, having inherited the abnormal X chromosome from their father. The daughters of these carriers then have a 50 percent chance of transmitting the disease to their sons, and a 50 percent chance that their daughters will also be carriers. From a careful history, family trees should be constructed. Until recently these have provided the basis for genetic counseling in this disease. If a careful history is obtained, over two-thirds of patients will have a positive family history.[83] The major problem is to counsel the daughters of known carriers and other female relatives in the hemophilic family. Curiously, many potential carriers do not seek information until they are pregnant.

Using assays of factor VIII clotting activity, it was learned that statistically the levels of factor VIII were lower in obligatory carriers than in a control population. However, the levels ranged from 0.02 to 2.0 U/ml, with a mean value of 0.5 U/ml.[168,169] In a small number of possible carriers in whom the level of coagulant factor VIII was low ($<$ 0.30 U/ml), this test was predictive, but in the group as a whole it was of little value.

The situation was improved greatly by the production of an antibody to factor VIII which was prepared in the rabbit (factor VIIIR:AG).[1] In the hemophilic population, the level of factor VIIIR:AG was normal or increased despite low levels of coagulant factor VIII (factor VIII:C). In obligatory carriers of hemophilia the factor VIIIR:AG levels were then shown to be normal or slightly higher than normal, with relatively less factor VIII:C. In normal control women, the levels of factor VIII:C measured by a clotting assay were proportional to the concentration of factor VIIIR:AG.[170] It was thus possible to distinguish over 90 percent of obligatory carriers from normal women while misclassifying only 1 percent of normal women as carriers. This methodology was further validated in a study of the daughters of known carriers.[171] At least 18 other research groups have now reported their findings and confirmed the principle of the test, although the detection rate has varied from 70 percent[172] to 100 percent.[173] In these initial studies there were no guidelines for standardization between centers. These are now set out in the *Bulletin of the World Health Organization* (1977), [174] which includes a section on statistical handling of the data based on discriminant analysis.[173,175,176]

Use of the relationship of factor VIIIR:AG to factor VIII:C is now the established method of carrier identification. Because the levels of factor VIII:C depend on X chromosome function, extreme inactivation of the chromosome in somatic cells could result in values of factor VIII:C within the normal range, thus making these carriers unidentifiable by this method. It is not surprising, therefore, that 10–20 percent of carriers may give normal results.[172] Some of these differences, however, are related to variations in techniques in laboratory methods, different standards, and different statistical handling. In addition, the results of some studies may have been influenced by the fact that the carriers took oral contraceptive or were pregnant.

*Christmas disease* is inherited in the same way as classic hemophilia, as an X chromosome-linked disorder. Detection of carriers is much less satisfactory than in classic hemophilia, since in most families the disorder is CRM negative (CRM⁻), that is, the titer of coagulant factor IX and of proteins detected by specific antibodies against this factor are proportionately reduced. In a group of twelve obligate carriers of Christmas disease studied at University Hospitals of Cleveland, seven could be distinguished from normal women because the coagulant titer of factor IX was 50 percent or less, at a level that misidentified 5 percent of normal women as carriers. Similar data have been recorded by others.[7,177–181]

In a minority of families with Christmas disease the defect is CRM positive (CRM$^+$), that is, the plasma contains a nonfunctional variant of factor IX. Unlike classic hemophilia, in most series relatively few obligate carriers of CRM positive Christmas disease could be identified by the relative excess of factor IX, as measured immunologically (factor IXR:Ag), compared to coagulant factor IX (factor IX:C).

### Prenatal Diagnosis of Classic Hemophilia and Christmas Disease

Because of the X-linked transmission of both of these diseases, the chance that a pregnant carrier's male fetus will be affected is 1 in 2 and the severity of the defect will be characteristic of the family. In addition, one-half of the female fetuses will be carriers. As these females do not present a clinical problem of bleeding in their lifetime, no action is required.

Amniocentesis should be carried out at the 12th–14th week of pregnancy only in those women who have had a complete explanation of what is involved. Amniocentesis is a relatively safe procedure, and culture of fetal cells allows a diagnosis of the sex to be made. No further action is required if the fetus is female. If a male fetus is present, some women may elect to abort all such fetuses, recognizing that one-half will be normal. If facilities are available, however, it is now possible to recognize classic hemophilia in utero. Upon agreement of the pregnant woman and her spouse, fetoscopy and fetal sampling are undertaken, allowing the selective abortion of affected male fetuses. Success of such a technique depends on obtaining pure fetal blood[182,183] and the availability of carefully standardized assays of factors VIII or IX. Fetoscopy is carried out under sedation and local anesthesia.[184] The site of introduction of the trocar and cannula is selected after a real-time ultrasound scan has been performed. Fetal blood samples should be taken from an umbilical vessel just above the placental insertion of the cord. From this site, pure fetal blood can be obtained from the lumen of the vessel. Hemostasis is good even in a hemophilic fetus, and the chance of entering the intervillous space and producing feto-maternal hemorrhage is low.[182,185] Confirmation that the sample is of fetal origin is carried out by analysis of the red cells on a combined cell counter and particle-size analyzer (Coulter Channelyzer). The fetal red cells have a much higher mean corpuscular volume (MCV); also, successive samples have a constant hematocrit, thus excluding dilution with amniotic fluid.

Fetal blood should be analyzed for levels of factors VIII:C, IX:C, VIIIR:AG, and VIIIC:AG. Mibasham and Rodeck[184] have examined 47 fetuses in a total of 46 pregnancies. Of these, 32 were shown to have normal assay values, using bioassay of factor VIII:C and immunoradiometric assays (IRMA) for factor VIII:C:AG. Their results were confirmed at birth, giving a 100 percent success rate for the technique. Classic hemophilia was diagnosed in 14 of the 47 fetuses at risk, and the diagnosis was confirmed in 10 available abortuses. These results have been confirmed by other investigators using similar techniques.[185a]

Detection of fetuses with Christmas disease is not as advanced as for classic hemophilia because the number of pregnancies available for study is small and the fetal level of factor IX and related vitamin-dependent factors is normally very low. Initial results suggest that this technique will also be of value in the detection of factor IX deficiency. With the advent of a sensitive IRMA assay for factor IX:C:AG, the sensitivity of the test should be increased despite the problem posed by families who are CRM positive in whom the test cannot be applied.[186]

The incidence of side effects from the procedure is low and the results appear to warrant the time, effort, and cost involved for those families who have made the decision to embark on it and who are prepared to terminate an affected fetus.

Despite the availability of accurate diagnostic tests, we have found resistance to their use in our patients. In an international survey of genetic counseling, we have found that patients have a surprising unwillingness to undergo diagnostic procedures, and up to 25 percent will reject amniocentesis because of the possible implications of the result. Even in those who have undergone termination, 40 percent have severe regrets about their decision.[187]

### Classic Hemophilia and Christmas Disease in Females

Classic hemophilia has been found in a small number of females, but the incidence is not as great as suggested by early authors due to confusion with other genetic disorders and deficiencies in the assay system.[188,189] The most common cause is interbreeding, usually in a family in which an affected male and a carrier female are involved.[190,191] The result is that the affected female hemophilic child will have one abnormal X chromosome from its father and another from its mother. Homozygous female hemophiliacs can also be found in breeding colonies of hemophilic dogs.[192,193]

A kindred in which the transmission of the disease through 3 generations of females has been ascribed to an autosomal dominant trait has been described.[194] Their plasma factor VIII:C levels were reduced, with a proportional reduction in factor VIIIC:AG, and these values ranged from 3 to 5 percent of normal. All other clotting tests were normal. It is not clear whether the mutated gene in this kindred is on the X chromosome or an autosome because of the limited amount of genetic information. It seems likely, however, that the phenotype resulted from mutation of a regulatory gene because of the dominance of the phenotype and because factors VIII:C and VIII:C:AG were reduced proportionately.[195]

A hemophilialike disease has also been recorded in a small number of females as a result of chromosomal abnormalities: 45 XX/45 X mosaicism,[196] 46 XY karyotype,[197] deleted X chromosome,[198] and inactive X isochromosome.[199]

Typical Christmas disease has also been detected in females, either because of interbreeding[200] or because the daughter of a carrier had an X chromosomal deletion.[201]

Rarely, instances of classic hemophilia or Christmas disease in females appear to have arisen from extreme lyonization, that is, the random inactivation of virtually all normal X chromosomes during fetal development of an obligate carrier.

### Gynecological and Obstetric Bleeding in Carriers of Classic Hemophilia

It is well recognized that the factor VIII:C level in hemophilic carriers has a mean value of 0.5 U/ml,[202] but in some it may be sufficiently low to produce clinical bleeding problems. Although this is usually manifested only after surgery or trauma, menstruation and childbirth in these females often presents with excess bleeding, which, however, is not usually a problem. The probable reason for the low complication rate from bleeding during pregnancy is that the factor VIII:C levels almost always rise above 0.5 U/ml.[171,203,204] In our own series of 10 pregnancies in hemophilic carriers with initial low levels of factor VIII:C, two had miscarriages with no hemorrhagic problems, one had an ectopic pregnancy with massive bleeding, and one had a threatened abortion which was treated prophylactically with concentrate and eventually resulted in a normal birth.

Management of such pregnant hemophilic carriers requires close collaboration of the obstetrician with the hemophilia center, and supervision should start prior to pregnancy. At antenatal visits, factor VIII:C should be measured and, if this remains low as term approaches, arrangements should be made for factor VIII concentrate to be available and for delivery to take place in a hospital. It has been our policy to infuse concentrate only after placental separation to avoid the risk of transmitting hepatitis to the fetus. Bleeding problems in the postpartum period are rare, but hematoma formation may occur at the site of episiotomy.

### Gynecological and Obstetric Bleeding in Carriers of Christmas Disease

Bleeding in women who are carriers of Christmas disease (factor IX deficiency) is well recognized and appears to be more common than in carriers of classic hemophilia.[205] Little has been found in the general literature about the obstetric care of such patients.[205] In our own population of Christmas disease carriers, four in number, who had a long history of excess bleeding and low factor IX levels, there was a total of seven pregnancies. Antepartum hemorrhage occurred in three of the seven. All cases were treated with factor IX concentrate, and none had fetal death. Postpartum hemorrhage occurred in two of the seven deliveries, and a third patient developed a perineal hematoma.

When the patients were monitored during pregnancy, there seemed to be a variable rise in factor IX activity, but half of the patients did not reach a level of 0.2 U/ml and consequently were at risk from bleeding. It is our policy to have these women deliver in the hospital and, after placental separation, to be given a prophylactic dose of factor IX concentrate.

## Replacement of Factors in Classic Hemophilia and Christmas Disease

As early as 1840, Lane[207] described successful blood transfusion in a hemophiliac. However, it was not until 1911 that Addis[208] showed the value of blood transfusion. Later, Payne and Steen,[209] in 1929, demonstrated that plasma therapy was superior to whole blood. Transfusion of whole blood is of little value in correcting the hemostatic defect and barely raises the level of the deficient factor; it should be used only when anemia must be corrected urgently and is best given in the form of packed cells. With modern concentrates of plasma, the following principles should be followed.

### Principles of Replacement Therapy with Plasma and Concentrates

Hemostasis can be secured in uncomplicated hemophilia and Christmas disease by the infusion of adequate amounts of plasma concentrates. The total amount required for an infusion depends on the following: (1) the basic level of AHF (factor VIII) or Christmas factor (factor IX) in the patient's plasma, (2) the severity of the injury or the extent of surgery, (3) the site of bleeding, (4) the presence of inhibitors, (5) the integrity of the other components involved in hemostasis, (6) the plasma volume of the patient, (7) the potency of the material to be used, and (8) the biological half-life of this material.

It is critical, therefore, that all of these factors be examined in the overall care of the bleeding episode and that the end result be checked by measuring the level of factor achieved in the patient's plasma about 15 minutes after the end of each infusion. When major surgery is to be undertaken, a level of 0.6–1.0 U/ml should be achieved and maintained until healing is well established from the wound and all drainage tracks. For less major procedures and in spontaneous bleeding, a lower level of clotting factor can be maintained (0.4–0.6

U/ml), and for minor bleeding a level of 0.2–0.4 U/ml is adequate.[210] It seems likely that in the past 10 years, excessive amounts of plasma concentrates have been given with little evidence of improvement in outcome. Such therapy is obviously wasteful and expensive and increases the patient's exposure to viruses. Studies are currently underway to determine the lowest permissible plasma level of concentrate which will produce hemostasis in spontaneous joint bleeding.

The biological half-life of factor VIII is about 8–12 hours in the plasma; claims that some concentrates have longer half-lives have not been substantiated. The biological half-life of factor IX is about 18–24 hours. Factor VIII remains primarily in the intravascular space and factor IX equilibrates with the extravascular space, giving a lower than predicted recovery.

Various formulas have been devised for assessing the dosage of concentrates. These are of some value, but the final determinant is the level achieved in the patient and his clinical hemostatic response.

### Antihemophilic Factor Concentrates

Treatment of clotting disorders by replacement with plasma or plasma products has depended on the development of a widespread system of blood banking, widespread plasma fractionation facilities, and research on plasma fractions. In the late 1940s, plasma was available only in limited amounts and was sufficient to provide low levels of factor replacement. This was satisfactory in the short term, but continued therapy often led to hypervolemia and heart failure. In addition, when hemophilia was to be treated, the plasma had to be prepared and infused soon after donation because of the short half-life of the AHF. Freezing of plasma provided a partial solution to this problem, but in general this treatment was wasteful and unsatisfactory.

*Plasma.*   Until 1964, fresh-frozen plasma (FFP) was the main therapeutic material used in the treatment of hemophilia. It was used almost exclusively for in-patient management and contained variable amounts of factor VIII, that is, up to 0.5 U/ml. To ensure hemostasis in an adult, a volume of about 1.5–2.0 liters was required, and possibly repeated within 24 hours. Such a use of scarce resources was extremely wasteful. Now plasma is used only in patients with rare disorders for which no concentrates are readily available.

*Cohn fraction I and Blombäck fraction I-0.*   Cohn fraction I is an 8 percent ethanol precipitate prepared from fresh plasma. Before the advent of cryoprecipitate, this concentrate, which contained approximately 50 U of factor VIII/g protein, was widely used in hemophilic surgery.[211] It was, however, expensive to prepare, and was rapidly superseded by Blombäck fraction I-0, which doubled the purity to 100 U of factor VIII/g protein.[143,211a] The main protein contained in both of these fractions is fibrinogen (60 percent of total protein in Cohn fraction I and 85 percent in Blombäck fraction I-0).

*Cryoprecipitate.*   A major advance in the practical management of hemophilia followed the observation of Pool and Robinson[212] that fibrinogen and factor VIII remained insoluble after thawing of frozen plasma. Harvesting of this cold-insoluble cryoprecipitate, using simple apparatus in a regional blood bank, radically altered management of hemophilia.[213,214] Cryoprecipitate produced by this method contains 50–80 percent of the starting factor VIII in a volume of about 10 ml.[215–218] Cryoprecipitate is also rich in fibrinogen, containing 3–10 times the amount found in starting plasma.[216,219] It may thus have a place in therapy for fibrinogen-depleted states. In addition, there are small amounts of other coagulation factors and trace amounts of albumin and globulins.[115] Successful therapy has now been widely reported in many clinical situations.[215-221] The advantages of cryoprecipitate are the simplicity of preparation, ease of administration, relatively low cost, and by selection of donors, reduced risk of hepatitis. It is, therefore, the treatment of choice in the mild hemophiliac who has not been exposed to plasma products and has no immunity against hepatitis viruses.

The main disadvantage of the use of cryoprecipitate alone is the variability of the preparation from one unit to another. Also, all preparations contain small amounts of trapped red cells or red cell fragments which may be antigenic. In our patients, 12 percent developed blood group antibodies.[115] Cryoprecipitate is the starting material for most of the modern fractionation methods, and because of the variability of the harvesting of factor VIII (varying sixfold among individuals), investigation was carried out by the National Heart, Lung and Blood Institute.[222,222a] The following steps were identified as critical for the final yield of factor VIII: (1) type of anticoagulant, (2) mixing during phlebotomy, (3) time and temperature of storage, (4) freezing temperature of plasma, (5) thawing temperature, and (6) freezing temperature of the resulting cryoprecipitate.[222-224]

Various ways have been sought to increase the factor VIII content of donor plasma by prior exercise and by infusion of des-amino-D-arginine vasopressin (DDAVP) (page 216). Such methods, however, have little place in routine use. With optimal technology, it should be possible to recover 500 U/liter of donor plasma, and each bag of cryoprecipitate should contain at least 100 U of factor VIII coagulant activity on the average.

The cost of production of cryoprecipitate is similar to that of concentrates in both the United States and the United Kingdom.[225-227]

*Intermediate and high-purity factor VIII concentrates.*    Cryoprecipitates are the starting material for these concentrates.[228] After any retained protein contaminants are washed out with a glycine-ethanol-citrate buffer, the cryoprecipitates are redissolved and adsorbed with aluminum hydroxide to remove the vitamin K-dependent factors.[229] The final product is freeze-dried and contains about 500 U of factor VIII/g protein. Such intermediate concentrates are rich in fibrinogen, which may make reconstitution a problem and limit the concentration achieved in solution to about 15 U of factor VIII/ml. An additional step involving precipitation with polyethylene glycol gives a product with approximately 1500 U of factor VIII per gram of protein, with a final factor VIII concentration of 30 U/ml.[230] With increasing purification, the amount of factor VIII lost in the process increases and the yield falls; hence, the purer the material, the more expensive in terms of financial cost and lost factor VIII. The higher-purity materials contain virtually no albumin and have significantly decreased amounts of α- and β-globulins. The main β-globulin which is still present is cold-insoluble globulin (fibronectin).[231] All high-purity materials also contain blood group alloantibodies as well as the other factor VIII activities.[232] Trace amounts of the chemicals used in the purification process are also present (aluminum is present at 1 μ/ml and polyethylene glycol at 1.5 ng/ml). Some materials contain minute amounts of heparin at concentrations of 1 U/ml.[225]

A persistent problem in the United States has been a discrepancy between the labeled potency of lyophilized factor VIII preparations and the amount obtained by direct assay of the reconstituted material. In general, the latter values may be as much as 40 percent less than those recorded on the label. In a study at University Hospitals of Cleveland, one source of this error has been identified. The manufacturers of factor VIII concentrates compare their material to a lyophilized standard prepared by the World Health Organization. This standard overstates the titer of factor VIII:C by two-thirds compared to the titer of a pool of 24 normal plasmas.

*Infusion of factor VIII into a hemophiliac.* Infusion of a factor VIII concentrate into a hemophilic patient (with no inhibitor) results in a rapid rise in factor VIII levels. This is followed by a rapid decrease and then an exponential decay in factor VIII levels. The first phase probably represents a time of equilibration of intravascular and extravascular factor VIII, and the second phase the degradation of the active coagulant site on the protein. The biological half-life of the decay phase is about 12 hours. The evidence is that the values recorded for the half-lives of a variety of factor VIII products produced from a variety of sources are similar,[228,233–235] although some authors have suggested a lower in vivo recovery with more highly purified materials.[236] Fibrinogen is present in the alcohol, ether, and polyethylene glycol fractionated materials and is present in much lower amounts in the high-potency glycine-precipitated concentrate. As the half-life of fibrinogen is longer than that of factor VIII, the result of prolonged therapy is a rise in the plasma level of fibrinogen, which may become very high. The significance of this high fibrinogen level is not clear, but it induces rouleaux formation and increases blood plasma viscosity.[237–239] It may also interfere with blood grouping procedures and increase the erythrocyte sedimentation rate markedly, a pitfall for the unwary.[115] Other proteins may also be present, and after massive infusion these may produce unusual biochemical abnormalities.[134]

### Complications of Therapy with Plasma and Factor VIII Concentrates

*Hypervolemia.* Before the advent of efficient concentrates, overloading of the circulation and heart failure were commonplace, even in fit young patients, due to the large volumes of plasma required to produce hemostasis. Plasma is now rarely used except in some of the rare bleeding disorders. If it is to be given repeatedly, a high dose of diuretics may be given prophylactically to control fluid overload.

*Allergic reactions.* Acute allergic reactions with plasma concentrates are relatively uncommon but can be life-threatening when they occur.[240–244] If allergic reactions do occur with every infusion of plasma, it is probably worthwhile to check the Gm and immunoglobulin A (IgA) groups of the donors and the recipient; however, little is known about this type of reaction.[154,245–247] Usually, such reactions present with mild symptoms such as urticaria or bronchospasm, which respond to steroids, antihistamines, or subcutaneous epinephrine (adrenaline). Rarely, the reaction may be severe, leading to rapid death. Some of these "allergic" reactions may be associated with complement activation and generation of the anaphylatoxin C3a.[248]

In patients with a history of reactions, it is our practice to administer prophylactically a small dose of an antihistamine. Care must be exercised, as these drugs have an antiplatelet action.[249] A variety of minor "allergic" reactions with nausea, headache, vertigo, tachycardia, and hypotension may be associated with the presence of small amounts of biologically active contaminants of concentrates such as bradykinin.

*Alloantibodies.* Hemolytic anemia may be produced in hemophilic patients of blood groups A or B if intensive therapy with concentrates is used.[232,241,250] The lyophilized concentrates currently used may contain up to 30 times the alloagglutinin level of plasma and, due to their long half-life, accumulation of these agglutinins occurs and may produce the biochemical and clinical signs of hemolysis. This condition is associated with a fall in hemoglobin level, a rise in the reticulocyte count, and a positive direct Coombs' test. Treatment with concentrates should be stopped, and hemolysis will settle rapidly. If hemostatic cover must be continued, type-specific single-donor units of cryoprecipitate should be given; if red cells are needed for transfusion purposes, washed red cells of group O should be used.

*Hepatitis after infusion of plasma products.*    With the advent of blood transfusion and the more general use of plasma products, it soon became apparent that a type of hepatitis might be transmitted[251-256] and that the risk increased with the number of units of blood given.[257] The Australia antigen has been found in all the fractions of blood used therapeutically in hemophilia and Christmas disease,[258] but the risk depends on the particular plasma fraction used; for example, the risk following administration of fibrinogen-rich concentrates may be as much as 35 times greater than that of whole blood. Because it is necessary to prepare modern concentrates from pools of plasma, the patient's exposure to the various viruses is high.

In theory, testing of every donor unit of blood should reduce the incidence of hepatitis,[259-261] but this has not totally eliminated the problem. The incidence of clinical jaundice varies from 2 to 30 percent of cases.[262-266] It is clear that such reports of clinical jaundice represent only the tip of the iceberg of virus hepatitis. In serial studies after infusion of concentrates, up to 70 percent of patients have had enzyme disturbance diagnostic of hepatitis.[267-270] In more recent studies, 90 percent of severely affected hemophiliacs have had abnormally high aspartate transaminase levels.[271]

The frequent exposure of hemophilic patients to hepatitis B virus (HBV) is evidenced by the high incidence of positive tests for HBV antibody. In our own severely affected patients who have been multiply transfused, the incidence is over 90 percent for the antibody to hepatitis B surface antigen (HBs-Ab); this is confirmed in other studies.[272]

In a small number of patients, there is persistence of HBs-Ag. In our own patients, this affects 3–5 percent of the severely afflicted patients and has been found in up to 17 percent of patients in other studies.[255,256,273,274] Patients with persistence of HBs-Ag have also been shown to have biochemical and histological evidence of liver impairment. When a sensitive test of liver function is employed (bromsulfthalein retention test), 30 percent of a group of multiply tranfused hemophiliacs have had abnormal retention.

It now seems probable, however, that HBV is not the main virus implicated in these cases of hepatitis. It is not common for HBV to cause prolonged abnormality of liver function except in patients in whom HBs antigen is detectable in the blood. Occasional patients do harbor HBV in the liver and have negative blood HBS-Ag, but they almost always have antibody to the virus core (anti-HBc). The low incidence of acute HBV infection in hemophilia is probably related to the high incidence of anti-Hbs virus in the blood.[275]

It is now established that there are other transmissible agents capable of causing posttransfusion hepatitis, and that these are responsible for 90 percent of this disease.[276-278] There is good evidence that more than 1 virus is involved in this non-A, non-B hepatitis. The acute illness is clinically mild, with an incubation period of 6–70 days, and is clinically similar in course to hepatitis A and B. There is clinical and epidemiological evidence to support the view that two types of non-A, non-B hepatitis exist and are associated with factor VIII infusions.[265,279,280] One type is associated with U.S. commercial concentrates and the second with U.K. factor VIII and European materials.[280a] This difference is probably related to variations in the methods of fractionation of the plasma. The attack rate associated with U.S. commercial concentrates is about 15 percent in patients receiving their first infusion of concentrate; this attack rate has remained constant over the past 5 years.[277]

Up to 40 percent of patients with hemophilia on regular factor VIII therapy have persistent abnormalities in liver function.[270] Most of these patients are asymptomatic and have no clinical stigmata of chronic liver disease. In addition, there is often no previous history of an acute infection. It is only with the advent of liver biopsy in certain selected centers that the true incidence of structural abnormalities in this group has become apparent.[272,281–283a] In the United Kingdom, about one-half of such patients have evidence of chronic liver disease or cirrhosis; the extent of the histologic abnormality bears no relationship to the abnormality of the enzymes, and indeed, normal biochemistry may be associated with gross pathology.[261,284] When biopsies are performed in patients with persistent elevation of transaminases, however, the incidence of histologic abnormalities rises up to 95 percent.

There is no evidence from current studies that other factors in the concentrates are toxic, and there is no evidence of hypersensitivity in the etiology of liver disease. About 5 percent of United Kingdom hemophiliacs are asymptomatic carriers of HBV. The carrier state of non-A, non-B hemophilia has been recognized, but no accurate data are available due to difficulties in testing.[285]

Most severe hemophiliacs, therefore, are exposed to a high risk of hepatitis from factor VIII and IX concentrates. They have about a 20–30 percent chance of resultant chronic hepatitis due to non-A, non-B viruses and a small risk from HBV.[272,278]

Use of corticosteroids in chronic liver disease with hemophilia is not well established, but there is little evidence of prolongation of the life span; indeed, it has been suggested that steroids may exacerbate the disease in HBs-Ag-positive patients.[286,287] As many of these patients are young,[261] long-term corticosteroids would seem to be unjustified and will result in stunting of growth.

As treatment of the established disease is unsatisfactory, how can this serious potential hazard of liver damage be avoided in the future? Replacement therapy has so improved the quality of life for hemophilic patients that it would be impossible to reduce the supply of plasma products to them. In the mildly affected patients, it is possible to use DDAVP to stimulate the production of factor VIII in the short term, and this is often sufficient to cover minor surgery. The Blood Tranfusion Service now has a policy of testing all donations of blood for HBV. This has led to a reduction in hepatitis transmission, but due to the insensitivity of the testing method and the size of the plasma pool necessary to prepare concentrates, the risk of hepatitis is still great.

As children are more liable to hepatic damage from these viruses and are more likely to develop the HBs-Ag carrier state,[287a] it seems wise to treat them initially with cryoprecipitate made from individual donors with a proven record of donations.[269,272,288,289] The additional expense and inconvenience are justified in this susceptible group.

In the short term, the most important objective is to ensure that the pool of blood donors is properly screened and, if possible, that panels of volunteers for plasmapheresis are established. In the long term, one must hope that isolation and identification of the various viruses will lead to the preparation of adequate vaccines.[290,291] Failing this, manufacturers of the concentrates must find some method of killing the viruses present in the concentrates. An alternate virus-free factor VIII may eventually be produced by cell or *Escherichia coli* cultures after genetic transformation.

*Animal AHF Preparations in Hemophilia*

At a time when adequate amounts of human factor VIII concentrate were not available, alternate sources of supply were considered.[292] A variety of animal plasmas were investigated, and a potent concentrate of AHF was prepared from pig and cow blood.[293,294] These were successfully infused into hemophilic patients and enabled major surgical procedures to be undertaken with good hemostasis.[103]

These crude preparations of porcine and bovine AHF were available commercially as a freeze-dried concentrate with a factor VIII activity approximately 100 times greater than that of human plasma. The animal protein was, however, antigenic, and after 10–12 days of therapy, the response to the infusion fell as antibodies developed. In addition, the preparations contained platelet agglutinins,[295] and thrombocytopenia was noted after use.[103,296,297] The thrombocytopenia is caused by a direct effect of the animal factor VIII molecule on human platelets, which has been localized to the factor VIIIR:Ag fraction.[157,158,298–300]

Separation of the factor VIII:C subcomponent is now possible using polyelectrolytes,[301] and a commercial concentrate of porcine factor VIII:C is now under trial. To date, over 100 courses of treatment have been administered to 46 patients. Most of these patients have been treated because of factor VIII inhibitors. The response to treatment depends on the degree of cross-reactivity of the antihuman factor VIII with porcine factor VIII and on the strength of the inhibitor.[302] Dosages of 20–50 U/kg of body weight have been given and repeated every 8 hours. Most of the patients studied have received human factor VIII prior to the animal product. The animal product also seems to increase inhibitor titers, although this tendency is less marked than after administration of human clotting factors.

Adverse reactions such as pyrexia, chills, skin rash, nausea, and headache respond to hydrocortisone or an antihistamine. Severe allergic reactions are also reported, and it is wise to administer a test dose of 100 U prior to treatment. With the substantial reduction in the levels of factor VIIIR:Ag, no significant effect on platelets has been found.

This concentrate would seem to have a place in the management of patients with inhibitors (page 205 and Chapter 7).

*Replacement Therapy in Christmas Disease*

Christmas factor (factor IX) is much more stable than factor VIII in vitro, and blood anticoagulated with acid-citrate-dextrose, when stored at 4°C, retains up to 80 percent of its original factor IX activity at 3 months. Outdated plasma might therefore be used for therapy except for the danger of hypervolemia. Dried plasma has a lower but more variable content of factor IX, as significant amounts are lost in the drying process; it is therefore not recommended. Fresh frozen plasma (FFP) retains its factor IX activity well and was once the mainstay of replacement therapy. It still has a role, if no other materials are available, for short-term use.

The first concentrates for use in factor IX deficiency were prepared from ethylenediaminotetraacetate (EDTA)-anticoagulated plasma adsorbed with tricalcium phosphate, eluted with citrate, and dried with ethanol.[303] This product was rich in prothrombin, factor VII (proconvertin), Stuart factor, and factor IX (antihemophilic factor B), and was accordingly named *PPSB*. A variety of concentrates have therefore been prepared, using different anticoagulants, precipitates, and adsorbents.

The starting material most commonly used now is the supernate from the production of cryoprecipitate; diethylaminoethyl(DEAE)-cellulose is used as the adsorbent.[304,305] The adsorbed vitamin K-dependent factors are eluted with phosphate or citrate buffers.

The final product is lyophilized. It contains relatively little factor VII but has approximately equal number of units of factors II, IX, and X. These factor IX concentrates are stable in the lyophilized state, store well, and are easy to reconstitute in a small volume of distilled water. After infusion there is rapid intravascular equilibration, but only about 50 percent of the injected material can be identified in the plasma 10 minutes after its injection, suggesting that another extravascular compartment exists which must be involved.[304,306,307]

The decay curve of infused factor IX is biphasic; for the first shorter phase it gives a biological half-life of 5 hours and for the second phase about 24 hours.[307] Similar results have been obtained with a variety of factor IX concentrates no matter how prepared.

As with hemophilia, the dose required is calculated on the basis of the severity of the defect, the rise of the factor IX level required, and the recovery predicted. In all cases of surgery, the postinfusion rise should be measured by assay. For major surgery a postinfusion value of 0.5–0.8 U/ml is necessary; for more minor procedures, 0.2–0.4 U/ml is satisfactory.

### Adverse Effects of Factor IX Concentrates

*Hepatitis.* In surveys of Christmas disease patients, serologic markers of previous infection with hepatitis are found in almost all severely affected patients who have been multiply transfused.[308,308a] This is in keeping with the high incidence of serum hepatitis and non-A, non-B hepatitis.

In patients who have not had previous exposure, transfusion of factor IX concentrates produces clinical hepatitis in about 60 percent of cases.[211a] This is probably a result of the pool size of the plasma used, as well as a reflection of the methodology used in the preparation.

*Thrombotic complications with factor IX complex.* As a result of the preparative procedures, some of the zymogens in factor IX concentrates become activated, and the level of factors IXa and Xa may be about 10 ng/ml.[309] Numerous studies have described thrombotic complications following surgery,[310–315] mainly deep vein thrombosis and pulmonary embolism. Recently, a case of acute myocardial infarction has been described in a patient with an inhibitor,[316] and an acute case of disseminated intravascular coagulation in a patient receiving a high dosage of factor IX following an elective knee joint replacement[317] (Chapter 8).

It has been suggested that in patients with chronic liver disease there is impairment of hepatic clearance of activated material, but this has never been substantiated.

In laboratory testing, many of these concentrates shorten the clotting time of plasma in the activated partial thromboplastin time, indicating the presence of activated materials.[318] In vivo, there may be a fall in the platelet count and the factor VIII level, and a rise in fibrin(ogen)-related antigens and fibrinopeptide A values.[317,319–322] The incidence of such reactions, however, is low, and the materials used seem generally to be safe and reliable[323,324] when used at the recommended dosage.

## Therapy for von Willebrand's Disease

Patients with this disease have a capillary-type bleeding defect characterized by persistent capillary bleeding from mucous surfaces and persistent bleeding after trauma (Chapter 6). In the original description by von Willebrand (1926),[22] the patients were shown to have ecchymoses with normal platelet counts. The major defects in factor VIII, platelet function, and bleeding time are described elsewhere (Chapter 6). Attention must then be paid to correction of both the factor VIII level and the bleeding time.[325,326] This has conventionally been done by infusion of factor VIII concentrates. It is, however, known that infusion of normal plasma or serum and hemophilic plasma restores normal factor VIII coagulant levels and factor VIIIR:Ag levels, and also corrects the bleeding time.[1,326] It is not clear if separate factors moderate these changes in human von Willebrand's disease. Accordingly, cryoprecipitate seems to be clinically satisfactory[215] and corrects, in many patients, the bleeding time and factor VIII level. This regimen seems to be more effective than the use of concentrates,[327-329] which produce erratic results at best.

Menorrhagia is a frequent problem in the female von Willebrand's disease patient. Some success has been claimed for the use of oral contraceptives and long-term use of inhibitors of fibrinolysis such as epsilon aminocaproic acid (EACA) or tranexamic acid (AMCA). Occasionally, cryoprecipitate may be required for prophylaxis, for example, at the time of examinations.

### Gynecological and Obstetric Bleeding in Patients with von Willebrand's Disease

Despite the lifelong nature of the bleeding tendency, major gynecological and antenatal problems seem to be rare and are related to the severity of the primary hemostatic defect. Of 3 patients with severe von Willebrand's disease examined by us during 5 pregnancies, 2 had to be treated for late postpartum hemorrhage despite the use of prophylactic cryoprecipitate. A total of 30 pregnancies have been described.[204,330,331,332] Of these, postpartum hemorrhage was described in 30 percent, usually occurring late. Many of these patients had had prophylactic plasma or cryoprecipitate, but hemostasis was not ensured for a prolonged period. This high incidence of postpartum bleeding is surprising, as the factor VIII:C level is thought to increase toward term. On review of 11 pregnancies which were carefully monitored, however, the factor VIII:C level remained abnormal (below 0.2 U/ml) at 40 weeks in one-half of the patients, as did the bleeding time.

The policy should therefore be to monitor factor VIII:C levels and bleeding times frequently during pregnancy. In those patients in whom the defects are not corrected spontaneously, an infusion of cryoprecipitate should be given prophylactically.

## Self-Treatment and Prophylaxis of Classic Hemophilia and Christmas Disease

With the advent of effective, safe, and stable concentrates, it has been proved possible to institute programs of self-therapy by patients in their own home or office. Already a massive literature has been developed in this area, covering the selection of patients, type and storage of concentrates, methods of teaching self-infusion, and complications and benefits of these programs.[333-335]

There can be little doubt now of the effectiveness of such regimens. They dramatically reduce the number and severity of bleeding episodes, shorten the duration of immobility and pain, reduce the amount of time lost from school, and improve the employability of patients.[336-338] Some doubt remains about their influence on the prevention of long-term joint disease, as well as about the causation of chronic liver disease and perhaps other long-term toxic features which may not yet be apparent.

Before being accepted into a self-therapy program, both the patient and his family require assessment for motivation and understanding of the disease. A period of education is usually required to ensure that the patient is familiar with the early signs of bleeding into various organs and with the technical aspects of the preparation and infusion of the concentrate. We have found that the most difficult factor is the reconstitution of concentrate. If necessary, parents of young children must be taught these techniques. Venipuncture is best demonstrated in the center and for the first few weeks is done under supervision. We require the patient to keep a diary of events, including the volume, unitage, and effects of each infusion. Special arrangements may need to be made for safe disposal of used syringes and needles, and advice given about storage of concentrates at home and in the office.[339] Appropriate literature is available from local and national hemophilia societies and the World Federation of Hemophilia.

The average number of units of concentrate given tends to increase gradually over the first few years of treatment; in the United Kingdom, it had risen by 1980 to 23,000 U per patient per year. It has been estimated that self-therapy results in financial savings.[226] Similar findings have come from studies in the United States, but the average dose of factor VIII has been 40,000 U/year/patient on self-therapy.[340] Even at this level of cost, there is recognition of the favorable cost/benefit result by the federal government.[341]

In an attempt to reduce the usage of factor VIII products, studies have been set up to examine the minimum effective dose of factor VIII concentrate for hemophiliacs on home therapy.[342,343] It seems likely that substantial savings of factor VIII can be made. These authors report that a dose as low as 5.7 U/kg controlled 85 percent of bleeds when the infusion was self-administered soon after the onset of symptoms.

Recently, a variety of complications have been observed in the United States in patients with classic hemophilia enrolled in home therapy programs. These problems raise serious questions about the use of lyophilized concentrates of factor VIII or IX. At least 17 cases of *Pneumocystis carinii* pneumonia or other opportunistic infections have been reported to the Centers for Disease Control.[344] These patients had the laboratory characteristics of the acquired immunodeficiency syndrome observed in some homosexuals. Further, in vitro studies in several centers have demonstrated similar changes in more than one-half of asymptomatic hemophiliacs who self-administer lyophilized factor VIII, that is, a relative decrease in T4 (helper) cells, a relative increase in T8 (suppressor) cells, impaired lymphocyte proliferation upon addition of phytohemagglutinins, and a decrease in natural killer activity.[345,345a] These changes have not yet been seen in patients treated with cryoprecipitates but inverted T4/T8 ratios have been detected in patients treated with factor IX concentrate.[345b] Moreover, a number of patients have had a syndrome resembling chronic idiopathic thrombocytopenic purpura, sometimes complicated by compensated hemolytic anemia (Evans' syndrome).[346] Of 100 patients receiving home therapy with lyophilized factor VIII in northern Ohio, 2 have had *Pneumocystis carinii* pneumonia, 2 have had lethal chronic hepatitis, 1 has had fatal Burkitt's lymphoma (another disorder seen in homosexuals), and 3 have had idiopathic thrombocytopenic purpura, all during 1982. These patients challenge our assumptions of the efficacy of lyophilized factor VIII as prepared in the United States.

## Treatment of Patients with Antibodies to Clotting Factors

There is as yet no agreement among clinicians on the best method of treating patients with antibodies to AHF (factor VIII)[347] (Chapter 7). Approximately 5–10 percent of patients with severe classic hemophilia will be so affected.[234,263,347–350] This occurs most often in severely affected patients. Most of these antibodies are IgG immunoglobulins and will destroy the factor VIII coagulant activity of infused concentrates. In hemophilia, two distinct patterns of behavior of these antibodies have emerged. In about two-thirds of the cases, the antibody level rises after exposure to factor VIII:C infusion and falls off over a period of weeks or months in accordance with the three week half-life of IgG. Reexposure to even minute amounts of factor VIII produces an anamnestic response, with a rapid rise in antibody titer which reaches a peak about two weeks later. These patients are the "high responders." The antibody titer is usually greater than 10 Bethesda U/ml and may rise to many thousands of units. In the other one-third of patients, the antibody circulates at low levels, with little or no rise in titer after factor VIII infusion. These patients are the "low responders." The antibody titer tends to be low and to remain below 5 Bethesda U/ml. Even if repeated doses of factor VIII are given, the antibody titer rises only slightly, and any rise is inconsistent. The distinction between high and low responders is not absolute, as some patients will show anamnestic responses only erratically.[349]

These antibodies are active only against factor VIII:C and seem not to react with other proteins or other parts of the factor VIII molecule. They cross-react with bovine and porcine factor VIII, but to a lesser degree than with human factor VIII.

It is not clear why some hemophiliacs develop antibodies and others, with the same severity of defect and the same or greater exposure to factor VIII, do not. There is some evidence that this group of patients may be defined by genetic factors,[348] as evidenced by the appearance in several members of families[351] and in twins.[352]

### Reduction of Antibody Level

The objective is to reduce the level of antibody by repeated plasmapheresis or plasma exchange. These procedures may provide temporary hemostasis; an infusion of factor VIII is given immediately afterward when the antibody titer is at its lowest.[121,353-357] The antibody tends to reappear rapidly in the circulation, presumably due to readsorption from the extravascular compartment. Repeated plasmapheresis may be effective in controlling the anamnestic response.[358]

### Transfusion of Factor VIII

Opinion is divided over the use of factor VIII in patients with antibodies. The more conservative clinicians tend to withhold factor VIII in the hope that the antibody level will remain low and that, if a life-threatening bleed occurs, it will be much easier to treat. Others will treat the known low responders with factor VIII, with the expectation that the antibody titer will not rise;[359] however, some low responders do become high responders.[349] Animal factor VIII cross-reacts with the antihuman antibody but is only about one-quarter as sensitive. These products thus may have a place in management (page 000).

### Prothrombin–Complex Preparations

Attempts have been made to bypass the site of action of the inhibitor on factor VIII:C. A variety of prothrombin–complex concentrates have been tried in individual hemophilic patients with antibodies over the past 10 years.[360-363] These preparations contain the vitamin K-dependent clotting factors, factors II, VII, IX, and X, in varying proportions. Anecdotal reports suggest that these preparations may be of value, as in many instances bleeding which was previously uncontrollable by other methods has been halted.[360,362,364-368] The initial preparations were batches which, fortuitously, were found to have been activated during preparation and were made available for investigational use. A variety of preparations have now been provided by commercial sources,[368] and over 400 episodes of treatment of hemophilic patients with antibodies have been documented in the literature. Concentrates have been used for almost every type of serious hemophilic bleeding, internally and externally, and for emergency and elective surgery. The consensus is that in these uncontrolled situations, treatment is of value; however, caution must be used, as negative results tend not to be published. Nonetheless, in a randomized crossover study, significant improvement followed treatment of acute hemarthrosis with prothrombin–complex concentrates at a dose of 500 U of factor IX.[368a] Although this study was double-blind, some of the participating physicians have told us that patients could distinguish between the prothrombin–complex concentrates and the placebo, making interpretation difficult.

The active principle of prothrombin–complex preparations is unknown, but presumably it is one or more *activated* components, such as activated factors II, VII, IX, and X. Intravenous administration is rapidly followed by shortening of the partial thromboplastin time, which may remain normal for 12–24 hours. There appears, however, to be no clear relationship between the observed laboratory correction of the defect and the cessation of bleeding. As the manufacturers of the early products reduced the content of activated clotting factors in order to decrease the risk of thromboembolism in Christmas disease patients, it was noted that the concentrates were no longer as effective in treating inhibitor patients.[368a,369]

An activated product, Autoplex, produced by controlled activation, is now available (from Hyland Laboratories), and clinical studies suggest its efficacy.[368,369a,370]

### Factor VIII Inhibitor Bypassing Activity (FEIBA)

This material is claimed to have antibody bypassing activity, but the active principle has eluded investigators despite intensive search.[371,372] A double-blind study of FEIBA against prothrombin–complex (Prothromplex-Immuno) in classic hemophilia patients with inhibitors has now been reported.[373] The authors studied joint, muscle, and open bleeding, and compared single doses of FEIBA (100 U/kg) with single doses of Prothromplex (50 U/kg) using randomized pairs of joints for comparison. Only patients who fulfilled the following criteria were admitted: (1) the inhibitor titer should have been at least 5 Bethesda U; (2) the patient should have been a high responder with more than one bleed per month in the preceding year, should have had no stigmata of liver disease, and should have been prepared to be admitted during the evaluation. Significant benefit resulted from the use of FEIBA, as judged by subjective appraisal by the patient and by joint mobility.

The place of such treatments in management is not yet proven. Further controlled studies are required to prove their clinical efficacy, resolve the dilemma of the assay method, establish unitage, monitor procoagulant side effects, and justify the high costs of the preparations.

Following the use of both FEIBA and prothrombin–complex preparations, there have been reports of anamnestic responses with a rise in antibody titers,[374–377] which may also negate the use of plasmapheresis and factor VIII preparations.

### Treatment of Antibodies by Immunosuppression

Repeated attempts have been made to suppress the immunologic response to factor VIII by the use of steroids, cyclophosphamide, or azathioprine.[310,378,379,379a] As yet, the place of such measures is not clear, but in certain selected patients successful results have been claimed. However, the long-term effects and the possibility of carcinogenesis make this an unpopular choice of treatment.

## PROTHROMBIN DEFICIENCY

The hereditary functional deficiency of prothrombin is a rare coagulation defect, with fewer than 30 cases recorded.[380] In congenital deficiency the concentration ranges from 0.01 to 0.1 U/ml.

Congenital prothrombin deficiency is inherited as an autosomal recessive trait, and several instances of consanguinity have been recorded. In some patients the coagulant deficiency is paralleled by a deficiency of antigens related to prothrombin, whereas in others such antigens can be detected.[380a] The diagnosis is suggested by a long prothrombin time and is established by specific assays. In both homozygotes and heterozygotes, bleeding may occur from mucous membranes or after trauma or surgery; females may have menorrhagia. Bleeding tends to be much milder in heterozygotes. A large number of genetic variants have been recorded, and were summarized in 1977 by Bloom.[381]

The half-life of prothrombin is long, approximately 4 days,[382,383] but in concentrates some molecules are probably in a degraded form and may have a shorter half-life. Plasma would seem to be a satisfactory treatment in this situation and could be given twice per week if needed. If concentrations are used to correct the defect, the levels should be monitored by assays.

## FACTOR V DEFICIENCY (PARAHEMOPHILIA, LABILE FACTOR OR PROACCELERIN DEFICIENCY)

Factor V deficiency is a rare hereditary bleeding disorder, with only about 60 families so far described.[384,385,385a] It is probably transmitted as an autosomal recessive trait, although some authors consider it to be partially dominant.[169,386] The genetic transmission has been complicated by the frequency of reported cases of consanguinity.[387,388] In retrospect, it is not clear in many cases whether these patients were truly deficient or had a functionally incompetent variant of factor V. A variety of other congenital abnormalities have been found in association, such as skeletal, renal, and cardiovascular abnormalities.[389] Factor V deficiency generally presents as a mild bleeding disorder, often in childhood. Homozygotes tend to bleed more severely. Epistaxis is the most common problem, but this is usually controlled by local pressure. Bleeding also occurs from cuts and dental extractions, and menorrhagia is common in affected females. Hematoma and hemarthrosis are rare. Bleeding can be controlled by the infusion of fresh plasma; the half-life in the plasma is about 35 hours.[390,391] The level of factor V which is necessary to achieve hemostasis is not certain but is in the range of 0.05–0.15 U/ml.

In deficiency of factor V, the prothrombin time is long. Assay of factor V depends on the availability of deficient plasma from an affected patient or the use of oxalated plasma exhausted of factor V activity by prolonged incubation.

## FACTOR VII (SERUM PROTHROMBIN CONVERSION ACCELERATOR, SPCA, OR PROCONVERTIN) DEFICIENCY

Factor VII "deficiency," whether due to the presence of an incompetent form of factor VII or to true deficiency, is a rare hereditary bleeding disorder with fewer than 100 recorded cases. It is probably inherited as an autosomal recessive trait.[392,393] The prothrombin time is long, and the diagnosis is made by specific assay for factor VII. Symptomatic patients are usually homozygous but are not always severely affected. Factor VII deficiency has also been associated with congenital hyperbilirubinemia (Gilbert's disease) or Dubin-Johnson syndrome.[394–396] Hemarthrosis, menorrhagia, gastrointestinal bleeding, and epistaxis are the main bleeding problems recorded in these patients. [393,397] Some patients remain asymptomatic. Rarely is hemorrhage found in the neonatal period; a few reports exist of umbilical bleeding. Intracranial bleeding has not been recorded.[398] The severity of the clinical bleeding tendency does not necessarily follow closely the recorded level of the assayed factor, which may be related to the presence of variants of the molecule.[399,400] Levels of 0.05–0.3 u/ml have been suggested by various authors as necessary for hemostasis. Factor VII deficiency combined with a qualitative platelet defect has also been recorded.[401]

Factor VII is very stable and can be replaced by stored blood, plasma, or a factor IX concentrate containing factor VII.

Because of the short biological half-life of factor VII (5 hours), replacement therapy in this group must be given at least 3 times every 24 hours. This leads to excessively high levels of the other vitamin K-dependent factors, with perhaps a consequent risk of thrombosis. Deep vein thrombosis and pulmonary embolism have been recorded in this situation.[312] It may be possible to produce a factor VII concentrate easily and cheaply for this very small group of patients.[402]

## DEFICIENCY OF FACTOR X (STUART-PROWER FACTOR)

Deficiency of factor X is an extremely rare hereditary deficiency, described originally in two families, the Stuarts[403] and the Prowers,[404] in whom the prothrombin time was abnormally long. The diagnosis is made by specific assay. In most patients the clotting is abnormally long in the presence of Russell's viper venom, which contains an activator of factor X. The disorder occurs in both sexes and is transmitted as an autosomal recessive trait. It may be manifested in the first few days of life by bleeding from the umbilical cord. Subsequent hemorrhagic problems are similar to those of hemophilia. Bleeding is more troublesome in homozygotes. On occasion, a prolonged bleeding time may be recorded.[405]

In the laboratory, a large number of variants of factor X have been recorded in both homozygotes and heterozygotes.[406–409a] Because of the long biological half-life of factor X (30–50 hours),[410,411] plasma is a safe and effective method of treatment. Concentrates of factor IX complex can also be given.[408,410] The level of factor X is not controlled in factor IX concentrates; accordingly, the level of factor X achieved in the patient's plasma must be constantly monitored by assay.

## PLASMA THROMBOPLASTIN ANTECEDENT (PTA, FACTOR XI) DEFICIENCY

Over 100 cases of PTA deficiency have been recognized since its original description. The disease is inherited as an autosomal recessive trait, and homozygotes tend to have excess bleeding. The bleeding tendency is usually mild, and only about one-third to one-half of the patients have a significant tendency to hemorrhage.[412] Bleeding usually follows trauma or a surgical procedure. In those patients who do bleed spontaneously, epistaxis and menorrhagia may be troublesome. The disorder is more common in Jewish individuals, especially in those of Eastern European descent.[413,414] It has been estimated that about 1 in 1000 of Ashkenazi Jews in Israel are homozygous for this trait.[415]

In the laboratory, the activated partial thromboplastin time is abnormally long and prothrombin time is normal. Specific assays distinguish PTA deficiency from other defects of the intrinsic pathway. The levels of recorded PTA in patients vary widely from 0.01 to 0.2 U/ml.[413,414] There seems to be no close correlation with the tendency to bleed,[416] and patients with a severe deficiency have been recorded to be only mildly affected by bleeding.[417,418] In addition, occasional patients have been described with prolongation of the bleeding time.[419] The biochemical nature of the defect is poorly understood, but in our study of 10 patients with a severe deficiency of PTA, no cross-reacting material was found using a heterologous antibody.[420]

Treatment of bleeding episodes is rarely necessary but should be carried out as already described: Plasma or the supernate from cryoprecipitate product is usually satisfactory even for major surgery.[215]

## CONGENITAL DISORDERS OF FIBRINOGEN

### Congenital Afibrinogenemia

Afibrinogenemia was originally described by Rabe and Salomon[421] in 1920; about 100 cases have now been recorded. The condition is probably inherited as an autosomal recessive trait, and there is often a history of consanguinity in the parents. Surprisingly, more cases have been recorded in males than females. The affected persons are homozygotes who, despite having extremely low levels of fibrinogen, may not have major bleeding problems. Umbilical bleeding in the neonatal period is rare; bleeding usually follows trauma or surgery, and females may have menorrhagia.

Joint bleeding has been rare, whereas cerebral hemorrhage has been recorded as a cause of death. The disease, however, is generally remarkably mild. The bleeding time may be prolonged and slightly lower platelet counts have been recorded[422] in association with abnormal platelet function tests.[423–425]

Bleeding responds to infusion of plasma or other sources of fibrinogen (cryoprecipitate), and because of the long half-life of fibrinogen (4–6 days) these may be required only twice a week. Antibodies against fibrinogen may, however, develop and shorten the half-life of the infused fibrinogen.[426] Paradoxically, thromboembolism may follow treatment.[427]

### Hypofibrinogenemia

Hypofibrinogenemia is probably the heterozygous state of afibrinogenemia and is occasionally found in the parents of such patients. The fibrinogen is apparently normal in structure. There are rarely major bleeding problems. The concentration of fibrinogen in these patients ranges from 10 to 50 mg/dl.

## Dysfibrinogenemia

Dysfibrinogenemia describes a qualitative defect in the fibrinogen molecule.[428] Many variants have been described, each named for the city in which the defect was noted. The abnormality has been identified chemically in only a few cases, in which a single amino acid substitution has been detected; in some patients the level of circulating fibrinogen is reduced. The functional defects attributed to the abnormal fibrinogen are usually recognized by the presence of a long thrombin time in patients with inexplicably long prothrombin or partial thromboplastin times. In most cases, either the release of fibrinopeptides is impaired or fibrin polymerization is defective, but other abnormalities are also seen.

Bleeding tends to be mild and usually occurs from the mucous membranes, with epistaxis, menorrhagia, and excess bleeding after surgery or trauma. Bleeding from the umbilicus may be the presenting feature in neonates. After surgery, some patients have a tendency to wound dehiscence, and during pregnancy there is a high incidence of placental bleeding with abortion. Paradoxically, there is also a tendency to thrombosis, perhaps because of lack of the antithrombin action of normal fibrin.[429]

Treatment follows the same principles as for afibrinogenemia. It has not been needed in any of the patients we have studied.

## FACTOR XIII (PLASMA TRANSGLUTAMINASE PRECURSOR) DEFICIENCY

Factor XIII is the precursor of the enzyme transglutaminase, which covalently bonds fibrin monomers. Numerous reports of congenital deficiency now exist[429a,430,431] following the original description of the condition.[432] Over 100 patients have now been described, and the condition has been recently reviewed.[433,434] The mode of inheritance is still in doubt. The great preponderance of male patients suggests the possibility that in some cases the disorder is sex linked.[435,436] Consanguinity has been described in the parents of more than one-half of the female patients, and the possibility remains that in most families transmission may be due to an autosomal recessive trait.[437] Homozygotes present with lifelong bleeding, which may start from the umbilical cord, and prolonged bleeding after trauma or surgery is common. During childhood, the patients bruise easily and excessively, and suffer subcutaneous and intramuscular hematomas. Delayed wound healing may also be a feature,[430] perhaps because factor XIII has an action on fibroblasts which may be mediated through other proteins.[438] A higher than normal rate of abortion may be found. Hemorrhage into the central nervous system seems to occur more commonly than in other genetic coagulation defects.

Because of the long half-life of factor XIII (4–7 days) and the small amounts required to achieve normal hemostasis (0.05 U/ml), prophylactic fresh frozen plasma can be administered every few weeks or on demand at the time of trauma.[439] As yet, there has been no evidence of the appearance of antibodies with such long-term prophylaxis.[440]

The diagnosis of factor XIII is indicated by the solubility of clots in 5 $M$ urea or 1 percent monochloroacetic acid. This screening procedure is rather insensitive because as little as one percent of factor XIII will result in insolubility of the fibrin. Accurate determination of enzyme levels is now possible using simple rate assays. These include the incorporation of labeled primary amines such as putrescine or fluorescent dansylcadaverine.[441]

## HAGEMAN TRAIT, PLASMA PREKALLIKREIN DEFICIENCY, AND HIGH MOLECULAR WEIGHT KININOGEN DEFICIENCY

Three hereditary defects of the early stages of the intrinsic pathway of thrombin formation are unaccountably asymptomatic despite major alterations in clotting assays.[442] These disorders, Hageman trait (the functional deficiency of Hageman factor or factor XII), plasma prekallikrein deficiency (Fletcher trait), and high molecular weight kininogen deficiency (Fitzgerald, Williams, or Flaujeac trait) come to attention because the whole blood clotting time and partial thromboplastin time are unusually long, although the subjects have no evidence of a hemorrhagic tendency; the prothrombin time is normal. The diagnosis is established by specific assays. No therapy has been required.

*Hageman trait* has been recognized, in Ohio, in at least 1 in 500,000 individuals. The disorder is almost always inherited as an autosomal recessive trait. The heterozygous condition, present in at least 1 in 300 persons, is the most common cause of modest prolongation of the activated partial thromboplastin time in apparently normal individuals. Rarely, the disorder is inherited in an autosomal dominant manner. The plasma of most patients appears to be devoid of protein immunologically recognizable as Hageman factor, but in two families plasma contained antigens related to this agent, as though an abnormal variant of the protein were present. *Plasma prekallikrein deficiency* is a much rarer defect. Two varieties have been recognized. A true deficiency is observed in American blacks. In whites, usually of Mediterranean origin, the plasma contains antigens related to plasma prekallikrein. *High molecular weight kininogen deficiency* is even more unusual. Besides the deficiency of high molecular weight kininogen, there may be a more or less complete deficiency of low molecular weight kininogen. Both plasma prekallikrein deficiency and high molecular weight kininogen deficiency are inherited as autosomal recessive traits.

## HERITABLE COMBINED COAGULATION FACTOR DEFICIENCIES

Kindreds containing individuals with to or more coagulation factor deficiencies have been described in a wide variety of combinations (Table 5-1). These disorders are quite rare; none of the combined defects other than factor V/VIII deficiency has been reported in more than five kindreds.

Combined factor V and factor VIII:C deficiency (earlier described as hemophilia-parahemophilia) has been reported in over 20 kindreds.[390,443–445] In some cases, this disorder has been associated with a variably prolonged bleeding time. In addition to the much greater than expected incidence of this combination,[446] transmission of the disorder via a single hereditary defect in most kindreds is suggested by repeated autosomal transmission of a factor V/VIII:C abnormality unaccompanied by the abnormalities of von Willebrand's disease (Chapter 6). In addition, some patients seem to possess reduced levels of a plasma inhibitor of activated protein C[447] (Chapter 2). Deficiency of such an inhibitor could ac-

**Table 5-1**
Reported Combined Coagulation
Factor Deficiencies

| |
|---|
| V and VIII:C* |
| II, VII, IX and X (varying combinations)* |
| VII and VIII |
| VII and IX |
| VIII and X |
| VIII and IX |
| VIII and XI |
| VIII and XII |
| VIII and fibrinogen |
| IX and XI |
| XI and XII |
| XII and XIII |
| VIII, IX and XI |

*Evidence for a single pathogenic defect described.

count for the observed combined defects. Not all kindreds with factor V/VIII deficiency exhibit deficient inhibitor,[448] and apparently coincident inheritance of parahemophilia and classic hemophilia has been reported.[449]

Two unrelated patients[450,451] and 2 affected siblings[452] have had lifelong deficient activity of prothrombin and 1 or more of the other vitamin K-dependent factors (VII, IX, and X). In all 4 patients, defective coagulation factor function appeared to result from inadequate posttranslational carboxylation (Gla residue formation) of these factors (Chapter 2). The patients differed in the degree of correction of this defect that followed administration of large doses of vitamin $K_1$. Two other patients exhibited similar deficiencies, but Gla residue formation was not examined. For each of these very rare combined deficiencies, a single congenital or hereditary defect in coagulation factor Gla residue formation seems likely.

For all other reported congenital and hereditary combined factor deficiencies (Table 5-1), there is as yet no identified basis for a single genetic defect. Accordingly, distinction of kindreds whose combined deficiency states reflect a single underlying defect from those whose deficiency states reflect the coincidence of two or more such defects of individual coagulation factors can only be inferred from patterns of inheritance. Since usually only a few generations and a small number of family members have been studied, these distinctions remain speculative. A recent extensive review suggests a provisional classification of these combined abnormalities.[446]

## PAIN IN BLEEDING DISORDERS

Pain plays a major part in the life of the bleeder. The acute pain of bleeding, usually into joints or muscles, is easily controllable with adequate amounts of analgesia. Often, however, this may require the use of morphine or similar analgesics and presents the ever-increasing problem of drug abuse.

Of more concern is the chronic pain of the degenerative hemophilic joint disease which is of low grade but persistent quality. It is our experience that abuse of drugs usually starts in an attempt to control it. Anti-inflammatory drugs have a place in management, but care must be taken to avoid the use of those with a potent antiplatelet action. In particular, aspirin and phenylbutazone should be avoided, as they may produce life-threatening hemorrhage which is difficult to treat.[112,113] Dihydrocodeine, paracetamol, choline magnesium trisalicylate, mefenamic acid, or pentazocine may be of value in pain control but may be abused by patients.

We have recently undertaken long-term studies of transcutaneous electrical nerve stimulation (TES)[453] to control the pain of hemophilic joints. The early results are promising and possibly will reduce the amount of analgesic required in individual patients. Such a method has been used with success in rheumatoid arthritis and experimental pain in humans.[454,455]

In a similar vein, various psychological techniques have been employed for pain control, that is, self-regulation techniques which consist of progressive muscular relaxation, meditative breathing, and guided imagery.[456] Such techniques must, however, be properly supervised in hemophilia centers.

If pain in the joints becomes sufficiently severe, joint replacement must be considered. To date, we have replaced 5 knee joints because of recurrent, overwhelming pain.

## CORTICOSTEROIDS IN COAGULATION DISORDERS

The theoretical basis for the administration of steroids for hemophilia is that patients with Cushing's syndrome are known to have an elevated level of plasma AHF,[457] and patients with a variety of diseases who are given corticosteroids have a significant rise in AHF levels. Uncontrolled studies have suggested that benefit may be produced in patients with hemophilia given large intravenous doses of steroids, with reduction of spontaneous bleeding as well as bleeding after dental extraction.[152,458] However, in a controlled trial of steroids in a group of hemophilic children, only a very slight rise of plasma AHF was recorded in some individuals, and no significant alteration was produced in the bleeding tendency.[151] In a double-blind controlled trial of low-dose prednisolone (7.5 mg/day in adults and 3 mg/day in children),[459] only a slight reduction in bleeding was found; this has been confirmed.[460] Long-term use of such drugs cannot be recommended in view of the potential side effects.

Steroids have been used in the treatment of hemarthrosis in patients with hemophilia. In one study, unlimited replacement with AHF was given and the factor levels were kept between 0.15 and 0.2 U/ml. In a second study, a single dose of replacement therapy was given and the AHF level was raised initially to 0.4–0.5 U/ml. Steroid therapy was prednisolone 1 mg/pound of body weight/day, with an upper limit of 80 mg/day for 3 days and then half of the initial dose for a further 2 days. The criterion of success was return of the joint to its prehemarthrosis condition. In the unlimited therapy study there was a significant reduction in the amounts of AHF required in the steroid-treated group. In the single-dose study there was a significant decrease in the number of steroid-treated joints which failed to respond. No long-term benefits were found, but it seems that short-term steroids reduced the severity of symptoms and joint bleeding and controlled the inflammatory response.

The mechanisms by which steroids act in bleeding disorders are not yet clear. There is usually a slight rise in plasma AHF levels, but probably of more importance is the increase in capillary resistance.[461] In patients with inhibitors there is some evidence of bene-fit after steroid use, but this is short-lived.[462] Against all of these minor benefits must be weighed the real hazards of long-term steroid therapy, especially in growing children.

## USE OF FIBRINOLYTIC INHIBITORS IN BLEEDING DISORDERS

Theoretically, there is reason to suppose that there is a balance between blood coagu-lation and fibrinolysis. Attempts have therefore been made over the past 15 years to alter this balance by inhibiting the fibrinolytic process with drugs which inhibit either plasmino-gen activation or plasmin. Two such drugs have been used in clinical practice, epsilon aminocaproic acid (EACA) and tranexamic acid (Cyclokapron). Most studies have been carried with EACA, which was discovered first. Subsequently, however, Cyclokapron was favored because of its significantly greater potency and fewer side effects.[463]

### Epsilon Aminocaproic Acid (EACA)

EACA is a protease inhibitor, with its greatest activity against plasminogen activators. At a concentration of $10^{-4}$ $M$ it will inhibit spontaneous generation of fibrinolytic activity in blood; at higher concentrations ($5 \times 10^{-2}$ $M$), it will inhibit formed plasmin.

With a standard dose of 6 g/day, it is possible to achieve a level of approximately $10^{-3}$ $M$ in plasma and other body fluids. It is thus possible to achieve a level which will preserve the fibrin of a hemostatic plug in a blood vessel. In other areas, such as the uterus, kidney, and cerebrospinal fluid, much higher concentrations may be achieved. This local effect is the basis of EACA use in menorrhagia, after prostatectomy, and after subarach-noid bleeding. Side effects include nausea, vomiting, diarrhea, faintness, and impotence. With large doses and long-term administration, muscle weakness and necrosis have been documented.[464,465]

### Tranexamic Acid (Cyclokapron)

Tranexamic acid, not available in the United States, is many times (up to 100-fold) more potent than EACA and at a concentration of $10^{-6}$ $M$ will inhibit the activation of plasminogen.[466] It requires a higher concentration to inhibit plasmin, and therefore has theoretical advantages over EACA. Side effects of treatment are rare and are significantly less troublesome than those seen with EACA.[467] Occasional alimentary side effects have been recorded, mainly nausea, vomiting, and diarrhea.

### Possible Side Effects of Fibrinolytic Inhibitors on the Renal Tract

Up to 90 percent of an orally administered dose of EACA or tranexamic acid will appear unaltered in the urine within 24 hours. Urine is rich in the physiological activator of fibrinolysis, urokinase, which is produced by renal cells and which maintains patency of the renal tract by promoting the lysis of fibrinous deposits.[468,469] Inhibition of this protective lytic mechanism may result in accumulation of clot in the urinary tract, possibly producing urinary colic, obstruction, and renal failure.[144,469,470] Death has resulted from renal failure as a result of obstruction due to unlysable fibrin.[444] In the event of such a problem, the patient may require hemodialysis or peritoneal dialysis during the acute anuric phase, while attempts are made to remove the obstruction either by instrumentation or by instillation of large amounts of activators.[471,472] In the event that renal function does not improve, renal transplantation may be required.

### Use in Dental Surgery

See page 192, this chapter.

### Use in Spontaneous Bleeding

Therapy with EACA or tranexamic acid in hemophilia with a view to reducing the number of episodes is theoretically attractive. Numerous clinical trials have been carried out in a double-blind controlled fashion with contradictory results,[472a,473–475] perhaps because some patients know whether they are receiving the medication or a placebo. Some trials have suggested a slight clinical reduction of bleeding and of factor VIII utilization, but against this must be weighed the long-term effects,[476] and there would seem to be no justification on current evidence for this therapy.

### Use in Joint Disease

It is well accepted that the synovium of joints produces an activator of plasminogen in large amounts. In hemophilia this activator may potentiate bleeding, and in clinical studies it has been suggested that bleeding is reduced by the use of EACA.[477]

## USE OF VASOPRESSIN AND ITS ANALOGUES IN HEMOPHILIA

The plasma level of factor VIII can be raised in normal people by stimulation of $\beta_2$-receptors and by vasopressin and some of its analogues.[478] Because of the side effects of vasopressin, notably contraction of smooth muscle in the uterus, gastrointestinal tract, and blood vessels, it has not found a place in treatment of hemophilia. The synthetic analogue desamino-8-arginine vasopressin (DDAVP), has no vasopressor activity but retains its antidiuretic action and stimulates release of plasminogen activator,[479] factor VIII,[480–485] and prostacyclin[486] from the endothelium. This agent is of value in patients with mild classic hemophilia and von Willebrand's disease.

The mechanism by which DDAVP produces its action on the endothelium is unknown. The indications are that DDAVP releases presynthesized molecules of factor VIIIR:Ag and plasminogen activator from the endothelium, and there is evidence that this factor VIII is identical to that which circulates in the plasma under normal conditions.[485,486a]

DDAVP should be given by the intravenous route to produce a rise in factor VIII,[481,482] although with more potent preparations now available, it may be taken by a nasal instillation, with a variable rise in factor VIII levels.[487] The response to an intravenous injection of DDAVP is dose related up to approximately 0.3 μg/kg body weight.[480,488] The result is a rise in the plasma levels of all AHF activities, that is, factors VIII:C, VIIIR:Ag, VIII:C:Ag, and VIII:VWF, all of which reach a maximum at 30 minutes.[481,483,484] In the mildly affected patient, a fourfold rise in levels of AHF can be expected above the starting basal level.[484] This response is sufficient to allow the performance of minor surgery without recourse to plasma products. The response, however, is not invariable, and in patients about to have surgery, a trial dose should be given the day prior to the operation to ensure that the patient will respond. In a severely affected hemophiliac, administration of DDAVP may result in a rise of all factor VIII activities except for factor VIII:C; therefore, DDAVP is of no value in this situation.[481]

In von Willebrand's disease, the response to DDAVP is variable and depends on the type of disease and the basal level of the factor VIII activities. Infusion of DDAVP does not increase the low level of factor VIII of type I (homozygous) von Willebrand's disease.[488a] In type II (intermediate) von Willebrand's disease with prolonged bleeding times, infusion of DDAVP increases factor VIII activities. This is usually associated with a reduction in bleeding time.[481,489]

Thus, in patients with mild hemophilia and in most patients with von Willebrand's disease in whom the various factor VIII activities are detectable in the basal state, infusion of DDAVP will temporarily correct the patient's hemostatic defect.

The therapeutic use of DDAVP to promote hemostasis should be accompanied by the administration of tranexamic acid to inhibit the induction of fibrinolysis. In addition, the patient must be observed for skin flushing, tachycardia, and a fall in blood pressure, which are probably due to liberation of prostacyclin from the endothelium.[486] Occasionally, patients may retain fluid due to the antidiuretic effect of DDAVP, and this may be sufficient to produce hypertension.[488]

Repeated use of DDAVP over a few days results in tachyphylaxis, presumably as a result of depletion of factor VIII stores. Hemostasis can therefore be ensured only for minor procedures (e.g., dental extraction) in which healing is complete within a few days. Perhaps the most important aspect of its potential use is the avoidance of plasma products in the group of mildly affected hemophilic patients who are highly susceptible to hepatitis if given factor VIII concentrates.

## PSYCHOLOGICAL AND SOCIAL PROBLEMS OF PATIENTS

Since the original descriptions of hemophilia, physicians have realized that psychological factors seemed to play a role in the initiation of bleeding and that often acute stress would provoke a bleed.[27] As medical management has improved, the psychosocial impact of these bleeding disorders has been highlighted and investigated in an attempt to determine the etiological factors.[111,490–494] It is often impossible to distinguish cause from effect in individual cases.[495]

The social problems of the patient usually start with deficient education due to absence from school. In our own studies in Scotland, many of the pupils were sent to schools for the physically and mentally handicapped. Those who attended schools for normal children had frequent absences because of bleeds, missing up to one-quarter of their educational time; the result was poor academic performance and poor grades on leaving school.[496–499]

The result of deficient schooling leads to difficulty in obtaining and holding down an adequate job. In local and national studies in the United Kingdom, the unemployment rate for hemophiliacs was 18 percent compared to an average rate of 6 percent for the general population. When the severely affected patients alone were surveyed in Scotland, an unemployment rate of almost 50 percent was found.[338,499] The problems of unemployment supplement the existing psychological factors and produce psychosomatic symptoms and frank psychosis.[499]

Perhaps the major impact is on the family of the hemophilic child.[337,500,501] The parents are subject to overwhelming emotions of guilt and recrimination, anxiety and anger; the end result is often marital friction, overprotection of the child by the mother, and relative neglect of the other siblings. The problems of the sisters become apparent only when they themselves are diagnosed as carriers.

A variety of frank psychiatric syndromes have been recorded in these patients, with behavioral disturbances manifested early as risk taking, alcoholism, drug dependence, and suicide. Depression, anxiety states, and phobias stunt normal relationships and inhibit normal development.[101,109,301,490,499,502]

There is evidence that with the advent of home care programs in the last 5 years, some of the social and psychological problems of hemophiliacs are improving.[338,502,503]

## REFERENCES

1. Zimmerman TS, Ratnoff OD, Powell AE: Immunologic differentiation of classic hemophilia (factor VIII deficiency) and von Willebrand's disease. J Clin Invest 50:244–254, 1971
2. Bertina RM, Linden IK van: Factor IX Zutphen. A genetic variant of blood coagulation factor IX with an abnormally high molecular weight. J Lab Clin Med 100:695–704, 1982
3. Bertina RM, Linden IK van: Factor IX Deventer—evidence for the heterogeneity of hemophilia $B_m$. Thromb Haemost 47:136–140, 1982
4. Brown PE, Hougie C, Roberts HR: The genetic heterogeneity of hemophilia B. N Engl J Med 283:61–64, 1970
5. Chung KS, Madar DA, Goldsmith JC, et al: Purification and characterization of an abnormal factor IX (Christmas factor) molecule. J Clin Invest 62:1078–1085, 1978
5a. Roberts HR, Grizzle JE, McLester WD, et al: Genetic variants of hemophilia B: Detection by means of a specific PTC inhibitor. J Clin Invest 47:360–365, 1968
6. Hougie C, Twomey JJ: Hemophilia $B_m$: A new type of factor IX deficiency. Lancet 1:698–700, 1967
7. Panicucci F, Sagripanti A, Conte B, et al: Characterization of heterogeneity of haemophilia B for the detection of carriers. Haemostasis 9:310–318, 1980
8. Study to Evaluate Supply-Demand Relationships for AHF and PTC Through 1980. US Dept of Health, Education and Welfare publication No. (NIH) 77–1274, 1980
9. Hardisty RM, Ingram GIC: Bleeding Disorders, Investigation and Management. Philadelphia, FA Davis, 1965
10. Essien EM: Haemorrhagic disorders. Part I: Tropical Africa. Clin Haematol 10:917–932, 1981
11. Forbes CD, MacKay N, Khan AA: Christmas disease and haemophilia in Kenya. Trans R Soc Trop Med Hyg 60:777–781, 1966
12. Khan AA, Forbes CD: Haemophilia in East Africa, (abstract). East Afr Med J 43:566, 1966
13. Merskey C: Bantu haematology and coagulation. Leech 28:45–51, 1958
14. Trowell HC: Case of haemophilia in a Muganda. East Afr Med J 17:464–465, 1941
15. Prentice CRM, Ratnoff OD: Genetic disorders of blood coagulation. Semin Hematol 4:93–132, 1967
16. Biggs R, Macfarlane RG (eds): Treatment of Haemophilia and Other Coagulation Disorders. Philadelphia, FA Davis, 1966
17. Ratnoff OD, Margolius A Jr.: On the epidemiology of hemophilia and Christmas disease. N Engl J Med. 256:845–846, 1957
18. Duckert F, Koller F: The old Swiss haemophilia families of Tenna and Wald, in Brinkhous KM, Hemker HC (eds): Handbook of Hemophilia. Amsterdam, Excerpta Medica, 1975, pp 21–29
19. Kasili EG, Kariithi MW: Hereditary bleeding disorders as seen at the Kenyatta National Hospital, Nairobi, Kenya. Trop Doct 9:76–80, 1979

20. Wall RL, McConnell JL, Moore D, et al: Christmas disease, color blindness and the blood group Xg[a]. Am J Med 43:214–226, 1967
21. Yoshida K: Haemophilia and related disease. Acta Haematol Jap 24:109–139, 1961
22. Willebrand EA von: Hereditare pseudohemofili. Finska Läkaresällsabits Handlingar 67:7–12, 1926
23. Bloom AL: Inherited disorders of blood coagulation, in Bloom AL, Thomas DP (eds): Haemostasis and Thrombosis. Edinburgh, Churchill Livingstone, 1981, pp 321–370
24. Ingram GIC, Jones VR, Hershgold EJ, et al: Factor VIII activity and antigen, platelet count and biochemical changes after adrenoreceptor stimulation. Br J Haematol 35:81–100, 1977
25. Prentice CRM, Forbes CD, Smith SM: Rise of factor VIII after exercise and adrenaline infusion measured by immunological and biological techniques. Thromb Res 1:493–505, 1972
26. Rizza CR: Effect of exercise on the level of antihaemophilic globulin in human blood. J Physiol 156:128–135, 1961
27. Legg JW: A Treatise on Haemophilia, Sometimes Called the Hereditary Haemorrhagic Diathesis. London, Lewis, 1872
28. Ratnoff OD, Lewis JH: Heckathorn's disease: Variable functional deficiency of antihemophilic factor (factor VIII). Blood 46:161–173, 1975
29. Davis T: Case of hereditary haemorrhaea. Edinburgh Med Surg J 25:291–293, 1826
30. Dubois E: Observation remarquable d'hemorrhophile. Gaz med Paris 6:43–47, 1838
31. Reinert H: "Uber Hämophilie" Inaugural dissertation. Gottingen, WF. Kaestner 1869, p. 12
32. Assman R: Die Hämophilie. Inaugural dissertation. Berlin, G. Lange, 1869
33. Lemp H: "De haemophilie nonnulla" quoted in Schmidt's Jahrbücher der in-und ausländischen Gesammten. Medicin 117:330–332, 1863
34. König F: Die Gelenkerkrankungen bei Blutern mit besonderer Berücksichtigung der Diagnose. Samml klinisher Vortrage Volkman, NF, Chirurgie, nr 11:233–242, 1892
35. Collins DH: Haemophilia, in The Pathology of Articular and Spinal Diseases, London, Edward Arnold, 1949.
36. DePalma AF, Cotler JM: Hemophilic arthropathy. Arch Surg 72:247–250, 1956
37. Key JA: Hemophilic arthritis (bleeder's joints). Ann Surg 95:198–225, 1932
38. Swanton MC: The pathology of hemarthrosis in hemophilia, in Brinkhous KM (ed): Hemophilia and Hemophilioid Diseases. Chapel Hill, NC, University of North Carolina Press, 1957, pp 219–224
39. Swanton MC: Hemophilic arthropathy in dogs. Lab Invest 8:1269–1277, 1959
40. Ali AM, Gandy RH, Britten MI, et al: Joint haemorrhage in haemophilia: Is full advantage taken of plasma therapy? Br Med J 3:828–831, 1967
41. Duthie RB, Rizza CR: Rheumatological manifestations of the haemophilias. Clin Rhemat Dis 1:53–93, 1975
41a. Biggs R, Matthews JM: in Biggs R, Macfarlane RG (eds): Treatment of Haemophilia and Other Coagulation Disorders. Oxford, Blackwell Scientific Publications, 1966, pp 129–143
42. Favreau JC, Laurin CA: Joint effusions and flexion deformities. Can Med Assoc J 88:575–576, 1963
43. Forbes CD, James W, Prentice CRM, et al: A comparison of thermography, radio-isotope scanning and clinical assessment of the knee joints in haemophilia. Clin Radiol 26:41–45, 1975
44. Henkel L, Watmough D: Die Thermographie in der Orthopädie. Z Orthop 106:817–830, 1969
45. Forbes CD, Greig WR, Prentice CRM, et al: Radioisotope knee joint scans in haemophilia and Christmas disease. J Bone Joint Surg 54B:468–475, 1972
46. Alarçon-Segovia D, Trujeque M, Tovar E, et al: Scintillation scanning of joints with technetium 99m. Arthritis Rheum 10:626, 1967 (abstract)
47. Whaley K, Pack AI, Boyle JA, et al: The articular scan in patients with rheumatoid arthritis:

A possible method of quantitating joint inflammation using radio-technetium. Clin Sci 35:547–552, 1968

48. Green FA, Hays MT: Joint scanning: Mechanism and application. Arthritis Rheum 12:299, 1969 (abstract)

49. Mowat AG, Disney TF, Vaughan JH: Articular scanning and external counting in experimental synovitis in the guinea pig. Ann Rheum Dis 30:183–186, 1971

50. Mainardi CL, Levine PH, Werb Z, et al: Proliferative synovitis in hemophilia: Biochemical and morphologic observations. Arthritis Rheum 21:137–144, 1978

51. Ahlberg Å: Haemophilia in Sweden VII. Incidence, treatment and prophylaxis of arthropathy and other musculo-skeletal manifestations of haemophilia A and B. Acta Orthop Scand (suppl 77):3–132, 1965

52. Arnold WD, Hilgartner MW: Hemophilic arthropathy. J Bone Joint Surg 59A:287–305, 1977

53. Pavlov H, Goldman AB, Arnold WD: Haemophilic arthropathy in the joints of the hands and feet. Br J Radiol 52:173–180, 1979

54. Jordan HH: Hemophilic Arthropathies. Springfield, Ill, Charles C. Thomas, 1958, pp 12–20

55. Petterson H, Ahlberg A, Nilsson IM: A radiologic classification of hemophilic arthropathy. Clin Orthop 149:153–159, 1980

56. Wood K, Omer A, Shaw MT: Haemophilic arthropathy. Br J Radiol 42:498–505, 1969

57. Boldero JL, Kemp HS: The early bone and joint changes in haemophilia and similar blood dyscrasias. Br J Radiol 39:172–180, 1966

58. Houghton GR: Joint surgery in haemophilia, in Forbes CD, Loew GDO (eds): Unresolved Problems in Haemophilia. Lancaster, England, MTP Press, 1982, pp 217–233

59. Houghton GR, Duthie RB: Orthopaedic problems in haemophilia. Clin Orthop 138:197–216, 1979

60. Ahlberg Å, Pettersson H: Synoviorthesis with radioactive gold in hemophiliacs. Acta Orthop Scand 50:513–517, 1979

61. Gamba G, Grignanai G, Ascari E: Synoviorthesis versus synovectomy in the treatment of recurrent haemophilic haemarthrosis: long-term evaluation. Thromb Haemost 45:127–129, 1981

62. Goodfellow JW: Editorial. He who hesitates is saved. J Bone Joint Surg 62(B):1–2, 1980

63. London JT, Kattlove H, Louie JS, et al: Synovectomy and total joint arthroplasty for recurrent hemarthroses in the arthropathic joint in hemophilia. Arthritis Rheum 20:1543–1545, 1977

64. Marmor L: Total knee replacement in haemophilia. Clin Orthop 125:192–195, 1977

65. Arden GP: Total joint replacement, in Arden GP, Ansell BM (eds): Surgical Management of Juvenile Chronic Polyarthritis. New York, Grune & Stratton, 1978, pp 125–160

66. McCollough NC III, Enis JE, Lovitt J, et al: Synovectomy or total replacement of the knee in hemophilia. J Bone Joint Surg 61A:69–75, 1979

67. Small M, Steven MM, Freeman PA, et al: Total knee arthroplasty in haemophilic arthritis. J Bone Joint Surg (Br)65:163–165, 1983

68. Post M, Telfer MC: Surgery in hemophilic patients. J Bone Joint Surg 57A:1136–1145, 1975

69. Hopf F: Quoted by Grandidier L (1839), in Schmidts Jahrbücher der in-und ausländischen gessamter Med 28:171, 1839

70. Hartmann JR, Diamond LK: Haemophilia and related haemorrhagic disorders. Practitioner 178:179–190, 1957

71. Wilkinson JF, Nour-Eldin F, Israëls MCG, et al: Haemophilia syndromes. A survey of 267 patients. Lancet 2:947–950, 1961

72. Forbes CD, King J, Prentice CRM, et al: Serum enzyme changes after intramuscular bleeding in patients with haemophilia and Christmas disease. J Clin Pathol 25:1034–1037, 1972

73. Woods CG: The management of musculo-skeletal problems in the haemophilias, in Duthie RB, Matthews JM, Rizza CR, et al (eds): The Haemophiliac. Oxford, Blackwell Scientific Publications, 1972, pp 1–174

74. Forbes CD, Moule B, Grant M, et al: Bilateral pseudotumors of the pelvis in a patient with Christmas disease with notes on localization by radioactive scanning and ultrasonography. Am J Roentgenol Rad Ther Nucl Med 121:173–176, 1974

75. Nowotny C, Niessner H, Thaler E, et al: Sonography: A method for localization of haematomas in hemophiliacs. Hemostasis 5:129–135, 1976

76. Wallis J, Van Kaick G, Schimf K, et al: Ultrasound diagnosis of muscle haematomas in haemophiliac patients. F Ront Nukl 134:153–156, 1981

77. Bayer WL, Shea JD, Curiel DC, et al: Excision of a pseudocyst of the hand in a hemophiliac (PTC-deficiency). J Bone Joint Surg 51A:1423–1427, 1969

78. Gunning AJ: The surgery of haemophilic cysts, in Biggs R, Macfarlane RG (eds): Treatment of Haemophilia and Other Coagulation Disorders. Oxford, Blackwell Scientific Publications, 1966, pp 262–278

79. Wessler S, Avioli LV: Changes in surgical management of hemophiliacs. Pseudotumor of the ilium. JAMA 206:2292–2296, 1968

80. Chen YF: Bilateral hemophilic pseudotumors of the calcaneus and cuboid treated by irradiation. Case report J Bone Joint Surg (Am) 47:517–521, 1965

81. Fraenkel GJ, Taylor KB, Richards WCD: Haemophilic blood cysts. Br J Surg 46:383–392, 1959

82. Silber R, Christensen WR: Pseudotumor of hemophilia in a patient with PTC deficiency. Blood 14:584–590, 1959

83. Ramgren O: A clinical and medico-social study of haemophilia in Sweden. Acta Med Scand (suppl 379):1–190, 1962

84. Pappas AM, Barr JS, Salzman EW, et al: The problem of unrecognized ''mild hemophilia.'' Survival of a patient after disarticulation of the hip. JAMA 187:772–774, 1964

85. Becker F: Sarkom-vortauschende sog. Resorptionsgeschwulst bei Hamophilie. Zentralb Chir 69:1133–1137, 1942

86. Nelson MG, Mitchell ES: Pseudo-tumour of bone in hemophilia. Acta Hamatol 28:137–144, 1962

87. Starker L: Knochenusur durch ein hämophiles subperiostales Hämatom. Mitt Grenzgeb Med Chir 31:381–415, 1919

88. Abell JM, Bailey RW: Hemophilic pseudotumor: Two cases occurring in siblings. Arch Surg 81:569–581, 1960

89. Fraenkel GJ, Taylor KB, Richards WCD: Haemophilic blood cysts. Br J Surg 46:383–392, 1959

90. Valderrama JAF de, Matthews JM: The haemophilic pseudotumour or haemophilic subperiosteal haematoma. J Bone Joint Surg 47B:256–265, 1965

91. Valderrama JAF de: The haemophilic blood cysts, in Brinkhous KM, Hemker HC (eds): Handbook of Hemophilia. Amsterdam, Excerpta Medica, 1975, pp 425–433

92. Gilbert MS: Hemophilic pseudotumour, in Brinkhous KM, Hemker HC (eds): Handbook of Hemophilia. Amsterdam, Excerpta Medica, 1975, pp 435–446

93. Kerr CB: Management of Haemophilia. Glebe NSW, Australian Medical Publication Co, 1963

94. McMahon JS, Blackburn CRM: Haemophilia pseudo-tumour: A report of a case treated conservatively. Aust NZ J Surg 29:129–134, 1960

95. Steel WM, Duthie RB, O'Connor, BT: Haemophilic cysts. Report of five cases. J Bone Joint Surg, 51B:614–626, 1969

96. van Creveld S, Kingma MJ: Subperiosteal haemorrhage in haemophilia A and B. Acta Paediatr (Uppsala) 50:291–296, 1961

97. Brant EE, Jordan HH: Radiologic aspects of hemophilic pseudotumours in bone. Am J Roentgenol 115:525–539, 1972

98. Horwitz H, Simon N, Bassen FA: Haemophilic pseudotumour of the pelvis Br J Radiol 32:51–54, 1959

99. Muller JH: Uber die Rontgentherapie von sog. Resorptiongeschwulsten bei Hamophilia. Strahlentherapie 72:281–285, 1942

100. Britten AFH, Salzman EW: Surgery in congenital disorders of blood coagulation. Surg Gynecol Obstet 123:1333–1358, 1966

101. Grandidier L: Die Hämophilie oder die Blüterkrankheit nach eigenen und fremden. Beobachtungen monographisch Bearbeitet, O. Wigand, Leipzig, 1855

102. Stuart J, Davies SH, Cumming RA, et al: Haemorrhagic episodes in haemophilia: A 5-year prospective study. Br Med J 2:1624–1626, 1966

103. Macfarlane RG, Mallam PC, Witts LJ, et al: Surgery in haemophilia. The use of animal antihaemophilic globulin and human plasma in thirteen cases. Lancet 2:251–259, 1957

104. Walker W: Peptic ulcer in a haemophiliac treated by gastrectomy. Lancet 1:749–751, 1955

105. Carron DB, Boon TH, Walker FC: Peptic ulcer in the haemophiliac and its relation to gastrointestinal bleeding. Lancet 2:1036–1039, 1965

106. Nour-Eldin F: Longevity of haemophiliacs, Br Med J 1:824, 1961 (letter)

107. Forbes CD, Barr RD, Prentice CRM, et al: Gastrointestinal bleeding in haemophilia. Q J Med n.s. 42:503–511, 1973

108. Agle DP: Psychiatric studies of patients with hemophilia and related states. Arch Intern Med 114:76–82, 1964

109. Early DF: Psychosis in association with haemophilia. Br J Psychiatry 105:243–246, 1959

110. Browne WJ, Mall MA, Kane RP: Psychosocial aspects of hemophilia. A study of 28 hemophilic children and their families. Am J Orthop 30:730–740, 1960

111. Mattsson A, Gross S: Social and behavioural studies on hemophilic children and their families. J Pediatr 68:952–964, 1966

112. Kaneshiro MM, Mielke CH Jr, Kasper CK, et al: Bleeding time after aspirin in disorders of intrinsic clotting. N Engl J Med 281:1039–1042, 1969

113. Mielke CH Jr., Britten AFH: Use of aspirin or acetaminophen in hemophilia. N Engl J Med 282:1270, 1970 (letter)

114. Forbes CD, Prentice CRM: Mortality in haemophilia—A United Kingdom survey, in JC Fratantoni, DL Aronson, (eds): Unsolved Therapeutic Problems in Hemophilia. DHEW Publication No. (NIH) 77-1089, Washington, DC 1977, pp 15–22

115. Forbes CD, Davidson JF: Management of coagulation defects. Clin Haematol 2:101–127, 1973

116. van Trotsenburg L: Neurological complications of haemophilia, in Brinkhous KM, Hemker HC (eds): Handbook of Hemophilia. Amsterdam, Excerpta Medica, 1975, pp 389–404

117. Denton RL, Gourdeau R: Electroencephalographic patterns in haemophilia. Bibl Haematol 34:135–138, 1970

118. Forbes CD, Renfrew S: Electroencephalography in haemophilia and Christmas disease. Haemostasis 4:36–39, 1975

119. Travis RL, Mitchell OC, Youmans JR, et al: Intracranial surgery in hemophilia: Use of a potent antihemophilic factor concentrate. Am Surg 34:602–604, 1968

120. Davies SH, Turner JW, Cumming RA, et al: Management of intracranial haemorrhage in haemophilia. Br Med J 2:1627–1630, 1966

121. Edson JR, McArthur JR, Branda RF, et al: Successful management of a subdural hematoma in a hemophiliac with an anti-factor VIII antibody. Blood 41:113–122, 1973

122. Ferguson GG, Barton, WB, Drake CG: Subdural hematoma in hemophilia. Successful treatment with cryoprecipitate. Case report. J Neurosurg 29:524–528, 1968

123. Friedman H, Guerry R, Wilkins RH: Intracerebral hematoma in a hemophiliac. Combined surgical and factor VIII treatment. JAMA 215:791–792, 1971

124. Potter JM: Head injury and haemophilia. Acta Neurochir 13:380–387, 1965

125. Blaauw G, Schenk VWD: Cervical cord tumour in two haemophilic brothers. J Neurol Sci 14:409–416, 1971

126. Schenk VWD: Haemorrhages in spinal cord with syringomyelia in a patient with haemophilia. Acta Neuropathol 2:306–308, 1963

127. Douglas AS, McAlpine SG: Neurological complications of haemophilia and Christmas Disease. Scott Med J 1:270–273, 1956

128. Jones RK, Knighton RS: Surgery in hemophiliacs with special reference to the central nervous system. Ann Surg 144:1029–1034, 1956

129. Sumner DW: Spontaneous spinal extradural hemorrhage due to hemophilia. Report of a case. Neurology 12:501–502, 1962

130. Harvie A, Lowe GDO, Forbes CD, et al: Intraspinal bleeding in haemophilia. Successful treatment with factor VIII concentrate. J Neurol Neurosurg Psychiatry 40:1220–1223, 1977

131. Silverstein A: Neuropathy in hemophilia. JAMA 190:554–555, 1964

132. Lyons JB: Femoral nerve lesion in haemophilia. J Irish Med Assoc 32:110–111, 1953

133. Duthie RB, Matthews JM, Rizza C, et al: Peripheral nerve lesions, in The Management of the Musculo-Skeletal Problems in the Haemophilias. Oxford, Blackwell Scientific Publications, 1972, pp 63–74

134. Forbes CD, King I, McNicol GP: Duplication of LDH-1 in a patient receiving multiple transfusions. Clin Chem 17:948–949, 1971

135. Ikkala E: Haemophilia. A study of its laboratory, clinical, genetic and social aspects based on known haemophiliacs in Finland. Scand J Clin Lab Invest 12(suppl 46):1–144, 1960

136. Davidson CS, Epstein RD, Miller GF, et al: Hemophilia. A clinical study of forty patients. Blood 4:97–119, 1949

137. Biggs R, Matthews JM: The treatment of haemorrhage in von Willebrand's disease and the blood level of factor VIII (AHG). Br J Haematol 9:203–214, 1963

138. Forbes CD, Prentice CRM: Renal disorders in haemophilia A and B. Scand J Haematol (suppl 30):43–50, 1977

139. Prentice CRM, Lindsay RM, Barr RD, et al: Renal complications in haemophilia and Christmas Disease. Q J Med 40:47–61, 1970

140. Albert DJ, Zimmerman TS, Mahoney SA, et al: Hemophilia (Factor VIII deficiency), hematuria and urological intervention. J Urol 103:421–424, 1970

141. Forbes CD, Craig JA, Prentice CRM, et al: Rupture of the ureter due to crushing injury in a boy with severe haemophilia. Br J Surg 58:931–934, 1971

142. Barkhan P: Haematuria in a haemophiliac treated with e-aminocaproic acid, Lancet 2:1061, 1964, (letter)

143. Blombäck M, Nilsson IM: Treatment of hemophilia A with human anti-hemophilic globulin. Acta Med Scand 161:301–321, 1958

144. Hilgartner MW: Intrarenal obstruction in haemophilia. Lancet 1:486, 1966 (letter)

145. Beck P, Evans KT: Renal abnormalities in patients with haemophilia and Christmas disease. Clin Radiol 23:349–354, 1972

146. Wright FW, Matthews JM, Brock LG: Complications of hemophilic disorders affecting the renal tract. Radiology 98:571–576, 1971

147. Goudemand M, Parquet-Gernez A, Deconninck B: Les incidents urinaires du traitement des hématuries des hemophiles par l'acide epsilon-amino caproique. Lille Med 13:408–412, 1968

148. Marcinski A, Kaniewska A, Byszy-Laube B, et al: Radiodiagnostic des hémorragies rénale et périrénales dans l' hémophilie, Ann Radiol 15:27–32, 1972

149. Wright FW, Matthews JM, Brock LG: Complications of hemophilic disorders affecting the renal tract. Radiology 98:571–576, 1971

150. Dalinka MK, Lally JF, Rancier LF, et al: Nephromegaly in hemophilia. Radiology 115:337–340, 1975

151. Canale VC, Hilgartner MW, Smith HC: Effect of corticosteroids on factor VIII level. J Pediatr 71:878–880, 1967

152. Abildgaard CF, Simone JV, Schulman I: Steroid treatment of hemophilic hematuria. J Pediatr 66:117–119, 1965

153. Gourdeau R, Denton RL: Steroids and hemophilia. Bibl Hematol 34:65–68, 1970

154. Prentice CRM, Izatt MM, Adams JF, et al: Amyloidosis associated with the nephrotic syndrome and transfusion reactions in a haemophiliac. Br J Haematol 21:305–311, 1971

155. Wardle EN: Immunoglobulins and immunological reactions in haemophilia. Lancet 2:233–234, 1967

156. Goudemand M, Delmas-Marsalet Y, Parquet-Gernez A, et al: L'utilisation des fractions anti-hemophiliques d'orgine animale dans l'hemophilie. Presse Med 76:197–200, 1968

157. Forbes CD, Prentice CRM: Aggregation of human platelets by purified porcine and bovine antihaemophilic factor. Nature (New Biol) 241:149–150, 1973

158. Forbes CD, Prentice CRM: Aggregation of human platelets by commercial porcine and bovine fibrinogen preparations. Haemostasis 1:156–160, 1973

159. Keidan SE, Lohoar E, Mainwaring D: Acute anuria in a haemophiliac due to transfusion of incompatible plasma. Lancet 1:179–182, 1966

160. Koene RAP, Gerlag PGG, Jansen JLF, et al: Successful haemodialysis and renal transplantation in a patient with haemophilia A. Proc Eur Dial Transplant Assoc 14:401–406, 1977

161. Gomperts ED, Malekzadeh MH, Fine RN: Dialysis and renal transplant in a hemophiliac. Thromb Haemost 46:626–628, 1981

162. Lucas ON, Carroll RT, Finkelmann A, et al: Tooth extractions in hemophilia. Control of bleeding without use of blood, plasma or plasma fractions. Thromb Diath Haemorrh 8:209–220, 1962

163. Walsh PN, Rizza CR, Matthews JM, et al: Epsilon-aminocaproic acid therapy for dental extractions in haemophilia and Christmas disease: A double-blind controlled trial. Br J Haematol 20:463–475, 1971

164. Cooksey, MW, Perry CB, Raper AB: Epsilon-aminocaproic acid therapy for dental extractions in haemophiliacs. Br Med J 2:1633–1634, 1966

165. Forbes CD, Barr RD, Reid G, et al: Tranexamic acid in control of haemorrhage after dental extraction in haemophilia and Christmas disease. Br Med J 2:311–313, 1972

166. Reid WO, Lucas ON, Francisco J, et al: The use of epsilon-aminocaproic acid in the management of dental extractions in the hemophiliac. Am J Med Sci 248:184–188, 1964

167. Tavenner RWH: Epsilon-aminocaproic acid in the treatment of haemophilia and Christmas disease with special reference to the extraction of teeth. Br Dent J 124:19–22, 1968

168. Rapaport SI, Patch MJ, Moore FJ: Antihemophilic globulin levels in carriers of hemophilia A. J Clin Invest 39:1619–1625, 1960

169. Veltkamp JJ, Drion EF, Loeliger EA: Detection of the carrier state in hereditary coagulation disorders. Thromb Diath Haemorrh 19:403–422, 1968

170. Zimmerman TS, Ratnoff OD, Littel AS: Detection of carriers of classic hemophilia using an immunologic assay for antihemophilic factor (factor VIII). J Clin Invest 50:255–258, 1971

171. Bennett B, Ratnoff OD: Changes in antihemophilic factor (AHF, factor VIII) procoagulant activity and AHF-like antigen in normal pregnancy and following exercise and pneumoencephalography. J Lab Clin Med 80:256–263, 1972

172. Bouma BN, van der Klaauw MM, Veltkamp JJ, et al: Evaluation of the detection rate of hemophilia carriers. Thromb Res 7:339–350, 1975

173. Ratnoff OD, Jones PK: The laboratory diagnosis of the carrier state for classic hemophilia. Ann Intern Med 86:521–528, 1977

174. WHO Report: Methods for the detection of haemophilia carriers: A memorandum. Bull WHO 55:675–702, 1977

175. Prentice CRM, Forbes CD, Morrice S, et al: Calculation of predictive odds for possible carriers of haemophilia. Proceedings of the IXth Congress, World Federation of Haemophilia, Istanbul, 1974, pp 34–36

176. Wahlberg T: Carriers and non-carriers of haemophilia A: Multivariate analysis of pedigree data, blood coagulation variables and bleeding symptoms. Doctoral thesis, Karolinska Institute, 1981, 1–39

177. Graham JB, Flyer P, Elston RC, et al: Statistical study of genotype assignment (carrier detection) in hemophilia B. Thromb Res 15:69–78, 1979

178. Kasper CK, Osterud B, Minami JY, et al: Hemophilia B: Characterization of genetic variants and detection of carriers. Blood 50:351–366, 1977

179.  Orstavik KH, Veltkamp JJ, Bertina RM, et al: Detection of carriers of haemophilia B. Br J
      Haematol 42:293–301, 1979
180.  Pechet L, Tiarks CY, Stevens J, et al: Relationship of factor IX antigen and coagulant in
      hemophilia B patients and carriers. Thromb Haemost 40:465–477, 1978
181.  Thompson AR: Factor IX antigen by radioimmunoassay in heterozygotes for hemophilia B.
      Thromb Res 11:193–203, 1977
182.  Rodeck CH: Fetoscopy guided by real-time ultrasound for pure fetal blood samples, fetal
      skin samples and examination of the fetus *in utero*. Br J Obstet Gynaecol 87:449–456, 1980
183.  Rodeck CH, Campbell S: Sampling pure fetal blood by fetoscopy in second trimester of
      pregnancy. Br Med J 2:728–730, 1978
184.  Mibashan RS, Rodeck CH: Prenatal diagnosis of haemophilia A and Christmas disease, in
      Forbes CD, Lowe GDO (eds): Unsolved Problems in Haemophilia. Lancaster, England, MTP
      Press, 1982, pp 203–212
185.  Mibashan RS, Peake IR, Rodeck CH, et al: Dual diagnosis of prenatal haemophilia A by
      measurement of fetal factor VIIIC and VIIIC antigen (VIII CAg). Lancet 2:994–997, 1980
185a. Firshein SI, Hoyer LW, Lazarchick J, et al: Prenatal diagnosis of classic hemmophilia. N
      Engl J Med 300:937–941, 1979
186.  Holmberg L, Gustavii B, Cordesius E, et al: Prenatal diagnosis of hemophilia B by an
      immunoradiometric assay of factor IX. Blood 56:397–401, 1980
187.  Forbes CD, Markova I: An international survey of genetic counselling in haemophilia. Ethics
      Sci Med 6:123–126, 1979
188.  Bulloch W, Fildes P: Haemophilia: Treasury of Human Inheritance, Parts V and VI. Eugenic
      Laboratory Memoirs XII. London, Dulan, 1911
189.  De La Chapelle A, Ikkala E, Nevanlinna MR, et al: Haemophilia A in a girl. Lancet 2:578–580,
      1961
190.  Merskey C: The occurrence of haemophilia in the human female. Q J Med 20:299–312, 1951
191.  Ulutin ON, Müftüğlu A, Palamar S: Haemophilia A in a girl with female sex chromatin pattern.
      Thromb Diath Haemorrh 14:65–73, 1965
192.  Graham JB, Barrow EM: The pathogenesis of hemophilia. An experimental analysis of the
      anticephalin hypothesis in hemophilic dogs. J Exp Med 106:273–292, 1957
193.  Graham JB, Brinkhous KM, Dodds WJ: Canine and equine hemophilia, in Brinkhous
      KM, Hemker HC (eds): Handbook of Hemophilia. Amsterdam, Excerpta Medica, 1975,
      pp 119–139
194.  Graham JB, Barrow ES, Roberts HR, et al: Dominant inheritance of hemophilia A in three
      generations of women. Blood 46:175–188, 1975
195.  Graham JB: Genetics of factor VIII, in Forbes CD, Lowe GDO (eds): Unresolved Problems
      in Haemophilia. Lancaster, England, MTP Press, 1982, pp 183–199
196.  Gilchrist GS, Hammond D, Melnyk J: Hemophilia A in a phenotypically normal female with
      XX/XO mosaicsm. N Engl J Med 273:1402–1406, 1965
197.  Nilsson IM, Bergman S, Reitalu J, et al: Haemophilia A in a ''girl'' with male sex-chromatin
      pattern. Lancet 2:264–266, 1959
198.  Samama M, Perrote C, Houissa R, et al: Hemophilie à feminine avec deletion d'une partie du
      bras long d'un chromosome X. Pathol-Biol suppl 25:10, 1977
199.  Mori PG, Pasino M, Rosanda Vadala C, et al: Haemophilia 'A' in a 46, X, i(Xq) female. Br
      J Haematol 43:143–147, 1979
200.  Hashmi KZ, MacIver JE, Delamore IW: Christmas disease in a female. Lancet 2:965–966,
      1978
201.  Bithell TC, Pizarro A, MacDiarmid WD: Variant of factor IX deficiency in female with 45,
      X Turner's syndrome. Blood 36:169–179, 1970
202.  Kerr CB, Preston AE, Barr A, et al: Inheritance of factor VIII, in Hunter RB, Wright IS,
      Koller F, et al (eds): Genetics and the Interaction of Blood Clotting Factors. Thrombosis
      Diath Haemorrh, Suppl., 173-179, 1965

203.  Hathaway WE, Bonnar J: Perinatal Coagulation. Monographs in Neonatology. New York, Grune & Stratton, 1978, pp 107

204.  Hill C, Taylor JJ: Von Willebrand's Disease in Obstetrics and Gynaecology. J Obstet Gynaecol Br Common 75:453–458, 1968

205.  Cook IA, Douglas AS: Demonstrable deficiency of Christmas factor in two sisters. Br Med J 1:479–482, 1960

206.  Clark KGA: Haemophilic woman. Lancet 1:1388–1389, 1973 (letter)

207.  Lane S: Haemorrhagic diathesis. Successful transfusion of blood. Lancet 1:185–188, 1840

208.  Addis T: The pathogenesis of hereditary hemophilia. J Pathol Bacteriol 15:427–452, 1911

209.  Payne WW, Steen RE: Haemostatic therapy in haemophilia. Br Med J 1:1150–1152, 1929

210.  Nilsson IM, Blomback M, Ramgren O: Haemophilia in Sweden VI: Treatment of haemophilia A with the human antihaemophilic factor preparation (fraction 1-0). Acta Med Scand (suppl 379):61–110, 1962

211.  Alexander B, Landwehr G: Studies of hemophilia II. The assay of antihemophilic clot promoting principle in normal human plasma with some observations on the relative potency of certain plasma fractions. J Clin Invest 27:98–105, 1948

211a. Boklan BF: Factor IX concentrate and viral hepatitis, Ann Intern Med 74:298, 1971 (letter)

212.  Pool JG, Robinson J: Observations on plasma banking and transfusion procedures for haemophilic patients using a quantitative assay for antihaemophilic globulin (AHG). Br J Haematol 5:24–30, 1959

213.  Hershgold EJ, Pool JG, Pappenhagen AR: The potent antihemophilic globulin concentrate derived from a cold insoluble fraction of human plasma: Characterization and further data on preparation and clinical trial. J Lab Clin Med 67:23–32, 1966

214.  Pool JG, Hershgold EJ, Pappenhagen AR: High potency antihaemophilic factor prepared from cryoglobulin precipitate. Nature 293:312, 1964

215.  Bennett E, Dormandy K: Pool's cryoprecipitate and exhausted plasma in the treatment of von Willebrand's disease and factor-XI deficiency. Lancet 2:731–732, 1966

216.  Forbes CD, Hunter J, Barr RD, et al: Cryoprecipitate therapy in haemophilia. Scott Med J 14:1–9, 1969

217.  Pool JG, Shannon AE: Production of high-potency concentrates of antihemophilic globulin in a closed-bag system. N Engl J Med 273:1443–1447, 1965

218.  Prentice CRM, Breckenridge RT, Forman WB, et al: Treatment of haemophilia (factor VIII deficiency) with human antihaemophilic factor prepared by the cryoprecipitate process. Lancet 1:457–460, 1967

219.  Brown DL, Hardisty RM, Kosoy MH, et al: Antihaemophilic globulin: Preparation by an improved cryoprecipitation method and clinical use. Br Med J 2:79–85, 1967

220.  Djerassi I, Bhanchet P, Hsieh Y, et al: Clinical use of cold precipitated antihemophilic globulin (factor VIII, CPAG). Transfusion 5:533–538, 1965

221.  Hattersley PG: The treatment of classic hemophilia with cryoprecipitates. JAMA 198:243–247, 1966

222.  Burka ER, Harker LA, Kasper CK, et al: A protocol for cryoprecipitate production. Transfusion 15:307–311, 1975

222a. Burka ER, Puffer T, Martinez J: The influence of donor characteristics and preparation methods on the potency of human cryoprecipitate. Transfusion 15:323–328, 1975

223.  Kasper CK, Myhre BA, McDonald JD, et al: Determinants of factor VIII recovery in cryoprecipitate. Transfusion 15:312–322, 1975

224.  Slichter SJ, Counts RB, Henderson R, et al: Preparation of cryoprecipitated factor VIII concentrates. Transfusion 16:616–626, 1976

225.  Aronson DL: Factor VIII (antihemophilic globulin). Semin Thromb Hemost 6:12–27, 1979

226.  Carter F, Forbes CD, Macfarlane JD, et al: Cost of management of patients with haemophilia. Br Med J 2:465–467, 1976

227. Carter F, MacFarlane J, Forbes CD, et al: Costing cryoprecipitate for haemophilia. Br Med J 2:256, 1975

228. Verstraete M, Vermylen J: Laboratory and clinical evaluation of concentrate for treatment of haemophilia. Acta Clin Belg 30:437–448, 1975

229. Johnson AJ, Karpatkin MH, Newman J: Clinical investigation of intermediate- and high-purity antihaemophilic factor (factor VIII) concentrates. Br J Haematol 21:21–41, 1971

230. Johnson AJ, Newman J, Howell MB, et al: Two large scale procedures for purification of human antihemophilic factor (AHF). Blood 28:1011, 1966 (abstract)

231. Aronson DL, Finlayson JS: Direct and indirect effects of chronic plasma protein infusion, in Fratantoni J, Aronson DL (eds): Unresolved Therapeutic Problems in Hemophilia. US Dept of Health, Education and Welfare publication No. (NIH) (77-1089). 1977, pp 93–101

232. Rosati LA, Barnes B, Oberman HA, et al: Hemolytic anaemia due to anti-A in concentrated antihemophilic factor preparations. Transfusion, 10:139–141, 1971

233. Abildgaard CF, Simone JV, Corrigan JJ, et al: Treatment of hemophilia with glycine-precipitated factor VIII. N Engl J Med 275:471–475, 1966

234. Shulman NR, Marder VJ, Hiller MC: A new method for measuring minimum in-vivo concentrations of factor VIII applied in distribution and survival studies and in detecting factor VIII inhibitors, in Brinkhous KM (ed) The Hemophilias: Chapel Hill, NC, University North Carolina Press, 1964, pp 29–43

235. Weiss AE, Webster WP, Strike LE, et al: Survival of transfused factor VIII in hemophilic patients treated with epsilon aminocaproic acid. Transfusion 16:209–214, 1976

236. Smith CM, Miller GE, Breckenridge RT: Factor VIII concentrates in outpatient therapy. JAMA 220:1352–1354, 1972

237. Dintenfass L, Forbes CD: Viscosity of blood in patients with myocardial infarction, haemophilia and thyroid disease. Effect of fibrinogen, albumin and globulin. Biorheology 10:457–462, 1973

238. Dintenfass L, Forbes CD: Artificial thrombus formation and blood viscosity in haemophilia A and Christmas disease Haemostasis 2:223–234, 1974

239. Dintenfass L, Forbes CD: Effect of fibrinogen on aggregation of red cells and on apparent viscosity of artificial thrombi in haemophilia, myocardial infarction, thyroid disease, cancer and control systems. Effect of ABO groups. Microvasc Res 9:107–118, 1975

240. Ahrons S, Glavind-Kristensen S, Drachmann O, et al: Severe reactions after cryoprecipitated human factor VIII. Vox Sang 18:182–184, 1970

241. Burman D, Hodson AK, Wood CBS, et al: Acute anaphylaxis, pulmonary oedema, and intravascular haemolysis due to cryoprecipitate. Arch Dis Childhood 48:483–485, 1973

242. Eyster ME, Bowman HS, Haverstick JN: Adverse reactions to factor VIII infusions, Ann Intern Med 87:248, 1977 (letter)

243. Maycock W d'A, Evans S, Vallet I, et al: Further experience with a concentrate containing human antihaemophilic factor. Br J Haematol 9:215–235, 1963

244. Rizza CR, Matthews JH: Management of the haemophilic child. Arch Dis Child 47:451–462, 1972

245. Kernoff PBA, Bowell PJ: Gm types and antibodies in multitransfused haemophiliacs. Br J Haematol 24:443–450, 1973

246. McVerry BA, Machin SJ: Incidence of allo-immunisation and allergic reactions to cryoprecipitate in hemophilia. Vox Sang 36:77–80, 1979

247. Rabiner SF, Telfer MC, Fajardo R: Home transfusion of hemophiliacs. JAMA 221:885–887, 1972

248. Veroust P, Veroust F, Adam C: Immunological studies in haemophilia: Complement levels and circulating immune complexes. Seventeenth Congress of the International Society of Haematology—Abstracts 1:213, 1978

249. Thomson C, Forbes CD, Prentice CRM: A comparison of the effects of antihistamines on platelet function. Thromb Diath Haemorrh 30:547–556, 1973

250. Seeler HA: Hemolysis due to anti-A and anti-B in factor VIII preparations. Arch Intern Med 130:101–103, 1972

251. Barnet RN, Fox RA, Snavely JG: Hepatitis following the use of irradiated human plasma. JAMA 144:226–228, 1950

252. Brightman IJ, Korns RF: Homologous serum jaundice in recipients of pooled plasma. JAMA 135:268–272, 1947

253. James G, Korns RF, Wright AW: Homologous serum jaundice associated with use of irradiated plasma: A preliminary report. JAMA 144:228–229, 1950

254. Propert SA: Hepatitis after prophylactic serum, Br Med J 2:677–678, 1938 letter

255. Seeff LB, Hoofnagle J: Acute and chronic liver disease in hemophilia, in Fratantoni JC, Aronson DL (eds): Unsolved Therapeutic Problems in Hemophilia. US Dept of Health, Education and Welfare publication No. (NIH), 77–1089, 1976, pp 61–72

255a. Seef LB, Wright EC, Zimmerman HJ: Post transfusion hepatitis 1973–75. A Veterans Administration Cooperative Study, in Vyas GN, Cohen SN, Schmid R (eds): Viral Hepatitis: A Contemporary Assessment of Etiology, Epidemiology, Pathogenesis and Prevention. Philadelphia, Franklin Institute Press, 1978, pp 371–381

256. Spurling N, Shone J, Vaughan J: The incidence, incubation period and symptomatology of homologous serum jaundice. Br Med J 2:409–412, 1946

257. Allen JG, Sayman WA: Serum hepatitis from transfusions of blood. Epidemiologic study. JAMA 180:1079–1085, 1962

258. Schroeder DD, Mozen MM: Australia antigen: Distribution during Cohn ehtanol fractionation of human plasma. Science 168:1462–1464, 1970

259. Alter HJ, Holland PV, Schmidt PJ: Hepatitis-associated antigen. To test or not to test? Lancet 2:142–143, 1970

260. Craske J: The epidemiology of factor VIII and IX associated hepatitis in the U.K., in Forbes CD, Lowe GDO (eds): Unresolved Problems in Haemophilia. Lancaster, England, MTP Press, 1982, p 5

261. Goldfield M, Black HC, Bill J, et al: The consequences of administering blood pretested for Hbs Ag by third generation techniques: A progress report. Am J Med Sci 270:335–342, 1975

262. Biggs R: Jaundice and antibodies directed against factors VIII and IX in patients treated for haemophilia or Christmas disease in the United Kingdom. Br J Haematol 26:313–329, 1974

263. Craske J, Dilling N, Stern D: An outbreak of hepatitis associated with intravenous injection of factor-VIII concentrate. Lancet 2:221–223, 1975

264. Cronberg S, Belfrage S, Nilsson IM: Fibrinogen-transmitted hepatitis. Lancet 1:967–969, 1963

265. Kasper CK, Kipnis SA: Hepatitis and clotting-factor concentrates, JAMA 221:510, 1972 (letter)

266. Preston FE, Triger DR, Underwood JCE: Experience of liver disease in haemophilia, in Forbes CD, Lowe GDO (eds): Unresolved Problems in Haemophilia. Lancaster, England, MTP Press, 1982, pp 41–45

267. Hampers CL, Prager D, Senior JR: Post-transfusion anicteric hepatitis. N Engl J Med 271:747–754, 1964

268. Levine PH, McVerry BA, Attock B, et al: Health of the intensively treated hemophiliac with special reference to abnormal liver chemistries and splenomegaly. Blood 50:1–9, 1977

269. Manucci PM, Capitanio A, del Ninno E, et al: Asymptomatic liver disease in haemophiliacs. J Clin Pathol 28:620–624, 1975

270. Mirick GS, Ward R, McCollum RW: Modification of post-transfusion hepatitis by gamma globulin. N Engl J Med 273:59–65, 1965

271. Thomas HC, Bamber M, Kernoff, PBA: Clinical, immunological and histological aspects of non-A, non-B hepatitis in haemophiliacs, in Forbes CD, Lowe GDO (eds): Unresolved Problems in Haemophilia. Lancaster, England, MTP Press, 1982, pp 27–36

272. Enck RE, Betts RF, Brown MR, et al: Viral serology (hepatitis B virus, cytomegalovirus, Epstein-Barr virus) and abnormal liver function tests in transfused patients with hereditary hemorrhagic diseases. Transfusion 19:32–38, 1979

273. Seeler RA, Mufson MA: Development and persistence of antibody to hepatitis associated (Australia) antigen in patients with hemophilia. J Infect Dis 123:279–283, 1971

274. Kunst VAJM, Rosier JGMC: Au antigen in at-risk patients. Lancet 1:423–424, 1970 (letter)

275. Kim HC, Said P, Ackley AM, et al: Prevalence of type B and non-A non-B hepatitis in hemophilia. Relationship to chronic liver disease. Gastroenterology 79:1159–1164, 1980

276. Alter HJ, Purcell RH, Feinstone SM, et al: Non-A non-B hepatitis: A review and interim report of an ongoing prospective study, in Vyas GN, Cohen SN, Schmid R (eds): Viral Hepatitis: A Contemporary Assessment of Etiology, Epidemiology, Pathogenesis and Prevention. Philadelphia, Franklin Institute Press, 1978, pp 359–369

277. Craske J, Spooner RJD, Vandervelde EM: Evidence for the existence of at least two types of factor-VIII-associated non-B transfusion hepatitis, Lancet 2:1051, 1978 (letter)

278. Knodell RG, Conrad ME, Ishak KG: Development of chronic liver disease after acute non-A, non-B post-transfusion hepatitis. γ Globulin prophylaxis in its prevention. Gastroenterology 72:902–909, 1977

279. Tsiquaye KN, Zuckerman AJ: New human hepatitis virus, (letter). Lancet 1:1135–1136, 1979

280. Zuckerman AJ: The three types of human viral hepatitis. Bull WHO 56:1–20, 1978

280a. Craske J, Kirk P, Cohen B, et al: Commercial factor VIII associated hepatitis, 1974–5, in the United Kingdom. A retrospective survey. J Hyg (Lond) 80:327–336, 1978

281. Lesesne HR, Morgan JE, Blatt PM, et al: Liver biopsy in hemophilia A. Ann Intern Med 86: 703–707, 1977

282. Manucci PM, Ronchi G, Rota L, et al: A clinicopathological study of liver disease in haemophiliacs. J Clin Pathol 31:779–783, 1978

283. Preston FE, Triger DR, Underwood JCE, et al: Percutaneous liver biopsy and chronic liver disease in haemophiliacs. Lancet 2:592–594, 1978

283a. Spero JA, Lewis JH, Fisher SE, et al: The high risk of chronic liver disease in multitransfused juvenile hemophilic patients. J Pediatr 94:875–878, 1979

284. Schimpf K, Zimmermann K, Rüdel J, et al: Results of liver biopsies, rate of icteric hepatitis, and frequency of anti-HG_S and HB_S-antigen in patients of the Heidelberg hemophilia center, Thromb Haemost 38:340, 1977 (abstract)

285. Tabor E, Seeff LB, Gerety RJ: Chronic non-A non-B hepatitis carrier state. Transmissible agent documented in one patient over a six-year period. N Engl J Med 303:140–143, 1980

286. Berk PD, Jones EA, Plotz PH: Corticosteroid therapy for chronic active hepatitis. Ann Intern Med 85:523–525, 1976

287. Plotz PH: Asymptomatic chronic hepatitis. Gastroenterology 68:1629–1630, 1975 (editorial)

287a. Gerety RJ, Schweitzer, IL: Viral hepatitis type B during pregnancy, the neonatal period and infancy. J Pediatr 90:368–374, 1977

288. Counts RB: Serum transaminase and serum HBs Ab in hemophiliacs treated exclusively with cryoprecipitate, in Fratantoni JC, Aronson D (eds): Unresolved Therapeutic Problems in hemophilia. US Dept of Health, Education and Welfare publication No. (NIH) 77-1089. Government Printing Office, 1977, pp 77–79

289. Hasiba UW, Spero JA, Lewis JH: Chronic liver dysfunction in multitransfused hemophiliacs. Transfusion 17:490–494, 1977

290. Howard CR: The development of hepatitis B vaccines and antiviral therapy, in Forbes CD, Lowe GDO (eds): Unresolved Problems in Haemophilia. Lancaster, England, MTP Press, 1982, pp 55–67

291. Zuckerman AJ: Priorities for immunisation against hepatitis B. Br Med J 284:686–688, 1982

292. Macfarlane RG, Biggs R, Bidwell E: Bovine antihaemophilic globulin in the treatment of haemophilia. Lancet 1:1316–1319, 1954

293. Bidwell E: The purification of bovine antihaemophilic globulin. Br J Haematol 1:35–45, 1955

294. Bidwell E: The purification of antihaemophilic globulin from animal plasma. Br J Haematol 1:386–389, 1955

295. Sharp AA, Bidwell E: The toxicity and fate of injected animal antihaemophilic globulin. Lancet 2:359–362, 1957

296. Nossel HL, Archer RK, Macfarlane RG: Equine haemophilia: Report of a case and its response to multiple infusions of heterospecific AHG. Br J Haematol 8:335–342, 1962

297. Rizza CR, Biggs R: Blood products in the management of haemophilia and Christmas disease, in Poller L (ed): Recent Advances in Blood Coagulation. London, Churchill, 1969, pp 179–195

298. Bottecchia D, Vermylen J: Factor VIII and human platelet aggregation. Br J Haematol 34:303–311, 1976

299. Brinkhous KM, Thomas BD, Ibrahim SA, et al: Plasma levels of platelet aggregating factor/von Willebrand factor in various species. Thromb Res 11:345–355, 1977

300. Forbes CD, Barr RD, McNicol GP, et al: Aggregation of human platelets by commercial preparations of bovine and porcine antihaemophilic globulin. J Clin Pathol 25:210–217, 1972

301. Middleton S: Polyelectrolytes and preparation of factor VIIIC, in Forbes CD, Lowe GDO (eds): Unresolved Problems in Haemophilia. Lancaster, England, MTP Press 1982, pp 109–118

302. Mayne EE, Madden M, Crothers IS, et al: Highly purified porcine factor VIII in haemophilia A with inhibitors to factor VIII, Br Med J 282:318, 1981 (letter)

303. Didisheim P, Loeb J, Blatrix C, et al: Preparation of a human plasma fraction rich in prothrombin, proconvertin, Stuart factor, and PTC and a study of its activity and toxicity in rabbits and man. J Lab Clin Med 53:322–330, 1959

304. Dike GWR, Bidwell E, Rizza CR: The preparation and clinical use of a new concentrate containing factor IX, prothrombin and factor X and a separate concentrate containing factor VII. Br J Haematol 22:469–490, 1972

305. Middleton SM, Bennett IH, Smith JK: A therapeutic concentrate of coagulation factors II, IX and X from citrated factor VIII depleted plasma. Vox Sang 24:441–456, 1973

306. Bidwell E, Booth JM, Dike GWR, et al: The preparation for therapeutic use of a concentrate of factor IX containing also factors II, VII, and X. Br J Haematol 13:568–580, 1967

307. Zauber NP, Levin J: Factor IX levels in patients with hemophilia B (Christmas disease) following transfusion with concentrates of factor IX or fresh frozen plasma (FFP). Medicine (Balt) 56:213–224, 1977

308. Hoofnagle JH, Aronson D, Roberts HR: Serologic evidence of hepatitis B infection in patients with hemophilia B. Thromb Diath Haemorrh 33:606–609, 1975

308a. Faria R, Fiumara N: Hepatitis B associated with konyne. N Engl J Med 287:358–359, 1972

309. Hultin MB: Activated clotting factors in prothrombin complex concentrates, Blood 54:1028–1037, 1979

310. Blatt PM, Lundblad RL, Kingdon HS, et al: Thrombogenic materials in prothrombin complex concentrates. Ann Intern Med 81:766–770, 1974

311. Gershwin ME, Gude JK: Deep vein thrombosis and pulmonary embolism in congenital factor VII deficiency. N Engl J Med, 288:141–142, 1973

312. Kasper CK: Post-operative thromboses in hemophilia B. N Engl J Med 289:160, 1973 (letter)

313. Machin SJ, Miller BR: Thrombosis and factor-IX concentrates, Lancet 1:1367, 1978 (letter)

314. Marchesi SL, Burney R: Prothrombin-complex concentrates and thromboses. N Engl J Med 290:403–404, 1974 (letter)

315. Yates AJ, Harvie A, Lowe GDO, et al: Mandril-grown graft for vascular access in Christmas disease. Br Med J 2:1108–1109, 1976

316. Fuerth JH, Mahrer P: Myocardial infarction after factor IX therapy. JAMA 245:1455–1456, 1981

317. Small M, Lowe GDO, Douglas JI, et al: Factor IX thrombogenicity: in vivo effects on coagu-

lation activation and a case report of disseminated intra-vascular coagulation. Thromb Haemost 48:76–77 1982

318.  Kingdon HS, Lundblad RL, Veltkamp JJ, et al: Potentially thrombogenic materials in factor IX concentrates. Thromb Diath Haemorrh 33:617–631, 1975

319.  Edson JR: Prothrombin complex concentrates and thromboses. N Engl J Med 290:403, 1974 (letter)

320.  Nossel HL, Kaplan KL, Spanondis K, et al: The generation of fibrinopeptide A in clinical blood samples: Evidence for thrombin activity. J Clin Invest 58:1136–1144, 1976

321.  Preston FE, Winfield D, Malia R, et al: Serial changes in the coagulation system following clotting factor concentrate infusion. Thromb Diath Haemorrh 34:475–482, 1975

322.  Vigano S, Cattaneo M, Gervasori W, et al: Increased fibrinopeptide A after prothrombin complex concentrates, Thromb Haemost 42:63, 1970 (abstract)

323.  Lane JL, Rizza CR, Snape TJ: A five year experience of the use of factor IX type DE(1) concentrate for the treatment of Christmas disease at Oxford. Br J Haematol 30:435–446, 1975

324.  Prowse CV, Cash JD: The use of factor IX concentrates in man: A 9-year experience of Scottish concentrates in the South-East of Scotland. Br J Haematol 47:91–104, 1981

325.  Biggs R, Matthews JM: The treatment of haemorrhage in von Willebrand's disease and the blood level of factor VIII (AHG). Br J Haematol 9:203–214, 1963

326.  Cornu P, Larrieu MJ, Caen J, et al: Transfusion studies in von Willebrand's disease: Effect on bleeding time and factor VIII. Br J Haematol 9:189–202, 1963

327.  Blatt PM, Brinkhous KM, Culp HR, et al: Antihemophilic factor concentrate therapy in von Willebrand disease. Dissociation of bleeding time factor and ristocetin-cofactor activities. JAMA 236:2770–2772, 1976

328.  Chediak JR, Telfer MC, Green D: Platelet function and immunologic parameters in von Willebrand's disease following cryoprecipitate and factor VIII concentrate infusion. Am J Med 62:369–376, 1977

329.  Nilsson IM, Hedner U: Characteristics of various factor VIII concentrates used in treatment of haemophilia A. Br J Haematol 37:543–557, 1977

330.  Telfer MC, Chediak J: Factor-VIII-related disorders and their relationship to pregnancy. J Reprod Med 19:211–222, 1977

331.  Evans PC: Obstetric and gynaecologic patients with von Willebrand's disease. Obstet Gynaecol 38:37–43, 1971

332.  Walker EH, Dormandy KM: The management of pregnancy in von Willebrand's disease. J Obstet Gynaecol Br Common 75:459–463, 1968

333.  Levine PH, Britten AFH: Supervised patient-management of hemophilia. A study of 45 patients with hemophilia A and B. Ann Intern Med 78:195–201, 1973

334.  Rabiner SF, Telfer MC: Home transfusion for patients with hemophilia A. N Engl J Med 283:1011–1015, 1970

335.  Rizza CR, Spooner JD: Home treatment of haemophilia and Christmas disease: Five years' experience. Br J Haematol 37:53–66, 1977

336.  Ingram GIC, Dykes SR, Creese AL, et al: Home treatment in haemophilia: Clinical, social and economic advantages. Clin Lab Haematol 1:13–27, 1979

337.  Markova I, Forbes CD: Haemophilia: A study into social and psychological problems. Health Bull (Edinburgh) 37:24–29, 1979

338.  Stuart J, Forbes CD, Jones P, et al: Improving prospects for employment of the haemophiliac. Br Med J 280:1169–1172, 1980

339.  Jones P, Fearns M, Forbes CD, et al: Haemophilia A—home therapy in the United Kingdom, 1975–76. Br Med J 1:1447–1450, 1978

340.  Aledort L, Diaz M: The cost of care, in Forbes CD, Lowe GDO (eds): Unresolved Problems in Haemophilia. Lancaster, England, MTP Press, 1982, pp 79–86

341.  Aledort LM, Goodnight SH: Hemophilia treatment: Its relationship to blood products, in Brown EM (ed): Progress in Hematology. New York, Grune & Stratton, 1981, 12:125–143

342.  Harris RI, Stuart J: Low dose factor VIII in adult with haemophilic arthropathy. Lancet 1:93–94, 1979

343.  Stirling ML, Prescott RJ: Minimum effective dose of intermediate factor-VIII concentrate in haemophiliacs on home therapy. Lancet 1:813–814, 1979

344.  *Pneumocystis carinii* pneumonia among persons with hemophilia A. Morbid Mortal Weekly Rep 31:365–367, 1982

344.  *Pneumocystis carinii* pneumonia among persons with hemophilia A. Morbid Mortal Weekly Rep 31:365–367, 1982

345.  Menitove JE, Aster RH, Casper JT, et al: T-lymphocyte subpopulations in patients with classic hemophilia treated with cryoprecipitate and lyophilized concentrates. N Engl J Med 308:83–86, 1983

345a. Lederman MM, Ratnoff OD, Scillian JJ, et al: Impaired cell-mediated immunity in patients with classic hemophilia. N Engl J Med 308:79–83, 1983

345b. deShazo RD, Andes WA, Nordberg J, et al: An immunologic evaluation of hemophiliac patients and their wives. Ann Int Med 99:159–164, 1983

346.  Ratnoff OD, Menitove JE, Aster RH, et al: Coincident classic hemophilia and ''idiopathic'' thrombocytopenic purpura in patients under treatment with concentrates of antihemophilic factor (factor VIII). N Engl J Med 398:439–442, 1983

347.  Bloom AL: Clotting factor concentrates for resistant haemophilia. Br J Haematol 40:21–27, 1978

347a. Barr RD, Forbes CD, McNicol CP, et al: Inhibitors of antihaemophilic globulin (factor VIII) and various spontaneous anti-coagulants. An account of six cases with a review of the literature. Coagulation 2:323–331, 1969

347b. Biggs R: Haemophilia treatment in the United Kingdom from 1969 to 1974. Br J Haematol 35:487–504, 1977

348.  Allain J-P, Frommel D: Antibodies to factor VIII. V. Patterns of immune response to factor VIII in hemophilia A. Blood 47:973–982, 1976

349.  Kasper CK: Management of inhibitors to factor VIII, Progress in Haematology. 12:143–165, 1981

350.  Shapiro SS, Hultin M: Acquired inhibitors to the blood coagulation factors. Semin Thromb Hemost 1:336–385, 1975

351.  Frommel D, Allain J-P: Genetic predisposition to develop factor VIII antibody in classic haemophilia. Clin Immunol Immunopathol 8:34–38, 1977

352.  European study group of factor VIII antibody: Development of factor VIII antibody in haemophilic monozygotic twins. Scand J Haematol 23:64–68, 1979

353.  Hall M: Haemophilia complicated by an acquired circulating anticoagulant: A report of three cases. Br J Haematol 7:340–348, 1961

354.  Mibashan RS: Management of patients with inhibitors: Replacement therapy (including plasmapheresis). Workshop on Inhibitors of Factor VIII and IX. Vienna, Facultas-Verlag, 1977, p 64

355.  Pintado T, Taswell HF, Bowie EJW: Treatment of life-threatening hemorrhage due to acquired factor VIII inhibitor. Blood 46:535–541, 1975

356.  Roberts HR, Scales MB, Madison JT, et al: A clinical and experimental study of acquired inhibitors to factor VIII. Blood 26:805–818, 1965

357.  Strauss HS: Acquired circulating anticoagulants in hemophilia A. New Engl J Med 281:866–873, 1969

358.  Cobcroft R, Tamagnini G, Dormandy KM: Serial plasmapheresis in a haemophiliac with antibodies to F VIII. J Clin Pathol 30:763–765, 1971

359.  Rizza CR: Management of patients with inherited blood coagulation defects, in Bloom AL,

Thomas DP (eds): Haemostasis and Thrombosis. Edinburgh, Churchill Livingstone, 1981, pp 371–388

360. Fekete LF, Holst SL, Pecetoom F, et al: "Auto-factor" IX concentrate: A new therapeutic approach to the treatment of haemophilia A patients with inhibitors, abstracted. Proceedings of the XIVth International Congress of Haematology, Sao Paulo, Brazil, 1972, (abstract 295)

361. Kelly P, Penner JA: Antihemophilic factor inhibitor: Management with prothrombin complex concentrates. JAMA 236:2061–2064, 1976

362. Kurczynski EM, Penner JA: Activated prothrombin concentrate for patients with factor VIII inhibitors. N Engl J Med 291:164–167, 1974

363. Penner JA: Therapeutic approaches to inhibitors: Vitamin K-dependent factor concentrates, in Seligsohn U, Rimon A, Horoszowski H (eds): Haemophilia. New York, Alan R Liss, 1981, pp 97–105

364. Abildgaard CF, Britton M, Harrison J: Prothrombin complex concentrate (Konyne) in the treatment of hemophilic patients with factor VIII inhibitors. J Pediatr 88:200–205, 1976

365. Lowe GDO, Harvie A, Forbes CD, et al: Successful treatment with prothrombin complex concentrate of postoperative bleeding in a haemophiliac with a factor VIII inhibitor. Br Med J 2:1110–1111, 1976

366. Stenbjerg S, Jorgensen J: Activated FIX concentrate (FEIBA) used in the treatment of haemophilic patients with antibody to FVIII. Acta Med Scand 203:471–476, 1978

367. Sultan U, Brouet JC, Debre P: Treatment of inhibitors to factor VIII with activated prothrombin concentrate. N Engl J Med 291:1087, 1974 (letter)

368. Abilgaard CF: Use of activated prothrombin complex in factor VIII inhibitors, in Forbes CD, Lowe GDO (eds): Unresolved Problems in Haemophilia. Lancaster, England, MTP Press, 1982, pp 133–142

368a. Lusher JM, Shapiro SS, Palascak JE, et al: Efficacy of prothrombin complex concentrates in hemophiliacs with antibodies to factor VIII. A multicenter therapeutic trial. N Engl J Med 303:421–425, 1980

369. Penner J, Kelly P: Factor VIII inhibitors: Therapeutic response to prothrombin complex concentrates, Thromb Haemost 38:339, 1977 (abstract)

369a. Abildgaard CF, Penner JA, Watson-Williams EJ: Anti-inhibitor coagulant complex (Autoplex) for treatment of factor VIII inhibitors in hemophilia. Blood 56:978–84, 1980

370. Hoots WK, Snyder MS, McMillan CS: Effects of activated prothrombin complex concentrate (APCC) for craniospinal hemorrhage in classic hemophiliacs with factor VIII inhibitors. Pediatr Res 14:535, 1980 abstract

371. Mariani G, Romoli D, Salvitti C, et al: In vivo activation of the extrinsic pathway by FEIBA, Thromb Haemost 42:365, 1979 (abstract)

372. Middleton S, Forbes CD, Prentice CRM: Thrombogenic potential of factor IX concentrates. Comparison of tests. Thromb Haemost 40:574–576, 1979

373. van Geylswijk JL: The effect of activated prothrombin-complex concentrate (FEIBA) on joints and muscle bleedings in patients with haemophilia A with an inhibitor to factor VIII, in Forbes CD, Lowe GDO (eds): Unresolved Problems in Haemophilia. Lancaster, England, MTP Press, 1982, pp 93–97

374. Allain J-P, Krieger GR: Prothrombin-complex concentrate in treatment of classical haemophilia with factor-VIII antibody. Lancet 2:1203, 1975 (letter)

375. Kasper CK, Feinstein DI: Rising factor VIII inhibitor titers after Konȳne, factor IX complex. N Engl J Med 295:505–506, 1976

376. Lechner K, Nowotny CH, Krinninger B, et al: Effect of treatment with activated prothrombin complex concentrate (FEIBA) on factor VIII-antibody level. Thromb Haemost 40:478–485, 1978

377. Manucci PM, Bader R, Ruggeri, ZM: Concentrates of clotting factor IX, Lancet 1:41, 1976 (letter)

378. Dormandy KM, Sultan Y: The suppression of factor VIII antibodies in haemophilia. Pathol Biol 23(suppl):17–23, 1975

379. Hultin MB, Shapiro SS, Bowman HS: Immunosuppressive therapy of factor VIIII inhibitors. Blood 48:95–108, 1976

379a. Hultin M: Management of inhibitors by immunosuppression, in Seligsohn U, Rimon A, Horoszowski H (eds): Haemophilia. Castle Hill Publications, London, 1981, pp 107–112

380. Owen CA, Henriksen RA, McDuffie FC, et al: Prothrombin Quick: A newly identified dysprothrombinemia. Mayo Clin Proc 53:29–33, 1978

380a. Shapiro SS, McCord S: Prothrombin, in Spaet TH (ed): Progress in Hemostasis and Thrombosis, New York, Grune & Stratton Volume 4, 1978, pp 177–209

381. Bloom AL: Immunological detection of blood coagulation factors in haemorrhagic disorders, in Hoffbrand AV, Brain MC, Hirsh J (eds): Recent Advances in Haematology. Edinburgh, Churchill Livingstone, 1977, pp 387–411

382. Biggs R, Denson KWE: The fate of prothrombin and factors VII, IX, and X transfused to patients deficient in these factors. Br J Haematol 9:532–547, 1963

383. Loeliger EA, Hensen A: On the turnover of factors II, VII, IX, and X under pathological conditions. Thromb Diath Haemorrh (suppl 13):195–200, 1964

384. Melliger EJ, Duckert F: Major surgery in a subject with factor V deficiency. Cholecystectomy in a parahaemophilic woman and review of the literature. Thromb Diath Haemorrh 25:438–446, 1971

385. Owren PA: Parahaemophilia. Haemorrhagic diathesis due to absence of a previously unknown clotting factor. Lancet 1:446–448, 1947

385a. Seeler RA: Parahemophilia. Factor V deficiency. Med Clin North Am 56:119–125, 1972

386. Kingsley CS: Familial factor V deficiency: The pattern of heredity. Q J Med 23:323–329, 1954

387. Kagami M, Morita H: Parahemophilia, the report of one family from Japan. Acta Haematol 35:102–112, 1966

388. Mitterstieler G, Müller W, Geir W: Congenital factor V deficiency. A family study. Scand J Haematol 21:9–13, 1978

389. deVries A, Matoth Y, Shamir Z: Familial congenital labile factor deficiency with syndactylism. Acta Haematol 5:129–142, 1951

390. Alexander B, Goldstein R: Parahemophilia in three siblings (Owren's disease). With studies on certain plasma components affecting prothrombin conversion Am J Med 13:255–272, 1952

391. Webster WP, Roberts, HR, Penick GD: Hemostasis in factor V deficiency. Am J Med Sci 248:194–202, 1964

392. Alexander B, Goldstein R, Landwehr G, et al: Congenital SPCA deficiency: A new hitherto unrecognized defect with hemorrhage rectified by serum and serum fractions. J Clin Invest 30:596–608, 1951

393. Marder VJ, Shulman NR: Clinical aspects of congenital factor VII deficiency. Am J Med 37:182–194, 1964

394. Levanon M, Rimon S, Shani M, et al: Active and inactive factor VII in Dubin-Johnson syndrome with factor VII deficiency, hereditary factor-VII deficiency and on coumadin administration. Br J Haematol 23:669–677, 1972

395. Seligsohn U, Shani M, Ramot B: Gilbert syndrome and factor-VII deficiency, Lancet 1:1398, 1970 (letter)

396. Seligsohn U, Shani M, Ramot B, et al: Dubin-Johnson syndrome in Israel. II. Association with factor VII-deficiency. Q J Med 39:569–584, 1970

397. Zimmerman R, Ehlers G, Ehlers W, et al: Congenital factor VII deficiency: A report of four new cases. Blut 38:119–125, 1979

398. Matthay K, Koerper MA, Ablin AR: Intracranial hemorrhage in congenital factor VII deficiency. J Pediatr 94:413–415, 1979

399. Girolami A, Fabris F, Dal Bo Zanon R, et al: Factor VII Padua: A congenital coagulation disorder due to an abnormal factor VII with a peculiar activation pattern. J Lab Clin Med 91:387–395, 1978

400. Girolami A, Falezza G, Patrassi G, et al: Factor VII Verona coagulation disorder: Double heterozygosis with an abnormal factor VII and heterozygous factor VII deficiency. Blood 50:603–610, 1977

401. Ly B, Solum NO, Vennerød AM, et al: A syndrome of factor VII deficiency and abnormal platelet release reaction. Scand J Haematol 21:206–214, 1978

402. Dike GWR, Griffiths D, Tadman AJ: Factor VII concentrate. Thromb Haemost 37:572–574, 1977 (letter)

403. Hougie C, Barrow EM, Graham B: Stuart clotting defect 1. Segregation of an hereditary hemorrhagic state from a heterogeneous group heretofore called 'stable factor' (SPCA, proconvertin, factor VII) deficiency. J Clin Invest 36:485–496, 1957

404. Telfer TP, Denson KWE, Wright DR: A 'new' coagulation defect. Br J Haematol 2:308–316, 1956

405. Bounameaux V: Coagulopathies avec temps de saignement prolongé. Thromb Diath Haemorrh 9:417–426, 1963

406. Denson KWE, Lurie A, DeCataldo F, et al: The factor-X defect: Recognition of abnormal forms of factor X. Br J Haematol 18:317–327, 1970

407. Fair DS, Plow EF, Edgington TS: Combined functional and immunochemical analysis of normal and abnormal human factor X. J Clin Invest 64:884–894, 1979

408. Girolami A, Molaro G, De Marco L: Factor X survival and therapeutic factor X levels in the abnormal factor X (factor X Friuli) coagulation disorder. Acta Haematol 52:223–231, 1974

409. Lechner K, Mähr G, Margariteller P, et al: Factor X Vorarlberg. A new variant of hereditary factor X deficiency, Haemost 42:58, 1979 (abstract)

409a. Girolami A, Molaro G, Lazzarin M, et al: A 'new' congenital haemorrhagic condition due to the presence of an abnormal factor X (factor X Friuli): A study of a large kindred. Br J Haematol 19:179–192, 1970

410. O'Leary D, Ruyman NF, Conrad M: Therapeutic approaches to factor X deficiency with emphasis on the use of a new clotting factor concentrate (Konyne). J Lab Clin Med 77:23–32, 1971

411. Roberts HR, Lechler E, Webster WP, et al: Survival of transfused factor X in patients with Stuart disease. Thromb Diath Haemorrh 13:305–313, 1965

412. Conrad FG, Breneman WL, Grisham DB: A clinical evaluation of plasma thromboplastin antecedent (PTA) deficiency. Ann Intern Med 62:885–898, 1965

413. Leiba H, Ramot B, Many A: Heredity and coagulation studies in ten families with factor XI (plasma thromboplastin antecedent) deficiency. Br J Haematol 11:654–665, 1965

414. Rapaport SI, Proctor RR, Patch MJ, et al: The mode of inheritance of PTA deficiency: Evidence for the existence of major PTA deficiency and minor PTA deficiency. Blood 18:149–165, 1961

415. Seligsohn U: High gene frequency of factor XI (PTA) deficiency in Ashkenazi Jews. Blood 51:1223–1228, 1978

416. Rimon A, Schiffman S, Feinstein DI, et al: Factor XI activity and factor XI antigen in homozygous and heterozygous factor XI deficiency. Blood 48:165–174, 1976

417. Edson JR, White JG, Krivit W: The enigma of severe factor XI deficiency without hemorrhagic symptoms. Distinction from Hageman factor and "Fletcher factor" deficiency: Family study and problems of diagnosis. Thromb Diath Haemorrh 18:342–348, 1967

418. Todd M, Wright IS: Factor XI (PTA) deficiency with no hemorrhagic symptoms. Case report. Thromb Diath Haemorrh 11:187–194, 1964

419. Nossel HL, Niemitz J, Sawitsky A: Blood PTA (factor XI) levels following plasma infusion. Proc Soc Exp Biol Med 115:896–897, 1964

420. Forbes CD, Ratnoff OD: Studies on plasma thromboplastin antecedent (factor XI), PTA deficiency, and inhibition of PTA by plasma, pharmacologic inhibitors and specific antiserum. J Lab Clin Med 79:113–127, 1972

421. Rabe F, Salomon E: Ueber Faserstoffmangel im Blut bein einem Falle von Hämophilie. Deutches Arch Klin Med 132:240–244, 1920

422. Flute PT: Disorders of plasma fibrinogen synthesis. Br Med Bull 33:253–259, 1977

423. Bang NU, Heidenreich RO, Matsuda M: Plasma protein requirements for human platelet aggregation. Throm Diath Haemorrh (suppl 42):37–41, 1970

424. Nachman RL, Marcus AJ: Immunological studies of proteins associated with the subcellular fractions of thrombasthenic and afibrinogenemic platelets. Br J Haematol 15:181–189, 1968

425. Weiss H, Rogers J: Fibrinogen and platelets in the primary arrest of bleeding: Studies in two patients with afibrinogenemia. N Engl J Med 285:369–374, 1971

426. deVries A, Rosenberg T, Kochwa S, et al: Precipitating antifibrinogen antibody appearing after fibrinogen infusions in a patient with congenital afibrinogenaemia. Am J Med 30:486–494, 1961

427. Egbring R von, Andrassy K, Egli H, et al: Diagnostische und therapeutische Probleme bei congenitaler Afibrinogenäe mie. Blut 22:175–201, 1971

428. Bloom AL: Inherited disorders of blood coagulation, in Bloom AL, Thomas DP (eds): Haemostasis and Thrombosis. Edinburgh, Churchill Livingstone, 1981, pp 321–370

429. Liu CY, Nossel HL, Kaplan KL: The binding of thrombin by fibrin. J Biol Chem 254:10421–10425, 1979

429a. Amris CJ, Ranek L: A case of fibrin-stabilizing factor (FSF) deficiency. Thromb Diath Hemorrh 14:332–340, 1965

430. Duckert F, Jung E, Schmerling DH: A hitherto undescribed congenital haemorrhagic diathesis probably due to fibrin stabilizing factor deficiency. Thromb Diath Haemorrh 5:179–186, 1960

431. Losowsky MS, Hall R, Goldie W: Congenital deficiency of fibrin-stabilising factor. Lancet 2:156–158, 1965

432. Laki K, Lóránd L: On the solubility of fibrin clots. Science 108:280, 1948

433. Lorand L, Losowsky MS, Miloszewski KJM: Human factor XIII: Fibrin stabilizing factor. Progr Hemost Thromb 5:245–290, 1980

434. Losowsky MS, Miloszewski KJA: Factor XIII. Br J Haematol 37:1–5, 1977

435. Hampton JW, Bird RM, Hammarsten DM: Defective fibrinase activity in two brothers. J Lab Clin Med 65:469–474, 1965

436. Ratnoff OD, Steinberg AG: Fibrin cross-linking and heredity. Ann NY Acad Sci 202:186–189, 1972

437. Hampton JW, Cunninghan GR, Bird RM: The pattern of inheritance of defective fibrinase (factor XIII). J Lab Clin Med 67:914–921, 1966

438. Beck EA, Duckert F, Ernst M: The influence of fibrin stabilizing factor on the growth of fibroblasts in vitro and wound healing. Thromb Diath Haemorr 6:485–491, 1961

439. Ikalla E, Myllylä G, Nevanlinna HR: Transfusion therapy in factor XIII (FSF) deficiency. Scand J Haematol 1:308–312, 1964

440. Hampton JW, Garrison D: Fibrinogen and fibrin stabilizing factor. Med Clin North Am 56:133–143, 1972

441. Lorand L, Lockridge OM, Campbell LK, et al: Transamidating-enzymes II. A continuous fluorescent method suited for automating measurements of factor XIII in plasma. Anal Biochem 44:221–231, 1971

442. Ratnoff OD, Saito H: Surface-mediated reactions, in Piomelli S, Yachnin S (eds): Current Topics in Hematology, vol. 2. New York, Alan R Liss, 1979, pp 1–57

443. Breederveld K, van Royen EA, Cate JW: Severe factor V deficiency with prolonged bleeding. Thromb Diath Haemorrh 32:538–548, 1974

444. Gobbi F: Use and misuse of aminocaproic acid. Lancet 2:472–473, 1967 (letter)

445. O'Brien JR: Factor V in blood coagulation *in vitro,* and a report of a case of factor-V deficiency. Br J Haematol 4:210–219, 1958

446. Soff GA, Levin J, Bell WR: Familial multiple coagulation factor deficiencies. Sem. in Thromb Hemost 7:112–169, 1981

447. Marlar RA, Griffin JH: Deficiency of protein C inhibitor in combined factor V/VIII deficiency disease. J Clin Invest 66:1186–1189, 1980

448. Canfield WM, Kisiel W: Evidence of normal functional levels of activated protein C inhibitor in combined factor V/VIII deficiency disease. J Clin Invest 70:1260–1272, 1982

449. Gobbi F, Ascari E, Barbieri U: Congenital combined deficiency of factor VIII (anti-haemophilic globulin) and factor V (proaccelerin) in two siblings. Thromb Diath Haemorrh 17:194–204, 1967

450. Chung K-S, Bezeaud A, Goldsmith JC, et al: Congenital deficiency of blood clotting factors II, VII, IX and X. Blood 53:776–787, 1979

451. Johnson CA, Chung KS, McGrath KM, et al: Characterization of a variant prothrombin in a patient congenitally deficient in factors II, VII, IX and X. Br J Haematol 44:461–469, 1980

452. Goldsmith GH Jr, Pence RE, Ratnoff OD, et al: Studies on a family with combined functional deficiencies of vitamin K-dependent coagulation factors. J Clin Invest 69:1253–1260, 1982

453. Wang JK: Stimulation produced analgesia. Mayo Clin Proc 51:28–30, 1976

454. Mannheimer C, Carlsson CA: The analgesic effect of transcutaneous electrical nerve stimulation (TNS) in patients with rheumatoid arthritis. A comparative study of different pulse patterns. Pain 6:329–334, 1979

455. Woolf CJ: Transcutaneous electrical nerve stimulation and the reaction to experimental pain in human subjects. Pain 7:115–127, 1979

456. Varni JW, Gilbert A, Dietrich SL: Behavioral medicine in pain and analgesia management for a hemophilic child with a factor VIII inhibitor. Pain 11:121–126, 1981

457. Ozsoylu S, Strauss HS, Diamond LK: Effects of corticosteroids on coagulation of the blood. Nature 195:1214–1215, 1962

458. Trieger N, McGovern JJ: Evaluation of coricosteroids in hemophilia. N Engl J Med 266:432–437, 1962

459. Bennett AE, Ingram GIC: A controlled trial of long-term steroid treatment in haemophilia. Lancet 1:967–70, 1967

460. Katsumi O: New aspects on the treatment of hemophilia. Nagoya J Med Sci 28:179–195, 1966

461. Kramar J: Stress and capillary resistance (capillary fragility). Am J Physiol 175:69–74, 1953

462. Blackburn EK: The clinical management of haemophilia and allied disorders, in Poller L (ed): Recent Advances in Blood Coagulation. London, Churchill, 1969, pp 155–178

463. Verstraete M (ed): Haemostatic Drugs. A Critical Appraisal. The Hague, Martinus Nijhoff, Medical Division, 1975, p 118

464. Frank MM, Sergent JS, Kane MA, et al: Epsilon aminocaproic acid therapy of hereditary angioneurotic edema. N Engl J Med 286:808–812, 1972

465. Korsan-Bengsten K, Ysander L, Blohmé G, et al: Extensive muscle necrosis after long-term treatment with aminocaproic acid (EACA) in a case of hereditary periodic edema. Acta Med Scand 185:341–346, 1969

466. Dubber AHC, McNicol GP, Douglas AS: Aminomethylcyclohexane carboxylic acid (AMCHA), a new synthetic fibrinolytic inhibitor. Br J Haematol 11:237–245, 1965

467. Gebauer D, Heigel K: Therapeutische Beeinflussung der Hämophilie durch AMCHA. Med Klin 64:378–382, 1969

468. McNicol GP, Fletcher AP, Alkjaersig N, et al: The absorption, distribution and excretion of $\epsilon$-aminocaproic acid following oral or intravenous administration to man. J Lab Clin Med 59:15–24, 1961

469.  McNicol GP, Fletcher AP, Alkjaersig N, et al: Use of epsilon aminocaproic acid, a potent inhibitor of fibrinolytic activity, in the management of postoperative hematuria. J Urol 86:829–837, 1961

470.  Stark SN, White JG, Langer L Jr., et al: Epsilon aminocaproic acid therapy as a cause of intrarenal obstruction in haematuria of haemophiliacs. Scand J Haematol 2:99–107, 1965

471.  Köstering H, Grabner FM, Henning HB, et al: Peritonealdialyse und locale Thrombolyse bei Hämophilie A mit postrenalem Nierenvarsagen. Z Urol Nephrol 65:341–346, 1972

472.  Sultan Y, Larrieu M-J, Meyer D: Acide epsilon aminocaproique et hématuries des hémophiles. Trois cas d'obstruction rénale unilatérale passagère. Bibl Haematol 26:100–106, 1966

472a.  Bennett AE, Ingram GIC, Inglis PJ: Anti-fibrinolytic treatment in haemophilia: A controlled trial of prophylaxis with tranexamic acid. Br J Haematol 24:83–88, 1973

473.  Gordon AM, McNicol GP, Dubber AHC, et al: Clinical trial of epsilon aminocaproic acid in severe haemophilia. Br Med J 1:1632–1635, 1965

474.  Mainwaring D, Keidan SE: Fibrinolysis in haemophilia: The effect of $\epsilon$-aminocaproic acid. Br J Haematol 11:682–688, 1965

475.  Strauss HS, Kevy SV, Diamond LK: Ineffectiveness of prophylactic epsilon aminocaproic acid in severe hemophilia. N Engl J Med 273:301–304, 1965

476.  Ratnoff OD: Epsilon aminocaproic acid—a dangerous weapon. N Engl J Med 280:1124–1125, 1969

477.  Storti E, Traldi A, Tosatti E, et al: Synovectomy, a new approach to haemophilic arthropathy. Acta Haematol 41:193–205, 1969

478.  Gader AMA, Clarkson AR, Cash JD: The plasminogen activator and coagulation factor VIII responses to adrenaline, noradrenaline, isoprenaline and salbutamol in man. Thromb Res 2:9–16, 1973

479.  Cash JD, Gader AMA, Mulder JL, et al: Structure-activity relations of the fibrinolytic response to vasopressins in man. Clin Sci Mol Med 54:403–409, 1978

480.  Lowe GDO, Pettigrew A, Middleton S, et al: DDAVP in haemophilia, Lancet 2:614, 1977 (letter)

481.  Ludlam CA, Peake IR, Allen N, et al: Factor VIII and fibrinolytic response to deamino-8-D-arginine vasopressin in normal subjects and dissociate response in some patients with haemophilia and von Willebrand's disease. Br J Haematol 45:499–511, 1980

482.  Manucci, PM, Ruggeri ZM, Pareti FI, et al: 1-Deamino-8-D-arginine vasopressin: A new pharmacological approach to the management of haemophilia and von Willebrand's disease. Lancet 1:869–872, 1977

483.  Manucci PM, Ruggeri ZM, Pareti FI, et al: DDAVP in haemophilia. Lancet 2:1171–1172, 1977 (letter)

484.  Manucci PM, Rota L, Benvenuti C, et al: Clinico-pharmacological studies of factor VIII response after DDAVP, Thromb Haemost 42:309, 1979 (abstract)

485.  Nilsson IM, Mikaelsson M, Vilhardt H, et al: DDAVP factor VIII concentrate and its properties in vivo and in vitro. Thromb Res 15:263–271, 1980

486.  Belch JJF, Small M, McKenzie F, et al; DDAVP stimulates prostacyclin production. Thromb Haemost 47:122–123, 1982

486a.  Prowse CV, Sas G, Gader AMA, et al: Specificity in the factor VIII response to vasopressin infusion in man. Br J Haematol 41:437–447, 1979

487.  Warrier IA, Khalifa AS, Lusher JH: Intranasal DDAVP in patients with von Willebrand's disease and hemophilia A, Pediatr Res 15:590, 1981 (abstract)

488.  Lowe GDO, Harvie A, Forbes CD, et al: DDAVP in haemophilia. Br Med J 4:1110, 1976 (letter)

488a.  Nilsson IM: Report of the working party on factor VIII-related antigens. Thromb Haemost 39:511–520, 1978

489.  Schmitz-Huebner U, Balleisen L, Arends P, et al: DDAVP-induced changes in factor VIII-

related activities and bleeding time in patients with von Willebrand's syndrome. Haemostasis 9:204–213, 1980

490. Agle DP, Mattson A: Psychiatric and social care of patients with hereditary hemorrhagic disease. Mod Treat 5:111–124, 1968

491. Editorial: Life as a haemophiliac. Br Med J 2:567–568, 1968

492. Katz AH: Hemophilia—A Study in Hope and Reality. Springfield, Ill, Charles C Thomas, 1970

493. Markova I, Lockyer R, Forbes CD: Haemophilia: A survey on social issues. Health Bull (Edinburgh) 35:177–182, 1977

494. Mattsson A, Gross S: Adaptational and defensive behaviour in young hemophiliacs and their parents. Am J Psychiatry 122:1349–1356, 1966

495. Chilcote RR, Baehner RL: Atypical bleeding in hemophilia: Application of the conversion model to the case study of a child. Psychosom Med 42:221–230, 1980

496. Boon RA, Roberts DF: The social impact of haemophilia. J Biosoc Sci 2:237–264, 1970

497. Bronks IG, Blackburn EK: A socio-medical study of haemophilia and related states. Br J Preventive Soc Med 22:68–72, 1968

498. Dietrich S: Modern management of haemophilia and its implications for educational programs. J School Health 43:81–83, 1973

499. Markova I, Lockyer R, Forbes CD: Self-perception of employed and unemployed haemophiliacs. Psychol Med 10:559–565, 1980

500. Bruhn JG, Hampton JW, Philips BU: A psycho-social study of married hemophiliacs and their wives and hemophiliac adolescents and their parents. J Psychosom Res 15:293–303, 1971

501. Markova I, MacDonald K, Forbes CD: Integration of haemophilic boys into normal schools. Child Care Health Dev 6:101–109, 1980

502. Agle D: Home care—Psychological benefits and hazards, in Aledort L, Manucci PM (eds): Clinical Problems Related to Haemophilia. Scand J Haematol Suppl 30 65–69, 1977

503. Forbes CD, Markova I, Stuart J, et al: To tell or not to tell: Haemophiliacs' views on their employment prospects. Int J Rehabil Res 5:13–18, 1982

Barry S. Coller

# 6

# Von Willebrand's Disease

In 1924 a 5-year-old girl from the Åland Islands off the coast of Finland was brought to the Deaconess Hospital in Helsinki, where she was evaluated for a severe bleeding disorder by Dr. Erich von Willebrand.[1] After investigating the patient and 65 other members of her family, von Willebrand concluded that she had a new bleeding disorder that differed from hemophilia in its three cardinal manifestations: (1) the affected individuals suffered primarily from mucocutaneous hemorrhage rather than hemarthrosis or deep muscle hemorrhage; (2) the inheritance was consistent with autosomal dominant rather than X-linked recessive transmission; and (3) in contrast to the normal bleeding times found in hemophiliacs, these patients had consistently prolonged bleeding times. Von Willebrand knew that thrombocytopenia could cause a prolonged bleeding time, and so he determined the platelet counts in these patients. When the counts were found to be normal, he concluded that the patients were suffering from a qualitative disorder of platelet function, in particular, thrombus formation. He went on to develop an in vitro apparatus for measuring "thrombus" formation in blood pumped to and fro in a glass capillary and showed that the blood of his patients behaved abnormally. What he could not determine was whether the abnormality in platelet function was intrinsic or extrinsic to the platelet.[1]

A series of infusion studies over the next several decades[2-8] suggested that the major abnormality responsible for the failure of hemostasis resided in the plasma of these patients and not their platelets: (1) plasma from normals but not from patients with von Willebrand's disease corrected the prolonged bleeding time; (2) normal platelets did not correct the bleeding time; (3) platelets from patients with von Willebrand's disease were effective in achieving hemostasis in patients with thrombocytopenia due to aplastic anemia.

In 1953 3 separate groups reported that patients with von Willebrand's disease had reduced levels of factor VIII (antihemophilic factor) coagulant activity (VIII:C).[9-11] Although this tended to blur the clear distinction between von Willebrand's disease and classic hemophilia, the observation that infusion of plasma obtained from the blood of classic hemophiliacs corrected the bleeding time defect in patients with von Willebrand's disease clearly showed that the factor VIII coagulant activity and the bleeding time correction factor were separate and distinct. Despite this finding, some association of these factors was suggested from the observation that both cryoprecipitate and Cohn fraction I-O, two crude plasma fractions rich in factor VIII coagulant activity, were able to shorten the bleeding time in von Willebrand's disease. With further refinements in purification of factor VIII coagulant activity, the linkage between these activities was shown to have limits since "high potency" factor VIII concentrates appear to have less von Willebrand factor activity than factor VIII coagulant activity.[12] These observations have important therapeutic implications since cryoprecipitate remains the treatment of choice for virtually all patients with von Willebrand's disease.

## PLATELET FUNCTION

Despite von Willebrand's initial demonstration of abnormal thrombus formation by platelets in von Willebrand's disease, most early attempts to define an in vitro abnormality in platelet physiology or function were unsuccessful. Normal results were found in clot retraction, platelet factor 3 (PF 3) availability, platelet adhesion to connective tissue, platelet electrophoretic mobility, and platelet aggregation induced by adenosine diphosphate (ADP), epinephrine, thrombin, or connective tissue.[13,14] Subsequent studies, however, identified 3 different assays in which von Willebrand's disease blood behaved abnormally: platelet retention by a column of glass beads,[15,16] ristocetin-induced platelet aggregation,[17] and ex vivo interaction of platelets with the subendothelial surface of segments of blood vessels.[18]

When normal or hemophilic blood is passed through a column containing small glass beads, a very high percentage of platelets are retained in the column. When von Willlebrand's disease blood is similarly tested, the percentage of platelets retained in the column is much less than normal. The results of correction experiments with this test were in accord with the conclusions from the earlier infusion studies since normal or hemophilic plasma or cryoprecipitate corrected the defect, whereas the plasma of patients with von Willebrand's disease did not. Conversely, antibodies directed against von Willebrand factor inhibited normal retention. Although the term *adhesiveness* was originally applied to this test, in fact, both adhesion of platelets to the beads and aggregation of platelets to each other contribute to the total retention of platelets within the column, and so the term *retention* is preferred. Studies of the mechanism of this test indicate that the initial adhesion of platelets to the glass beads requires fibrinogen but not von Willebrand factor, whereas the subsequent interaction between these glass-adherent platelets and flowing platelets is dependent on both von Willebrand factor and ADP.[19] In this assay, therefore, the von Willebrand factor appears to be mediating platelet–platelet interactions rather than platelet–surface interactions. Since factors other than von Willebrand factor are required for normal platelet retention, this test is not specific for von Willebrand's disease. It is, however, quite sensitive, with virtually all patients with clinically evident disease showing significant decreases when the assay is performed according to the standardized procedures now available.[20]

Ristocetin, an antibiotic similar in structure, mechanism of action, and antimicrobial spectrum to vancomycin, was introduced into clinical practice in the late 1950s. Soon thereafter, it was noted to produce thrombocytopenia in recipients and was, therefore, removed from clinical use. Approximately a decade later, ristocetin was shown to aggregate normal platelets in vitro but to cause little or no aggregation of von Willebrand's disease platelets.[17] As with platelet retention, this defect could be corrected with normal or hemophilic plasma or cryoprecipitate, and the aggregation of normal platelets could be inhibited by antibodies against von Willebrand factor. Simply washing normal platelets free of plasma von Willebrand factor made them unresponsive to ristocetin; adding back normal plasma (or purified von Willebrand factor) restored the aggregation, thus permitting the development of a quantitative assay.[21] Since this assay appeared to correlate well with bleeding time correction in vivo, it was originally termed a *von Willebrand factor assay,* but as exceptions to this relationship are known, it is preferable to refer to it as a measure of ristocetin cofactor activity (VIII:RCo). The subsequent observation that platelets fixed with formaldehyde could still be clumped by the combination of ristocetin and normal plasma not only facilitated the performance of the assay but also emphasized the relatively passive role played by the platelet.[22] Ristocetin is thus unlike ADP, epinephrine, collagen, and thrombin, all of which require intact energy metabolism to obtain platelet aggregation. For this reason, this reaction is better termed *agglutination* than *aggregation* so as to liken it to immune agglutination of red blood cells. Although the platelet functions in a passive role with regard to energy metabolism, there is an absolute requirement that the platelet contain an intact ristocetin-dependent receptor to which the von Willebrand factor can bind.[23,24] This receptor is easily degraded by a variety of proteases and is absent from the platelets of patients with the Bernard-Soulier syndrome, a congenital inherited bleeding disorder (see Chapter 4).[25] Platelets from the latter patients do not aggregate with ristocetin (even though their plasma contains normal amounts of VIII:RCo), do not bind von Willebrand factor in the presence of ristocetin, are not retained normally by glass bead columns, and do not interact normally with subendothelial surfaces ex vivo.[26] Several groups have identified a specific deficiency of the platelet membrane glycoprotein identified as GPIb in patients with Bernard-Soulier syndrome, allowing a tentative identification of this glycoprotein as the von Willebrand factor receptor.[25,26] Additional support for this identification comes from studies employing monoclonal antibodies,[27,27a] but some observations appear to be at odds with this hypothesis.[28]

The molecular mechanism responsible for ristocetin-induced platelet agglutination has been studied intensively. Multiple lines of evidence point to a primary role for electrostatic interactions.[29-33] According to a current working hypothesis, positively charged ristocetin binds to the platelet surface, reducing the surface charge and in some way permitting the von Willebrand factor to bind to its receptor. The latter, by virtue of its multiple binding sites and large size (see below), can act as a bridge between platelets and agglutinate them. Interestingly, the binding of von Willebrand factor has also been shown to be associated with a decrease in the platelet's surface charge, which may operate in addition or as an alternative to the bridging mechanism in facilitating agglutination.[32] Additional support for a mechanism that emphasizes the importance of ristocetin's positive charge comes from studies showing that a variety of structurally unrelated polycations can substitute for ristocetin under appropriate circumstances.[34,35] Most recently, certain snake venoms have been found that can substitute for ristocetin,[36] but certain patients may show a discordance between their response to ristocetin and the venoms;[36a] a claim that ristocetin-induced agglutination correlates better with clinical symptoms than venom-induced agglutination has been made.[36a] A preliminary report indicates that the platelets from patients with Bernard-Soulier syndrome are agglutinated by the snake venoms, whereas platelets from patients with Glanzmann's thrombasthenia (see Chapter 4) are not.[36b] This suggests that the von Willebrand factor is not binding to GPIb when platelets are stimulated with the venoms and it raises the possibility that the binding is occurring to the GPIIb/IIIa complex.

To simulate more closely the in vivo condition and to permit the differentiation between initial platelet adhesion to a surface and the subsequent platelet–platelet aggregation, an ex vivo morphometric technique was developed. In this assay, blood is passed over a segment of rabbit aorta that was previously denuded of endothelial cells. After the perfusion is completed the wall of the rabbit aorta is examined microscopically. Under the appropriate conditions of anticoagulation and shear forces, the platelets in von Willebrand's disease blood adhere and aggregate abnormally. These abnormalities can be corrected, at least in part, with von Willebrand factor.[18,37]

## Biochemistry of the von Willebrand Factor and Its Relationship to Factor VIII Coagulant Activity

Normal human von Willebrand factor has been purified by several different laboratories, and although some controversy remains, there is general agreement on the fundamental aspects of its structure.[20,38,39] As purified in vitro, von Willebrand factor shows the unusual characteristic of being composed of a series of macromolecules of extremely high molecular weight (estimated to be between 1 and $15 \times 10^6$).[40–43] When disulfide bonds are reduced, each of these macromolecules appears to consist of a single glycoprotein subunit with a molecular weight of approximately 230,000. The macromolecules thus result from the covalent association of varying numbers of these subunits via disulfide bonds. Approximately 5 percent of the glycoprotein's weight is composed of carbohydrate, at least some of which is exposed on the surface.[44–48] The organization of the basic subunits into the macromolecular aggregate appears to be quite complex.[43,49,50] It is important to emphasize how enormous these molecules are since the largest ones are considerably larger than some virus particles. In addition, since the molecules are made up of the joining together of multiple identical subunits, it is likely that many more than one platelet binding site is present on the surface of the molecule at any one time. These two molecular features, large size and multiple binding sites, make the von Willebrand factor an ideal bridging molecule as discussed above, with regard to its platelet cofactor function. One might well liken these features of the von Willebrand factor to those of another well-known agglutinating molecule, immunoglobulin M (IgM). With this in mind, it is not surprising that the higher molecular weight forms are able to bind to platelets at lower concentrations of ristocetin and are more effective in mediating ristocetin-induced platelet agglutination. There are other differences between the high and low molecular weight forms, including the ability to be precipitated after freezing and slow thawing of plasma (cryoprecipitation) and survival after injection in vivo.[51–54] It is important to appreciate this molecular weight-dependent heterogeneity when interpreting the results of assays based on immunologic as opposed to platelet agglutination activity, since one may have low molecular weight material that is immunologically active but does not support platelet agglutination well.

Both endothelial cells and megakaryocytes have been reported to synthesize von Willebrand factor.[55,56] As endothelial cells in culture actually release the factor into the culture medium, it is presumed that they do the same thing in vivo, and thus they are believed to be the major source of plasma von Willebrand factor. Recent biochemical studies of endothelial cells grown in culture indicate that the vWf subunit of Mr 230,000 is derived from a larger precursor and that the formation of the multimers occurs before the protein leaves the surface of the endothelial cells.[56a,56b] Von Willebrand factor is detectable in the subendothelium in vivo, where it may be derived from the overlying endothelial cells or from the deposition of plasma von Willebrand factor.[57,58] The von Willebrand factor synthesized by megakaryocytes appears to be localized in platelet α-granules.[59] The multimeric structure of platelet von Willebrand factor appears to differ somewhat from plasma von Willebrand factor in that it contains a subpopulation of multimers of higher Mr.[59a] On stimulation, platelet-associated von Willebrand factor is released.[60] When thrombin is the stimulus, von Willebrand factor becomes exposed on the platelet surface in a reaction that probably requires the GPIIb/IIIa complex.[59a,60a,60b] Although there are insufficient data to precisely define the importance of platelet von Willebrand factor, two observations make it difficult to assign it a central role in hemostasis: (1) plasma alone can correct, at least temporarily, the bleeding of patients with von Willebrand's disease whose platelets are devoid of von Willebrand factor and whose platelets do not take the infused von Willebrand up into α-granules, and (2) infusion of normal platelets into patients with severe von Willebrand's disease does not correct the long bleeding time. Platelets may also have surface-associated von Willebrand factor, but technical limitations have prevented a definitive resolution of this issue.[60a,60b]

Since the early observations that patients with von Willebrand's disease have reduced levels of factor VIII coagulant activity (VIII:C), there has been considerable interest in the interrelationship between this clotting activity and the von Willebrand factor. This interest was further stimulated by the paradoxical finding that infusion of plasma or cryoprecipitate into patients with von Willebrand's disease results in a delayed and persistent rise in VIII:C,[24] a response that contrasts sharply to the abrupt rise and decline of VIII:C found in patients with classic hemophilia. The paradox became even more intriguing when it was noted that infusion of hemophilic plasma, devoid of VIII:C, into patients with von Willebrand's disease also resulted in delayed and prolonged increases in VIII:C coagulant activity. When antibodies to the von Willebrand factor became available ("factor VIII-related antigen," VIIIR:Ag),[61] it was shown that the coagulant activity was still rising when the von Willebrand factor antigen was decreasing.[62]

Although some controversy persists, the weight of experimental data currently available supports the following working hypothesis: (1) The von Willebrand factor and the factor containing VIII:C are separate molecules. The molecular structure of the former was described above. The molecular structure of the latter is in doubt since there have been only preliminary reports of purification of the human molecule,[63,63a–d] and there is a lack of agreement on the molecular weight of the protein(s). (2) The von Willebrand factor and VIII:C proteins circulate as a stable complex in plasma and remain complexed in vitro when subjected to many of the commonly used purification techniques. (3) A rough estimate of the plasma level of von Willebrand factor is 5–10 μg/ml, whereas that of VIII:C is 0.2 μg/ml. If one assumes a mean molecular weight of $6 \times 10^6$ for von Willebrand factor, then there is 1 molecule of VIII:C for every 1–2 molecules of von Willebrand factor or 1 molecule of VIII:C for every 30–60 von Willebrand factor subunits. (4) The gene(s) coding for the von Willebrand factor multimers are on an autosomal chromosome, whereas those coding for VIII:C are on the X chromosome. (5) The X-dependent gene(s) required for the production of VIII:C is normal in patients with von Willebrand's disease. (6) The von Willebrand factor may stimulate the synthesis of VIII:C and/or prolong the survival of VIII:C by forming a complex which resists catabolism and/or inactivation.[64] (7) The infusion of the von Willebrand factor present in normal or classic hemophilic plasma into a patient with von Willebrand's disease thus elicits the synthesis of VIII:C and/or protects the VIII:C that is being made. It can be postulated that a single von Willebrand factor molecule may have the capacity to complex with many VIII:C molecules. Thus, even though the von Willebrand factor protein concentration decreases soon after infusion, the remaining protein may be able to carry an increasing amount of the newly synthesized or catabolism-protected VIII:C.

**Table 6-1**

Assays Commonly Employed in the
Evaluation of von Willebrand's Disease

Bleeding time
Platelet retention
Activated partial thromboplastin time
VIII:C
VIIIR:Ag
   Electroimmunoassay (Laurell)
   Immunoradiometric assay
   Radioimmunoassay
Enzyme-linked immunosorbent assay (ELISA)
   Crossed antigen-antibody electrophoresis
   Multimer analysis by agarose gel electrophoresis
Ristocetin-induced platelet aggregation
VIII:RCo

It should be appreciated that the above hypothesis is based primarily on inferential data and doubtless will require modification as more direct information becomes available.

## PREVALENCE

The variability of clinical and laboratory manifestations of von Willebrand's disease has made it difficult to establish its true prevalence. Estimates of 3–4[65] and 7[66] per 100,000 population have been made in the United Kingdom and Lausanne, Switzerland, respectively. For comparison, the prevalence of classic hemophilia (the functional deficiency of VIII:C) was found to be twice that of von Willebrand's disease in the United Kingdom study, but only about 70 percent of that of von Willebrand's disease in Switzerland. Several large series have been reported, including 40 patients from Iran (22 families),[67] 100 patients from Italy (57 families),[68] 37 patients from France (24 families),[13] and 26 patients from Sweden (20 families).[69] In these series the percentage of patients categorized as having severe disease ranged widely (10–61 percent), probably reflecting different biases of ascertainment and diagnostic criteria. A recent study of severe von Willebrand's disease (<1 percent von Willebrand factor antigen) in Europe and Israel found the incidence to range from 0.5 to 3.1 per million population, with Scandinavian countries tending to have the highest rates.[69a]

## LABORATORY EVALUATION

The laboratory tests most commonly employed in the evaluation of patients thought to have von Willebrand's disease are listed in Table 6-1. Several considerations must be emphasized: (1) von Willebrand's disease is a heterogeneous disorder and thus, although easily diagnosed in its severe forms, may be very difficult to distinguish from normal when mild; (2) there is considerable variation in the values obtained in a single individual from time to time, and thus a firm diagnosis may require repeated study; (3) several of the assays lack the precision of such commonly performed tests as the prothrombin time and thus must be interpreted cautiously; (4) intercurrent conditions such as pregnancy, stress, chronic disease, recent exercise, diabetes, and perhaps even cigarette smoking may significantly affect the results of some of the laboratory tests; (5) confirmation by study of family members is always desirable and may be crucial when studies are equivocal; and (6) in the author's opinion, the risk of transmitting hepatitis precludes the use of plasma infusion for the sole purpose of establishing the diagnosis.

## Bleeding Time

The bleeding time remains the single most important diagnostic test for von Wille-brand's disease since, despite exceptions, clinical symptoms probably correlate better with this test than with any of the others. Virtually all patients with severe von Willebrand's disease will have quite prolonged bleeding times using the template modification of the Ivy technique.[70] Patients with mild disease usually have less prolonged bleeding times and on occasion may have borderline or even normal values. In this latter group, it is especially important to repeat the bleeding time since one should hesitate to make the diagnosis of von Willebrand's disease in a patient with a repeatedly normal bleeding time unless there is compelling supportive evidence. Interestingly, when the bleeding time is performed on the earlobe according to the Duke technique,[71] the difference between normals and patients with von Willebrand's disease is not as great as with the Ivy technique.[72,73] A larger percentage of patients with the disorder thus may give borderline or normal results with this method. Moreover, in patients with severe von Willebrand's disease, there may be difficulty in stopping the bleeding from the earlobe. As a result, the Ivy technique is preferred because of its sensitivity and safety. The increased sensitivity may be a draw-back when the bleeding time is used to monitor therapy, however, since it has been shown that therapy sufficient to correct the Duke bleeding time usually is sufficient to maintain hemostasis even though the Ivy bleeding time may remain prolonged.[72] Ratnoff and Bennett reported on another bleeding time technique involving the puncture of the tip of the middle finger.[74] The technique appears to be as sensitive as the Ivy technique and has the advantage of avoiding scar formation, thus facilitating patient cooperation with serial studies. This method does not show improvement in von Willebrand's disease patients under stress or during pregnancy despite increases in the VIII:C, VIIIR:Ag (von Willebrand factor antigen), and platelet retention.

## Platelet Retention Test

Although not universally held, it is the author's belief that when performed according to the Bowie technique with meticulous blood handling, this assay is extremely sensitive to the von Willebrand's disease defect.[20] It is of considerable benefit, therefore, when the diagnosis is equivocal.[75] It is not, however, specific for von Willebrand's disease, and its performance does require considerable technical skill. These last two considerations have led to its abandonment in many laboratories.

## Activated Partial Thromboplastin Time

Since the majority of patients with von Willebrand's disease have reduced levels of VIII:C, it is not surprising that prolongation of the activated partial thromboplastin time is commonplace. The sensitivity of this assay for a reduction in VIII:C varies considerably with the reagents and method employed, but will almost always be significantly prolonged at values below 30 percent of normal. Almost all of the severely affected and most of the moderately affected patients thus will have prolonged times, with the exception of those patients who have variants of von Willebrand's disease in which there is a discrepancy between the VIII:C and von Willebrand factor levels. Mildly affected patients, however, may not have prolonged times, and thus this test is not sensitive for the detection of von Willebrand's disease.

## VIII:C

The values of VIII:C, the coagulant property of antihemophilic factor (factor VIII), are reduced below the normal range sometime during the course of the disease in the vast majority of patients with von Willebrand's disease (e.g., in 98 of the 100 patients reported from Italy,[68] 36 of the 40 from Iran,[67] and all 37 from France[14]). Mildly affected patients, however, and even severely affected patients with variants of von Willebrand's disease may have normal VIII:C levels.[76–80] Moreover, and perhaps more importantly, considerable variability exists when a single patient is studied serially. For example, in a recent study of mildly affected individuals in which 50 patients from 25 families were tested on multiple occasions, only 64 of the 202 samples analyzed had abnormally low VIII:C levels; only 18 of the 50 patients, however, failed to have at least 1 abnormal value.[81] Thus, there is a clear need to repeat this assay in borderline cases and to define carefully the normal range of values in each laboratory.

## VIIIR:Ag (Von Willebrand Factor Antigen)

Quantification of VIIIR:Ag is commonly performed by Laurell electroimmunoassay,[61] radioimmunoassay, or immunoradiometric assay (IRMA).[82] Since the von Willebrand factor is not a single molecular species, and since each assay relies upon certain physical as well as immunologic features of the molecules (e.g., the Laurell technique relies on movement through a gel and thus may favor smaller molecules), some differences between the assays are to be expected. In general, all of the assays give abnormal results in the vast majority of patients. The radioimmune assays are, however, more sensitive than the electroimmunoassay and may be able to detect immunologic variations of the von Willebrand factor molecule.[82] With the IRMA assay, 89 of the 100 Italian patients gave reduced values,[68] as did 36 of the 40 Iranian patients (4 patients' plasmas showed abnormal reactivity, and so no value could be assigned).[67] The electroimmunoassay also identified the 36 abnormal Iranian patients, but it gave normal values for the 4 patients with abnormal reactivity.[67] The electroimmunoassay was also used in the study designed to assess variability of test results in mild von Willebrand's disease; although only 130 of the 202 samples had decreased VIIIR:Ag, 43 of the 50 patients had at least one abnormal value.[81]

## VIII:RAg by Crossed Immunoelectrophoresis[83,84]

Theoretically, this technique is designed first to separate proteins on the basis of their molecular charge and then to identify them immunologically. It is performed by first electrophoresing the sample in agarose gel in a horizontal direction and then localizing the proteins by electrophoresing the separated antigens at 90° to the first dimension into a gel containing specific antiserum. As the antigen moves into the antibody-containing gel, the protein is precipitated and can be easily detected. In practice, however, it is the size of the von Willebrand factor protein rather than its molecular charge that appears to determine its mobility in the first dimension. The most anodal von Willebrand factor multimers (fastest-moving ones) thus are the smallest, and the ones closest to the sample placement well are the largest. Normal plasma and cryoprecipitate give similar patterns, with the major portion of the molecules moving slowly. Some variants of von Willebrand's disease are characterized by a selective decrease in the larger forms of the von Willebrand factor protein, and the plasmas from these patients demonstrate increased anodal mobility in the assay.

## Multimer Analysis by Agarose Gel Electrophoresis

This more specialized technique involves electrophoresis of plasma through agarose and identification of multimeric forms by overlaying the gel with radiolabeled antibody to von Willebrand factor.[43] It gives a more precise description of the molecular weights of the multimeric forms present than does crossed immunoelectrophoresis. Although this technique is available in only a few clinical laboratories at present, samples can be sent to commercial laboratories for analysis.

## Ristocetin-Induced Platelet Aggregation

The addition of ristocetin to platelet-rich plasma results in platelet aggregation.[17] At certain concentrations of ristocetin, the response occurs in two waves, with the second wave apparently dependent on the platelet release reaction since it can be inhibited by aspirin. The initial wave, however, is independent of the release reaction and is, at least in part, a function of the level of von Willebrand factor in the plasma; it is decreased or absent in most patients with von Willebrand's disease.[21] Attempts to quantify the reaction have relied on assessment of either the initial slope of the response at a fixed concentration of ristocetin or the minimum concentration of ristocetin needed to achieve a certain slope or extent of aggregation. For the results to be even semiquantitative, however, careful attention must be paid to such variables as pH, the stirring mechanism, and the platelet count.[29] Moreover, the use of the patient's own platelets introduces a variable that cannot be controlled for easily, and thus any platelet alteration that affects the platelet receptor for von Willebrand factor or the release reaction may affect the total aggregation obtained. Even under the best circumstances, this assay has limitations as a screening test, since a significant percentage of patients with mild von Willebrand's disease will have normal aggregation. Moreover, patients with a specific variant of von Willebrand's disease, the type IIb form (see below), have increased ristocetin-induced aggregation. In the Italian study, 70 percent of the patients had decreased, 18 percent had normal, and 12 percent had increased ristocetin-induced aggregation when assessed by the minimum concentration of ristocetin required to achieve a 30 percent increase in light transmission.[68,85]

## VIII:RCo

To overcome some of the variables involved in ristocetin-induced aggregation of platelet-rich plasma, a quantitative assay was developed based on a comparison of the ability of dilutions of normal or test plasma to restore the aggregation of von Willebrand's disease platelet-rich plasma.[86] Since the time of the original studies, the assay has evolved in several steps: (1) Simply washing normal platelets was found to free them of sufficient plasma

**Table 6-2**

Identification of Heterozygous von Willebrand Patients
by Conventional Methods

|                        | Sensitivity (%)* | Specifictiy (%)† |
|------------------------|------------------|------------------|
| Symptoms alone         | 65               | 77               |
| Bleeding time alone    | 27               | 97               |
| VIII:C alone           | 15               | 97               |
| VIIIR:Ag alone         | 27               | 100              |
| VIII:RCo alone         | 42               | 100              |
| At least 1 abnormal test | 58             | 93%              |

Adapted from Miller CH, Graham JB, Goldin LR, et al: Genetics of classic von Willebrand's disease II. Optimal assignment of the heterozygous genotype (diagnosis) by discriminant analysis. Blood 54:137–148, 1979. With permission.
*Sensitivity is defined as the percentage of patients having the disorder whose test results are abnormal.
†Specificity is defined as the percentage of individuals who do not have the disorders whose test results are normal.

VIII:RCo, so that they no longer responded to ristocetin alone; they could then substitute for von Willebrand's disease platelets. (2) Platelets fixed in a low concentration of formaldehyde were found to be able to substitute for fresh platelets,[22] with the assay adapted so that either timed macroscopic agglutination or the initial slope of agglutination could be employed for quantification. (3) Lyophilized, fixed platelets were found to be able to substitute for fresh or fixed platelets.[87] Although methodologic and standardization problems remain, there is general agreement that this is the most useful in vitro assay in the diagnosis of von Willebrand's disease since, at least in patients who have not been transfused, it seems to correlate best with the bleeding time.[86,88]

Two recent studies offer some insight into the problems involved in making the diagnosis of heterozygous von Willebrand's disease with the currently available techniques. Miller et al.[89,90] obtained data on 181 members of 2 extended families with von Willebrand's disease. By pedigree analysis they were able to identify 26 individuals who were transmitters of the disease (i.e., they had both an affected predecessor and an affected descendent) and who could, therefore, be reasonably presumed to be heterozygotes for von Willebrand's disease. Interestingly, only 65 percent of these individuals had significant clinical symptoms as judged by a detailed questionnaire. More disturbing, however, was the finding that 23 percent of the normal controls (unrelated spouses of the patients) also were judged to have positive bleeding histories. Since the clinical history is the screening test most commonly employed in deciding whether to evaluate patients further, the implications of these estimates of sensitivity (65 percent) and specificity (77 percent) are grave given that the frequency of the gene in the normal population is probably no more than 10 in 100,000. For example, in applying these data to a population of 100,000, 7 patients with von Willebrand's disease would have clinical symptoms (65 percent of the 10 expected patients), and 22,998 of the normals (23 percent of 99,990) would have clinical symptoms. Thus, only 7 out of 23,006, or 0.03 percent of those individuals with symptoms, would have heterozygous von Willebrand's disease, whereas a full 35 percent of the patients with heterozygous von Willebrand's disease would still remain undetected. A similar analysis was applied to the laboratory tests used in the diagnosis von Willebrand's disease; the sensitivities and specificities for detecting the heterozygous state are shown in Table 6-2. Although

**Table 6-3**
Correlation between the Number of Times Patients with von Willebrand's
Disease Were Tested for VIII:C, VIIIR:Ag, VIII:RCo, and Bleeding Time
and the Number of Patterns of Normal and Abnormal Results Obtained

| No. of Times Tested | No. of Patterns* | | | | | |
|---|---|---|---|---|---|---|
| | 1 | 2 | 3 | 4 | 5 | 6 |
| 2 | 5 | 7 | | | | |
| 3 | 3 | 1 | 2 | | | |
| 4 | 1 | 3 | 3 | 4 | | |
| 5 | | 4 | 4 | 1 | 3 | |
| 6 | 2 | 1 | 1 | | | |
| 7 | 1 | | | | 2 | 1 |

Adapted from Abildgaard CF, Suzuki Z, Harrison J, et al: Serial studies in von Willebrand's disease: Variability versus "variants." Blood 56:712–716, 1981. With permission.
*With four assays performed and each assay scored as either normal or abnormal, a total of 16 patterns of normal/abnormal results are possible.

this study indicated that 42 percent of heterozygous patients will fail to have even a single abnormal test, the author suspects that most coagulationists do not believe that it is this difficult to diagnose the disorder as it is found in the general population. Miller et al. also analyzed the number of abnormal tests in the "affected" patients in these families (i.e., those individuals with at least 1 abnormal test). They found that 15 percent had all 4 tests abnormal, 13 percent had 3 abnormal tests, 20 percent had 2 abnormal tests, and 52 percent had only a single abnormal test.

Some data on the constancy of laboratory findings in von Willebrand's disease are also available. In the above-mentioned study,[89,90] 22 individuals from the family were subsequently retested. Although the results of only 18 of the 140 repeat assays (13 percent) were significantly different from the initial results, this was sufficient to require reclassification of 5 of the 22 individuals (23 percent) from affected to unaffected or vice versa. Abildgaard et al.[81] performed serial studies of bleeding time, VIII:C, VIIIR:Ag and VIII:RCo on 50 individuals from 25 families. The number of patterns of positive and negative results they observed is shown in Table 6-3. Note that only 11 of the 50 patients consistently demonstrated the same pattern. As expected, Table 6-3 also shows that the number of patterns observed increased when the number of times the patients were tested increased.

Although these studies emphasize the difficulties involved in evaluating patients who may have von Willebrand's disease, several points should be emphasized: (1) Almost by definition, patients with clinically severe von Willebrand's disease will have strongly positive histories; these patients also usually have severe laboratory abnormalities, especially in VIII:RCo activity, and so the diagnosis can be confirmed with ease. (2) Although the overall specificity of a bleeding history taken by questionnaire may not be great, the specificity of certain symptoms (such as repeated spontaneous epistaxis from both nostrils requiring packing, cautery, and transfusion) is unquestionably much greater.[91] (3) Although a considerable number of heterozygotes may not be detected using the bleeding history as a screening test, the risk of excessive hemorrhage is probably considerably less in these patients than in severely affected patients, and thus the clinical impact of this insensitivity is probably less than one might initially think. This insensitivity, however, may make the genetics in a single family more difficult to analyze since an asymptomatic heterozygous parent may be mistaken for normal and thus the inheritance may be misinterpreted as autosomal recessive. (4) As we learn more about the specific biochemical defects in the different subgroups of von Willebrand's disease, our diagnostic accuracy is certain to improve as, for example, with studies to define the molecular weights of the multimers present. (5) The coagulationist can expect that a significant fraction of patients sent for evaluation of an abnormal bleeding history will have no detectable abnormality.

## Clinical Symptoms

Details of the clinical symptoms found in a single large Swedish family (42 affected individuals)[92] and 37 cases from 24 families reported from France[13] are summarized in Table 6-4. Epistaxis is not only the most common symptom but also the most common first symptom, with 16 of the 37 French patients presenting this way. Gingival bleeding, easy bruising, and menorrhagia in women, are the next most common symptoms. Bleeding after tonsillectomy and gastrointestinal hemorrhage also occur; the latter can be a very serious problem since it is often difficult to identify the bleeding site, and the response to therapy is unpredictable. The specificity of the above symptoms for von Willebrand's disease (or some other coagulation disorder) depends in large part on the frequency and severity of the symptoms as well as the circumstances surrounding them. One needs to inquire, therefore, whether epistaxis is (1) only from a single nostril (in which case it is more likely related to an anatomical defect), (2) confined to episodes of coryza, (3) associated with forced-air heating systems (which may dry the nasal mucosa), or (4) spontaneous or occurring only after trauma (patients may not even be aware of the trauma they produce when they pick their nose). The duration of the epistaxis and the method required to stop it (direct pressure, packing, cautery) may give additional insight into the severity of the symptoms, especially if the patient required medical assistance. Perhaps the most specific historical indicator of the severity of epistaxis is whether or not the patient required transfusions to stop the bleeding or replace the blood lost. Questions that may help in evaluating gingival bleeding include the following: (1) Is the bleeding spontaneous (is there blood on the patient's pillowcase upon rising), or does it occur only with tooth brushing? (2) What type of toothbrush bristle (soft or firm) is used? (3) Is the patient known to have gingival disease? Bruising is often a difficult symptom to evaluate because a significgant number of individuals (predominantly women) with no obvious hemostatic defects have excessive bruising and because patients show considerable individual variation in deciding what constitutes "excessive" bruising. Differentiating points that may be helpful include frequency, size, spontaneity (inquire as to potentially overlooked minor trauma), and location (if present on the back or trunk, they are more likely to be spontaneous than if confined to the extremities). An index of the severity of menorrhagia may be obtained by inquiring whether the patient has been told that she became anemic as a result (and was given iron therapy); transfusions were required; birth control pills were prescribed to suppress menses; or hysterectomy or radiation sterilization was performed. It is difficult to quantify blood loss during menstruation by the history when none of the above objective criteria are met. Inquiry as to whether the patient considers her periods excessive when compared to those of family members or friends may be helpful. The number of pads or tampons used seems not to be helpful in determining the severity since patients vary greatly in their hygienic practices. It may be more useful to ask about the number of days during which the patient has heavy flow and the total number of days of an average menstrual period; if the former

**Table 6-4**
Frequency of Symptoms in Patients with von Willebrand's Disease

| | Sweden | | | | France | | | |
|---|---|---|---|---|---|---|---|---|
| | Male (12) | | Female (30) | | Male* (18) | | Female* (19) | |
| | No. | Percent | No. | Percent | No. | Percent | No. | Percent |
| Epistaxis | 8 | 67 | 16 | 53 | 25 | | | 68 |
| Gingival bleeding | 2 | 17 | 10 | 33 | 15 | | | 41 |
| Tonsillar hemorrhage | — | | — | | 3 | | | 8 |
| Easy bruising and hematomas | 2 | 17 | 16 | 53 | 11 | | | 30 |
| Gastrointestinal bleeding | 1 | 8 | 2 | 7 | 4 | | | 11 |
| Prolonged bleeding with cuts and trauma | 2 | 17 | 12 | 40 | — | | | — |
| Bleeding after tooth extraction | 6 | 50 | 16 | 53 | — | | | — |
| Postoperative bleeding | 1 | 8 | 7 | 23 | — | | | — |
| Menorrhagia | | | 13 | 43 | 11 | | | 30 |
| Postpartum hemorrhage | | | 7 | 23 | — | | | — |
| Postabortion hemorrhage | | | 2 | 7 | — | | | — |
| Hemarthrosis, spontaneous or posttraumatic | | | 1 | 3 | 3 | | | 8 |
| Other (lip, tongue, postvaccination, lung) | | | 1 | 3 | 2 | | | 5 |

Combined data from Silver J, Nilsson IM: On a Swedish family with 51 members affected by von Willebrand's disease. Acta Med Scand 175:636–637, and Larrieu MJ, Caen JP, Meyer DO, et al: Congenital bleeding disorders with long bleeding time and normal platelet count. II. Von Willebrand's disease (report of thirty-seven patients). Am J Med 45:354–372, 1968. With permission of the publishers.

*The data for both sexes are pooled.

is more than 3 and/or the latter more than 6 or 7, the author usually considers the patient to have menorrhagia. Needless to say, gynecologic causes of menometrorrhagia should be considered and specifically inquired about, especially the presence of fibroid tumors.

Prolonged bleeding after dental extraction was common in the Swedish family but was not mentioned in the French series. Although this is a very common hemostatic challenge, patients often fail to volunteer this information, and so specific inquiry should be made. The extent of the hemostatic challenge, however, differs significantly with the location of the tooth and whether it was deciduous or permanent. Inquiry as to whether packing, suturing, or transfusion was required to stop the bleeding may help to assess the patient's diathesis. Similarly, prolonged bleeding from cuts and trauma is a fairly common complaint amoung affected patients. Questions concerning shaving habits (did the patient switch from a blade razor to an electric razor because of prolonged oozing?) may highlight such a problem. Surgical procedures and severe trauma are probably the most demanding assaults on the hemostatic system; thus, it is not altogether surprising that patients with mild forms of the disease may be undetected in their youth, only to be discovered later on when exposed to these stresses. In one of the French patients, in fact, the diagnosis was made at the age of 67 after a severe traumatic hematoma. By careful attention to historical details, the author believes that it is possible to improve significantly on the reported 77 percent specificity for the clinical history.

Several additional aspects of clinical symptomatology need to be stressed: (1) Spontaneous hemarthroses are rare and occur only in patients with very low VIII:C levels. (2) There is a tendency for symptoms to decrease significantly after adolescence, especially in women. (3) Postpartum hemorrhage is very variable and may even vary in different deliveries in the same woman.[93,94,94a] (4) Only a small fraction of affected patients have severe bleeding symptoms, and death as a result of bleeding is extremely rare at present; uncontrollable gastrointestinal hemorrhage may be the lethal event.

## GENETICS

Many studies have documented an autosomal dominant pattern of inheritance in von Willebrand's disease, and this is considered the usual pattern. In an extensive study from Sweden,[95] the penetrance was estimated as 73–90 percent but the expression varied dramatically even within families. The risk of an affected parent having a child with clinically manifest disease was 40 percent, and the risk of having a severely affected child was 4 percent regardless of the severity of the parents' symptoms. Several reports have suggested that von Willebrand's disease may also be inherited as an autosomal recessive trait since unaffected consanguineous parents have had severely affected children.[96] For example, 17 of 100 cases recently reported from Italy were believed to fall into this category.[68] There is, however, considerable difficulty in making general statements about inheritance for the following reasons: (1) There is great variability in the clinical and laboratory expression of the disease, with a significant fraction of obligate heterozygotes not manifesting the disease. An "unaffected" parent may thus be harboring the same gene as an "affected" parent; as a result, the traditional genetic concepts of dominant and recessive fail to convey their intended information. (2) As is becoming increasingly apparent, von Willebrand's disease is not, in fact, the result of a single well-defined defect; rather, it is a syndrome characterized by a functional deficiency. That deficiency can result from a variety of defects acting in concert with a series of other genetically controlled factors that affect the expression of the defect. (3) Pedigrees of individual families that seem to have both dominant and recessive modes of transmission have been reported, raising the possibility of more complex inheritance patterns, as for example, with double heterozygosity.[76]

## PATTERNS OF VON WILLEBRAND'S DISEASE

The newer techniques that permit evaluation of the structure of the von Willebrand factor molecule have shown heterogeneity in the abnormalities found in different patients. This has allowed for a subdivision of von Willebrand's disease into different types. Since these techniques are new and only a small number of patients have been studied in detail, the following formulation must be considered tentative, and will undoubtedly be revised.

### Type I

This type is characterized by a concordant reduction in all of the factor VIII–von Willebrand factor complex activities. It can, perhaps, be further subdivided into those patients who apparently inherited the disorder in an autosomal recessive manner and thus are presumably homozygotes (or perhaps double heterozytes) and those who inherited it in an autosomal dominant fashion and thus are presumably heterozygotes.[96] The homozygous patients are almost always severely affected clinically and have virtually undetectable levels of plasma, platelet, and endothelial cell VIIIR:Ag and VIII:RCo. Very low but still measurable levels of VIII:C are usually present. Consanguinity is common, and careful study of the parents often reveals normal levels of VIII:C but decreased levels of VIIIR:Ag and VIII:RCo. These patients are at risk of developing anti-von Willebrand factor antibodies when infused with plasma fractions, and these antibodies may complicate their therapy (see below).[97] Fifty-five percent of the 40 Iranian patients[67] and 17 percent of the Italian patients[68] were thought to fall into this category. Since even the highly sensitive immunologic tests usually fail to detect any VIIIR:Ag in the plasma of such patients, it was generally believed that these patients had a quantitative defect related to either decreased synthesis or increased destruction of the von Willebrand factor protein. Recently, techniques employing radiolabeled anti-VIIIR:Ag antibodies have increased the sensitivity of the assays and permitted the subdivision of the apparently homozygous patients into 3 categories: (1) no detectable von Willebrand factor protein by any technique, (2) detectable protein with abnormal electrophoretic migration, and (3) detectable protein with normal migration.[98] The frequency of each of these types remains uncertain.

The apparently heterozygous type I patients usually have moderate to severe clinical symptoms, but rarely as severe as those of the presumed homozygotes. Analysis of their plasma and platelets shows that all of the multimeric forms of the von Willebrand factor protein are present, but the total amount of protein is reduced.[43] Preliminary biochemical analysis failed to find a significant difference in the structure of the von Willebrand factor in these patients.[99]

### Type II

This type is characterized by discordant reductions in the factor VIII–von Willebrand factor complex activities, with VIII:RCo being more reduced than VIII:C or VIIIR:Ag.[100] At least 3 subgroups have been recognized. In type IIa, the patients may have mild to severe clinical symptoms, and the inheritance is most compatible with autosomal dominant transmission. Ristocetin-induced aggregation of platelets in platelet-rich plasma is reduced, as is VIII:RCo. The crossed antigen-antibody immunoelectrophoresis of plasma reveals increased anodal mobility, which has been shown to be due to a reduction in the higher molecular weight multimers.[43] Analysis of platelet von Willebrand factor protein shows the same abnormalities as those of the plasma protein.[43] Preliminary biochemical analysis failed to reveal significant differences in the structure of the von Willebrand factor protein.[99] At least one report indicates that these patients may have a decreased amount of carbohydrate associated with their von Willebrand factor protein,[101] but the frequency with which this occurs is controversial.[102,102a] Interestingly, VIIIR:Ag values may be higher by electroimmunoassay than by immunoradiometric analysis,[82] perhaps related to the smaller molecules' ease of movement through the gel; in fact, the abnormal size distribution may invalidate quantification of VIIIR:Ag by the latter technique since the antigen behaves aberrantly in this assay.[82,100] The VIIIR:Ag that remains in the supernatant after normal plasma is cryoprecipitated, and that is similarly enriched in the lower molecular weight forms of von Willebrand factor, also behaves aberrantly in the immunoradiometric assay.[82,100]

The distinguishing characteristic of the type IIb patients is the ability of their platelets to aggregate in response to much lower concentrations of ristocetin than do normal platelets.[43,85] Despite this, and perhaps somewhat ironically, when the plasma from these patients is tested for VIII:RCo in an assay employing washed normal platelets, their values are low or at best borderline (e.g., of the 12 Italian patients, 3 had values below 20 percent, 2 were between 20 and 30 percent, 5 had values between 30 and 40 percent, and only 2 had values between 40 and 50 percent).[68] Plasma VIIIR:Ag in these patients is selectively reduced in the higher molecular weight forms, not unlike the situation in the type IIa variant. Two features however, clearly separate these 2 entities: (1) the platelet von Willebrand factor protein in the type IIb variant appears to contain all of the molecular weight forms, including the higher ones,[43] and (2) in accord with the aggregation data, the plasma von Willebrand factor protein in type IIb binds to platelets at lower concentrations of ristocetin than does normal von Willebrand factor (in comparison, in type IIa very little von Willebrand factor protein binds to platelets, even in the presence of high concentrations of ristocetin).[43,85] Clinically, this disorder appears to be inherited as an autosomal dominant trait and is characterized by a prolonged bleeding time and moderately severe disease. In the patients reported from Italy, the investigators concluded that their platelets were not responsible for the increased von Willebrand factor binding since the same increased binding could be demonstrated using patient plasma and normal platelets.[68] It is clear that there is additional heterogeneity within each of the von Willebrand disease subtypes noted above as evidenced by a recent comprehensive study.[102b] The therapeutic implications of these findings is still under investigation.

In addition to type IIa, type IIb and platelet-type or pseudo-von Willebrand's disease, patients with von Willebrand disease-related phenotypes have been reported who do not fit the above classification. Two severely affected patients have been reported to have prolonged bleeding times and a discordant reduction in VIII:RCo compared to VIII:C and VIIIR:Ag. Unlike the patients in the above groups, however, these patients did not have a selective loss of the high molecular weight multimers as judged by crossed antigen-antibody electrophoresis and gel chromatography. Interestingly, when their von Willebrand factor proteins were purified, they were found to be deficient in carbohydrate;[103] subsequent biochemical studies confirmed the importance of the von Willebrand factor's carbohydrate moiety in mediating its platelet cofactor role.[44-47] A patient with similar clinical and laboratory findings and indirect evidence of a carbohydrate abnormality of his von Willelbrand factor has also been reported by another group.[36a] Finally, using an improved method for multimer resolution, a patient with clinical and laboratory features of type IIa von Willebrand's disease was found to have a unique multimeric pattern. It was proposed that this may represent a different disease entitity.[103a]

### "Platelet"-type von Willebrand's Disease (Pseudo-von Willebrand's Disease)

There are now several reports of patients with platelets that appear to bind the high molecular weight forms of the von Willebrand factor excessively, leaving their plasma with both a reduced amount of the protein and a disproportionately large fraction of low molecular weight multimers. Clinically, these patients have a bleeding disorder that is similar to von Willebrand's disease, but as the defect is thought to be primarily in the platelet and not in the von Willebrand factor, it has been termed *platelet-type* or *pseudo-von Willebrand's disease*.[104-107] The patients have increased ristocetin-induced platelet aggregation at low concentrations of ristocetin. In addition, variable degrees of thrombocytopenia and increases in platelet size have been reported in association with this disorder. The most striking finding is that cryoprecipitate can induce aggregation of some, if not all, of these patients' platelets when added to citrated platelet-rich plasma. This last feature permits easy separation of these patients from those with type IIb von Willebrand's disease.

### THE DEFECT IN VON WILLEBRAND'S DISEASE

As already indicated, both megakaryocytes and endothelial cells are believed to be able to synthesize von Willebrand factor. Although not universally accepted,[108] the weight of evidence supports the idea that plasma von Willebrand factor derives from endothelial cell synthesis. The role of the von Willebrand factor associated with platelets (and presumably derived from megakaryocytes) is less clear. The finding of minor differences in the structure of platelet and plasma VIII:RAg raised the possibility that these proteins are under separate genetic control;[109] however, a concordant absence of both platelet and plasma von Willebrand factor has been found in some patients with severe von Willebrand's disease,[110-112] making this unlikely. The structural differences observed may have resulted from proteolytic degradation, or perhaps differences in the processing of the same genetic information.

With the foregoing in mind, it is possible to advance a scheme to identify the sites at which alterations may result in an abnormal von Willebrand factor protein and a von Willebrand disease phenotype[113] (Fig. 6-1). These include (1) an abnormality in the primary structure of the subunit protein; (2) a regulatory abnormality affecting transcription, messenger ribonucleic acid (mRNA) processing or translation; (3) a posttranslational defect in glycosylation; (4) a posttranslational defect in multimer formation or precursor processing; (5) a defect in release; (6) a defect in interconversion of multimers; (7) a defect in von Willebrand factor catabolism; and (8) a defect in binding to subendothelium or platelets. It must be stressed that we have very little information on the mechanism of multimer formation by disulfide bond formation, and it remains controversial whether there is a dynamic equilibrium between multimers of different sizes in plasma.[56a,56b,113a-c]

This scheme emphasizes the complexity of the control of circulating von Willebrand

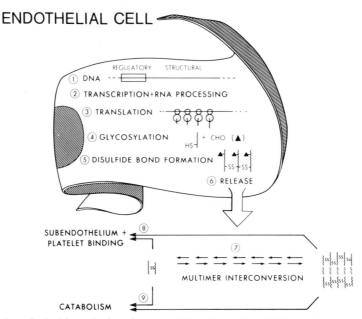

**Fig. 6-1.** Steps in the biosynthesis, release, and disposition of von Willebrand factor derived from endothelial cells.

factor levels and the many different sites at which abnormalities can result in the appearance of the same phenotype. It is humbling to realize that with our current information it is impossible to identify definitely the precise abnormality in any of the types of von Willebrand's disease described to date. Two recent findings are of interest with regard to the pathogenesis of the von Willebrand's disease defect. In support of the hypothesis that there is an endothelial cell defect in at least some forms of the disease, it was found that a patient with homozygous von Willebrand's disease failed to show a rise in both plasma VIIIR:Ag and plasminogen activator (a substance previously identified as deriving from the endothelium) when infused with the drug 1-deamino 8-D-arginine vasopressin (DDAVP; see below).[65] In another study, based on only a small group of patients, an apparent association between mitral valve prolapse and von Willebrand's disease was found, leading the authors to speculate on the presence of a generalized mesenchymal defect.[114] Two subsequent studies have addressed this same question; one study confirmed an increased incidence of mitral valve prolapse in patients with von Willebrand's disease, but the other found no such increase.[114a,114b]

## MECHANISM OF BLEEDING IN VON WILLEBRAND'S DISEASE AND THERAPY FOR BLEEDING EPISODES

Unlike classic hemophilia, in which the excellent correlation between clinical symptoms and the laboratory assessment of disease severity has permitted careful titration of therapy and accurate prediction of clinical response, the therapy of von Willebrand's disease remains more empirical and necessarily more controversial. This results from the variability of response to therapy and, more importantly, from the lack of a universally accepted assay for measuring the response. Ultimately, the uncertainly stems from both the variability of the disorder itself and our lack of understanding of the precise role of von Willebrand factor in hemostasis.

The weight of current evidence suggests that the von Willebrand factor is involved in the adhesion of platelets to the subendothelium.[18] In this model, the von Willebrand factor is thought to be present on the subendothelial surface that is exposed when there is endothelial injury, either as a result of prior abluminal deposition by the previously overlying endothelial cells or by the binding of plasma von Willebrand factor to subendothelial elements after endothelial damage.[57,58,115] Once the von Willebrand factor is present on the subendothelium, platelets will adhere to this immobilized form of the protein. It should be pointed out, however, that in the absence of ristocetin, platelets do not interact with von Willebrand factor in vitro or in vivo, and so some alteration of the von Willebrand factor upon immobilization must be postulated. Moreover, in both the ristocetin-induced aggregation and the platelet retention phenomena, the von Willebrand factor appears to mediate platelet–platelet interactions and not platelet adhesion; even in the ex vivo morphometric assay, in which a defect in platelet adhesion in von Willebrand's disease has been most convincingly demonstrated, recent data support a role for von Willebrand factor in platelet–platelet interactions.[37] Complicating the issue is the observation that the role of von Willebrand factor appears to depend on the shear rate in both the platelet retention and ex vivo morphometric systems, with the defect due to a deficiency of von Willebrand factor much more apparent at high rather than low shear.[116] This shear dependence may influence the sites at which clinical hemorrhage occurs. Recently, both ADP and thrombin have been shown to induce the binding of von Willebrand factor to platelets under certain conditions.[117,117a] Studies on patients with thrombasthenia and with monoclonal antibodies specific for sites on the platelet membrane indicate that von Willebrand factor binds primarily, if not exclusively, to the glycoprotein IIb–IIIa complex when stimulated with these agents; this is in sharp contrast to the binding induced by ristocetin, which occurs exclusively to glycoprotein Ib.[117b–d] The recent observation that fibrinogen competes effectively with von Willebrand factor for binding to thrombin-treated platelets[117c] casts doubt on the physiologic significance of this phenomenon since there is so much more fibrinogen than von Willebrand factor in plasma.

Several general principles of therapy seem to be well supported:

1. Patients with very low levels of VIII:C are at high risk of developing the same types of bleeding (soft tissue and joint) as hemophiliacs, and it is reasonable to try to achieve the same VIII:C levels one would try to achieve in hemophiliacs for the same type of hemorrhage.[3,95] This is easier to accomplish in patients with von Willebrand's disease since one can anticipate that the VIII:C response will last much longer (up to 48 hours) than it does in hemophilic patients (about 12 hours). Thus, an VIII:C more than 25 percent of normal (0.25U/ml, where 1 U is defined as the amount of VIII:C in 1 ml of normal plasma) has been maintained with 10–15 ml/kg/day of plasma or 1.0–1.5 bags of cryoprecipitate [where 1 bag is the amount of cryoprecipitate obtained from the plasma in a 1 unit (about 500 ml) blood donation] per 10 kg body weight per day.

2. Mucosal bleeding may not be controlled even though high levels of VIII:C are obtained. In this case, control seems to correlate best with shortening of the bleeding time and, to a lesser extent, with improvement in the VIII:RCo (with the caveat that a lack of correlation with VIII:RCo has also been reported).[88,97] The technique used for the bleeding time is crucial, however, since the template modification of the Ivy technique may not be corrected even though the patient achieves good clinical hemostasis, whereas the Duke

bleeding time correction appears to correlate better with clinical improvement.[72,73] It has been proposed that reducing the Duke bleeding time to about 10 minutes is sufficient for control of minor bleeding episodes such as epistaxis and superficial injuries, whereas it should be reduced to about 5 minutes for more severe hemorrhage or in preparation for surgical procedures.[95]

3. Cryoprecipitate is the preferred replacement therapy, although fresh or fresh frozen plasma may be substituted if the former is not available and the patient can tolerate the fluid load.[2,4,7,8] High-potency factor VIII concentrates should not be used because the currently available preparations have been reported to be ineffective in controlling mucosal bleeding.[12] Perhaps this is because these preparations do not contain the high molecular weight von Willebrand factor multimers (as judged by several techniques) and have relatively little VIII:RCo.[118-120] As one might anticipate, there is also considerable variability in the bleeding time correcting ability of different cryoprecipitate preparations, resulting most likely from variations in the donors' levels of von Willebrand factor and the specifics of the techniques employed in their preparation. This variability makes it quite difficult to establish firm guidelines concerning therapy. In vitro assessment of the material to be infused by VIII:RCo assay has not permitted a reliable prediction of clinical response, although evidence of loss of the higher molecular weight multimers seems to identify products that are ineffective.[118-120] Thus, it is still necessary to maintain an empiric approach. Recommendations made by Nilsson[95] are given in Table 6-5 based on the VIII:C content of cryoprecipitate. Since there are approximately 100 U VIII:C per bag of cryoprecipitate, dividing the dose by 100 will give a reasonable estimate of the number of bags of cryoprecipitate needed. For example, on the day of major surgery in a patient with severe von Willebrand's disease, the dose would be 3 bags for every 10 kg of body weight. It should be emphasized that it is necessary to administer therapy for a considerable period of time after major surgical procedures and postpartum since delayed bleeding may occur in these situations.

4. Epsilon aminocaproic acid, which at low concentrations prevents the conversion of plasminogen to plasmin and at high concentrations inhibits plasmin directly, has been used effectively in reducing the bleeding associated with dental extraction in hemophilacs and is probably also effective in patients with von Willebrand's disease.[95] One should be certain that the patient is not having diffuse intravascular coagulation and is not pregnant before administering it. According to one regimen, it should be administered at a dose of 50–100 mg/kg by either the intravenous or oral route just prior to the procedure, three hours thereafter, and then every 6 hours for the next week. If gastrointestinal distress or faintness occurs, the dose can be reduced. Others have used 4 g every 4 hours for all adults with good results.

5. In an attempt to avoid the complications of plasma and its fractions, the synthetic analogue of vasopressin, 1-deamino 8-D-arginine vasopressin (DDAVP), has been administered intravenously to hemophilic and von Willebrand's disease patients at a dose of 0.2–0.5 μg/kg in an attempt to increase the VIII:C and von Willebrand factor.[121-123] The drug is diluted in 30 ml of normal saline and infused over 15–20 minutes; more rapid infusion often results in an increase in heart rate and mild facial flushing. Water retention and hyponatremia have been reported,[124] but these complications are apparently rare and can be easily monitored. In early studies, infusions were often repeated at 12- to 24-hour intervals, but resistance to therapy with repeated doses has been noted and this clearly limits the response. The response to DDAVP in von Willebrand's disease is quite variable, and although there appears to be some relationship between the type of von Willebrand's disease

**Table 6-5**

Recommended Treatment in von Willebrand's Disease

| | Desired Values for: | | | Severe Cases: Dose VIII:C/d* (U/kg/Body Weight) | Mild Cases: Dose VIII:C/d* (U/kg/Body Weight) |
|---|---|---|---|---|---|
| | VIII:C (%) | Duke Bleeding Time (Minutes) | Duration of Treatment | | |
| Major surgical operations Tonsillectomy Gastrectomy Cholecystectomy Hysterectomy | 40–70% during operation and the first postoperative days, 30–40% until about the seventh day, afterward 10–15% until healed | <5 | 2–3 weeks | Days 1–2, 20–40; days 3–8, 10–20; days 8, 5–10 | Days 1–2, 15–30; days 3–8, 5–15 |
| Minor surgical operations Tooth extraction Appendectomy Herniorrhaphy | 20–50% during operation, then about 15% for 6–8 days | <5 | 6–8 days | Day 1, 15–20; days 2–8, 5–10 | Day 1, 5–15; days 2–8, 5 |
| Delivery | As for major surgery | | 2–4 weeks | As for major surgery | As for major surgery |
| Severe hemorrhagic conditions Gastrointestinal bleeding Severe menorrhagia Head injury Intracranial hemorrhage Postoperative hemorrhage | 20–50% | <5 | About 7 days | 15–20 | 5–15 |
| Minor bleeding episodes Superficial injuries Nose bleeding | 15–20% | <10 | 2–5 days | 5–10 | 0–5 |

Adapted from Nilsson IM: Haemorrhagic and Thrombotic Disease. New York, Wiley, 1971, p. 100. With permission.

*d = day

and the response, for practical purposes it is not yet possible to predict the response of a given individual. In general, patients with severe type I disease tend to have little or no response with regard to VIIIR:Ag, VIII:RCo, or bleeding time, although they may have some VIII:C response. Patients with mild type I disease and most patients with type IIa may have quite significant responses, with the increase in VIII:RCo usually less dramatic than that of VIII:C or VIIIR:Ag. Bleeding time correction has been very variable, which may be accounted for by differences in technique. The role of DDAVP in the management of patients with type IIb von Willebrand's disease is quite controversial. Although increases in VIIIR:Ag, VIII:RCo, and VIII:C have been reported,[125-128] a recent report of DDAVP-induced thrombocytopenia in association with intravascular platelet aggregates suggests that DDAVP may be contraindicated.[128a] The presumed mechanism is release of abnormal high molecular forms of von Willebrand factor that can then cause direct platelet agglutination. Support for this hypothesis comes from studies showing an increase in high molecular weight forms of von Willebrand factor[128] and the ability of plasma obtained from such patients after DDAVP infusion to agglutinate normal platelets in vitro.[128a] Thus, although DDAVP appears to be promising in the management of selected patients with the more mild forms of von Willebrand's disease, the unpredictability of the response and the rapid development of resistance make it far from ideal therapy; its proper role in the management of patients remains to be determined.

It is interesting to note a report in which the child of a patient with von Willebrand's disease had normal levels of VIII:C, VIIIR:Ag, and VIII:RCo in cord blood, but was found at 6 months of age to have abnormally low levels of all of these factors as well as evidence of a decrease in the high molecular weight multimers.[129] The authors suggested that the vasopressin administered to the mother at the time of delivery may have resulted in the increased levels of the factors and thus complicated the diagnosis.

6. Patients with severe von Willebrand's disease may develop antibodies that precipitate von Willebrand factor; this complication requires special management.[97] Infusion with cryoprecipitate results in little or no increase in VIII:RCo and only a minimal increase in VIIIR:Ag. The VIII:C increase, although greater than that of the VIII:RCo or VIIIR:Ag, is usually blunted and fails to show the characteristic delayed rise. Anamnestic antibody responses often occur after therapy, and patients have been shown to have circulating immune complexes during this time. Side effects such as lumbar and abdominal pain and hypotension can occur soon after cryoprecipitate infusion is begun, and these may be severe. Intravenous hydrocortisone (0.3–0.5 g) has been reported to decrease but not abolish these reactions. Control of soft tissue bleeding (hemarthroses and muscle hematomas) is usually adequate, presumably reflecting the increase in VIII:C, but mucosal bleeding is only poorly controlled, presumably reflecting the poor VIII:RCo response.

7. Observations of patients treated with oral contraceptives and patients during pregnancy suggest that estrogens increase VIII:C and VIIIR:Ag in all but the most severely affected patients; VIII:RCo and bleeding time improvements, however, are much more variable.[74,93,94,130] In some patients, the increase in VIIIR: Ag may be confined to the smaller molecular weight multimers, thus accounting for the discrepancy in functional activities.[131] From a practical standpoint, a recent review of the literature[94] indicates that intrapartum or immediate postpartum hemorrhage is rare if the patient's VIII:C has risen to more than 50 percent before delivery, regardless of the bleeding time or VIII:RCo. Since these values return to prepregnancy levels rapidly after delivery and since hemorrhage may occur for as long as one month postpartum, very careful follow-up of these patients is required. The estrogen effect may account for the general improvement in mu-

cosal bleeding noted during pregnancy and in women who are treated with oral contraceptives to suppress their menses. This effect underscores the difficulty of establishing the diagnosis of von Willebrand's disease when the patient is first seen during pregnancy or while on estrogen therapy.

## REFERENCES

1. Jorpes EJ: E. A. von Willebrand och von Willebrands sjukdom. Nord Med 67:729–732, 1962
2. Nilsson IM, Blombäck M, Jorpes EJ, et al: Von Willebrand's disease and its correction with human plasma fraction I-O. Acta Med Scand 159:179–188, 1957
3. Biggs R, Matthews JM: The treatment of haemorrhage in von Willebrand's disease and the blood level of factor VIII (AHG). Br J Haematol 9:203–214, 1963
4. Cornu P, Larrieu MJ, Caen J, et al: Transfusion studies in von Willebrand's disease: Effect on bleeding time and factor VIII. Br J Haematol 9:189–203, 1963
5. Stefanini M, Dameshek W: The Hemorrhagic Disorders. New York, Grune & Stratton, 1955, pp 56–59
6. Schulman I, Smith CH, Erlandson M, et al: Vascular hemophilia. Pediatrics 18:347–361, 1956
7. Weiss HJ: The use of plasma and plasma fractions in the treatment of a patient with von Willebrand's disease. Vox Sang 7:267–280, 1962
8. Perkins HA: Correction of the hemostatic defects in von Willebrand's disease. Blood 30:375–380, 1967
9. Alexander B, Goldstein R: Dual hemostatic defect in pseudohemophilia. J Clin Invest 32:551, 1953 (abstract)
10. Larrieu MJ, Soulier JP: Deficit en facteur antihemophilique a chez une fille, associé a un trouble du saignement. Rev Hematol 8:361–370, 1953
11. Quick AJ, Hussey CV: Hemophilic condition in the female. J Lab Clin Med 42:929–930, 1953 (abstract)
12. Green D, Potter EV: Failure of AHF concentrate to control bleeding in von Willebrand's disease. Am J Med 60:357–360, 1976
13. Larrieu MJ, Caen JP, Meyer DO, et al: Congenital bleeding disorders with long bleeding time and normal platelet count. II. Von Willebrand's disease (report of thrity-seven patients). Am J Med 45:354–372, 1968
14. Weiss HJ: Von Willebrand's disease—diagnostic criteria. Blood 32:668–679, 1968
15. Zucker, MB: In vitro abnormality of the blood in von Willebrand's disease correctable by normal plasma. Nature (Lond) 197:601–602, 1963
16. Salzman EW: Measurement of platelet adhesiveness. A simple in vitro technique demonstrating an abnormality in von Willebrand's disease. J Lab Clin Med 62:724–735, 1963
17. Howard MA, Firkin BG: Ristocetin—a new tool in the investigation of platelet aggregation. Thromb Diath Haemorrh 26:362–369, 1971
18. Tschopp TB, Weiss HG, Baumgartner HR: Decreased adhesion of platelets to subendothelium in von Willebrand's disease. J Lab Clin Med 83:296–300, 1974
19. McPherson J, Zucker MB: Platelet retention in glass bead columns: Adhesion to glass and subsequent platelet–platelet interactions. Blood 47:55–67, 1976
20. Gralnick HR, Coller BS, Shulman NR, et al: Factor VIII. Ann int Med 86:598–616, 1977
21. Weiss HL, Rogers J, Brand H: Defective ristocetin-induced platelet aggregation in von Willebrand's disease and its correction by factor VIII. J Clin Invest 52:2697–2707, 1973
22. Allain JP, Cooper HA, Wagner RH, et al: Platelets fixed with paraformaldehyde: A new reagent for assay of von Willebrand factor and platelet aggregating factor. J Lab Clin Med 85:318–328, 1975
23. Kao K-J, Pizzo SV, McKee P: Demonstration and characterization of specific binding sites for factor VIII/von Willebrand factor on human platelets. J Clin Invest 63:656–664, 1979

24. Morisato DK, Gralnick HR: Selective binding of the factor VIII/von Willebrand factor protein to human platelets. Blood 55:9–15, 1980

25. Phillips DR: An evaluation of membrane glycoproteins in platelet adhesion and aggregation, in Spaet TH (ed): "Progress in Hemostasis and Thrombosis, vol. 5. New York, Grune & Stratton, 1980, pp 81–109

26. George JN, Reimann TA: Inherited disorders of the platelet membrane: Glaanzmann's thrombasthenia and Bernard-Soulier disease, in Colman RW et al (eds): Textbook of Hemostasis and Thrombosis. Philadelphia, JB Lippincott, 1982, pp 496–506

27. Ruan C, Tobelem G, McMichael AJ, et al: Monoclonal antibody to human platelet glycoprotein I. II. Effects on human platelet function. Br J Haematol 49:511–519, 1981

27a. Coller BS, Peerschke EI, Scudder LE, et al: Studies with a murine monoclonal antibody that abolishes ristocetin-induced binding of von Willebrand factor to platelets: Additional evidence in support of GPIb as a platelet receptor for von Willebrand's factor. Blood 61:99–110, 1983

28. George JN, Reimann TA, Moake JL, et al: Bernard-Soulier disease: A study of four patients and their parents. Br J Haematol 48:459–467, 1981

29. Coller BS, Franza Br Jr, Gralnick HR: The pH dependence of quantitative ristocetin-induced platelet aggregation: Theoretical and practical implications—a new device for maintenance of platelet-rich plasma pH. Blood 47:841–854, 1976

30. Howard MA: Inhibition and reversal of ristocetin-induced platelet aggregation. Thromb Res 6:489–499, 1975

31. Kirby EP, Mills DCB: The interaction of bovine factor VIII with human platelets. J Clin Invest 56:491–502, 1975

32. Coller BS, Gralnick HR: Studies on the mechanism of ristocetin-induced platelet agglutination: Effects of structural modification of ristocetin and vancomycin. J Clin Invest 60:302–312, 1977

33. Coller BS: The effects of ristocetin and von Willebrand factor on platelet electrophoretic mobility. J Clin Invest 61:1168–1175, 1977

34. Rosborough TK, Swaim WR: Abnormal Polybrene-induced platelet agglutination in von Willebrand's disease. Thromb Res 12:937–942, 1978

35. Coller BS: Polybrene-induced agglutination and reduction in electrophoretic mobility: Enhancement by von Willebrand factor and inhibition by vancomycin. Blood 55:276–281, 1980

36. Brinkhous KM, Read MS, Reddick RL, et al: Pathophysiology of platelet-aggregating von Willebrand factor: Applications of the venom coagglutinin vWf assay. Ann NY Acad Sci 370:191–204, 1981

36a. Howard MA, Salem HH, Thomas KB, et al: Variant von Willebrand's disease type B revisited. Blood 60:1420–1428, 1982

36b. Salem HH, Howard MA, Perkins J, et al: Botrocetin induced platelet agglutination. Blood 60:204a, 1982 (abstract)

37. Turitto VT, Weiss HJ, Baumgartner HR: Altered thrombus formation distinct from defective platelet adhesion in von Willebrand's disease. Circulation 62:III-106, 1980 (abstract)

38. Hoyer LW: The factor VIII complex: Structure and function. Blood 58:1–13, 1981

39. McKee PA, Andersen JC, Switzer ME: Molecular structural studies of human factor VIII. Ann NY Acad Sci 240:8–33, 1974

40. Zimmerman TS, Roberts J, Edgington TS: Factor-VIII-related antigen: Multiple molecular forms in human plasma. Proc Natl Acad Sci USA 72:5121–5125, 1975

41. Fass DN, Knutson GJ, Bowie EJW: Porcine Willebrand factor: A population of multimers. J Lab Clin Med 91:307–320, 1978

42. Hoyer LW, Shainoff JR: Factor-VIII-related protein circulates in normal human plasma as high molecular weight multimers. Blood 55:1056–1059, 1980

43. Ruggeri ZM, Zimmerman TS: Variant von Willebrand disease. Characterization of two sub-

types by analysis of multimeric composition of factor VIII/von Willebrand factor in plasma and platelets. J Clin Invest 65:1318–1325, 1980

44. Legaz ME, Schmer G, Counts RB, et al: Isolation and characterization of human factor VIII (antihemophilic factor). J Biol Chem 248:3946–3955, 1973

45. Gralnick HR: Factor VIII/von Willebrand factor protein: Galactose, a cryptic determinant of von Willebrand factor activity. J Clin Invest 62:496–499, 1978

46. Sodetz JM, Pizzo SV, McKee P: Relationship of sialic acid to function and in vivo survival of human factor VIII/von Willebrand factor protein. J Biol Chem 252:5538–5546, 1977

47. Sodetz JJ, Paulson JC, Pizzo SV, et al: Carbohydrate on human factor VIII/von Willebrand factor: Impairment of function by removal of specific galactose residues. J Biol Chem 253:7202–7206, 1978

48. Ratnoff OD, Kass L, Lang PD: Studies on the purification of antihemophilic factor (factor VIII). II. separation of partially purified antihemophilic factor by gel filtration of plasma. J Clin Invest 48:957–962, 1969

49. Counts RB, Paskell SL, Elgee SK: Disulfide bonds and the quaternary structure of factor VIII/von Willebrand factor. J Clin Invest 62:702–709, 1978

50. Ruggeri ZM, Zimmerman TS: The complex multimeric composition of factor VIII/von Willebrand factor. Blood 57:1140–1143, 1981

51. Doucet-deBruine MHM, Sixma JJ, Over J, et al: Heterogeneity of human factor VIII. II. Characterization of forms of factor VIII binding to platelets in the presence of ristocetin. J Lab Clin Med 92:96–107, 1978

52. Over J, Bouma BN, Van Mourik JA, et al: Heterogeneity of human factor VIII. I. Characterization of factor VIII present in the supernatant of cryoprecipitate. J Lab Clin Med 91:32–46, 1978

53. Over J, Sixma JJ, Doucet-de Bruïne MHM, et al: Survival of $^{125}$iodine-labelled factor VIII in normals and patients with classic hemophilia. Observations on the heterogeneity of human factor VIII. J Clin Invest 62:223–234, 1978

54. Gralnick HR, Williams SB, Morisato DK: Effect of the multimeric structure of the factor VIII/von Willebrand factor protein on binding to platelets. Blood 58:387–397, 1981

55. Jaffe EA, Hoyer LW, Nachman RL: Synthesis of von Willebrand factor by cultured human endothelial cells. Proc Natl Acad Sci USA 71:1906–1909, 1974

56. Nachman R, Levine R, Jaffe, EA: Synthesis of factor VIII antigen by cultured guinea pig megakaryocytes. J Clin Invest 60:914–921, 1977

56a. Wagner DD, Marder VJ: Biosynthesis of von Willebrand protein by human endothelial cells. Identification of a large precursor polypeptide chain. J Biol Chem 258:2065–2067, 1983

56b. Lynch DC, Williams R, Zimmerman TS, et al: Biosynthesis of the subunits of factor VIIIR by bovine aortic endothelial cells. Proc Natl Acad Sci 80:2738–2742, 1983

57. Rand JH, Sussman II, Gordon RE, et al: Localization of factor-VIII-related antigen in human vascular subendothelium. Blood 55:752–756, 1980

58. Sakariassen KS, Bolhuis PA, Sixma JJ: Human blood platelet adhesion to artery subendothelium is mediated by factor VIII-von Willebrand factor bound to subendothelium. Nature 279:636–638, 1979

59. Nachman RL, Jaffe EA: Subcellular platelet factor VIII antigen and von Willebrand factor. J Exp Med 191:1101–1113, 1975

59a. Fernanda Lopez Fernandez M, Ginsburg MH, Ruggeri ZM, et al: Multimeric structure of platelet factor VIII/von Willebrand factor: The presence of larger multimers and their re-association with thrombin-stimulated platelets. Blood 60:1132–1138, 1982

60. Kouts J, Walsh PN, Plow EF, et al: Active release of human platelet factor VIII-related antigen by adenosine diphosphate, collagen, and thrombin. J Clin Invest 62:1255–1263, 1978

60a. George JN, Onofre AR: Human platelet surface binding of endogenous secreted factor VIII-von Willebrand factor and platelet factor 4. Blood 59:194–197, 1982

61. Zimmerman TS, Ratnoff OD, Powell AE: Immunologic differentiation of classic hemophilia (factor VIII deficiency) and von Willebrand's disease with observations on combined deficiencies of antihemophilic factor and proaccelerin (factor V) and on an acquired circulating anticoagulant against antihemophilic factor. J Clin Invest 50:244–254, 1971

62. Bennett B, Forman WB, Ratnoff OD: Studies on the nature of antihemophilic factor (factor VIII). Further evidence relating the AHF-like antigens in normal and hemophilic plasmas. J Clin Invest 52:2191–2197, 1973

63. Fay PJ, Chavin SI, Marder VJ: Purification and characterization of the human factor VIII:C protein. Circulation 66(suppl 2):II-50, 1982 (abstract)

63a. Weinstein M, Fulcher C, Chute L, et al: Apparent molecular weight of purified human VIII:C compared with purified and plasma VIII:C antigen. Circulation 66(suppl 2):II-50, 1982 (abstract)

63b. Rotblat F, O'Brien DP, Middleton SM, et al: Purification and characterisation of human factor VIII:C. Thromb Haemostas 50:108, 1983 (abstract)

63c. Hamer RJ, Beeser-Visser NH, Sixma JJ: Purification of human factor VIII procoagulant protein. Thromb Haemostas 50:108, 1983 (abstract)

63d. Fulcher C, Gardner J, Griffin J, et al: Proteolysis of human factor VIII procoagulant protein with thrombin and activated protein C. Thromb Haemostas 50:351, 1983 (abstract)

64. Weiss HJ, Sussman II, Hoyer LW: Stabilization of factor VIII in plasma by the von Willebrand factor. J Clin Invest 60:390–404, 1977

65. Bloom AL: The von Willebrand syndrome. Semin Hematol 17:215–227, 1980

66. Bachman F: Diagnostic approach to mild bleeding disorders. Semin Hematol 17:292–305, 1980

67. Shoa'i I, Lavergne JM, Ardaillou N, et al: Heterogeneity of von Willebrand's disease: Study of 40 Iranian cases. Br J Haematol 37:67–83, 1977

68. Italian Working Group: Spectrum of von Willebrand's disease: A study of 100 cases. Br J Haematol 35:101–112, 1977

69. Nilsson IM, Blombäck M, Blombäck B: v. Willebrand's disease in Sweden, its pathogenesis and treatment. Acta Med Scand 164:263–278, 1959

69a. Mannucci PM, on behalf of the European Thrombosis Research Organization: Incidence of severe von Willebrand's disease in Western Europe and Israel. Thromb Haemostas 50:34, 1983 (abstract)

70. Mielke CH, Jr, Kaneshiro MM, Maher IA, et al: The standardized normal Ivy bleeding time and its prolongation by aspirin. Blood 34:204–215, 1969

71. Duke WW: The relation of blood platelets to hemorrhagic disease. JAMA 55:1185–1192, 1910

72. Borchgrevink CF, Egeberg O, Godal HC, et al: The effect of plasma and Cohn's fraction I on the Duke and Ivy bleeding times in von Willelbrand's disease. Acta Med Scand 173:235–242, 1963

73. Nilsson IM, Magnusson S, Borchgrevink C: The Duke and Ivy methods for determination of bleeding time. Thromb Diath Haemorrh 10:223–234, 1963

74. Ratnoff OD, Bennett B: Clues to the pathogenesis of bleeding in von Willebrand's disease. N Engl J Med 289, 1182–1183, 1973

75. Strauss HS, Bloom GE: Von Willebrand's disease. Use of a platelet-adhesiveness test in diagnosis and family investigation. N Eng J Med 273:171–181, 1965

76. Gralnick HR, Coller BS, Sultan Y: Studies of the human factor VIII/von Willebrand factor protein. III. Qualitative defects in von Willebrand's disease. J Clin Invest 56:814–827, 1975

77. Peake IR, Bloom AL, Giddings JC: Inherited variants of factor-VIII-related protein in von Willebrand's disease. N Engl J Med 291:113–117, 1974

78. Firkin B, Firkin F, Stott L: Von Willebrand's disease type B: A newly defined bleeding diathesis. Aust NZ J Med 3:225–229, 1973

79. Meyer D, Jenkins CSP, Dreyfus MD, et al: Willebrand factor and ristoceton. Br J Haematol 28:579–599, 1974

80. Bowie EJW, Fass DN, Olson JD, et al: The spectrum of von Willebrand's disease revisited. Mayo Clin Proc 51:35–41, 1976

81. Abildgaard CF, Suzuki Z, Harrison J, et al: Serial studies in von Willebrand's disease: Variability versus "variants." Blood 56:712–716, 1981
82. Girma J-P, Ardaillou N, Meyer D, et al: Fluid-phase immunoradiometric assay for the detection of qualitative abnormalities of factor VIII/von Willebrand factor in variants of von Willebrand's disease. J Lab Clin Med 93:296–939, 1979
83. Zimmerman, TS, Roberts J, Edgington TS: Factor-VIII-related antigen: Multiple molecular forms in human plasma. Proc Natl Acad Sci 72:5121–5125, 1975
84. Sultan Y, Simeon J, Caen JP: Electrophoretic heterogeneity of normal factor VIII/von Willebrand protein, and abnormal electrophoretic mobility in patients with von Willebrand's disease. J Lab Clin Med 87:185–197, 1976
85. Ruggeri ZM, Pareti FI, Mannucci PM, et al: Heightened interaction between platelets and factor VIII/von Willebrand factor in a new subtype of von Willebrand's disease. N Engl J Med 302:1047–1051, 1980
86. Weiss HJ, Hoyer LW, Rickles FR, et al: Quantitative assay of a plasma factor deficient in von Willebrand's disease that is necessary for platelet aggregation: Relationship to factor VIII procoagulant activity and antigen content. J Clin Invest 52:2708–2716, 1973
87. Brinkhous KM, Read MS: Preservation of platelet receptors for platelet aggregating factor/von Willebrand factor by air drying, freezing of lyophilization: new stable platelet preparations for von Willebrand factor assays. Thromb Res 13:591–597, 1978
88. Weiss HJ: Relation of von Willebrand factor to bleeding time. N Engl J Med 291:420, 1974 (letter)
89. Miller CH, Graham JB, Goldin LR, et al: Genetics of classic von Willebrand's disease. I. Phenotypic variation within families. Blood 54:117–136, 1979
90. Miller CH, Graham JB, Goldin LR, et al: Genetics of classic von Willebrand's disease. II. Optimal assignment of the heterozygous genotype (diagnosis) by discriminant analysis. Blood 54:137–145, 1979
91. Wahlberg TH, Blombäck M, Hall P, et al: Application of indicators, predictor and diagnostic indices in coagulation disorders. I. Evaluation of a self-administered questionnaire with binary questions. Meth Inform Med 19:194–200, 1980
92. Silwer J, Nilsson IM: On a Swedish family with 51 members affected by von Willebrand's disease. Acta Med Scand 175:627–643, 1964
93. Noller KL, Bowie EJW, Kempers RD, et al: Von Willebrand's disease in pregnancy. Obstet Gynecol 41:865–872, 1973
94. Telfer MC, Chediak, J: Factor-VIII-related disorders and their relationship to pregnancy. J Reprod Med 19:211–222, 1977
94a. Lipton RA, Ayromlooi J, Coller BS: Severe von Willebrand's disease during labor and delivery. JAMA 248:1355–1357, 1982
95. Nilsson IM: Haemorrhagic and Thrombotic Disease. New York, Wiley, 1971, pp 90–99
96. Ingram GIC: Classification of von Willebrand's disease. Lancet 2:1364–1365, 1978
97. Mannucci PM, Ruggeri ZM, Ciavarella N, et al: Precipitating antibodies to factor VIII/von Willebrand factor in von Willebrand's disease: Effects on replacement therapy. Blood 57:25–31, 1981
98. Zimmerman TS, Abildgaard CF, Meyer D: The factor VIII abnormality in severe von Willebrand's disease. N Engl J Med 301:1307–1310, 1979
99. Nachman RL, Jaffe EA, Miller C, et al: Structural analysis of factor VIII antigen in von Willebrand disease. Proc Natl Acad Sci USA 77:6832–6836, 1980
100. Sixma JJ, Over J, Bouma BN, et al: Predominance of normal low molecular weight forms of factor VIII in "variant" von Willebrand's disease. Thromb Res 12:929–935, 1978
101. Gralnick HR, Sultan Y, Coller BS: Von Willebrand's disease. Combined qualitative and quantitative abnormalities. N Engl J Med 296:1024–1030, 1977
102. Zimmerman TS, Voss R, Edgington TS: Carbohydrate of the factor VIII/von Willebrand factor in von Willebrand's disease. J Clin Invest 64:1298–1302, 1979

102a. DeMarco L, Shapiro SS: Properties of human asialo-factor VIII. A ristocetin-independent platelet-aggregating agent. J Clin Invest 68:321–328, 1981

103. Gralnick HR, Coller BS, Sultan Y: Carbohydrate deficiency of the factor VIII/von Willebrand factor protein in von Willebrand's disease variants. Science 192:56–59, 1976

103a. Ruggeri ZM, Nilsson IM, Lombardi R, et al: Aberrant multimeric structure of von Willebrand factor in a new variant of von Willebrand's disease (type IIC). J Clin Invest 70:1124–1127, 1982

104. Takahashi H: Studies on the pathophysiology and treatment of von Willebrand's disease. IV. Mechanism of increased ristocetin-induced platelet aggregation in von Willebrand's disease. Thromb Res 19:857–867, 1980

105. Weiss HJ, Meyer D, Rabinowitz R, et al: Pseudo-von Willebrand's disease. An intrinsic platelet defect with aggregation by unmodified human factor VIII/von Willebrand factor and enhanced adsorption of its high-molecular-weight multimers. N Engl J Med 306:326–333, 1982

106. Gralnick HR, Williams S, Shafer B, et al: Von Willebrand's disease with normal ristocetin-induced platelet aggregation: Abnormal platelets and abnormal factor VIII/von Willebrand factor protein. Blood 58:193a, 1981 (abstract)

107. Miller JL, Castella A: Platelet-type von Willebrand's disease: Characterization of a new bleeding disorder. Blood 60:790–794, 1982

108. Wall RT, Counts RB, Harker LA, et al: Binding and release of factor VIII/von Willebrand's factor by human endothelial cells. Br J Haematol 46:287–298, 1980

109. Nachman RL, Jaffe EA, Ferris B: Peptide map analysis of normal plasma and platelet factor VIII antigen. Biochem Biophys Res Commun 92:1208–1214, 1980

110. Coller BS, Hirschman RJ, Gralnick HR: Studies on the factor VIII/von Willebrand factor antigen on human platelets. Thromb Res 6:469–480, 1975

111. Howard MA, Montgomery DC, Hardisty RM: Factor-VIII-related antigen in platelets. Thromb Res 4:617–624, 1974

112. Meucci P, Peake IR, Bloom AL: Factor VIII-related activities in normal haemophilic and von Willebrand's disease platelet fractions. Thromb Haemost 40:288–301, 1980

113. Graham JB: Genetic control of factor VIII. Lancet 1:340–342, 1980

113a. Lynch DC, Williams R, Kirby E, et al: Mechanism of factor VIIIR (von Willebrand factor) synthesis by bovine endothelial cells. Clin Res 30:506A, 1982 (abstract)

113b. Harrison RL, McKee PA: Endothelial cell cytoplasmic von Willebrand factor is multimeric and functionally active. Circulation 66(suppl 3):II-176, 1982 (abstract)

113c. Wagner DD, Marder VJ: Biosynthesis of von Willebrand protein by human endothelial cells. Blood 60(suppl 1):244a, 1982 (abstract)

114. Pickering NJ, Brody JI, Barrett MJ: Von Willebrand syndromes and mitral-valve prolapse. N Engl J Med 305:131–134, 1981

114a. De Rosa V, Binetti G, Melandri G, et al: Mitral valve prolapse in patients with von Willebrand's disease. Thromb Haemostas 50:32, 1983 (abstract)

114b. White GC, II, McMillan CW, Roberts HR, et al: Normal incidence of mitral valve prolapse in patients with von Willebrand's disease. Thromb Haemostas 50:33, 1983 (abstract)

115. Legrand YJ, Fauvel F, Gurman N, et al: Microfibrils platelet interaction: Requirement of von Willebrand factor. Thromb Res 19:737–739, 1980 (letter)

116. Weiss HJ, Turitto VT, Baumgartner HR: Effect of shear rate on platelet interaction with subendothelium in citrated and native blood. I. Shear-dependent decrease of adhesion in von Willebrand's disease and the Bernard-Soulier syndrome. J Lab Clin Med 92:750–764, 1978

117. Fujimoto T, Ohara S, Hawiger J: Thrombin-induced exposure and prostacyclin inhibition of the receptor for factor VIII/von Willebrand factor on human platelets. J Clin Invest 69:1212–1222, 1982

117a. Fujimoto T, Hawiger J: Adenosine diphosphate induces binding of von Willebrand factor to human platelets. Nature 297:154–156, 1982

117b. Ruggeri ZM, Bader R, DeMarco L: Glanzmann's thrombasthenia: Deficient binding of von Willebrand factor to thrombin-stimulated platelets. Circulation 66(suppl 2):207, 1982 (abstract)

117c. Gralnick HR, Coller BS: Platelets stimulated with thrombin and ADP bind von Willebrand factor to different sites than platelets stimulated with ristocetin. Clin Res 31:482A, 1983 (abstract)

117d. Ruggeri ZM, de Marco L, Montgomery RR: Platelets have more than one binding site for von Willebrand factor Clin Res 31:322A, 1983 (abstract)

117e. Gralnick HR, Williams S, Coller B: Thrombin and ADP induced binding of vWf to platelets is related to glycoprotein GPIIb/IIIa. Thromb Haemostas 50:192, 1983 (abstract)

118. Nilsson IM, Holmberg L, Stenberg P, et al: Characteristics of the factor VIII protein and factor XIII in various factor VIII concentrates. Scand J Haematol 24:340–349, 1980

119. Weinstein M, Deykin D: Comparison of factor VIII-related von Willebrand factor proteins prepared from human cryoprecipitate and factor VIII concentrate. Blood 53:1095–1105, 1979

120. Ekert H, Chavin SI: Changes in electrophoretic mobility in human factor VIII-related antigen: Evidence for subunit structure. Br J Haematol 36:271–279, 1977

121. Mannucci PM, Pareti FI, Holmberg L, et al: Studies on the prolonged bleeding time in von Willebrand's disease. J Lab Clin Med 88:662–671, 1976

122. Ludlam CA, Peake IR, Allen N, et al: Factor VIII and fibrinolytic response to deamino-8-D-arginine vasopressin in normal subjects and dissociate response in some patients with haemophilia and von Willebrand's disease. Br J Haematol 45:499–511, 1980

123. Schmitz-Huebner U, Balleisen L, Arends P, et al: DDAVP-induced changes of factor VIII-related activities and bleeding time in patients with von Willebrand's syndrome. Haemostasis 9:204–213, 1980

124. Lowe G, Pettigrew A, Middleton S, et al: DDAVP in haemophilia. Lancet 2:614–615, 1977 (letter)

125. Theiss W, Schmidt G: DDAVP in von Willebrand's disease: Repeated administration and the behavior of the bleeding time. Thromb Res 13:1119–1123, 1978

126. Mennon C, Berry EW, Ockelford P: Beneficial effect of DDAVP on bleeding-time in von Willebrand's disease. Lancet 2:743–744, 1978 (letter)

127. Takahashi H, Sakuragawa N, Shibata A: Von Willebrand disease with an increased ristocetin-induced platelet aggregation and a qualitative abnormality of the factor VIII protein. Am J Hematol 8:299–308, 1980

128. Ruggeri ZM, Mannucci PM, Lombardi R, et al: Multimeric composition of factor VIII/von Willebrand factor following administration of DDAVP: Implications for pathophysiology and therapy of von Willebrand's disease subtypes. Blood 59:1272–1278, 1982

129. Weinger RS, Cecalupo AJ, Olson JD, et al: Neonatal von Willebrand's disease: Diagnostic difficulty at birth. Am J Dis Child 134:793–794, 1980

130. Alperin JB: Estrogens and surgery in women with von Willebrand's disease. Am J Med 73:367–371, 1982

131. Samama M, Lecrubier C, Conrad J, et al: Abnormal factor VIII-related-antigen, von Willebrand disease, and pregnancy. Lancet 1:151, 1976 (letter)

Sandor S. Shapiro

# 7

# Hemorrhagic Disorders Associated with Circulating Inhibitors

Disorders of hemostasis can result from inhibition of the normal hemostatic mechanism, as well as from deficiency of one of its components. Such inhibition occurs when antibodies against specific hemostatic components arise either as the result of replacement therapy in patients with coagulation factor deficiencies such as hemophilia A (classic hemophilia) or B (Christmas disease),[1] or spontaneously, in previously healthy individuals, in the presence or absence of accompanying disease.[2,3] Another commonly seen immunologic inhibitor, the so-called lupus anticoagulant,[4] can be a source of great difficulty in the diagnostic laboratory, despite the fact that it rarely causes a hemorrhagic diathesis. Hemorrhagic disorders may also arise because of the absence of one of the physiologically important plasma proteinase inhibitors, such as $\alpha_2$-antiplasmin[5] or activated protein C inhibitor.[6] Finally, in rare cases, acquired specific coagulation factor deficiencies may result from nonimmunologic mechanisms, such as the factor IX (Christmas factor) deficiency occurring in some individuals with massive nephrotic syndrome[7] or the factor X (Stuart factor) deficiency occurring in some individuals with amyloidosis.[8] This chapter will discuss the current concepts regarding pathogenesis, natural history, and treatment of such disorders. In each area the discussion will be selective and the bibliography limited to pertinent recent references. For a more complete treatment of each area, the reader should consult references 1–8.

## IMMUNOLOGIC INHIBITORS OF THE HEMOSTATIC MECHANISM

### Inhibitors Against Factors VIII and IX in Hemophilias A and B

One of the major complications of transfusion therapy in hemophilias A and B is the elicitation of an antibody to the infused coagulation factor. In hemophilia A this complication occurs in 5–10 percent of patients, whereas in hemophilia B it is seen in 1–3 per-

*Supported in part by NIH Grant HL-09163 from the National Heart, Lung and Blood Institute and by a grant from the Delaware Valley Chapter, National Hemophilia Foundation.

271

cent of patients.[1,9] In both diseases, the overwhelming majority of antibodies develop in patients with severe disease and factor VIII:C levels $\leq 0.03$ U/ml. Since severe disease occurs in approximately one-half of the patients with hemophilia A but in only one-third of those with hemophilia B, the prevalence of antibodies in patients with severe hemophilia A or B is not too dissimilar.[1] However, since hemophilia a is 5–6 times more common than hemophilia B, factor IX antibodies are actually encountered 5–10 times less frequently than factor VIII antibodies. As might be expected, data concerning factor IX antibodies are largely anecdotal, whereas it has been possible to collect a substantial amount of careful data on the occurrence and natural history of factor VIII antibodies. For this reason, the discussion to follow will be concerned largely with factor VIII antibodies in patients with hemophilia A.

Inhibitors to factor VIII in hemophilia A arise as a result of transfusion of factor VIII-containing materials, such as plasma, cryoprecipitate, or factor VIII concentrates. They react with the factor VIII coagulant portion of the factor VIII:C–von Willebrand factor complex, neutralizing factor VIII coagulant activity. Hemophiliacs with inhibitors have normal levels of factor VIII-related antigen (as measured with heterologous antiserum) and of ristocetin cofactor activity. The inhibitors are almost all immunoglobulins G (IgG) and are most frequently restricted in heterogeneity, usually composed of only a single light chain type and often showing a preponderance of a single IgG subtype.[10,11] Factor VIII antibody is measured by its ability to neutralize the coagulant activity of factor VIII when mixed with normal plasma or another source of factor VIII. A peculiarity of the neutralization reaction is the slowness with which factor VIII:C activity is neutralized in the test tube, this reaction commonly requiring at least 1.0–1.5 hours to complete. For this reason, laboratory tests are done with a minimum of two hours' incubation of patient plasma and factor VIII. Two methods are in common use, the so-called Bethesda[12] and the new Oxford[13] assays. In the Bethesda assay, patient plasma (or dilutions thereof) and a standard normal plasma are incubated at 37°C for two hours, after which factor VIII activity is measured. One Bethesda U/ml is that concentration which neutralizes 50 percent of the added factor VIII in two hours. In the new Oxford assay, patient plasma (or dilutions thereof) and factor VIII concentrate are incubated at 37°C for 4 hours, followed by factor VIII:C measurement. This incubation period was chosen because occasional inhibitors require more than 2 hours to neutralize factor VIII. One new Oxford U/ml is that concentration of inhibitor which neutralizes 50 percent of the added factor VIII in four hours. A recent comparative study of a series of antibody plasmas showed that the two methods classified the antibodies in the same order, although the results expressed in Bethesda units were about 20 percent higher than those expressed in new Oxford units.[14] Since the affinity of factor VIII antibodies for factor VIII seems to vary from patient to patient, both methods are somewhat arbitrary. Nevertheless, comparison of data would be much easier if all laboratories used the same technique.

Observations on inhibitor patients suggest that there may be at least two types of antibody response.[15,16] In most patients, high-titer antibodies occur ($>10$ Bethesda U/ml), making further replacement therapy with factor VIII impractical. If factor VIII therapy is withheld, antibody titers will drop over a variable period of months to years, but will rise again within 3–5 days of exposure to factor VIII, reaching peak levels within 10–20 days.[1] On the other hand, in a small group of inhibitor patients (10–25 percent), only low levels of antibodies arise (1–2 Bethesda U/ml), levels which tend not to increse after exposure to factor VIII. These patients can be placed on home therapy with factor VIII, albeit at slightly higher doses than would be used in an uncomplicated hemophiliac, and will respond well.

These two categories of response may not be biologically distinct, since low responders become high responders when exposed to high-intensity factor VIII therapy, such as might be required for an operative procedure.

A small percentage of factor VIII inhibitors arises in patients with mild hemophilia A who ordinarily receive little factor VIII. These inhibitors most frequently are seen following intensive factor VIII therapy, such as employed for operative procedures. The appearance of the inhibitor is associated with reduction of the circulating factor VIII:C and increased severity of the bleeding diathesis. These inhibitors, however, tend to be short-lived, usually disappearing within weeks to months of cessation of factor VIII therapy, and not recurring on subsequent treatment with more modest quantities of factor VIII. Inhibitors in severe hemophiliacs, on the other hand, tend to persist once formed, with only rare exceptions.[17,18]

The intensity and frequency of exposure to factor VIII in the hemophilic population are widely variable. It has been suggested that those individuals destined to form antibodies will have done so after a cumulative exposure to factor VIII of 50–100 days.[19] The American cooperative study found that, although one-third of antibodies were detected before age 10 and two-thirds before age 20, some multiply transfused hemopiliacs did not develop antibodies until well into adult life.[16,18] It is thus wise to measure factor VIII:C and factor VIII antibody levels on a regular basis in all hemophiliacs, at least once a year, and before any contemplated surgical procedure.

It is not clear why some, but not all, heavily transfused hemophiliacs become immunized to factor VIII:C. In a recently completed American study of the natural history of factor VIII antibodies in patients with hemophilia A, it was found that the occurrence of antibodies in brothers with this disease is nonrandom.[20] That is, hemophilic sibships in which more than one brother had an antibody or in which all brothers were antibody-free occurred more frequently than would have been predicted, on the basis of chance alone, from the overall frequency of factor VIII antibodies in the hemophilic population. Thus, some genetic factor, probably controlling a limb of the immunologic response, seems to be involved. Studies of histocompatibility antigens (HLA) in patients with and without antibodies have produced conflicting results. A European study of 57 multitransfused brothers from 26 families found no predictive significance to HLA markers,[21] whereas the American study[20] on 35 antibody formers and 105 hemophiliacs without antibodies showed a significantly decreased frequency of the HLA-A1 antigen in inhibitor patients (8.6 percent) as opposed to noninhibitor patients (36.2 percent). Although these data support the notion of a genetic component in antibody formation, they are not helpful in identifying patients at risk. A recent study has examined subtypes of complement components BF,C2, C4A, and C4B. The synthesis of these proteins is controlled by genes located, like the major histocompatibility locus, on chromosome 6.[22] It was found that a subtype of C4A was 2–3 times more frequent among antibody formers than among hemophiliacs without antibodies.[23] Although complement typing of patients with less than 0.03 U/ml of factor VIII:C thus can identify a subpopulation whose risk of antibody formation may be 1 in three, the goal of accurately identifying those patients prone to antibody formation has yet to be reached.

The management of a patient with a factor VIII antibody must be individualized.[24] A low responder may be treated for hemorrhagic episodes essentially like an uncomplicated hemophiliac. Similarly, surgery may be undertaken under cover of factor VIII, although it is important to bear in mind the possibility that the antibody level may increase to high titers 3–5 days following initiation of factor VIII therapy. High responders may be treated with factor VIII when their titers are below 5–10 Bethesda U/ml, with the expectation of normal hemostasis for at least 2–3 days. This period is generally adequate for the treatment of most serious hemorrhagic events. However, antibody titers will rise soon afterward making such an approach difficult for surgery, when 5–10 days of normal hemostasis are required. It is occasionally possible to combine this approach with plasmapheresis,[25,26] replacing withdrawn plasma with factor VIII concentrate, although the problem of the anamnestic response will still occur. Since factor VIII antibodies sometimes show striking species specificity, high-purity porcine factor VIII has been used successfully in several inhibitor patients.[27–30] The incidence of anamnestic rises in antibody titer after repeated use has been low.[28] Mild reactions, however, may occur,[29] and one severe anaphylactic reaction has been reported,[30] so that much more information will be required to assess this approach.

For these reasons, there has been great interest in the use of prothrombin complex concentrates (PCCs) in the treatment of patients with factor VIII antibodies. Although the active principle in these concentrates is still not known, their efficacy has been demonstrated in two controlled, double-blind studies in patients with hemophilia A and factor VIII antibodies. The American cooperative study of hemarthroses of the knee, ankle, and elbow demonstrated that single infusions of the so-called nonactivated PCCs, Konyne and Proplex, at a dose of 75 U/kg of factor IX, were effective in 50 percent of the bleeding episodes, as opposed to an albumin placebo.[31] The importance of the double-blind structure of the study was underscored by the finding that the albumin placebo was effective 25 percent of the time. Nevertheless, the difference between the drug and the placebo was highly statistically significant. A subsequent study compared an activated PCC, FEIBA (Immuno) to its nonactivated analogue.[32] The activated product was effective in approximately 65 percent of episodes, compared to 50 percent effectiveness for the nonactivated material. A recently completed study of the activated product Autoplex, compared with Proplex, showed no significant difference in the efficacy of the 2 products.[33] Activated products, therefore, seem only marginally more effective than their nonactivated counterparts. In view of the much greater cost of activated products, it seems reasonable to reserve them for patients not controlled by nonactivated PCCs, or patients with emergency, life-threatening bleeding. Clinical experience suggests that both types of product may be more effective when used several times, 4–8 hours apart.

In approximately 15 percent of treatments PCCs cause a rise in factor VIII antibody titer,[34] probably due to the presence in these preparations of factor VIII coagulant-related antigenic material,[35] but this response is not consistently seen in any particular patient or with specific lots of PCC. In order to decrease further the likelihood of antibody rises, when red cell replacement is necessary, it should be given in the form of 3 times washed red blood cells.[36] There have been occasional reports of thromboembolic complications or myocardial infarction after the use of PCCs,[24] primarily in patients receiving massive doses, much in excess of the recommended levels, or in patients with significant degrees of hepatic dysfunction (see Chapter 8).

Recently, attempts have been made to remove inhibitors by extracorporeal circulation over chromatographic columns of staphylococcal protein A bound to Sepharose.[37] These columns remove several subtypes of IgG and are not specific for coagulation factor antibodies. This novel approach is still in a preliminary stage, and it is too early to judge its effectiveness.

Two approaches have been used in an effort to eliminate established antibodies. Brackman et al.[38,39] have attempted to induce a stage of immunologic tolerance by treating patients with massive daily doses of factor VIII (75–100 U/kg/day), supplemented with large amounts of PCCs for periods of months to more than 1 year. Inhibitors eventually disappeared in 14 of 17 patients, but it is too early to know whether this state will be permanent in the face of continued rechallenge with factor VIII. The emotional and financial costs of this regimen are so great that careful documentation of its successful outcome must be achieved before it can be recommended for general use. In this regard, the recent report by Rizza and Matthews[40] is of great interest. These authors reported the long-term experience of the Oxford Haemophilia Centre in the treatment of bleeding episodes in 22 inhibitor patients with cryoprecipitate and factor VIII concentrates. The doses of factor VIII administered were much smaller than those given given by Brackman et al.[38,39] The 12 patients who required frequent treatment (once, up to several times monthly) showed a progressive decrease in antibody titer over the 3–5 years of observation. Perhaps some form of tolerance can be induced using frequent small infusions of factor VIII, if this regimen is continued long enough.

Attempts have also been made to eradicate factor VIII antibody-producing clones of lymphocytes through the use of a variety of immunosuppressive agents.[24] In general, such treatment has not been curative, although anamnestic responses may have been reduced in some patients. Occasionally, usually in individuals treated at the time of antibody detection or shortly thereafter, antibodies have disappeared after administration of drugs, particularly cyclophosphamide.[17] Since antibodies occasionally disappear spontaneously, however,[17,18] it is difficult to be certain that such cases represent cures.

Similar considerations apply to patients with hemophilia B and factor IX antibodies. Factor IX antibodies occur almost exclusively in patients with severe hemophilia B and tend to persist once elicited.[1] The few antibodies studied by immunologic techniques have all been IgG, but have shown greater heterogeneity than hemophilic factor VIII antibodies.[41,42] Factor IX antibodies are measured by techniques analogous to those used for factor VIII antibodies. However, antibody neutralization of factor IX activity is much more rapid than that seen with factor VIII, and the incubation period in the assay can be reduced to one hour. The approaches to treatment are similar to those outlined for patients with factor VIII antibodies. PCCs appear to be useful in this setting as well, although little of this experience has been published. Of course, when PCCs are used in hemophilia B patients with factor IX antibodies, an increase in antibody titer can be expected.[43]

## Inhibitors Against Factors VIII and IX in Nonhemophilic Individuals

Several hundred cases have been reported of factor VIII inhibitors occurring in nonhemophilic individuals, particularly in postpartum women, in patients with a variety of drug reactions and diseases with prominent immunological components, and in males and females with no apparent underlying disease.[1–3]

There are at least 33 reports in the literature of postpartum women who developed a hemorrhagic diathesis due to a factor VIII inhibitor.[1,41,44] The inhibitor generally occurred within weeks to months of delivery of a normal child of either sex. In all but a few instances, the affected women had no underlying disorder. The course has been highly variable: Most inhibitors have disappeared within 12–18 months, although some have been documented for as long as 11 years. In 9 women whose inhibitor had disappeared, a subsequent pregnancy was not associated with its reappearance.[1,44] In a 10th case, the inhibitor reappeared in a subsequent pregnancy.[3] The pathogenesis of postpartum inhibitors is not known. It has been suggested that allotypes of factor VIII may exist and that this syndrome results from maternal sensitization to a paternal allotype transmitted to the fetus, with subsequent cross-reaction with the mother's own factor VIII.[1] On the basis of available date,[44] this hypothesis is unlikely.

Factor VIII inhibitors have been reported in patients with lupus erythematosus, rheumatoid arthritis, and other autoimmune disorders,[1-3,45,46] in patients with a variety of dermatologic diseases,[1-3] in patients with malignancies, particularly lymphocytic disorders,[3,45,47] and in drug reactions, predominantly those related to penicillin and ampicillin,[1-3,45] as well as in individuals with no apparent underlying disease. [1-3,45,48] In nearly all cases, the inhibitor was discovered because of the onset of a hemorrhagic diathesis.

Factor VIII inhibitors in nonhemophilic individuals are almost all IgG immunoglobulins, but are more heterogeneous than the antibodies present in patients with hemophilia A, with respect to light chain type and heavy chain subtype.[10] In addition, although some nonhemophilic antibodies resemble those seen in hemophilia A with respect to factor VIII neutralization, many neutralize factor VIII with more complex kinetics.[45] Patients with antibodies of the latter kind frequently have measurable plasma factor VIII coexistent with measurable antibody titers.[45] Recent evidence suggests that some of these antibodies combine with factor VIII near, but not at, the coagulant active site, such that factor VIII–antibody complexes still retain some in vitro coagulant activity.[49] Such complexes may have limited in vivo activity, since nonhemophilic patients with factor VIII antibodies and plasma factor VIII levels of 0.04–0.19 U/ml have had episodes of spontaneous bleeding.[45] Spontaneous hemorrhage rarely occurs in uncomplicated hemophiliacs at similar factor VIII levels.

The course of the inhibitors is very variable.[3] In the absence of therapy, about one-third eventually disappear, usually within 12–18 months, but antibodies have disappeared spontaneously as long as 48 months after onset.[3] These results reflect a minority of patients who have not experienced any severe bleeding episodes. In patients with significant bleeding, corticosteroids and other immunosuppressive agents have been used. Treatment with corticosteroids alone may be effective in one-third of patients,[3,50] particularly in children and postpartum women.[3] Responses occur within 4–6 weeks, and frequently within 1–2 weeks. In an additional group of patients, corticosteroids may cause a decline in inhibitor levels.[3,50] In one large series, addition of azathioprine or cyclophosphamide to corticosteroids, frequently with a large intravenous bolus of factor VIII, resulted in the decline or disappearance of one-half of the inhibitors so treated.[3] This approach may be most beneficial in patients whose antibody titer is less than 10 Bethesda U/ml when treatment is initiated.[3,46] In sum, although these data are difficult to evaluate fully, it appears that 30–40 percent of all nonhemophilic inhibitors eventually disappear, either spontaneously or after drug therapy.

Treatment of bleeding can be accomplished either with factor VIII, if inhibitor titers are below 5–10 Bethesda U/ml, or with PCCs. Although it has been suggested that anamnestic rises in antibody titer should not occur in nonhemophiliacs, whose antibody production ought to be maximally stimulated by their continuous production of factor VIII, such rises definitely do occur.[1,47]

In contract to factor VIII inhibitors, the occurrence of factor IX inhibitors in nonhemophilic individuals has been reported only 9 times.[1,51,52] The inhibitors have arisen in settings similar to those seen with nonhemophilic factor VIII inhibitors.

## Inhibitors Against the von Willebrand Factor

Antibodies directed against the von Willebrand factor portion of the factor VIII:C–von Willebrand factor complex have been reported in 9 patients with severe congenital von Willebrand's disease as a result of transfusion therapy.[55-59] The antibodies, all polyclonal IgG, blocked ristocetin cofactor activity and, in 6 cases, [56-59] showed a precipitin reaction in gel diffusion against von Willebrand factor-related antigen. The antibodies did not react specifically with the coagulant portion of the VIII:C–von Willebrand factor complex. Results of therapy have been reported in 4 of these patients.[60] Cryoprecipitate infusions successfully raised VIII:C levels, perhaps accounting for the satisfactory response seen in joint or soft tissue hemorrhages. The bleeding time, however, was not corrected, and treatment of mucosal bleeding was unsatisfactory. In all instances, infusions were complicated by severe side effects, including lumbar and abdominal pain and hypotension. These effects were seen soon after infusion began and persisted for several hours. Corticosteroids were useful in ameliorating these symptoms. Indirect evidence suggests that these symptoms were due to the appearance in the circulation of large amounts of immune complexes.

A syndrome of acquired von Willebrand's disease has been reported on at least 24 occasions in the past 15 years.[61-77] Most of these individuals had an underlying lymphoproliferative or autoimmune disorder. Bleeding symptoms have generally been those seen in mild to moderate von Willebrand's disease. Characteristically, the bleeding time is prolonged and components of the factor VIII complex are depressed. Although infusion of cryoprecipitate often causes a rise in level of the factor VIII complex, the rise in transient at best. Electrophoretic studies have shown a relative lack of the highest molecular weight von Willebrand factor polymers in the plasma and preferential removal of these same polymers after cryoprecipitate infusion.[71,75,77] Despite the in vivo findings, it has been difficult to show inhibition of VIII:C or ristocetin cofactor activities in the test tube. In two studies, the addition of protein A-Sepharose to a mixture of patient and normal plasma resulted in removal of factor VIII complex activities after centrifugation, strongly suggesting that soluble IgG-factor VIII complexes had formed in the mixture.[72,77] In several cases the inhibitor has been characterized as an immunoglobulin,[62,64,65,67,70,74] and in several more an M component has been present,[72,77] although it has not proven to be the inhibitor.

In two patients the inhibitor disappeared after treatment, in one after radiation therapy for lymphoma[71] and in the other after surgical resection of a Wilms' tumor.[76]

## Inhibitors Against Other Coagulation Factors

Factor V (proaccelerin) inhibitors have been reported in 17 individuals,[1,41,78-80] only one of whom was congenitally deficient in factor V. In 11 of the remaining 16, the inhibitor appeared within 1–3 weeks of a surgical procedure. In at least 7 of these 11 cases, the postoperative course was complicated by sepsis. An additional nonsurgical patient had a recent unspecified infection that had been treated with tetracycline for three weeks. Two nonsurgical patients had tuberculosis; one of these had been treated with streptomycin. Streptomycin had also been administered in 5 of the 10 surgical patients, and 1 additional individual had a more remote history of 3 years of treatment with streptomycin for tuberculosis.

The presence of an inhibitor to factor V causes prolongation of the prothrombin, partial thromboplastin, and Russell's viper venom times. Plasma factor V is less than 10 percent, and usually is undetectable. Mixing of patient plama with normal plasma causes loss of factor V from the normal plasma.

Both IgG and IgM inhibitors have been reported. They tend to be of low titer and are usually associated with mild bleeding. Several patients, however, have exhibited a severe bleeding diathesis, and three have died of bleeding.[1,41] Of the remaining 14 inhibitors, at least 10 disappeared within 9 months of onset, 3 without any therapy and 7 after treatment with adrenocorticotropic hormone (ACTH), corticosteroids, or some form of immunosuppressive chemotherapy. It is thus not clear whether these drugs influenced the natural history of this disease.

If bleeding is severe enough to require treatment, fresh frozen plasma may be of benefit in some patients with low-titer inhibitors. Frequently, however, plasma treatment is ineffective. In one recently reported case, [80] platelet transfusions were associated with an excellent clinical response as well as with shortening of prolonged clotting tests, an increase in plasma factor V levels from 2–4 to 8–10 percent, and disappearance of the inhibitor. These effects lasted for 5–6 days. In contrast, infusion of fresh frozen plasma had no corrective effect. Whether these effects are due to the hemostatic action of the infused platelets[81] or to the removal of antibody by platelet-associated factor V[82] is not clear. In either case, this approach should be considered in factor V patients who are not responding to plasma infusions.

Specific inhibitors against coagulation factors other than factors VIII, IX, or V have rarely been reported. In many cases, they have occurred in patients with laboratory or clinical evidence of systemic lupus erythematosus (SLE). An inhibitor against factor VII has been reported only once, [83] in a 66-year-old man with a pulmonary neoplasm, no clinical evidence of SLE, but elevated titers of antinuclear antibody and positive lupus erythematosus preparations. The partial thromboplastin time was normal, but the prothrombin time was 20 seconds (control 12.2 seconds) and was not corrected by infusion of 2 Units of fresh frozen plasma. The inhibitor was probably an IgG, and the neutralization of factor VII in vitro was complete within 5 minutes. Specific assays for factors XII, XI, X, IX, VIII, and V were normal. Little bleeding was noted in this patient.

Two inhibitors against factor X have been reported,[84] but neither fulfills the criteria for a specific inhibitor. Both occurred in patients with leprosy. There was no evidence of amyloidosis (see the section on rapid in vivo disappearance of coagulative factors without in vitro evidence of an inhibitor). Neither patient had a bleeding diathesis. One of these patients had depressed levels of factors IX, XI, and XII, as well as factor X, and probably had a lupus anticoagulant (see the section on lupus anticoagulants). The other patient had low factor X in assays using Russell's viper venom, but not in assays using tissue thromboplastin. In addition, normal levels of factor X were measured immunologically. It is possible that this patient had a lupus anticoagulant, or that an antibody was present that combined with factor X and preferentially hindered its activation with Russell's viper venom, but not with tissue thromboplastin.

Inhibitors against factor XI (plasma thromboplastin antecedent PTA) have occurred in at least six patients with congenital factor XI deficiency, although only two of these have been reported,[1,85] and only one has been investigated by modern techniques.[85] This inhibitor was a polyclonal IgG with predominance of the IgG4 subclass. It was a high-titer antibody associated with unmeasurable levels of factor XI and moderately severe bleeding without antecedent trauma. Eleven factor XI inhibitors have been reported in individuals without congenital factor XI deficiency,[1,41,86–89] all females. Of these, nine had SLE,[1,41,86,89] one had rheumatoid arthritis and disseminated intravascular coagulation,[88] and one, a three-year-old child, developed an inhibitor following a respiratory infection. In most of these cases factor XII was also moderately depressed but this may have been an artifact of measurement. Inhibitory activity could be detected by mixing experiments in vitro in all cases but one,[89] in which evidence strongly suggested the presence of an IgG antibody combining with, but not neutralizing, factor XI. Presumably, the depressed level of factor XI in this patient (less than 2 percent) was due to rapid clearance of the factor

XI–antibody complex. Factor XII (Hageman factor) inhibitors have been reported only twice,[41,90] once in a male and once in a female. The female had SLE,[41] and the male had minimal-change glomerulonephritis.[90]

Hypoprothrombinemia has been noted in some patients with SLE and a lupus antico-agulant (see the section on lupus anticoagulants), but the mechanism is poorly understood. In those patients so studied, immunoreactive prothrombin and functional prothrombin levels were equally depressed. Despite lack of in vitro evidence of prothrombin neutralization, infusion of plasma or concentrates has not increased prothrombin levels.[91,92] In at least one case, hypoprothrombinemia was due to the presence of an antibody combining with, but not neutralizing, prothrombin, presumably resulting in rapid disappearance of the immune complex.[91] In another, the patient's plasma showed precipitin activity against purified thrombin, and the patient's gamma globulin fraction prolonged the thrombin time of normal plasma.[92] One other case of an antibody to prothrombin has been reported.[93] The patient was a 73-year-old woman, with no previous bleeding history, who bled after dental extraction. Her gamma globulin fraction bound to and neutralized the clotting and amidolytic activity of thrombin, and bound to prothrombin as well. As with the SLE patients, this patient's inhibitor cleared on treatment with corticosteroids and immunosuppressive chemotherapy.

Inhibitors against fibrinogen have been reported in 8 individuals.[1,94–96] Two have been patients with a probable diagnosis of congenital afibrinogenemia.[1] Two cases occurred in patients with SLE,[94] 1 occurred in a patient with chronic aggressive hepatitis, postnecrotic cirrhosis, and ulcerative colitis,[95] and one was found in a patient with Down's syndrome[96]; all 4 were females, 3 under the age of 15. Five of the antibodies were characterized as IgG, two of which[94] were restricted in their heterogeneity (one an $IgG_3\kappa$ and one an $IgG_1\lambda$). One antibody interfered with the rate of release of fibrinopeptide A from fibrinogen, although not with the enzymatic activity of thrombin.[96] Some patients have had a bleeding disorder, usually mild[1,95,96]; others have had no bleeding.[94] One antibody disappeared spontaneously within five months.[96] In the other cases, data are insufficient to document the natural history of the syndrome.

At least 10 cases have been reported of inhibitors interfering with the action of activated factor XIII, the enzyme covalently cross-linking the fibrin polymer.[1,41,97,98] Only one has occurred in an individual congenitally deficient in factor XIII. Inhibitors can be classified into 3 types:[98] those interfering with activation of factor XIII (type 1), those interfering with the enzymatic function of activated factor XIII (type II), and those directed against the cross-linking sites on fibrin, preventing access by the enzyme (type III). Bleeding, usually severe, has been present in all cases. Five patients had received isoniazid prior to inhibitor development,[1,41] and one developed the inhibitor as part of an SLE-like syndrome induced by the beta-adrenergic antagonist, practolol.[97] Plasma therapy has not been very successful, probably because of the high titer of the inhibitor in most cases.[1] There is no clear evidence that immunosuppressive therapy has been useful.[1] In 3 patients[1,97] drug withdrawal eventually resulted in disappearance of the inhibitor.

## Lupus Anticoagulants

The term *lupus anticoagulant* was coined by Feinstein and Rapaport [99] for a coagulation inhibitor, recognized since 1951, occurring in about 10 percent of patients with SLE, in persons with other diseases, and in individuals with no detectable underlying disorder. This subject has been reviewed recently,[91] and the reader is referred to that publication for greater detail.

At present, lupus anticoagulants are best defined as inhibitors which interfere to a variable degree with phospholipid-dependent coagulation tests, without inhibiting the activity of any specific coagulation factor.[91] Thus, the prothrombin time, partial thromboplastin time, Russell's viper venom time, and 1-stage coagulation factor assays based on these tests may all be abnormal. Prolongation of the partial thromboplastin and Russell's viper venom times are very common. Prolongation of the prothrombin time is less common, and a significantly prolonged prothrombin time should suggest the presence of hypoprothrombinemia, which may be present in as many as 25 percent of patients.[91] Severe hypoprothrombinemia (prothrombin below 20 percent) is very uncommon, however. Several tests have been used to identify lupus anticoagulants,[100] and their relative sensitivity is unknown. Whereas the prothrombin time is relatively insensitive and is not usually grossly prolonged, performance of this assay with diluted thromboplastin [101] forms the basis of a widely used screening test. However, not all lupus anticoagulants give abnormal results in this dilute thromboplastin system.[91] In our hands, the most useful assay has been the Russell's viper venom time, when performed with limiting amounts of venom and phospholipid.[100] In addition to an abnormal test, confirmation of the presence of an inhibitor requires demonstration of the inhibition of normal plasma coagulation tests in a mixture of patient and normal plasma. Because the inhibitor interferes with phospholipid-dependent tests, specific assays for coagulation factors, especially those based on the partial thromboplastin time, such as assays for factors XII, XI, IX, and VIII, may be artifactually low. Characteristically, clotting times in these assays approach normal the higher the dilution of patient plasma. This phenomenon has undoubtedly been responsible for some of the published reports of inhibitors directed against factors XI and XII in SLE.

Recent studies[91] have shown that most lupus anticoagulants in SLE and other conditions are immunoglobulins with specificity toward phospholipids carrying a net negative charge. These phospholipids—primarily phosphatidylserine, phosphatidylethanolamine, and phosphatidic acid—are very potent, in micellar form, in test tube coagulation by supporting prothrombin activation on their surfaces. Several lupus anticoagulants have now been shown to inhibit the binding of prothrombin to micelles containing anionic phospholipids.[91] This mechanism also explains the high correlation of false-positive serologic tests for syphilis with the presence of a lupus anticoagulant, since cardiolipin, the reagent most commonly used in these serologic tests, is itself an anionic phospholipid.[91] This mechanism, however, does not appear to explain all cases. First, at least one report suggests that the lupus anticoagulants may be a heterogeneous group of inhibitors against factors XII, XI, and X.[102] Second, patients on long-term chlorpromazine, who have a very high prevalence of lupus inhibitors,[103-105] have a very low prevalence of positive serologies,[105] suggesting that, despite the similarities in coagulation test results, the mechanism in this group of patients may be different.

Despite the abnormalities of coagulation tests, bleeding related solely to the presence of a lupus anticoagulant is rarely, if ever, seen.[91,106] In all probability, this is due to the fact that platelets are capable of supporting prothrombin conversion, and probably other analogous reactions. even in the presence of a lupus anticoagulant.[91] In keeping with this, substitution of washed platelets, treated with calcium ionophore, for phospholipid normalizes abnormal tests and usually gives rise to normal specific factor assays in cases where phospholipid-dependent assays are low. Correction of phospholipid-dependent tests by substitution of platelets is probably a good confirmatory test for most lupus anticoagulants;[100] a lupus anticoagulant that was neutralized by lysed, but not by intact, washed platelets has been described.[107] A recent case has been reported in which the anticoagulant inhibited prothrombin conversion in purified systems in the presence of either phospholipid or platelets.[108]

The most intriguing observation concerning patients with lupus anticoagulants, made by several authors, concerns the high prevalence of thromboembolic phenomena. When reported series are collected, 27 percent of patients are found to have had at least one thromboembolic episode, a figure three times higher than that reported for SLE patients without lupus anticoagulants.[91] Although the explanation for this is not known, it has recently been reported that plasma from patients with a thromboembolic history inhibits prostacyclin production by vascular tissue.[91,109] It will be of great interest to extend these studies to larger numbers of patients with SLE, with and without lupus anticoagulants.

## Rapid in Vivo Disappearance of Coagulation Factors without in Vitro Evidence of an Inhibitor

The inability to correct an isolated coagulation factor deficiency by the infusion of plasma or plasma fractions usually signifies the presence of an inhibitor. Corroboration is generally sought by in vitro mixing experiments: The suspected inhibitor plasma should prolong the coagulation tests of normal plasma. However, several situations exist in which in vitro inhibition cannot be demonstrated. For example, antibodies may be present which combine with a coagulation factor without neutralizing its activity. In such cases, immune complexes may be cleared rapidly, resulting in an isolated coagulation factor deficiency uncorrectable by plasma infusion. At least two cases of this type have been reported, both of which were described earlier in this chapter: one was an antibody to prothrombin,[91] the other an antibody to factor XI.[89] How frequently this phenomenon occurs is presently unknown.

The in vivo appearance of an inhibitor without in vitro corroboration can also occur due to nonimmunologic loss of a coagulation factor from the circulation. For example, factor IX deficiency has been seen in patients with the nephrotic snydrome and massive proteinuria due to the loss of factor IX in the urine.[7] Another example is the deficiency of factor X seen in some patients with amyloidosis.[8] Although several hemostatic defects have been seen in patients with amyloidosis, factor X deficiency appears to be due to the ability of amyloid fibrils from some individuals to bind factor X relatively specifically,[8,110,111] In both of these situations, infusion of plasma or concentrates produces less than the expected yield and half-life for the coagulation factor.

## BLEEDING SYNDROMES DUE TO ABSENCE OF PLASMA COAGULATION OR FIBRINOLYTIC ENZYME INHIBITORS

Bleeding disorders can arise due to the unopposed action of the fibrinolytic system and, possibly, of other enzymes capable of inactivating coagulation factors. The former situation occurs when the physiologic inhibitor of plasmin, $\alpha_2$-antiplasmin,[5] is absent. The latter condition is exemplified by the absence of the plasma inhibitor of activated protein C[6], which may give rise to the syndrome of combined factor V and factor VIII deficiency.

### $\alpha_2$-Antiplasmin Deficiency

$\alpha_2$-Antiplasmin is the major inhibitor of plasmin,[5] and is normally present in plasma at concentrations of 5–7 mg/dl.[112] It is probably synthesized in the liver, since patients with several forms of liver disease may have low levels of $\alpha_2$-antiplasmin, usually in the range of 1.5–5.0 mg/dl.[7] It may also be synthesized by megakaryocytes, since platelets contain this inhibitor.[113] Congenital deficiency of $\alpha_2$-antiplasmin has been reported in at least four kindreds, affecting both males and females. The disorder is transmitted autosomally, and homozygotes in three of the four kindreds[114,115,117] have had a severe hemorrhagic diathesis characterized by spontaneous hemarthroses, subcutaneous hemorrhage, and prolonged bleeding from cuts. The fourth kindred[115] consists of three sisters, all under five years of age, who had umbilical bleeding in the neonatal period and suffer primarily from gum bleeding, epistaxis, and subcutaneous hematomas after trauma. However, since spontaneous hemarthroses did not appear in the other homozygotes[114,115,117] until a slightly older age, it is too early to comment on the possible variability in the clinical manifestations of this disorder. Absence of $\alpha_2$-antiplasmin gives rise to rapid whole blood clot lysis[118] but, surprisingly, is not associated with hypofibrinogenemia or low levels of factors V or VIII.[114-117] In at least one kindred,[115] use of the fibrinolytic inhibitor tranexamic acid has been reported to be effective in controlling bleeding episodes. Of particular interest is the observation that heterozygotes with half-normal levels of $\alpha_2$-antiplasmin may have a mild hemorrhagic disorder, manifested by bleeding after surgery or tooth extractions and easy bruising after slight trauma.[115,117]

## Protein C Inhibitor Deficiency

Protein C is a vitamin K-dependent zymogen capable of being activated to a serine protease.[119,120] The active enzyme inactivates factors V and VIII in the presence of phospholipid and calcium ions.[121-123] Protein C activation is a physiologically significant reaction, since congenital deficiency of protein C is associated with a thrombotic disorder.[124] Plasma contains an inhibitor of activated protein C which is distinct from other known protease inhibitors.[6] In 4 unrelated cases of combined factor V and VIII deficiency, a bleeding disorder reported at least 30 times,[125,126] this inhibitory activity was undetectable.[6] This mechanism for a combined deficiency of 2 coagulation factors is very appealing, although a recent study of 4 other unrelated cases found normal levels of activated protein C inhibitory activity.[127]

## REFERENCES

1. Shapiro SS: Acquired inhibitors to the blood coagulation factors. Semin Thromb Hemost 1:336–385, 1975
2. Lechner K: Acquired inhibitors in non-hemophilic patients. Haemostasis 3:65–93, 1974
3. Green D, Lechner K: A survey of 215 non-hemophilic patients with inhibitors to factor VIII. Thromb Haemost 45:200–203, 1981
4. Shapiro SS, Thiagarajan P: Lupus anticoagulants. Prog Hemost Thromb 6:263–285, 1982
5. Lijnen HR, Collen D: Interactions of plasminogen activators and inhibitors with plasminogen and fibrin. Semin Thromb Hemostas 8:2–10, 1982
6. Marlar RA, Griffin JH: Deficiency of protein C inhibitor in combined factor V/VIII deficiency disease. J Clin Invest 66:1186–1189, 1980
7. Natelson EA, Lynch EC, Hettig RA, et al: Acquired factor IX deficiency in the nephrotic syndrome. Ann Intern Med 73:373–378, 1970
8. Greipp PR, Kyle RA, Bowie EJW: Factor-X deficiency in amyloidosis: A critical review. Am J Hematol 11:443–450, 1981
9. Eyster ME, Lewis JH, Shapiro SS, et al: The Pennsylvania Hemophilia Program 1973–1978. Am J Hematol 9:277–286, 1980
10. Allain JP, Gaillandre A, Lee, H: Immunochemical characterization of antibodies to factor VIII in hemophilic and nonhemophilic patients. J Lab Clin Med 97:791–800, 1981

11. Kavanagh ML, Wood CN, Davidson JF: The immunological characterization of human antibodies to factor VIII isolated by immuno-affinity chromatography. Thromb Haemost 45: 60–64, 1981

12. Kasper CK, Aledort LM, Counts RB, et al: A more uniform measurement of factor VIII inhibitors. Thromb Diath Haemorrh 34:869–872, 1975

13. Rizza CR, Biggs R: The treatment of patients who have factor VIII antibodies. Br J Haematol 24:65–82, 1973

14. Austen DEG, Lechner K, Rizza CR, et al: A comparison of the Bethesda and New Oxford methods of factor VIII antibody assay. Thromb Haemost 47:72–75, 1982

15. Allain JP, Frommel D: Antibodies to factor VIII. V. Patterns of immune response to factor VIII in hemophilia A. Blood 47:973–982, 1976

16. Gill FM, Shapiro SS, Poole WK, et al: The natural history of factor VIII inhibitors in patients with hemophilia A, a national cooperative study. I. Characteristics of the population. Submitted

17. Hultin MB, Shapiro SS, Bowman HS, et al: Immunosuppressive therapy of factor VIII inhibitors. Blood 48:95–108, 1976

18. McMillan CW, Shapiro SS, Lazerson J, et al: The natural history of factor VIII inhibitors in patients with hemophilia A, a national cooperative study. II. Observations on the initial development of factor VIII inhibitors. Submitted

19. Strauss HS: Acquired circulating anticoagulants in hemophilia A. N Engl J Med 281:866–873, 1969

20. Shapiro SS, Poole WK, Hemophilia Study Group: The natural history of factor VIII inhibitors in patients with hemophilia A, a national cooperative study. III. Evidence for genetic determinants of the immune response to factor VIII. Submitted

21. Frommel D, Allain JP, Saint-Paul E, et al: HLA antigens and factor VIII antibody in classic hemophilia. Thromb Haemost 46:687–689, 1981

22. Alper CA, Awdeh ZL, Raum D: Complement loci of the major histocompatibility complex, in Zaleski MB, Abeyounis CJ, Kano K (eds): Immunobiology of the Major Histocompatibility Complex. New York, Karger, 1981, pp 174–191

23. Raum D, Awdeh Z, Shapiro SS, et al: Major histocompatibility complex-linked immune response genes in man. Clin Res 30:508A, 1982. (abstract)

24. Kasper CK: Management of inhibitors to factor VIII. Prog Hematol 12:143–163, 1981

25. Wensley RT, Stevens RF, Bevin AM, et al: Plasma exchange and human factor VIII concentrate in managing haemophilia A with factor VIII inhibitors. Br Med J 281:1388–1389, 1980

26. Francesconi M, Korninger C, Thaler E, et al: Plasmapheresis: Its value in the management of patients with antibodies to factor VIII. Haemostasis 11:79–86, 1982

27. Mayne EE, Madden M, Crothers IS, et al: Highly purified porcine factor VIII in haemophilia A with inhibitors to factor VIII. Br Med J 282:318, 1981

28. Kernoff PBA, Thomas ND, Lilley PA, et al: Clinical experience with polyelectrolyte-fractionated porcine factor VIII concentrate in the treatment of haemophiliacs with antibodies to factor VIII. Br J. Haematol 49:131–132, 1981. (abstract)

29. Kernoff PBA, Tuddenham EGD: Reactions to low-molecular-weight porcine factor VIII concentrates. Br Med J 283:381–382, 1981

30. Erskine JG, Davidson JF: Anaphylactic reaction to low-molecular-weight porcine factor VIII concentrate. Br Med J 282:2011–2012, 1981

31. Lusher JM, Shapiro SS, Palascak JE, et al: Prothrombin complex concentrates in hemophiliacs with inhibitors— a multicenter therapeutic trial. N Eng J Med 303:421–425, 1980

32. Sjamsoedin LJM, Heijnen L, Manser-Bunschoten EP, et al: The effect of activated prothrombin-complex concentrate (FEIBA) on joint and muscle bleeding in patients with hemophilia A and antibodies to factor VIII, a double-blind clinical trial. N Eng J Med 305:717–721, 1981

33. Lusher J, Blatt PM, Penner JA, et al: Autoplex vs. Proplex: A controlled double-blind study of effectiveness in acute hemarthroses in hemophiliacs with inhibitors. Blood (in press)

34. Kasper CK, Hemophilia Study Group: Effect of prothrombin complex concentrates on factor VIII inhibitor levels. Blood 54:1358–1368, 1979

35. Onder O, Hoyer LW: Factor VIII coagulant antigen in factor IX complex concentrates. Thromb Res 15:569–572, 1979

36. Laurian Y, Girma JP, Allain JP, et al: Absence of anamnestic response after transfusion of washed red blood cells in haemophilia A patients with antibody to factor VIII. Scand J Haematol 28:233–237, 1982

37. Nilsson IM, Jonsson S, Sundqvist S, et al: A procedure for removing high titer antibodies by extracorporeal protein-A–sepharose adsorption in hemophilia: Substitution therapy and surgery in a patient with hemophilia B and antibodies. Blood 58:38–44, 1981

38. Brackmann HH, Etzel F, Hofmann P, et al: The successful treatment of acquired inhibitors against factor VIII. Thromb Haemostas 38:369, 1977 (abstract)

39. Brackman HH, Egli H: The treatment of haemophilia patients with inhibitors, in Seligsohn U, Rimon A, Horroszowski H (eds): Haemophilia, Tunbridge Wells, Castle House, 1981, pp 113–119.

40. Rizza CR, Matthews JM: Effect of frequent factor VIII replacement on the level of factor VIII antibodies in haemophiliacs. Br J Haematol 52:13–24, 1982

41. Shapiro SS: Antibodies to blood coagulation factors. Clin Haematol 8:207–214, 1979

42. Orstavik KH: Alloantibodies to factor IX in haemophilia B characterized by crossed immunoelectrophoresis and enzyme-conjugated antisera to human immunoglobulins. Br J Haematol 28:15–23, 1981

43. Penner JA, Kelly PE: Management of patients with factor VIII or IX inhibitors. Sem Thromb Hemostas 1:386–399, 1975

44. Coller BS, Hultin MB, Hoyer LW, et al: Normal pregnancy in a patient with a prior postpartum factor VIII inhibitor: With observations on pathogenesis and prognosis. Blood 58:619–624, 1981

45. Allain JP, Gaillandre A, Frommel D: Acquired haemophilia: Functional study of antibodies to factor VIII. Thromb Haemost 45:285–289, 1981

46. Green D, Schuette PT, Wallace WH: Factor VIII antibodies in rheumatoid arthritis. Effect of cyclophosphamide. Arch Intern Med 140:1232–1235, 1980

47. Waddell CC, Lehane DE, Zubler MA: Acquired factor VIII inhibitor in a patient with mycosis fungoides. Cancer 47:2901–2903, 1981

48. Herbst KD, Rapaport SI, Kenoyer DG, et al: Syndrome of an acquired inhibitor of factor VIII responsive to cyclophosphamide and prednisone. Ann Intern Med 95:575–578, 1981

49. Gawryl MS, Hoyer LW: Inactivation of factor VIII coagulant activity by two different types of human antibodies. Blood 60:1103–1109, 1982

50. Spero JA, Lewis JH, Hasiba U: Corticosteroid therapy for acquired factor VIII:C inhibitors. Br J Haematol 48:635–642, 1981

51. Miller K, Neeley JE, Krivit W, et al: Spontaneously acquired factor IX inhibitor in a nonhemophilic child. J Pediatr 93:232–234, 1978

52. Torres A, Lucia JF, Oliveros A, et al: Anti-factor IX circulating anticoagulant and immune thrombocytopenia in a case of Takayasu's arteritis. Acta Haematol 64:338–340, 1980

53. Sarji KE, Stratton RD, Wagner RH, et al: Nature of von Willebrand factor: A new assay and a specific inhibitor. Proc Natl Acad Sci USA 71:2937–2941, 1974

54. Stratton RD, Wagner RH, Webster WP, et al: Antibody nature of circulating inhibitor of plasma von Willebrand factor. Proc Natl Acad Sci USA 72:4167–4171, 1975

55. Egberg N, Blombäck M: On the characterization of acquired inhibitors to ristocetin induced platelet aggregation found in patients with von Willebrand's disease. Thromb Res 9:527–531, 1976

56. Mannucci PM, Meyer D, Ruggeri ZM, et al: Precipitating antibodies in von Willebrand's disease. Nature 262:141–142, 1976

57. Shoa'i I, Lavergne JM, Ardaillou N, et al: Heterogeneity of von Willebrand's disease. Study of 40 Iranian cases. Br J Haematol 37:67–83, 1977

58. Maragall S, Castillo R, Ordinas A, et al: Inhibition of Willebrand factor in von Willebrand disease. Thromb Res 14:495–501, 1979

59. Ruggeri ZM, Ciavarella N, Mannucci PM, et al: Familial incidence of precipitating antibodies in von Willebrand's disease: A study of four cases. J Lab Clin Med 94:60–75, 1979

60. Mannucci PM, Ruggeri ZM, Ciavarella N, et al: Precipitating antibodies to factor VIII/von Willebrand factor in von Willebrand's disease: Effects on replacement therapy. Blood 57:25–31, 1981

61. Simone JV, Cornet JA, Abildgaard CF: Acquired von Willebrand's syndrome in systemic lupus erythematosus. Blood 31:806–812, 1968

62. Ingram GIC, Kingston PJ, Leslie J, et al: Four cases of acquired von Willebrand's syndrome. Br J Haematol 21:189–199, 1971

63. Pool-Wilson PA: Acquired von Willebrand's syndrome and systemic lupus erythematosus. Proc R Soc Med 65:561–562, 1972

64. Ingram GIC, Prentice CRM, Forbes CD, et al: Low factor-VIII-like antigen in acquired von Willebrand's syndrome and response to treatment. Br J Haematol 25:137–140, 1973

65. Mant MJ, Hirst J, Gauldie J, et al: Von Willebrand's syndrome presenting as an acquired bleeding disorder in association with a monoclonal gammopathy. Blood 42:429–436, 1973

66. Leone G, Pola P, Guerrera G, et al: Sindrome di von Willebrand acquistita in corso di malattia disreattiva. Haematologica 59:212–220, 1974

67. Handin RI, Martin V, Moloney WC: Antibody-induced von Willebrand's disease: A newly defined inhibitor snydrome. Blood 48:393–405, 1976

68. Stabelforth P, Tamagnini GL, Dormandy KM: Acquired von Willebrand syndrome with inhibitors both to factor VIII clotting activity and ristocetin-induced platelet aggregation. Br J Haematol 33:565–573, 1976

69. Matsuda S, Acki I, Kikuchi M, et al: A case of acquired von Willebrand's syndrome associated with IgG myeloma. Rinsho Ketsueki 18:1007–1011, 1977

70. Wautier JL, Fusciardi J, Warnet A, et al: Syndrome de Willebrand acquis et angiodysplasie au cours d'une leucémie lymphoïde chronique. Nouv Presse Med 6:3733–3739, 1977

71. Joist HN, Cowan JF, Zimmerman TS: Acquired von Willebrand's disease: Evidence for a quantitative and qualitative factor VIII disorder. N Engl J Med 298:988–991, 1978

72. Zettervall O, Nilsson IM: Acquired von Willebrand's disease caused by a monoclonal antibody. Acta Med Scand 204:521–528, 1978

73. Gouault-Heilmann M, Dumond MD, Intrator L, et al: Acquired von Willebrand snydrome with IgM inhibitor against von Willebrand's factor. J Clin Pathol 32:1030–1035, 1979

74. McGrath KM, Johnson CA, Stuart JJ: Acquired von Willebrand disease associated with an inhibitor to factor VIII antigen and gastrointestinal telangiectasia. Am J Med 67:693–696, 1979

75. Meyer D, Frommel D, Larrieu MJ, et al: Selective absence of large forms of factor VIII/von Willebrand factor in acquired von Willebrand's syndrome. Response to transfusion. Thromb Haemost 42:285, 1979 (abstract)

76. Noronha PA, Hruby HA, Maurer HS: Acquired von Willebrand disease in a patient with Wilms tumor. J Pediatr 95:997–999, 1979

77. Gan TE, Sawers RJ, Koutts J: Pathogenesis of antibody-induced acquired von Willebrand syndrome. Am J Hematol 9:363–371, 1980

78. Feinstein DI: Acquired inhibitors of factor V. Thromb Haemost 39:663–674, 1978

79. Lust A, Bellon A: A circulating anticoagulant against factor V. Acta Clin Belg 33:62–65, 1978

80. Chediak J, Ashenhurst JB, Garlick I, et al: Successful management of bleeding in a patient with factor V inhibitor by platelet transfusions. Blood 56:835–841, 1980

81. Miletich JP, Majerus DW, Majerus PW: Patients with congenital factor V deficiency have decreased factor Xa binding sites on their platelets. J Clin Invest 62:824–831, 1978

82. Giddings JC, Shearn SAM, Bloom AL: The immunological localization of factor V in human tissue. Br J Haematol 29:57–65, 1975

83. Campbell E, Sanal S, Mattson J, et al: Factor VII inhibitor. Am J Med 68:962–964, 1980

84. Ness PM, Hymas PG, Gesme D, et al: An unusual factor-X inhibitor in leprosy. Am J Hematol 8:397–402, 1980

85. Stern DM, Nossel HL, Owen J: Acquired antibody to factor XI in a patient with congenital factor XI deficiency. J Clin Invest 69:1270–1276, 1982

86. DiSabatino CA, Clyne LP, Malawista SE: A circulating anticoagulant directed against factor XIa in systemic lupus erythematosus. Arthritis Rheum 22:1135–1138, 1979

87. Beck DW, Strauss RG, Kisker CT, et al: An intrinsic pathway inhibitor in a 3-year-old child. Am J Clin Pathol 71:470–472, 1979

88. Fischer DS, Clyne LP: Circulating factor XI antibody and disseminated intravascular coagulation. Arch Intern Med 141:515–517, 1981

89. Vercellotti GM, Mosher DF: Acquired factor XI deficiency in systemic lupus erythematosus. Thromb Haemost 48:250–252, 1982

90. Bateman D, Gokal R, Prescott R, et al: Minimal-change glomerulonephritis associated with circulating anticoagulant to factor XII. Br Med J 281:358, 1980

91. Shapiro SS, Thiagarjan P: Lupus anticoagulants, in Spaet T (ed): Progress in Hemostasis and Thrombosis, vol. 6. New York, Grune & Stratton, 1982, pp 263–285.

92. Struzik T, Haricki Z, Hawiger R, et al: Cryocoagulopathy with presence of immuno-antithrombin in the course of lupus erythematosus disseminatus. Acta Med Polonica 5:61–80, 1964

93. Scully MF, Ellis V, Kakkar VV, et al: An acquired coagulation inhibitor to factor II. Br J Haematol 50:655–664, 1982

94. Galanakis DK, Ginzler EM, Fikrig SM: Monoclonal IgG anticoagulants delaying fibrin aggregation in two patients with systemic lupus erythematosus (SLE). Blood 52:1037–1046, 1978

95. Hoots WK, Carrell NA, Wagner RH, et al: A naturally occurring antibody that inhibits fibrin polymerization N Engl J Med 304:857–861, 1981

96. Marciniak E, Greenwood MF: Acquired coagulation inhibitor delaying fibrinopeptide release. Blood 53:81–92, 1979

97. Milner GR, Holt PJL, Bottomley J, et al: Practolol therapy associated with a systemic lupus erythematosus-like syndrome and inhibitor to factor XIII. J Clin Pathol 30:770–773, 1977.

98. Lopaciuk S, Bykowska K, McDonagh JM, et al: Differences between Type I autoimmune inhibitors of fibrin stabilization in two patients with severe hemorrhagic disorder. J Clin Invest 61:1196–1203, 1978

99. Feinstein DI, Rapaport SI: Acquired inhibitors of blood coagulation, in Spaet TH (ed): Progress in Hemostasis and Thrombosis, vol. 1. New York, Grune & Stratton, 1972, pp 75–95.

100. Thiagarajan P, Shapiro SS: Lupus anticoagulants, in Colman RW (ed): Methods in Hematology: Disorders of Thrombin Formation Other Than Hemophilia. New York, Livingstone-Churchill, 1983

101. Schleider MA, Nachman RL, Jaffe EA, et al: A clinical study of the lupus anticoagulant. Blood 48:499–509, 1976

102. Coots MC, Miller MA, Glueck HI: The lupus inhibitor: A study of its heterogeneity. Thromb Haemost 46:734–739, 1981

103. Canoso RT, Hutton RA, Deykin D: A chlorpromazine-induced inhibitor of blood coagulation. AM J Hematol 2:183–191, 1977

104. Zucker S, Zarrabi MH, Romano GS, et al: IgM inhibitors of the contact activation phase of coagulation in chlorpromazine-treated patients. Br J Haematol 40:447–457, 1978

105. Zarrabi MH, Zucker S, Miller F, et al: Immunmologic and coagulation disorders in chlorpromazine-treated patients. Ann Intern Med 91:194–199, 1979

106. Zarrabi MH, Zucker S, Derman, et al: Lack of correlation between surgical bleeding and chlorpromazine (CPZ) induced inhibition of coagulation. A prospective study. Blood 58: 228a, 1981 (abstract)

107. Goldsmith GH, Saito H, Muir WA: Labile anticoagulant in a patient with lymphoma. Am J Haematol 10:305–311, 1981

108. Dahlbäck B, Nilsson IM, Frohm B: Inhibition of platelet prothrombinase activity by a lupus anticoagulant. Blood 62:218–225, 1983

109. Carreras LO, Vermylen JG: ''Lupus'' anticoagulant and thrombosis—possible role of inhibition of prostacyclin formation. Thromb Haemost 48:38–40, 1982

110. Furie B, Greene E, Furie BC: Syndrome of acquired factor X deficiency and systemic amyloidosis. In vivo studies of the metabolic fate of factor X. N Engl J Med 297:81–85, 1977

111. Furie B, Voo L, McAdam KPWJ, et al: Mechanism of factor X deficiency in systemic amyloidosis. N Engl J Med 304:827–830, 1981

112. Aoki N, Yamanaka T: The $\alpha_2$-plasmin inhibitor levels in liver disease. Clin Chim Acta 84:99–105, 1978

113. Plow EF, Collen D: The presence and release of $\alpha_2$-antiplasmin from human platelets. Blood 58:1069–1074, 1981

114. Aoki N, Saito H, Kamiya T, et al: Congenital deficiency of $\alpha_2$-plasmin inhibitor associated with severe hemorrhagic tendency. J Clin Invest 63:877–884, 1979

115. Kluft C, Vellenga E, Brommer EJP, et al: A familial hemorrhagic diathesis in a Dutch family: An inherited deficiency of $\alpha_2$-antiplasmin. Blood 59:1169–1180, 1982

116. Yoshioka A, Kamitsuji H, Takase T, et al: Congenital deficiency of $\alpha_2$-plasmin inhibitor in three sisters. Haemostasis 11:176–184, 1982

117. Miles LA, Plow EF, Donnelly KJ, et al: A bleeding disorder due to deficiency of $\alpha_2$-antiplasmin. Blood 59:1246–1251, 1982

118. Aoki N, Sakata Y, Matsuda M, et al: Fibrinolytic states in a patient with congenital deficiency of $\alpha_2$-plasmin inhibitor. Blood 55:483–488, 1980

119. Stenflo J: A new vitamin K-dependent protein: Purification from bovine plasma and preliminary characterization. J Biol Chem 251:355–363, 1976

120. Kisiel W: Human plasma protein C: Isolation, characterization and mechanism of activation by $\alpha$-thrombin. J Clin Invest 64:761–769, 1979

121. Esmon C, Comp P, Walker F: Functions for protein C, in Suttie J (ed): Vitamin K. Metabolism and Vitamin K-Dependent Proteins. Baltimore, University Park Press, 1980, pp 72–83

122. Vehar G, Davie E: Preparation and properties of bovine factor VIII (antihemophilic factor). Biochemistry 19:401–410, 1980

123. Marlar RA, Kleiss AJ, Griffin JH: Mechanism of action of human activated protein C, a thrombin-dependent anticoagulant enzyme. Blood 59:1067–1072, 1982

124. Griffin JH, Evatt B, Zimmerman TS, et al: Deficiency of protein C in congenital thrombotic disease. J Clin Invest 68:1370–1373, 1981

125. Soff GA, Levin J: Familial multiple coagulation factor deficiencies. I. Review of the literature: Differentiation of single hereditary disorders associated with multiple factor deficiencies from coincidental concurrence of single factor deficiency states. Semin Thromb Hemosas 7:112–148, 1981.

126. Hultin MB, Eyster ME: Combined factor V-VIII deficiency: A case report with studies of factor V and VIII activation by thrombin. Blood 58:983–985, 1981.

127. Canfield WM, Kisiel W: Evidence of normal functional levels of activated protein C inhibitor in combined factor V/VIII deficiency disease. J Clin Invest 70:1260–1272, 1982,

Oscar D. Ratnoff

# 8

# Disseminated Intravascular Coagulation

Disseminated intravascular coagulation (DIC), the widespread deposition of fibrin in small blood vessels, is a common feature of many disorders. This process may cause ischemic damage to tissues and organs. Paradoxically, however, a systemic bleeding tendency stemming from depletion of clotting factors often dominates the clinical picture, and few if any thrombi may be found post mortem. DIC is precipitated by activation of the clotting mechanisms diffusely within the bloodstream, but how this comes about is not always understood.

This chapter will review the experimental basis for the concept of DIC and present some illustrative clinical disorders. Other syndromes are discussed more appropriately elsewhere in this volume and will be mentioned only briefly. Additionally, note will be made of those diseases in which localized thrombosis leads to systemic hemostatic defects that mimic DIC, a distinction often blurred in the literature.

## EXPERIMENTAL DISSEMINATED INTRAVASCULAR COAGULATION

Our understanding of DIC ultimately derives from observations of de Blainville,[1] casually reported to the Paris Académie de Médecine in 1834. Intravenous injection of large amounts of brain tissue was fatal within two minutes; at autopsy, the blood vessels and chambers of the heart were filled with what looked like ordinary clotted blood. In modern terms, the brain tissue, rich in tissue thromboplastin, clotted the recipients' blood via the extrinsic pathway of thrombin formation.

Half a century later, Wooldridge,[2] an eccentric English physiologist, refined de Blainville's experiments by slowly infusing much smaller amounts of animal tissue—extracts of calf thymus or testes, or erythrocytic stroma. The recipients survived, but their blood was incoagulable; further injections of tissue seemed harmless. The signifiance of these critical experiments was not appreciated until 1921, when Mills[3] found that blood was incoagulable after the intravenous injection of lung tissue because it had been depleted of fibrinogen. This observation has since been repeated many times, using tissue thromboplastin,[4] thrombin,[5] or coagulant snake venoms[6,7] to "defibrinate" the animal.

When brain thromboplastin is infused slowly into dogs, the clotting time is modestly prolonged and the plasma acquires thrombin-inhibitory properties before the concentration of fibrinogen has appreciably decreased.[4,8] Additionally, the coagulant titers of other clotting factors, such as prothrombin,[8,9] proaccelerin (factor V),[9] antihemophilic factor (AHF, factor VIII),[10] and factor VII,[11] decrease and the animal becomes thrombocytopenic.[8] Under certain circumstances, evidence of enhanced plasma fibrinolytic activity emerges[11] and the plasma contains soluble intermediates of the formation of fibrin, or the degradation products of the digestion of fibrinogen or fibrin.[12]

Remarkably, as Wooldridge[2] had noted, gross thrombi are rare or absent in animals subjected to experimental DIC. Platelet-fibrin thrombi are demonstrable in the smallest blood vessels, particularly those of the lung, liver, and kidneys, but are often notably sparse. Two hypotheses, not mutually exclusive, have been proposed to explain the paucity of thrombi. A local fibrinolytic response may dissolve small thrombi.[13] Alternatively, the slow infusion of coagulants may result in incomplete polymerization of fibrin, which then circulates in the form of soluble polymers of fibrin monomer, or complexes of fibrin monomer with fibrinogen or with the products of the proteolysis of fibrinogen or fibrin.

When soluble fibrin monomers are infused into rabbits, fibrin clots may be deposited in glomerular capillaries, a process enhanced by administration of epsilon aminocaproic acid, which inhibits generation of the fibrinolytic enzyme, plasmin.[14] After experimental DIC has been induced, antigenic material related to fibrinogen can be identified immunologically in reticuloendothelial cells, but this technique does not distinguish among fibrinogen, fibrin, or their degradation products.[11,15] Blockade of the reticuloendothelial system enhances deposition of fibrinlike materials in the glomerular capillaries and elsewhere,[15,16] emphasizing the importance of the reticuloendothelial system for the "clearance" of these substances from the circulation.

A form of experimental DIC of interest because of its possible clinical relevance is that induced by endotoxin.[17] After a single intravenous injection of endotoxin into rabbits, only an occasional thrombus is found in the microcirculation of the lung, liver, spleen, or kidneys, but the plasma contains fibrin monomers, fibrinogen–fibrin complexes, or soluble fibrin polymers, as though fibrin formation were incomplete.[18] How endotoxin initiates intravascular fibrin formation is unclear. Although some endotoxins can activate Hageman factor (factor XII), this process alone will not initiate DIC.[19] Endotoxins, however, release clot-promoting agents from blood mononuclear cells, alter platelets, and damage vascular endothelial cells, all processes that may contribute to intravascular clotting.[17,20]

A second intravenous injection of endotoxin into rabbits 24 hours after the first is lethal, a process described as the generalized Shwartzman reaction. Cortisone or agents such as thorium dioxide that block the reticuloendothelial system can be substituted for the first injection, and in pregnant animals only one injection of endotoxin suffices. At autopsy, thrombosis of small blood vessels is widespread, and diffuse hemorrhagic renal cortical necrosis is particularly prominent. The glomerular capillaries are occluded with fibrin-like material.

One explanation for the generalized Shwartzman reaction is that in nonpregnant rabbits the reticulendothelial system phagocytizes the soluble fibrin intermediates that are induced by the first injection of endotoxin. Thus blocked, the reticuloendothelial system cannot clear the circulation of the fibrin that forms after the second injection of endotoxin, and thrombi are laid down in the microvasculature. Presumably pregnancy, cortisone, and thorium dioxide similarly prevent clearance of fibrin, so that a single injection of endotoxin is enough to induce the thrombotic lesions. Supporting this view are observations that the intravenous injection of tissue thromboplastin or thrombin results in glomerular lesions similar to those of the generalized Shwartzman reaction in pregnant mice and rabbits.[17]

## THE PATHOPHYSIOLOGY OF DISSEMINATED INTRAVASCULAR COAGULATION

Our understanding of DIC as a disease process is based upon the experimental observations detailed in the preceding paragraphs. Presumably in one way or another, a procoagulant gains access to the circulating blood, where it initiates reactions leading to the formation of fibrin throughout the circulation. The procoagulant is usually endogenous, but exogenous agents such as snake venoms and endotoxin may be responsible for DIC. Intravascular coagulation thus may be initiated by tissue thromboplastin or some analogous substance. Alternatively, endothelial injury, in some cases brought about by endotoxin, exposes clot-promoting subendothelial structures that may activate both the intrinsic and extrinsic pathways of thrombin formation, and bring about platelet adhesion, aggregation, and the release reaction. In either case, thrombin is generated, and this enzyme severs fibrinopeptides from fibrinogen; free fibrinopeptide A, cleaved from the A$\alpha$ chain of fibrinogen, is demonstrable in the plasma of patients with DIC.[21] Snake venoms may bring about thrombin generation or may directly release fibrinopeptide A from fibrinogen.

As fibrin monomers are generated in this way, they may form soluble complexes with themselves, with fibrinogen, or with the degradation products of fibrinolysis.[22–24] With further formation of fibrin monomers, this ''soluble fibrin'' may polymerize, and fibrin thrombi then form in the small blood vessels of kidneys, lungs, liver, skin, and elsewhere. Thrombosis is especially likely to take place under conditions of low blood flow, as in shock, with its accompanying hypoxia and acidosis. The deposited fibrin may be phagocytized by reticuloendothelial cells[16] or may undergo local fibrinolysis. Direct evidence of enhanced fibrinolytic activity is not a constant finding in blood drawn from patients with DIC, although rarely fibrinolytic activity is so prominent that it is difficult to distinguish DIC from primary fibrinolytic purpura.

The process of fibrinolysis is ordinarily attributed to activation of plasminogen either by tissue activators released from vascular endothelium or monocytes or by Hageman factor-dependent mechanisms. Proteases liberated by leukocytes or other cells, however, may contribute to the degradation of fibrin. The fibrinolytic enzymes seem not only to dissolve thrombi in the microvasculature but also to degrade the soluble fibrin monomer complexes. Either before or after this proteolysis, however, soluble fibrin monomers may be covalently linked by fibrin-stabilizing factor (factor XIII) that has been activated by the liberated thrombin[25]; such cross-linked soluble complexes have been demonstrated in patients undergoing DIC.[26] Whether unaltered fibrinogen undergoes significant proteolytic digestion is less clear. Fibrin(ogen) degradation products are probably principally responsible for inhibition of fibrin formation by the plasma of patients with DIC; they block the formation and action of thrombin,[27] especially the polymerization of fibrin.[28]

The immunologic methods used to detect the degradation products of the action of proteases upon fibrinogen and fibrin [fibrin(ogen) degradation or split products] are not specific; they also detect soluble forms of fibrin. Merskey's[29] term, fibrinogen–fibrin-related antigens (FRA), is therefore a more accurate name for these agents, and will be used in this chapter.

Concomitant with the consumption of fibrinogen in DIC, other changes in the hemostatic mechanisms take place similar to those observed in experimental animals. The titer of many clotting factors, including prothrombin, factor VII, Stuart factor (factor X), proaccelerin (factor V), AHF (factor VIII), Hageman factor (factor XII), plasma prekallikrein, and high molecular weight kininogen, may be reduced, as measured by coagulant assays.[30–38] Some of these agents may have been consumed in the process of thrombin generation, but this may be only a partial explanation for the reduced titers. For example, prekallikrein may be consumed by its conversion to kallikrein by Hageman factor-mediated reactions, and lowered coagulant titers of AHF and proaccelerin may result from their inactivation by thrombin, plasmin, or activated protein C. Particularly interesting is the demonstration that the coagulant titer of AHF (factor VIII:C) may be significantly less than the concentration of AHF-like antigens as measured by heterologous antiserum (factor VIIIR:Ag), as though the protein had been inactivated in vivo.[37]

Decreased titers of antithrombin III[37] and $\alpha_2$-antiplasmin[39] may also be found in DIC. Presumably, these inhibitors are bound to enyzmes activated during this syndrome.

Thrombocytopenia is frequent in DIC, and its presence has been used to distinguish this process from the much rarer syndrome of primary fibrinolysis. The decreased number of platelets has been attributed to their utilization in the formation of platelet-fibrin thrombi, to their clumping by thrombin and subsequent removal from the bloodstream, and to their adhesion and aggregation at sites where subendothelial structures have been exposed by endothelial injury. Thrombocytopenia is not diagnostic of DIC, as other causes are commonplace in the very situations in which this process occurs.[40]

When the incitant for DIC is envenoming by the bite of a snake whose venom directly transforms fibrinogen to fibrin, changes in other clotting factors are usually not observed and the platelet count need not be depressed; sometimes evidence that fibrinolysis has occurred is detected.[41,42]

In addition to changes in the hemostatic mechanisms, the blood in some patients with DIC may show striking changes in the morphology of erythrocytes, which appear to be fragmented.[43] The genesis of this microangiopathic hemolytic anemia is uncertain, but Bull et al.[44] demonstrated similar alterations when erythrocytes were forcibly filtered through a clot, as though the fibrin strands had chopped up the red cells and the membranes had then resealed.

## Hypo- and Afibrinogenemic States

DIC severe enough to cause a sharp decrease in the concentration of plasma fibrinogen may arise in many situations. In the most fulminant cases, such as the hemorrhagic disorders of parturition, the patient has sudden and often lethal generalized bleeding. The concentration of fibrinogen in plasma, which normally averages about 300 mg/dl in nonpregnant individuals, falls precipitously; indeed, this protein may be undetectable, a condition described as afibrinogenemia. The level of fibrinogen below which bleeding may occur seems to vary from patient to patient, presumably dependent upon other changes in the hemostatic mechanisms. A rule of thumb is that a hemorrhagic diathesis becomes apparent when the concentration of fibrinogen is 100 mg/dl or less. Patients with congenital afibrinognemia bleed only with trauma or menstruation. This indicates that other concomitant abnormalities must be present to explain the bleeding phenomena of DIC.

In fulminant DIC of short duration, such as amniotic fluid embolism or premature separation of the placenta, bleeding is most likely to occur from exposed wounds, such as those at the site of vascular puncture or the placental bed. Cutaneous hemorrhages, including ecchymoses, petechiae, and hematomas, may appear, and the patient may sustain hemorrhage into the central nervous system, the gastrointestinal or genitourinary tracts, or elsewhere. Death within a few hours of the onset of symptoms is more usually due to hypovolemic shock than to the ischemic changes that result from thrombosis of small blood vessels.

If DIC persists for more than a few hours, the patients's bleeding may extend to additional sites, such as the pleural or pericardial cavities, the respiratory tract, or even the joints; occasionally, the patient experiences epistaxis.[30] Acral cyanosis—a gunmetal gray to purplish discoloration of the fingers, the toes, and sometimes the ears and nose—may be prominent, particularly in patients with septicemia or hypotension.[30] Occasionally, the tips of the fingers may become gangrenous, as if the blood supply were occluded with thrombi. More rarely, bullae may be superimposed upon deep purple or black patches of bruising, particularly on the extremities. These bullae may then take on the appearance of superficial cutaneous gangrene, resembling the lesions of purpura fulminans (page 305). Evidence of occlusion of the blood supply to various organs, such as diffuse cerebral symptoms and other neurologic signs, and renal failure may supervene. We have seldom been certain whether renal failure was due to thrombosis or to the condition underlying the genesis of DIC.

In more chronic forms of severe DIC, such as may occur in patients with neoplasia, the predominant symptom is usually the enhanced bleeding tendency, with minimal evidence of ischemic damage.[30] Some patients, however, may have nonbacterial thrombotic endocarditis (marantic endocarditis), and this process may be complicated by embolization to the brain, coronary arteries, kidney, extremities, and elsewhere.[45] Particularly vexing in DIC, especially in patients with neoplasia, is the thrombosis of large arteries and veins and pulmonary embolism, which occur with disturbing frequency[29,30] (Chapter 10). This is certainly not surprising in the clinical setting in which DIC occurs. Minna et al[30] emphasized the frequency with which thrombosis arises along the path of venous or arterial catheters inserted to treat the patient's underlying condition.

In general, the treatment of DIC associated with hypo- or afibrinogenemia is primarily the treatment of the underlying disorder, whether it be antivenom after snakebite, emptying the uterus in disorders of parturition, or therapy in neoplasia. Transfusion of fibrinogen-rich plasma fractions, such as cryoprecipitates prepared for the care of hemophiliacs, may provide hemostasis, but possibly at the risk of fostering additional thrombosis and transmitting hepatitis. If the bleeding is life-threatening, temporary hemostasis may be provided by intravenous infusion of cryoprecipitate, which is rich in fibrinogen, at a dose of 1 bag/3kg of body weight. Theoretically, a more rational approach is the intravenous infusion of heparin in full therapeutic doses, as this agent inhibits the coagulant properties of activated Stuart factor (factor Xa) and thrombin.[29,46,47] Warfarin and its congeners seem to be of much less benefit. Heparin treatment is sometimes of great help in chronic forms of DIC, such as those associated with neoplasm or with retention of a dead fetus in utero. Unfortunately, heparin is often contraindicated during acute DIC because of the risk of bleeding into the central nervous system or from exposed wounds—for example, the site from which the placenta is expelled in patients with premature separation of the placenta. Its value in acute situations thus is limited to cases in which obvious sites of bleeding are not present. The administration of epsilon aminocaproic acid or tranexamic acid is contraindicated, as these agents block the activation of plasminogen and therefore may prevent the protective dissolution of thrombi.[48] Needless to say, appropriate treatment of shock, a common accompaniment of acute DIC, must be pursued vigorously. Moreover, in many disorders thrombotic lesions are localized to a particular organ rather than disseminated. In such situations, fibrinogen-related antigens and other hemostatic abnormalities may nonetheless be found in plasma, leading to the probably erroneous conclusion that the patient has undergone DIC. In such patients, treatment with heparin to halt the progress of fibrin deposition has usually been disappointing.

## Disseminated Intravascular Coagulation without Hypofibrinogenemia

Inspired by the writings of McKay[49] and others, investigators have proposed that many syndromes are associated with DIC that is not severe enough to deplete plasma fibrinogen. In these conditions, as varied as cirrhosis of the liver and preeclampsia, the deposition of fibrin in small blood vessels is inferred from the detection of fibrinogen-related antigens or fibrinopeptide A in plasma. This process can sometimes be established histologically, for example, by renal biopsy. Commonly, no other coagulative abnormalities are noted, but the concentration of fibrinogen, although within the normal range, may be less than would be anticipated in light of the underlying disease. In some patients, the presence of microangiopathic changes in erythrocytes raises the question of DIC.

The difficulty in interpreting the role of DIC in some situations is exemplified by the report of van Hulsteijn et al.[50] that fibrinopeptide A is increased in the plasma of patients with ''serious bacterial infections.'' This assay cannot reveal the source of the fibrinopeptide A, and therefore cannot distinguish DIC from extravascular generation of this peptide.

## LABORATORY DIAGNOSIS OF DISSEMINATED INTRAVASCULAR COAGULATION

In the more severe forms of DIC, the concentration of fibrinogen and other clotting factors may be reduced, the platelet count may be decreased, and, inconstantly, evidence of fibrinolysis may be present. These changes are similar to those observed in animal studies. The thrombin time, prothrombin time, and activated partial thromboplastin time may be prolonged, and fibrinogen-related antigens, including soluble forms of fibrin and the products of fibrinolysis [fibrin(ogen) degradation products], may be demonstrable.

The diagnosis of hypo- or afibrinogenemia is established by measurement of plasma fibrinogen. A qualitative test, suitable for rapid diagnosis during the hemorrhagic crises of parturition, is the addition of 1 ml of blood to 0.1 ml of bovine thrombin (1000 NIH U/ml), a procedure adapted from that of Page.[51,52] The mixture is allowed to stand for a minute or two. Except in severe hypofibrinogenemia, the tube will seem to be filled with clot. The tube is then gently tapped, causing the clot to shrink. The size of the clot is then estimated visually. In severe hypofibrinogenemia, the observer may falsely conclude that the clot has undergone immediate and total fibrinolysis, but careful examination will usually reveal a small nubbin of fibrin at the bottom of the tube.[53]

Quantitative determination of plasma fibrinogen is performed by converting it to fibrin by addition of thrombin and measuring the protein content of the washed clot.[54,55] Alternatively, fibrinogen can be assayed semiautomatically by measuring the turbidity that evolves when diluted plasma is mixed with thrombin and calcium ions.[56]

The thrombin time, that is, the clotting time of a mixture of plasma and thrombin, is nearly always prolonged in hypofibrinogenemic forms of DIC.[30,57] This test is influenced by the concentration of fibrinogen and by inhibitors of fibrin formation that may be present during DIC. The thrombin time is not an accurate measure of the concentration of fibrinogen in plasma, although it has been used for this purpose.

Particularly important in patients in whom the concentration of fibrinogen is not clearly diminished are tests for the presence of fibrinogen-related antigens. Soluble fibrin, intermediates in the formation of fibrin, such as polymers of fibrin monomer or complexes of fibrin monomer and fibrinogen or fibrin(ogen) degradation products, can be precipitated or gelled by addition of protamine sulfate[23,58] or ethanol.[22] More useful are immunologic tests that detect both soluble fibrin and fibrin(ogen) degradation products.[59] Among the many techniques described, we have found most advantageous the aggregation of latex particles coated with antiserum against human fibrinogen fragments D and E. A commercial kit, the Thrombo-Wellco test, marketed by the Burroughs Wellcome Company (Research Triangle, North Carolina) is highly satisfactory. A positive test is the aggregation of latex particles by plasma that has been diluted fivefold or more. The reagent reacts with both fibrin monomer and fibrin(ogen) degradation products and should not be considered specific for the latter. The degradation products of fibrin released into plasma can also be demonstrated by their unique property of clumping certain strains of Staphylococcus aureus.[60] A recent experimental technique identifies the presence in plasma of soluble fibrin or fibrin degradation products that still contain fibrinopeptide B.[61] Addition of thrombin to plasma extracts of patients with evidence of intravascular coagulation released antigens that reacted specifically with antibodies against fibrinopeptide B.

Among the many other tests used to determine the presence of DIC, mention should be made of the assay of fibrinopeptide A, which is released into plasma in abnormally high amounts through the action of thrombin upon fibrinogen.[21] Although this test provides direct evidence that coagulation has taken place, as noted earlier it does not prove conclusively that the clotting process is intravascular. Specific assays for clotting factors or inhibitors of clotting or fibrinolysis are seldom helpful in the care of patients. Similarly, thrombocytopenia is commonplace in DIC, but may be due not to this process but rather to the patient's underlying disease.

The blood smear should be routinely examined for the presence of microangiopathic changes. Distorted erythrocytes, however, are not universally found, and they are characteristic of thrombotic thrombocytopenic purpura and the hemolytic-uremic syndrome, whose relationship to DIC is disputed.

## SYNDROMES OF DISSEMINATED INTRAVASCULAR COAGULATION (Table 8-1)

### Normal Pregnancy and Childbirth

During normal pregnancy, the titers of many clotting factors increase; teleologically, perhaps these changes help to prevent exsanguination at childbirth. Probably the most significant change, recognized more than a century ago, is the rise in the concentration of fibrinogen, which reaches an average of 450 mg/dl in the last weeks of pregnancy, about 50 percent higher than the level in nonpregnant women. The titer of AHF (factor VIII)[62,63] and, less strikingly, those of the vitamin K-dependent clotting factors, [64,65] Hageman factor, (factor XII) and plasminogen also rise.[66–68] The genesis of these changes is unclear but

**Table 8-1**

Some Syndromes of Disseminated Intravascular Coagulation

---

Secondary to the introduction of extrinsic clot-promoting agents
    Amniotic fluid embolism
    Envenoming by poisonous snake
    Premature separation of the placenta
    Intrauterine retention of a dead fetus
    Malignancy (e.g., carcinoma of the prostate or pancreas, acute promyelocytic luekemia, etc.)
    Autoadministration of ascitic fluid
    Fat embolism
    Transfusion of concentrates of vitamin K-dependent clotting factors
Secondary to intravascular elaboration of clot-promoting agents
    Acute hemolytic processes (e.g., mismatched blood transfusion)
    Extracorporeal circulation
    Near-drowning in fresh water
Secondary to vascular injury
    Sepsis with gram-positive or gram-negative organisms, septic abortion, Waterhouse-Fredrichsen
        syndrome
    Infectious diseases (e.g., generalized herpes simplex, dengue, cytomegalic viremia, scrub typhus,
        Rocky Mountain spotted fever, miliary tuberculosis, bacterial endocarditis, trypanosomiasis)
    Heat stroke
    Traumatic shock, burns, head injury, surgical procedures
    Cardiac arrest
Pathogenesis uncertain
    Eclampsia
    Anaphylaxis
    Hypothermia
    Hepatic disease
    Hydatidiform mole

---

may be related to the increased titer of estrogens. The titers of fibrin-stabilizing factor (factor XIII)[69] and plasma thromboplastin antecedent (PTA, factor XI),[66,67] and spontaneous in vitro fibrinolytic activity[66,70] decrease. The platelet count is unaltered in normal pregnancy.[71] We have not been able to confirm the reported decrease in antithrombin III. In the last trimester, the titer of fibrinopeptide A in plasma is slightly elevated, as though local thrombin generation normally occurred at the placental site.[72]

During the course of normal childbirth, transient increases in plasma fibrinolytic activity, as measured in vitro, [71,73] and fibrinogen-related antigens may be detected.[73,74] At the same time, there are minor decreases in the concentration of fibrinogen and in the coagulant titers of Hageman factor[68] and AHF (factor VIII:C). This last change is unaccompanied by a decrease in the concentration of AHF-like antigens (factor VIIIR:Ag), as measured with heterologous antiserum.[75] The temptation is strong to assume that during normal childbirth a minor degree of DIC takes place. No significant alterations in prothrombin or the platelet count are found during normal parturition.

## Premature Separation of the Placenta

This complication occurs in about 0.5 percent of deliveries.[76] In 1901, DeLee[77] described a patient with this disorder in whom uterine bleeding was accompanied by manifestations of a generalized bleeding tendency. This phenomenon was explained by Dieckmann,[78] who detected severe hypofibrinogenemia in several patients; in about one-fourth of patients with premature separation of the placenta, the concentration of fibrinogen is less than 100 mg/dl.[79] In most instances, hypofibrinogenemia is demonstrable within about 8 hours of the onset of symptoms of abruption.[79]

Several hypotheses have been offered to explain the hypofibrinogenemia accompanying premature separation of the placenta. Dieckmann[78] proposed that fibrinogen was lost through hemorrhage and utilized in the formation of the retroplacental clot. Indeed, as much as 9 g or more of fibrinogen can be found in the uterus after premature separation, accounting for 50–75 percent of the loss of this protein.[80] A more likely explanation derives from the work of Obata[81] and others. Placental tissue is thromboplastic, and its intravenous infusion brings about defibrination in experimental animals. Schneider[82] and Page et al.[9] suggested that this was the course of events in women undergoing premature separation of the placenta. In agreement with this hypothesis, the titers of other clotting factors and the platelet count fall; the decrease in coagulant AHF is unaccompanied by a fall in the concentration of AHF-like antigens (factor VIIIR:Ag), as if this factor were inactivated during the course of DIC.[31,38,53,73,75,79,83] Other investigators have attributed the hypofibrinogenemia of premature separation of the placenta to fibrinolysis. Indeed, enhanced fibrinolytic activity, as measured in vitro, has been found, and fibrinogen-related antigens can be detected in increased concentration,[60,74,84] but this is not universal.[75] Whether increased fibrinolysis is secondary to DIC, whether it reflects concomitant shock, or whether it is an exaggeration of the normal changes observed at delivery is not certain. Supporting the view that hypofibrinogenemia is secondary to DIC is the fact that renal cortical necrosis was once a common complication of premature separation of the placenta. Deposits of thrombin may be found at autopsy in small blood vessels, particularly those of the lung, liver, and kidneys.[78,82]

Treatment of the hemorrhagic diathesis associated with premature separation of the placenta consists of correcting volume depletion with red cells and plasma and emptying the uterus. After delivery, the concentration of fibrinogen rises rapidly, at a rate of about 10 mg/dl/hr, and thus reaches hemostatically effective levels in 12 hours or less.[79] At one time, replacement of fibrinogen by the administration of concentrates of plasma rich in this protein was advocated. In most cases, however, this procedure is unnecessary and carries with it the immediate risk of furnishing more fibrinogen for thrombin formation. We have seen the late development of renal failure after infusion of fibrinogen, whether from hypovolemic shock or from deposition of fibrin in the renal vasculature. If the patient's hypofibrinogenemia seems so extreme that it must be treated, cryoprecipitates should provide prompt hemostasis (page 293). Heparin and inhibitors of plasmin generation such as epsilon aminocaproic acid have no place in the treatment of premature separation of the placenta.

## Amniotic Fluid Embolism

Amniotic fluid embolism is one of the few DIC syndromes in which the agent responsible for defibrination has been clearly identified. In this disorder, amniotic fluid is infused into the maternal bloodstream during parturition. Although the clinical picture was recognized earlier, amniotic fluid embolism was first delineated by Steiner and Lushbaugh.[85] The incidence of amniotic fluid embolism has been variously estimated at 1:8000–1:80,000 deliveries.[85,86] The typical patient is a multiparous woman 30 years old or more. Amniotic fluid embolism is said to be more frequent during tumultuous delivery. It has also occurred during cesarean section.

Just before, during, or after childbirth, the patient experiences sudden respiratory and circulatory failure that may be immediately fatal. This catastrophe appears to be due to the obstruction of the pulmonary circulation by amniotic fluid debris that is surrounded by platelet-fibrin thrombin.[38,85] A role for prostaglandins in the development of pulmonary hypertension has been proposed by Morgan[86] in his excellent review of amniotic fluid embolism.

In those patients who survive the immediate consequences of amniotic fluid embolism, and in some who do not display premonitory symptoms, uncontrollable uterine hemorrhage ensues within minutes or hours after delivery.[87] Soon, hallmarks of profound systemic hemostatic failure such as bleeding from vascular puncture sites or from the gastrointestinal tract become evident, and uterine atony may magnify uterine bleeding. The mortality from amniotic fluid embolism is said to be above 80 percent[86], despite its rarity, it is the principal cause of death in childbirth.

The course of events in amniotic fluid embolism seems reasonably certain. Amniotic fluid gains access to the maternal circulation through tears in the membranes; injury or rupture of the uterus may be overt.[86] The presence of amniotic fluid in the maternal circulation can be established during life by detection of amniotic debris such as desquamated fetal epithelial cells—"squames"—in the buffy coat of peripheral blood. At autopsy, squames or lanugo hairs are readily found in the pulmonary vessels. In the test tube, amniotic fluid or its contaminants are clot-promoting; some investigaters believe that it behaves more like a direct activator of Stuart factor (factor X) than like tissue thromboplastin.[88–90] The syndrome thus appears to be a counterpart of Wooldridge's classic experiments (page 289). The changes in peripheral blood are similar to those in experimental DIC, with decreases in the concentration of fibrinogen and other clotting factors, thrombocytopenia, the presence of inhibitory activity against the formation of fibrin, and enhanced fibrinolytic activity.[38,87,91]

Therapy must be directed primarily at relieving cardiopulmonary failure and hypovolemic shock. Although the administration of fibrinogen in the form of cryoprecipitates (page 293) and uterine packing may be helpful, the dismal mortality rate suggests that effective therapy has not yet been developed.

## Dead Fetus Syndrome

In 1901, DeLee[77] described a woman who bled severely from the uterus after delivery of a macerated dead fetus. He was impressed by the fact that the expelled blood was incoagulable. Many years later, Weiner et al.[92] related intrauterine fetal death in the second trimester of pregnancy to severe uterine hemorrhage at spontaneous delivery two or three months later. Each of their three patients had hypofibrinogenemia, and two had generalized bleeding. These patients were among 15 women in whom fetal death was related to Rh-isoimmunization. Subsequent experience indicated that the syndrome is independent of the cause of fetal death.

Hypofibrinogenemia in women with retention of a dead fetus is not unusual; it was detected in 5 of 28 women we studied.[93] Evidences of a hemorrhagic syndrome may appear within three weeks after apparent fetal death. The concentration of fibrinogen generally falls, but may ultimately reach a plateau at, for example, 100mg/dl, as though synthesis and utilization of fibrinogen were in balance. In some cases, the platelet count and the titers of other clotting factors are also decreased, but these changes are not invariable.

The pathogenesis of hypofibrinogenemia in women with a retained dead fetus can only be inferred. Therapeutic doses of heparin, which should inhibit the generation and action of thrombin, correct the fibrinogen deficiency as though the hemostatic defects were the result of chronic intravascular coagulation brought about by agents released from the products of conception.[94,95] In agreement with this view, the titer of fibrinogen-related antigens is increased after fetal death.[74]

The treatment of "dead fetus syndrome" is emptying of the uterus, which can usually be accomplished without transfusion of fibrinogen. The concentration of plasma fibrinogen soon rises to normal levels. Occasionally, the fetus can be delivered only by cesarean section. Once the diagnosis of fetal death has been established, prophylactic emptying of the uterus is appropriate. To prevent bleeding in the hypofibrinogenemic patient, heparin can be infused, as first suggested by Lerner et al.[95] Bonnar[38] recommends that hypofibrinogenemia be corrected by the intravenous administration of heparin, 1000 U/hr for 24–48 hours. Heparin therapy can then be discontinued and labor induced.

## Abortion

Septic abortion, usually the result of crude attempts to empty the uterus, may be complicated by severe hypofibrinogenemia presumably due to DIC.[96] In most instances, the uterus is infected with coliform organisms, *Clostridium perfringens*, or a mixture of organisms. The patient may have severe generalized bleeding and, besides hypofibrinogenemia, the typical laboratory abnormalities of DIC. In some patients, the red cells undergo fragmentation and gross intravascular hemolysis may ensue.[38,97]

Although some authors invoke endotoxemia to explain the occurrence of DIC in septic abortion, the organisms in some patients are not thought to produce endotoxins. More likely, clot-promoting substances are released into the circulation from infected uterine tissue, or intravascular clotting is secondary to damage to vascular endothelium. Therapy should be directed at the invariable shock and at the infection itself. Cryoprecipitates rich in fibrinogen (page 293) may provide temporary hemostasis. In a few cases, the administration of heparin to inhibit intravascular coagulation has been tried,[97,98] but the prognosis is grave.

The author has not seen severe DIC due to septic abortion since the legalization of abortion in the United States. Laboratory evidence of mild transient DIC is found after abortion by installation of hypertonic solutions into the amniotic sac, a procedure that may force amniotic fluid into the systemic circulation.[99–103] The changes are maximal at about the time of the induced abortion. Although the procedure is ordinarily of no consequence, rare patients may have hemorrhagic symptoms,[104–106] and a fatal outcome from cerebral hemorrhage has been reported.[107] Abortion using prostaglandins does not appear to induce DIC.[102,108]

## Hydatidiform Mole

Rarely, DIC has been identified in women with hydatidiform mole.[49] If the patient survives hemorrhage at the time of delivery, the bleeding defect quickly resolves.

## Preclampsia and Eclampsia

Interest in the relationship between toxemia of pregnancy and DIC was triggered by a report of the unusual coincidence in three cases of eclampsia, thrombocytopenia, an abnormally long thrombin time, and hemoglobinemia and hemoglobinuria attributed to intravascular hemolysis.[109] Two of the patients had impaired hepatic function. Although this complex has been described in other eclamptics, it is the exception rather than the rule.[110,111] Thrombocytopenia was present in 28 of 95 patients with eclampsia studied by Pritchard et al.,[112] and elevations of the thrombin time were common, but overt hemolysis was identified in only 2 of 118 patients. Indirect evidence of hemolysis, however, including elevated indirect serum bilirubin, reticulocytosis, nucleated red blood cells in peripheral blood, and disorted red cells, is more common.

Patients with eclampsia may exhibit such hallmarks of DIC as thrombocytopenia and decreased titers of clotting factors, but elevation of soluble fibrin or fibrinogen-related antigens is erratic.[112,113] Clinically significant hypofibrinogenemia is not observed unless some other causative factor, such as premature separation of the placenta, is present.

Similar but less impressive changes are seen in women with preeclampsia.[113,114] The life span of circulating platelets is decreased in severe preeclampsia,[115] and in some patients fibrinogen-related antigens may be detected.[27,116] The titer of AHF coagulant activity (factor VIII:C) may be relatively lower than the concentration of AHF-like antigens (factor VIIIR:Ag), as though this factor had been altered by intravascular generation of thrombin.[117] Among 13 patients with preeclampsia, 6 had evidence of a mild hemolytic process.[114]

The origin of the hematologic changes observed in preeclampsia and eclampsia remains unknown, as does the role of intravascular clotting in the evolution of the clinical symptoms. Histologically, fibrin deposition is found in the small blood vessels of the liver, kidney, and brain.[111,118,119] The analogy to thrombotic thrombocytopenic purpura and hemolytic-uremic syndrome is tempting but unsupported. McKay and Müller-Berghaus[48] drew a comparison between the renal lesions of eclampsia and the generalized Shwartzman phenomenon, but this is similarly speculative.

Specific therapy for the hematologic complications of preeclampsia and eclampsia is usually unnecessary. Treatment should be directed at the toxemia of pregnancy.

### Envenoming by Poisonous Snakes

The hemorrhagic disorders that follow envenoming are reviewed in Chapter 17. Some venoms contain ''hemorrhagins'' that produce extensive vascular endothelial damage, thus bringing about bleeding. Others contain enzymes that induce DIC through actions upon the blood-clotting mechanism. For example, the venom of *Ankistrodon rhodostoma,* the Malayan pit viper, severs fibrinopeptide A from the Aα chain of fibrinogen, converting it to fibrin monomer. That of *Echis carinatus,* the saw-scaled viper, changes prothrombin to thrombin, and the venom of the Russell's viper has the dual action of activating Stuart factor (factor X) and, like thrombin, enhancing the action of proaccelerin (factor V). The character of the coagulant enzymes, the coexistence of other venom constituents that influence the formation and destruction of clots, and the possible presence of hemorrhagins that damage endothelium or of hemolysins that might liberate clot-promoting erythrocytic stroma all influence the nature and course of the DIC that follows envenoming.[120,121]

### Thrombosis After Infusion of Concentrates of the Vitamin K-Dependent Clotting Factors

Lyophilized concentrates of the vitamin K-dependent clotting factors have been recommended for treatment of bleeding episodes in patients with acquired or hereditary deficiencies of these factors or for patients who have circulating anticoagulants against AHF (factor VIII). The use of these concentrates has been complicated by a high incidence of hepatitis and, less often, by thromboembolic events, particularly after surgery.[122] Additionally, severe and even lethal DIC has been described in patients with hereditary deficiencies of Stuart factor (factor X) or Christmas factor (factor IX), liver disease, or circulating anticoagulants. [123-126] Other patients have laboratory changes suggestive of mild DIC, including transient hypofibrinogenemia.[127-129] Myocardial infarction after the use of lyophilized concentrates has also been described.[125,130]

The observations imply that some concentrates of the vitamin K-dependent clotting factors may contain either active clot-promoting agents or substances that can trigger the release of endogenous procoagulants. The use of newer preparations is said to be less hazardous.

## Hemolytic Reactions

Among the agents that Wooldridge[2] used to induce DIC in his original experiments was erythrocytic stroma. That severe DIC may follow the transfusion of incompatible blood is therefore not unexpected; as little as 100 ml of mismatched blood may bring about sudden bleeding.[49,131] The patient may have hypofibrinogenemia, thrombocytopenia, and other evidence of DIC.[132-135] In lethal cases, thrombi may be found in small blood vessels.[49]

Therapy for patients who sustain transfusion reactions due to mismatching should be directed not only at the prevention of renal failure but also at potential or overt DIC. Unless contraindicated by the presence of open wounds, the patient should be treated with full doses of heparin and, if needed, cryoprecipitates, platelets, and fresh plasma.[136] Holland[137] raises the question, too, of whether heparin should be given prophylactically when a hemolytic reaction is anticipated.

Near drowning in fresh water produces a syndrome of intravascular hemolysis and DIC similar to that of mismatched transfusion.[138,139] Acidosis, hypoxemia, and cardiorespiratory depression may contribute to the intravascular clotting process. The treatment of near drowning should include the same measures used to correct defective hemostasis in patients who have had DIC after transfusion of mismatched blood, but the author knows of no evidence that heparin has been helpful in this situation.

McKay[49] reviewed evidence that other intravascular hemolytic syndromes, such as favism and paroxysmal nocturnal hemoglobinuria, might be complicated by DIC. But Mannucci et al.[140] found no evidence of DIC in individuals who had massive intravascular hemolysis induced by ingestion of fava beans. These authors postulated that additional factors, such as impaired reticuloendothelial function, must be present for hemolysis to lead to DIC. Further, Crosby and Stefanini,[141] describing hemolysis and DIC-like changes after transfusion of compatible blood to patients with paroxysmal nocturnal hemoglobinuria, pointed out that these complications did not arise if washed erythrocytes were infused. Perhaps, then, hemolysis and DIC in these patients occur because whole blood supplies components of complement. These studies raise the question of whether the immunologic reaction that results from mismatched blood transfusion and the profound shock of near-drowning are more important than hemolysis in the genesis of DIC in these syndromes.

## Head Injury

Traumatic brain damage is a well-recognized cause of massive DIC. Perhaps in these cases brain tissue, which is highly thromboplastic, enters the systemic circulation and initiates intravascular coagulation via the extrinsic pathway.[142] Among 13 individuals who sustained destruction of brain tissue from gunshot wounds or massive blunt trauma, Goodnight et al.[143] found four who had "striking clinical and laboratory evidence of hemostatic failure due to acute defibrination," with oozing from venipuncture and tracheostomy sites, bloody return from nasogastric tubes, and gross hematuria after bladder catheterization. The concentration of fibrinogen was 40 mg/dl or less in these patients. Deficiences of other clotting factors and thrombocytopenia were detected, and the diagnosis of DIC was supported by positive protamine gelation tests and the presence of fibrinogen-related antigens. Five other patients had less marked abnormalities that were thought to be sufficiently severe to contribute to intracranial bleeding. In contract, in an equal number of patients who had a head injury that caused loss of consciousness without evidence of brain destruction, neither symptoms nor laboratory evidence of defibrination were found. Similar findings have been recorded by other investigators.[142,144]

The management of the hemostatic defects associated with brain trauma is difficult. Replacement of fibrinogen with cryoprecipitate, repletion of other clotting factors with fresh frozen plasma or whole blood, and transfusion of platelets may be helpful.[143,145] Although the administration of heparin and epsilon aminocaproic acid has been recommended,[146] the former may enhance bleeding and the latter may prevent the dissolution of clots, thus leading to organ damage, particularly in the kidney.[146]

## Shock and Related Syndromes

Shock from whatever cause may be complicated by DIC. Vascular damage from tissue anoxia, infection, toxins, or anaphylaxis has been implicated in the genesis of this syndrome, which, in turn, may exaggerate bleeding and cause further tissue damage by thrombosis. Gross evidence of DIC may be demonstrable, including acral cyanosis and gangrene or patchy cutaneous gangrene of the extremities.[30,147] Hardaway[147] emphasized the role of acidosis secondary to tissue anoxia in enhancing the thrombotic tendency in hypovolemic shock.

Deposition of microthrombi in the pulmonary circulation after surgery or trauma may contribute to respiratory insufficiency, but pulmonary failure is seldom attributable to this process alone.[148] Bone, et al.[149] found gross evidence of DIC in one-fourth of a series of 30 patients with acute respiratory distress syndrome not associated with trauma or surgery. Each of the seven patients with DIC bled at sites of venipuncture, four had gastrointestinal bleeding, and two had petechiae, ecchymoses, or both. Six of the seven had acrocyanosis or ischemic necrosis of the fingers or extremities. Thrombi were found in the small blood vessels in all five patients who came to autopsy, and in the kidneys and skin in four. These observations raise the question of whether the acute respiratory distress syndromes are the result rather than the cause of thrombosis within the pulmonary microcirculation, but the issue is unresolved.[150] Widespread platelet thrombi have been found in newborn infants with respiratory distress syndrome, probably reflecting vascular damage secondary to hypoxia.[151–153]

Coagulation abnormalities suggestive of DIC may follow resuscitation after cardiac arrest.[154] Evidence of DIC is not found after myocardial infarction. Rarely, renal failure may complicate cardiogenic shock. In this situation, fibrinogen-related antigens are increased in serum and the platelet count is reduced, as though localized thrombosis may have occurred within the renal vasculature.[155]

Anaphylactic shock is said to induce defibrination.[29] In our experience, anaphylaxis after wasp sting released an inhibitor of thrombin into the circulation without causing hypofibrinogenemia.[156] The titers of other clotting factors, except Hageman factor (factor

XII) and AHF (factor VIII), were all reduced. Similar findings have been reported by others.[157,158] The syndrome thus has many features of DIC, but the mechanisms responsible are unclear.

## Burns

Hemorrhagic complications are frequent in patients who have suffered thermal injury. The most severely affected patients may have thrombocytopenia, hypofibrinogenemia, and decreased titers of plasminogen and clotting factors except AHF (factor VIII)[159,160] The turnover of platelets, fibrinogen, and plasminogen is abnormally rapid. Although these changes may be due to local consumption of clotting factors and platelets in the burned areas, microthrombi are found in biopsy specimens of undamaged skin[160,161] and modest elevations of the titer of fibrinogen-related antigens may be detected.[159,160,162]

The pathogenesis of DIC in burned patients is not clear. The acute hemolytic anemia found in some patients may be important (page 301), and concomitant septicemia or hypotension may contribute to the process. Although heparin therapy has been recommended, the evidence that this alleviates the hemostatic defects associated with severe burns is thin.

## Heat Stroke

Heat stroke is an often lethal syndrome in which individuals who have been exposed to high atmospheric temperatures are unable to control their body temperature despite cutaneous vasodilatation; sweating is sometimes, but not always, impaired or absent. A common feature is a generalized bleeding tendency, with ecchymoses, cutaneous and conjunctival petechiae, gastrointestinal and urinary tract hemorrhage, and bleeding from sites of vascular puncture. At autopsy in patients who die soon after the onset of heat stroke, microscopic hemorrhages are found in the brain and other organs, and widespread damage to tissue cells is evident.[49] Thrombosis of either small or large vessels is only occasionally found. In contrast, in patients who die more than 9 days after the onset of heat stroke, pulmonary embolism and myocardial infarction are commonplace.[163]

Shibolet et al.[164] related the hemorrhagic diathesis of heat stroke to severe hypo- or afibrinogenemia. The usual changes associated with DIC have been detected; the bleeding time is often prolonged. A likely explantation is that DIC is the result of widespread vascular endothelial damage.[165]

Besides the primary treatment of heat stroke, attention has been directed to correcting the hemostatic abnormality. The administration of heparin to halt the process of DIC has been suggested,[166] but has not been uniformly beneficial and may exaggerate the bleeding tendency. A more cautious approach would be the transfusion of cryoprecipitates to provide fibrinogen (page 293) and the administration of platelet concentrates, but the efficacy of these maneuvers is not certain.

## Hypothermia

Experimental hypothermia in dogs induces thrombocytopenia; deficiencies of fibrinogen, prothrombin, and factor VII; and increased fibrinolytic, antithrombin, and proaccelerin (factor V)-like activities.[167] Administration of heparin before and during hypothermia prevents the fall in fibrinogen. Similar changes have been observed in hypothermic newborns and adults in the few human cases that have been studied.[168–170] In a fatal case described by Mahajan et al.[171] rewarming seemed responsible for the induction of DIC. These authors pointed out that thrombosis of multiple organs is common after hypothermic death. Presumably, the initiating event is vascular injury from hypoxemia, acidosis, and hypotension, a process exacerbated by the hyperviscosity that accompanies this syndrome.

## Fat Embolism

After fractures of long bones or surgery to insert prosthetic joints, marrow fat droplets may enter the circulation and embolize to the lung, brain, and other organs, inducing respiratory failure and diffuse or focal cerebral symptoms.[172,173] Microthrombi may be found in the cerebral microcirculation at autopsy. Fat embolism has also been described in patients who have suffered severe burns, infections, or sickle cell crises, or who have undergone cardiopulmonary bypass surgery or renal transplantation.[173,174] In the setting of bone injury, petechiae of the skin (usually sparing the face), conjunctivae, buccal mucosa and palate may provide a clue to the diagnosis.

Riseborough and Herndon[175] reported that in patients with lower limb fractures who had a decrease in arterial $PO_2$ and may thus have sustained fat embolism, the platelet count was moderately reduced transiently, and the level of fibrinogen-related antigens was elevated. Bradford et al.,[176] too, observed thrombocytopenia, particularly in hypoxemic patients. Although these changes have been interpreted as evidence that fat droplets initiate DIC, it is equally likely that they are in part secondary to formation of thrombin in pulmonary vessels, as in experimental fat embolism.[177] DIC, if it occurs, may be secondary to the severe hypoxia and acidosis of cardiorespiratory failure. Although the thrombotic lesions of experimental fat embolism are inhibited by pretreatment with heparin,[177] therapy with anticoagulants is not of proven value.[178]

## Infectious Diseases

Some degree of DIC, as indicated by such laboratory changes as thrombocytopenia, decreased titers of clotting factors, and the presence of fibrinogen-related antigens in serum, is found in an extraordinary number of infectious diseases. Wilson et al.[179] believe that as many as two-thirds of all cases of DIC are precipitated by infection. Often, however, other explanations for the patients' laboratory changes are evident; for example, thrombocytopenia is common in many infectious processes, but is usually not due to DIC (Chapter 11). In those patients who have hypo- or afibrinogenemia, however, it is reasonable to assume that DIC has taken place.

The prototypic example of DIC with sepsis is *meningococcal bacteremia* with profound shock, cutaneous ecchymosis and petechiae, and, at autopsy, visceral petechiae particularly in the adrenal cortex, the classical Waterhouse-Friderichsen syndrome.[180] Such patients may exhibit all the laboratory features of severe DIC; at autopsy, thrombi can be demonstrated in the small blood vessels of the adrenal cortex, renal cortex, and sometimes other organs. These profound changes are not seen in all cases of meningococcemia, and their presence is a poor prognostic sign.

The temptation is strong to assume that the severe DIC associated with meningococcemia or sepsis with other gram-negative organisms such as *Escherichia coli, Pseudomonas aeruginosa,* or *Klebsiella* is the consequence of endotoxemia (page 290). But a similar syndrome has often been observed in patients with sepsis due to *Streptococcus pneumoniae, Staphylococcus aureus,* or *Clostridium perfringens.* Perhaps, then, DIC may be triggered by other bacterial toxins or by endothelial damage caused by the bacteria themselves. Alternatively, it may be secondary to hypoxemia and acidosis that result from bacteremic shock, or to the release of other cellular procoagulants.

Of particular interest is the DIC that accompanies the fulminant sepsis that may strike individuals who have asplenia without warning. The absence of a spleen may be congenital or the result of surgical excision or atrophy, as occurs in sickle cell disease.[181–183] Patients are catastrophically ill with a Waterhouse-Friderichsen-like syndrome of shock, renal failure, and cutaneous hemorrhage. The offending organism is almost always *Streptococcus pneumoniae,* but other agents may be implicated, among them, *Neisseria meningitides* and *Hemophilus influenzae.* Widespread petechiae, ecchymoses, and other manifestations of bleeding are prominent, and the patient exhibits the laboratory changes of severe DIC, including hypo- or afibrinogenemia. The mortality rate is high, death ensuing within hours of the onset of symptoms. How DIC is induced is conjectural; perhaps sepsis brings about vascular endothelial damage and in this way initiates intravascular clotting. The current practice of routine prophylaxis of splenectomized patients with pneumococcal vaccine[184] does not always prevent this complication.[185]

Therapy for DIC secondary to septicemia should be directed at the primary illness. Anticoagulant and antiplatelet medication has not been of proven value.

A sharp decrease in the concentration of fibrinogen in plasma is seen rarely in many other infectious processes (Table 8–1). Evidence of DIC without hypofibrinogenemia is much more common.

### Other Syndromes of DIC

This lengthy catalog by no means exhausts the list of syndromes that are associated with DIC. The significance of DIC in neoplasia, infectious disease, and cirrhosis is discussed further in Chapters 10, 11, and 14, respectively.

## SYNDROMES OF LOCALIZED INTRAVASCULAR COAGULATION*

### Purpura Fulminans

Purpura fulminans is a fortunately rare disorder in which cutaneous gangrenous patches appear suddenly in apparently healthy individuals, often a week or two or as long as a month after a banal infection such as scarlet fever, chicken pox, measles, or rubella, or after smallpox vaccination. It is a distinct entity, although the term purpura fulminans has been used loosely to describe similar lesions in such disorders as severe low-output cardiac failure, shock, septicemia, and peripheral embolism. Purpura fulminans occurs almost exclusively in children, in whom the lesions begin without warning as sharply demarcated blue-purple areas on the skin of the extremities or buttocks, or, less often, on the tip of the nose, the lobes of the ears, the malar region, the palate, the penis, or the scrotum.[186] The lesions vary in diameter from a few centimeters to 20 cm or more. Often they appear to be arranged symmetrically, but they do not follow a recognizable neural distribution. After a day or two, the patches turn black, bullae may appear, and the lesions become frankly gangrenous. The patients are febrile, hypotensive, and critically ill.

---

*See table 8-2

**Table 8-2**
Some Syndromes Associated with
Localized Intravascular Coagulation
_____

Purpura fulminans
Hemangiomatous lesions (e.g., gaint hemangioma,
    hemangioendotheliosarcoma, etc.)
Aneurysm of major arteries
Thrombotic thrombocytopenic purpura
Hemolytic-uremic syndrome
Renal disease, lupus erythematosus
Malignant hypertension
Rejection of renal transplants
_____

The gangrenous lesions result from thrombotic occlusion of the small blood vessels in the affected area; the vessels are the site of necrotizing vasculitis.[187,188] Larger vessels may be occluded with thrombi, and rarely the viscera may be gangrenous. The pathogensis of this bizarre disorder is unknown. Although some writers have likened the lesions to those of the Shwartzman or Arthus reactions, the author is not familiar with evidence supporting this interpretation.

Perhaps because clotting factors are consumed in the formation of thrombi, or because widespread vascular damage serves as an incitant to DIC, the patients may have a generalized bleeding diathesis, with epistaxes, petechiae, hematomas, and splinter hemorrhages of the fingers and toes; in addition, there may be visceral bleeding. Often the peripheral blood is depleted of platelets, fibrinogen, and other clotting factors, and the bleeding time may be abnormally long.[188–190] Red blood cells sometimes exhibit typical microangiopathic changes.

The course of purpura fulminans is erratic. Sometimes the patient dies in shock after two or three days, or he may survive, only to face amputation of the gangrenous areas. New lesions may appear over a period of several weeks.

The therapy for patients with purpura fulminans consists of the administration of heparin in full doses, as originally suggested by Little.[191] Hypovolemic shock, if present, should be treated. Surgery should be delayed as long as feasible, as far less tissue may need to be removed than at first seems necessary. If the patient survives, skin grafting of the excised areas may be required.

## Hemangiomatous Lesions

Giant hemangioma of infancy was first linked to the presence of a hemorrhagic tendency by Kasabach and Merritt,[192] whose two-month-old patient had a petechial rash, thrombocytopenia, and abnormally long bleeding and clotting times. Subsequently, other patients with giant hemangiomas were described who also had hypofibrinogenemia, deficiencies of other plasma clotting factors, and microangiopathic hemolytic anemia.[193–197] These changes seem to result from intravascular sequestration of platelets and fibrin within the relatively static blood in the vascular network of the tumor.[198] Perhaps, as has been suggested, continuous fibrinolysis and destruction of platelets within the tumor perpetuate the process, which may be secondary to impaired endothelial function.

A similar syndrome may be found with other vascular tumors in which stasis of blood flow is prominent, including Klippel-Trénaunay syndrome (cavernomatous hemangioma of a limb associated with varices and hypertrophy of soft tissue and bone),[199] hemangio-endothelioma of the spleen, liver, or other organs,[200,201] and hemangioendotheliosarcoma.[202]

Therapy for the hemorrhagic syndrome associated with these vascular tumors varies with their nature and location. Irradiation provided temporary relief of thrombocytopenia in Kasabach and Merritt's original case.[192] In others, surgical excision has been attempted, not always successfully. Heparin therapy to block the progression of thrombosis within the tumor may be helpful.[193]

## Aneurysm

Fine and his associates[203] described a 51-year-old hypertensive woman who sustained lethal dissecting aneurysm of the entire length of the aorta. She had hypofibrinogenemia, thrombocytopenia, and a prolonged bleeding time, and her serum was ''positive'' for fibrinogen-related antigens. The same changes have been described in other cases of dissecting, saccular, or fusiform aneurysms of the aorta or femoral arteries. Although the syndrome only occasionally produces a systemic hemorrhagic tendency, excessive bleeding may occur during and after surgical repair, contributing to morbidity and mortality.[204] The most likely explanation for the hemorrhagic tendency is local rather than disseminated deposition of fibrin and platelets within the lesion, but DIC manifested by fibrin deposition in glomerular capillaries may occur secondary to hemorrhagic shock.[205,206]

## Thrombotic Thrombocytopenic Purpura

Thrombotic thrombocytopenic purpura, first described by Moschcowitz,[207] is an acute, highly fatal syndrome of fever, changing neurologic signs and symptoms, severe thrombocytopenia, hemolytic anemia, and renal failure.[208–210] The red cells have striking microangiopathic changes, a defect observed only sporadically in classic DIC. At biopsy or autopsy, arterioles and capillaries are found to be occluded with hyaline material composed of platelets, fibrin, and, in some cases, immunoglobulins and complement.[211] The absence of perivascular inflammation or vascular necrosis is impressive, although proliferation of vascular endothelium and aneurysmal dilatation of arterioles may be prominent.[212]

A review of the reported cases suggests that more than one disorder is classified as thrombotic thrombocytopenic purpura. This may account for the variety of laboratory abnormalities observed and for the variable response of patients to therapy. A rather sterile argument concerns whether thrombotic thrombocytopenic purpura is a form of DIC. Although the lesions are widespread, laboratory changes of DIC are only sporadically found. A few patients may have increased titers of fibrinogen-related antigens or decreased concentrations of fibrinogen, but most do not display these abnormalities.[210,213] One current hypothesis is that the deposition of platelets and fibrin in the microvasculature is due to the presence of an agent in the patient's plasma that aggregates normal platelets and is cytotoxic for vascular endothelium; the cytotoxic agent may be an immunoglobulin.[214,215] Alternatively, Remuzzi et al.[216] have proposed that the patient's plasma lacks a factor that normally stimulates endothelial production of prostacyclin, which inhibits platelet aggregation. Perhaps supporting the concept that plasma contains an abnormal activator of platelet aggregation is the finding of Moak[217] that the plasma of patients with chronic relapsing thrombotic thrombocytopenic purpura contained very large multimers of that part of the AHF complex that supports ristocetin-induced platelet agglutination (factor VIII:RCo). During relapse, the concentration of the multimers decreased, as if these were consumed in the formation of intravascular platelet aggregates.

The beneficial effects of exchange transfusion of blood or plasma are consistent with all of the cited observations.[218,219] Such treatment sometimes provides dramatic relief of symptoms, and appears to be more effective than splenectomy or the administration of corticosteroids or antiplatelet agents such as aspirin or dipyridamole. (see Chapter 4)

## Hemolytic-Uremic Syndrome

In 1955, Gasser et al.[220] described five infants who died of renal failure within days after the onset of a symptom complex superficially resembling thrombotic thrombocytopenic purpura. The patients had microangiopathic hemolytic anemia, thrombocytopenia, bilateral renal cortical necrosis, and central nervous system disturbances. The predominance of renal failure and the relatively less prominent central nervous system findings are in contrast to the symptoms of thrombotic thrombocytopenic purpura, but whether this is a fundamental difference is uncertain.

The hemolytic-uremic syndrome begins acutely, often after a few days of nausea, vomiting, and high fever, or after an apparently ordinary respiratory infection. Most patients are healthy infants less than two years old, but adults have also been affected, including women who were pregnant or taking oral contraceptives.[221] Histologically, necrosis or infarction of glomeruli is found, along with deposition of fibrin-platelet thrombi in renal capillaries and arterioles.[222-224] About 10 percent of patients die, but this grim prognosis is better than that of the natural course of thrombotic thrombocytopenic purpura.

Thrombocytopenia is associated with a decreased platelet life span, and, as anticipated, in vitro aggregation of these cells is depressed during the azotemic phase.[225,226] Hypofibrinogenemia is rare, but the biological half-life of fibrinogen is decreased.[226] Although increased fibrinogen-related antigens are occasionally demonstrated, whether such patients truly have DIC can certainly be debated[227]; other hemostatic studies usually give normal results.[228] Treatment must be directed at the renal failure. Heparin or fibrinolytic therapy or the administration of antiplatelet drugs has been recommended, but have no proven value.[223,228]

## Extracorporeal Circulation

Although seldom a problem now, multiple coagulative defects were commonplace during extracorporeal circulation with early forms of apparatus. Hypofibrinogenemia, decreased titers of clotting factors, and thrombocytopenia were found, along with enhanced fibrinolytic activity.[49] Present-day equipment and techniques produce far fewer significant hemostatic abnormalities. An impressive fall in the platelet count and qualitative platelet abnormalities are still frequent, but these can be prevented by administration of prostacyclin during surgery.[229] Currently, the principal causes of bleeding during cardiopulmonary bypass surgery are the inadvertent administration of excessive amounts of heparin or its inadequate neutralization with protamine sulfate, or induced qualitative platelet changes.[230]

## Venous Thrombosis and Pulmonary Embolism

The formation of thrombi in major blood vessels consumes clotting factors, but this process does not significantly deplete the circulating blood. Localized thrombosis and pulmonary embolism, however, can be associated with release into the plasma of fibrinopeptide A, severed from fibrinogen, or fibrinogen-related antigens.[21,231-233]

Klein and Bell[234] described two patients with pulmonary emboli who developed DIC while being treated with heparin. Perhaps this phenomenon was related to the release by heparin of platelet coagulant activity in susceptible patients.

## Other Syndromes of Localized Intravascular Coagulation

An important pathologic process in many disorders is the local formation of fibrin-platelet thrombi. Under such circumstances, fibrinogen-related antigens may spill into the bloodstream, but DIC is rarely if ever found. Thus, patients with a variety of renal disorders characterized by glomerular deposition of fibrin-platelet aggregates may have increased titers of both plasma and urinary fibrinogen-related antigens.[233,235] In malignant hypertension, microangiopathic changes in red cells may be observed.[43] Similarly, increased fibrinogen-related antigens are sometimes found in rheumatoid arthritis or systemic lupus erythematosus, although in the latter this may be secondary to renal involvement.[59,236] Therapy with heparin or inhibitors of platelet aggregation alone or in combination has had doubtful efficacy in renal or hypertensive disease.[237–239]

During the initial weeks after renal transplantation, fibrinogen-related antigens are found in the urine; these reappear if the graft undergoes either reversible or irreversible rejection. If the transplant undergoes acute or hyperacute rejection, fibrinogen-related antigens may also be found in plasma, sometimes with microangiopathic red cell changes, thrombocytopenia, and other evidence of intravascular coagulation, including deposition of fibrin in other organs.[240–242] Histologically, the glomeruli may be the site of extensive thrombosis.[243] These changes, perhaps engendered by damage to renal endothelium by immune complexes, have led to the use of heparin, inhibitors of platelet aggregation, or both, but this therapy is not clearly superior to immunosuppression.[244]

## REFERENCES

1. de Blainville HMD: Injections de matière cérébrale dans les veines. Gaz Med Paris (ser 2) 2:524, 1834
2. Wooldridge LC: Ueber intravasculäre Gerinnungen. Arch Anat Physiol (Physiol Abt) 397–399, 1886
3. Mills CA: The action of tissue extracts in the coagulation of blood. J Biol Chem 46:167–192, 1921
4. Ratnoff OD, Conley CL: Studies on afibrinogenemia. II. The defibrinating effect on dog blood of intravenous injection of thromboplastic material. Bull Johns Hopkins Hosp 88:414–424, 1950
5. Mellanby J: Thrombase—its preparation and properties. Proc Royal Soc London Sect B 113:93–106, 1933
6. Martin CJ: On some effects upon the blood produced by injection of the Australian black snake *(Pseudoechis porphyriacus)*. J Physiol (Lond) 15:380–400, 1893
7. Mellanby J: The coagulation of blood. Part II. The action of snake venoms, peptone and leech extract. J Physiol (Lond) 38:441–503, 1909
8. Hartmann RC, Conley CL, Krevans JR: The effect of intravenous infusion of thromboplastin on ''heparin tolerance.'' J Clin Invest 30:948–956, 1951
9. Page EW, Fulton LD, Glendening MB: The cause of the blood coagulation defect following abruptio placentae. Am J Obstet Gynecol 61:1116–1122, 1951
10. Penick GD, Roberts HR, Webster WP, et al: Hemorrhagic states secondary to intravascular clotting. Arch Pathol 66:708–714, 1958
11. Izak G, Galewsky K: Studies on experimentally induced hypercoagulable state in rabbits. Thromb Diath Haemorrh 16:228–242, 1966
12. Kowalski E, Budzyński AZ, Kopeć M, et al: Circulating fibrinogen degradation pro-

ducts (FDP) in dog blood after intravenous thrombin infusion. Thromb Diath Haemorrh 13:12–24, 1965

13. Lewis JH, Szeto ILF, Bayer WL, et al: Leukofibrinolysis. Blood 40:844–855, 1972
14. Müller-Berghaus G, Róka L, Lasch HG: Induction of glomerular microclot formation by fibrin monomer infusion. Thromb Diath Haemorrh 29:375–383, 1973
15. Lee R, McClusky RJ: Immunochemical demonstration of the reticuloendothelial clearance of circulating fibrin aggregates. J Exp Med 116:611–618, 1962
16. Lee L: Reticuloendothelial clearance of circulating fibrin in the pathogenesis of the generalized Shwartzman reaction. J Exp Med 115:1065–1082, 1962
17. Müller-Berghaus G: Pathophysiology of generalized intravascular coagulation. Semin Thromb Hemostas 3:209–246, 1977
18. Shainoff JR, Page IH: Cofibrins and fibrin-intermediates as indicators of thrombin activity in vivo. Circ Res 8:1013–1022, 1960
19. Botti RE, Ratnoff OD: Studies on the pathogenesis of thrombosis: An experimental ''hypercoagulable'' state induced by the intravenous injection of ellagic acid. J Lab Clin Med 64:385–398, 1964
20. Hiller E, Saal JG, Riethmüller G: Procoagulant activity of activated monocytes. Haemostasis 6:347–350, 1977
21. Nossel HL, Yudelman I, Canfield RE, et al: Measurement of fibrinopeptide A in human blood. J Clin Invest 54:43–53, 1974
22. Godal HC, Abildgaard U: Gelation of soluble fibrin in plasma by ethanol. Scand J Haematol 3:342–350, 1966
23. Kidder WR, Logan LD, Rapaport SI, et al: The plasma protamine paracoagulation test: Clinical and laboratory evaluation. Am J Clin Pathol 58:675–686, 1972
24. Vermylen JG, Chamone DAF: The role of the fibrinolytic system in thromboembolism. Progr Cardiovasc Dis 21:255–266, 1979
25. Graeff H, Hafter R: Detection and relevance of crosslinked fibrin derivates in blood. Semin Thromb Hemostas 8:57–68, 1982
26. Estellés A, Gilabert J, Aznar J: Structure of soluble fibrin monomer complexes in obstetric patients. Thromb Res 28:575–579, 1982
27. Roszkowski D, Niewiarowska M, Bar-Pratkowska J: Fibrinogen derived coagulation inhibitors in obstetric cases of acute fibrinolysis. Thromb Diath Haemorrh 13:25–34, 1965
28. Latallo ZS, Fletcher AP, Alkjaesig N, et al: Inhibition of fibrin polymerization by fibrinogen degradation products. Am J Physiol 202:681–686, 1962
29. Merskey C: Defibrination syndrome, in Biggs R (ed): Human Blood Coagulation, Haemostasis and Thrombosis (ed 2). Oxford, Blackwell Scientific Publications, 1976, pp 442–535
30. Minna JD, Robboy SJ, Colman RW: Disseminated Intravascular Coagulation. Springfield, Ill, Charles C Thomas, 1974
31. Johnson JF, Seegers WH, Braden RG: Plasma Ac-globulin changes in placenta abruptio. Am J Clin Pathol 22:322–326, 1952
32. Saito H, Ratnoff OD, Pensky J: Radioimmunoassay of human Hageman factor (factor XII). J Lab Clin Med 88:506–514, 1976
33. Nossel HL: The contact system, in Biggs R (ed): Human Blood Coagulation, Haemostasis and Thrombosis (ed 2). Oxford, Blackwell Scientific Publications, 1976, pp 81–142
34. Saito H, Goldsmith G, Waldmann R: Fitzgerald factor (high molecular weight kininogen) clotting acting in human plasma in health and disease and in various animal plasmas. Blood 48:941–947, 1976
35. Saito H, Poon M-C, Vicic W, et al: Human plasma prekallikrein (Fletcher factor) clotting activity and antigen in health and disease. J Lab Clin Med 92:84–95, 1978
36. McDuffie FC, Giffin C, Niederinghaus R, et al: Prothrombin, thrombin and prothrombin fragments in plasma of normal individuals and of patients with laboratory evidence of disseminated intravascular coagulation. Thromb Res 16:759–773, 1979

37. Spero JA, Lewis JH, Hasibu U: Disseminated intravascular coagulation. Findings in 346 patients. Thromb Haemost 43:28–33, 1980

38. Bonnar J: Haemostasis and coagulation disorders in pregnancy, in Bloom AL, Thomas DP (eds): Haemostasis and Thrombosis. New York, Churchill Livingstone, 1981, pp 454–471

39. Aoki N: Natural inhibitors of fibrinolysis. Progr Cardiovasc Dis 21:267–286, 1979

40. Ockelford PA, Carter MB: Disseminated intravascular coagulation: The application and utility of diagnostic tests. Semin Thromb Hemostas 8:198–216, 1982

41. Bell WR, Pitney WR, Goodwin JF: Therapeutic defibrination in the treatment of thrombotic disease. Lancet 1:490–493, 1968

42. Prentice CRM, Edgar W, McNicol GP: Characterization of fibrin degradation products in patients on Ancrod therapy: Comparison with fibrinogen derivatives produced by plasmin. Br J Haematol 27:77–87, 1974

43. Brain MC: Microangiopathic hemolytic anemia. N Engl J Med 281:833–835, 1969

44. Bull BS, Rubenberg ML, Dacie JV, et al: Microangiopathic haemolytic anemia. Mechanisms of red cell fragmentation. In vitro studies. Br J Haematol 14:643–652, 1968

45. Sack GH, Levin J, Bell WR: Trousseau's syndrome and other manifestations of chronic disseminated coagulopathy in patients with neoplasms: Clinical, pathophysiologic and therapeutic features. Medicine 56:1–37, 1977

46. Verstraete M, Amery A, Vermylen C, et al: Heparin treatment of bleeding, letter. Lancet 1:446, 1963

47. Heene DL: Disseminated intravascular coagulation: Evaluation of therapeutic approaches. Semin Thromb Hemostas 4:291–317, 1977

48. McKay DG, Müller-Berghaus G: Therapeutic implications of disseminated intravascular coagulation. Am J Cardiol 20:392–410, 1967

49. McKay DG: Disseminated Intravascular Coagulation. An Intermediary Mechanism of Disease. New York, Hoeber, Harper & Row, 1965

50. Hulsteijn H van, Fibbe W, Bertina R, et al: Plasma fibrinopeptide A and beta-thromboglobulin in major bacterial infections. Thromb Haemostas 48:247–249, 1982

51. Page EW: Discussion of Kellogg, FS Hemorrhagic tendencies in toxemia of pregnancy: Practical evaluation and management. Obstet Gynecol Surv 3:746–757, 1948

52. Ratnoff OD, Pritchard JA, Colopy JE: Hemorrhagic states during pregnancy. N Engl J Med 253:63–69, 97–102, 1955

53. Jackson DP, Hartmann RC, Busby T: Fibrinogenopenia complicating pregnancy. Obstet Gynecol 5:223–247, 1955

54. Ratnoff OD, Menzie C: A new method for the determination of fibrinogen in small samples of plasma. J Lab Clin Med 37:316–320, 1951

55. Ogston D, Ogston CM, Bennett NB: Arterio-venous differences in the components of the fibrinolytic enzyme system. Thromb Diath Haemorrh 16:32–37, 1966

56. Mortazavi M, Jones PK: A semi-automated turbidimetric method for determination of plasma fibrinogen. Am J Clin Pathol 70:76–78, 1978

57. Merskey C, Johnson AJ, Kleiner CJ, et al: The defibrination syndrome. Clinical features and laboratory diagnosis. Br J Haematol 13:528–549, 1967

58. Seaman AJ: The recognition of intravascular clotting. The plasma protamine paracoagulation test. Arch Intern Med 125:1016–1021, 1970

59. Merskey C, Kleiner GJ, Johnson AJ: Quantitative estimation of split products of fibrinogen in human serum, relation to diagnosis and treatment. Blood 28:1–18, 1966

60. Lipiński B, Hawiger J, Jeljaszewicz J: Staphylococcal clumping with soluble fibrin monomer complexes. J Exp Med 126:979–988, 1967

61. Butler VP Jr, Weber DA, Nossel HL, et al: Immunochemical studies of antiserum to human fibrinopeptide-B. Blood 59:1006–1012, 1982

62. Kasper CK, Hoag MS, Aggeler PM, et al: Blood clotting factors in pregnancy: Factor VIII concentrations in normal and AHF-deficient women. Obstet Gynecol 24:242–247, 1964

63.  Bennett B, Ratnoff OD: Antihemophilic factor (AHF, factor VIII) procoagulant activity and AHF-like antigen in normal pregnancy, and following exercise and pneumoencephalography. J Lab Clin Med 80:256–263, 1972

64.  Pechet L, Alexander B: Increased clotting factors in pregnancy. N Engl J Med 265:1093–1097, 1961

65.  Nossel HL, Lanzkowsky P, Levy S, et al: A study of coagulation factor levels in women during labour and in their newborn infants. Thromb Diath Haemorrh 16:185–197, 1966

66.  Bonnar J, McNicol GP, Douglas AS: Fibrinolytic enzyme system and pregnancy. Br Med J 3:387–389, 1969

67.  Biland L, Duckert F: Coagulation factors in the newborn and his mother. Thromb Diath Haemorrh 29:644–651, 1973

68.  Hellgren M, Blombäck M: Studies on blood coagulation and fibrinolysis in pregnancy during delivery and in the puerperium. I. Normal condition. Gynecol Obstet Invest 12:141–154, 1981

69.  Coopland A, Alkjaersig N, Fletcher AP: Reduction in factor XIII (fibrin stabilizing factor) concentration during pregnancy. J Lab Clin Med 73:144–153, 1969

70.  Biezenski JJ, Moore HC: Fibrinolysis in normal pregnancy. J Clin Pathol 11:306–310, 1958

71.  Ratnoff OD, Colopy JE, Pritchard JA: The blood-clotting mechanism during normal parturition. J Lab Clin Med 44:408–415, 1954

72.  Royen EA van, Cate JW ten: Generation of a thrombin-like activity in late pregnancy. Thromb Res 8:487–491, 1976

73.  Kleiner GJ, Merskey C, Johnson AJ, et al: Defibrination in normal and abnormal parturition. Br J Haematol 19:159–178, 1970

74.  Bonnar J, Davidson JF, Pidgeon CF, et al: Fibrin degradation products in normal and abnormal pregnancy and parturition. Br Med J 3:137–140, 1969

75.  Bennett B, Oxnard SC, Douglas AS, et al: Studies on antihemophilic factor (AHF, factor VIII) during labor in normal women, in patients with premature separation of the placenta, and in a patient with von Willebrand's disease. J Lab Clin Med 84:851–860, 1974

76.  Golditch IM, Boyce NE: Management of abruptio placentae. JAMA 212:288–293, 1970

77.  DeLee JB: A case of fatal hemorrhagic diathesis with premature detachment of the placenta. Am J Obstet 44:785–792, 1901

78.  Dieckmann WJ: Blood chemistry and renal function in abruptio placentae. Am J Obstet Gynecol 31:734–745, 1936

79.  Pritchard JA, Brekken AL: Clinical and laboratory studies on severe abruptio placentae. Am J Obstet Gynecol 97:681–700, 1967

80.  Pritchard JA, Wright MR: Pathogenesis of hypofibrinogenemia in placental abruption. N Engl J Med 261:218–222, 1959

81.  Obata I: On the nature of eclampsia. J Immunol 4:111–139, 1919

82.  Schneider CL: "Fibrin embolism" (disseminated intravascular coagulation) with defibrination as one of the end results during placenta abruptio. Surg Gynecol Obstet 92:27–34, 1951

83.  Pritchard JA: Abruptio placentae and hypofibrinogenemia. Am J Obstet Gynecol 76:347–362, 1958

84.  Graeff H, Hugo R von: Fibrinogen derivatives in a case of abruptio placentae. Am J Obstet Gynecol 120:335–340, 1974

85.  Steiner PE, Lushbaugh CC: Maternal pulmonary embolism by amniotic fluid as a cause of obstetric shock and unexpected deaths in obstetrics. JAMA 117:1245–1254, 1340–1345, 1941

86.  Morgan M: Amniotic fluid embolism. Anaesthesia 34:20–32, 1979

87.  Weiner AE, Reid DE: The pathogenesis of amniotic-fluid embolism III. Coagulant activity of amniotic fluid. N Engl J Med 243:597–598, 1950

88.  Weiner AE, Reid DE, Roby CC: The hemostatic activity of amniotic fluid. Science 110:190–191, 1949

89. Rendelstein FD, Frischauf H, Deutsch E: Über die gerinnungsbeschleunigende Wirkung des Fruchtwassers. Acta Haematol 6:18–31, 1951

90. Yaffe H, Eldon A, Hornstein E, et al: Thromboplastic activity in amniotic fluid during pregnancy. Obstet Gynecol 50:454–456, 1977

91. Ratnoff OD, Vosburgh GJ: Observations on the clotting defect in amniotic-fluid embolism. N Engl J Med 246:970–973, 1952

92. Weiner AE, Reid AD, Roby CC, et al: Coagulation defects with uterine death from Rh isosensitization. Am J Obstet Gynecol 60:1015–1022, 1950

93. Pritchard JA, Ratnoff OD: Studies of fibrinogen and other hemostatic factors in women with intrauterine death and delayed delivery. Surg Gynecol Obstet 101:467–477, 1955

94. Phillips LL, Sciarra JJ: Hypofibrinogenemia with a dead fetus treated with intravenous heparin. Am J Obstet Gynecol 93:1161–1162, 1965

95. Lerner R, Margolin M, Slate WG, et al: Heparin in the treatment of hypofibrinogenemia complicating fetal death in utero. Am J Obstet Gynecol 97:373–378, 1967

96. Conley CL, Ratnoff OD, Hartmann RC: Studies on afibrinogenemia. I. Afibrinogenemia in a patient with septic abortion, acute yellow atrophy of the liver and bacteremia due to E. coli. Bull Johns Hopkins Hosp 88:402–413, 1951

97. Rubenberg ML, Baker LRI, McBride JA, et al: Intravascular coagulation in a case of *Clostridium perfringens* septicaemia: Treatment by exchange transfusion and heparin. Br Med J 4:271–274, 1967

98. Clarkson AR, Sage RE, Lawrence JR: Consumption coagulopathy and acute renal failure due to gram-negative septicemia after abortion. Complete recovery with heparin therapy. Ann Intern Med 70:1191–1199, 1969

99. Talbert LM, Adcock DF, Weiss AE, et al: Studies on the pathogenesis of clotting defects during salt-induced abortions. Am J Obstet Gynecol 125:656–662, 1973

100. Stander RW, Flessa HC, Glueck HI, et al: Changes in maternal coagulation factors after intra-amniotic injection of hypertonic saline. Obstet Gynecol 37:660–666, 1971

101. Royen EA van, Treffers RE, Cate JW ten: Hypertonic saline induced abortion as pathophysiologic model of low grade intravascular coagulation. Scand J Haematol 13:166–174, 1974

102. MacKenzie IZ, Sayers L, Bonnar J, et al: Coagulation changes during second-trimester abortion induced by intra-amniotic prostaglandin E$_2$ and hypertonic solutions. Lancet 2:1066–1069, 1975

103. Nossel HL, Wasser J, Kaplan KL, et al: Sequence of fibrinogen proteolysis and platelet release after intrauterine infusion of hypertonic saline. J Clin Invest 64:1371–1378, 1979

104. Beller FK, Rosenberg M, Kolker M, et al: Consumption coagulopathy associated with intra-amniotic infusion of hypertonic salt. Am J Obstet Gynecol 112:534–540, 1972

105. Brown FD, Davidson EC Jr, Phillips LL: Coagulation studies after hypertonic saline infusion for late abortions. Obstet Gynecol 39:538–543, 1972

106. Halbert DB, Buffington JS, Crenshaw C Jr, et al: Consumptive coagulopathy with generalized hemorrhage after hypertonic saline-induced abortion. A case report. Obstet Gynecol 39:41–44, 1972

107. Lemkin SR, Kattlove HE: Maternal death due to DIC after saline abortion. Obstet Gynecol 42:233–235, 1973

108. Bell WR, Wentz AC: Abortion and coagulation by prostaglandin. Intra-amniotic dinoprost tromethamine effect in the coagulation and fibrinolytic systems. JAMA 225:1082–1084, 1973

109. Pritchard JA, Weisman R Jr, Ratnoff OD, et al: Intravascular hemolysis, thrombocytopenia and other hematologic abnormalities associated with severe toxemia of pregnancy. N Eng J Med 250:89–98, 1954

110. Young J: Renal failure after utero-placental damage. Br Med J 2:715–718, 1942

111. Counihan TB, Doniach I: Malignant hypertension supervening rapidly on pre-eclampsia. J Obstet Gynaecol Br Empire 61:449–453, 1954

112. Pritchard JA, Cunningham FG, Mason RA: Coagulation changes in eclampsia: Their frequency and pathogenesis. Am J Obst Gynecol 124:855–864, 1976

113. Bonnar J, McNicol GP, Douglas AS: Coagulation and fibrolytic systems in pre-eclampsia and eclampsia. Br Med J 2:12–16, 1971

114. Pritchard JA, Ratnoff OD, Weisman R Jr: Hemostatic defects and increased red cell destruction in preclampsia and eclampsia. Obstet Gynecol 4:159–164, 1954

115. Rákóczi I, Tallián F, Bagdány S, et al: Platelet life-span in normal pregnancy and pre-eclampsia as determined by a non-radioisotope technique. Thromb Res 15:553–556, 1979

116. McKillop C, Howie PW, Forbes CD, et al: Soluble fibrinogen/fibrin complexes in pre-eclampsia. Lancet 1:56–58, 1976

117. Redman CWG, Denson KWE, Beilin LJ, et al: Factor-VIII consumption in pre-eclampsia. Lancet 2:1249–1252, 1977

118. Vassalli P, Morris RH, McCluskey RT: The pathogenic role of fibrin deposition in the glomerular lesions of toxemia of pregnancy. J Exp Med 118:467–478, 1963

119. Govan ADT: The histology of eclamptic lesions. J Clin Pathol 29(suppl 10):63–69, 1976)

120. deVries A, Cohen I: Hemorrhagic and blood coagulation disturbing action of snake venoms, in Poller L (ed): Recent Advances in Blood Coagulation. London, JA Churchill, 1969, pp 277–297

121. Tu AT: Venoms: Chemistry and Molecular Biology. New York, Wiley, 1977

122. Kasper CK: Postoperative thromboses in hemophilia B. N Engl J Med 289:403, 1974 (letter)

123. Blatt PM, Lundblad RL, Kingdon HS, et al: Thrombogenic materials in prothrombin complex concentrates. Ann Intern Med 81:766–770, 1974

124. Davey RJ, Shashaty GG, Rath CE: Acute coagulopathy following infusion of prothrombin complex concentrate. Am J Med 60:719–722, 1976

125. Lusher JM, Shapiro SS, Palascak JE, et al: Efficacy of prothrombin-complex concentrates in hemophiliacs with antibodies to factor VIII: A multicenter therapeutic trial. N Engl J Med 303:421–425, 1980

126. Small M, Lowe GDO, Douglas JT, et al: Factor IX thrombogenicity: In vivo effects on coagulation activation and a case report of disseminated intravascular coagulation. Thromb Haemostas 48:76–77, 1982

127. Cederbaum AI, Blatt PM, Roberts HR: Intravascular coagulation with use of human prothrombin complex concentrates. Ann Intern Med 84:683–687, 1976

128. Abilgaard CF, Penner JA, Watson-Williams EJ: Anti-inhibitor coagulant complex (Autoplex) for treatment of factor VIII inhibitors in hemophilia. Blood 56:978–983, 1980

129. Sjamsoedin LJM, Heijen L, Mauser-Bunschoten EP, et al: The effect of activated prothrombin-complex concentrate (FE1BA) on joint and muscle bleeding in patients with hemophilia A and antibodies to factor VIII. A double-blind clinical trial. N Engl J Med 305: 717–721, 1981

130. Fuerth JH, Mahrer P: Myocardial infarction after factor IX therapy. JAMA 245:1455–1456, 1981

131. Muirhead EE: Incompatible blood transfusions with emphasis on acute renal failure. Surg Gynecol Obstet 92:734–746, 1951

132. Conley CL: Untoward reactions from blood transfusion. Maryland J 1:547–552, 1952

133. Krevans JR, Jackson DP, Conley CL, et al: The nature of the hemorrhagic disorder accompanying hemolytic transfusion reactions in man. Blood 12:834–841, 1957

134. Langdell RD, Hedgpeth EM Jr: A study of the role of hemolysis in the hemostatic defect of transfusion reactions. Thromb Diath Haemorrh 3:566–571, 1959

135. Kluge A, Krah E, Schimpf K: Hämolytisch-hämorrhagischer Transfusions-Zwischenfall mit Koagulopathie infolge inkompletter Blutgruppen-Antikörper. Thromb Diath Haemorrh 21:472–481, 1969

136. Rock RC, Bove JR, Nemerson Y: Heparin treatment of intravascular coagulation accompanying hemolytic transfusion reactions. Transfusion 9:57–61, 1969

137.  Holland PV: Other adverse effects of transfusion, in Petz LD, Swisher SN (eds): Clinical Practice of Blood Transfusion. New York, Churchill Livingstone, 1981, pp 783–803
138.  Meyers A: Fibrin split products in the severely burned patient. Arch Surg 105:404–407, 1972
139.  Culpepper RM: Bleeding diathesis in fresh water drowning. Ann Intern Med 83:675, 1975 (letter)
140.  Mannucci PM, Lobina GF, Caocci L, et al: Effect on blood coagulation of massive intravascular hemolysis. Blood 33:207–213, 1969
141.  Crosby WH, Stefanini M: Pathogenesis of the plasma transfusion reaction with especial reference to the blood coagulation system. J Lab Clin Med 40:374–386, 1952
142.  Clark JA, Finelli RE, Netsky MG: Disseminated intravascular coagulation following cranial trauma. J Neurosurg 52:266–269, 1980
143.  Goodnight SH, Kenoyer G, Rapaport SI, et al: Defibrination after brain-tissue destruction. A serious complication of head injury. N Engl J Med 290:1043–1047, 1974
144.  Miner ME, Graham SH, Gildenberg PL: Disseminated intravascular coagulation fibrinolytic syndrome following head injury in children: Frequency and pragmatic implications. J Pediatr 100:687–691, 1982
145.  Editorial: Disseminated intravascular coagulation and head injury. Lancet 2:531, 1982
146.  Watts C: Disseminated intravascular coagulation. Surg Neurol 8:258–262, 1977
147.  Hardaway RM III: Syndrome of Disseminated Intravascular Coagulation with Special Reference to Shock and Hemorrhage. Springfield, Ill, Charles C Thomas, 1966
148.  Collins JA: Post-traumatic pulmonary insufficiency, in Zuidema GD, Rutherford RP, Ballinger WF II (eds): The Management of Trauma (ed 3). Philadelphia, WB Saunders Co, 1979, pp 114–147
149.  Bone RC, Francis PB, Pierce AK: Intravascular coagulation associated with the adult respiratory distress syndrome. Am J Med 61:585–589, 1976
150.  Rinaldo JE, Rogers RM: Adult respiratory-distress syndrome. Changing concepts of lung injury and repair. N Engl J Med 306:900–909,1982
151.  Hathaway WE, Mull MM, Pechet GS: Disseminated intravascular coagulation in the newborn Pediatrics 43:233–240, 1969
152.  Favara BE, Franciosi RA, Butterfield LJ: Disseminated intravascular and cardiac thrombosis of the neonate. Am J Dis Child 127:197–204, 1974
153.  Bleyl U: Morphologic diagnosis of disseminated intravascular coagulation: Histologic, histochemical and electromicroscopic studies. Semin Thromb Hemostas 3:247–267, 1977
154.  Mehta B, Briggs DK, Sommers SC, et al: Disseminated intravascular coagulation following cardiac arrest: A study of 15 patients. Am J Med Sci 264:353–363, 1972
155.  Krug H, Raszeja-Wanic B, Wochowiak A: Intravascular coagulation in acute renal failure after myocardial infarction. Ann Intern Med 81:494–497, 1974
156.  Ratnoff OD, Nossel HL: Wasp study anaphylaxis. Blood 61:132–139, 1983
157.  Smith PL, Kagey-Sobotka A, Bleeker ER, et al: Physiologic manifestations of human anaphylaxis. J Clin Invest 66:1072–1080, 1980
158.  Smith VT: Anaphylactic shock, acute renal failure and disseminated intravascular coagulation. Suspected complications of zomepirac. JAMA 247:1172–1173, 1982
159.  Caprini JA, Lipp V, Zuckerman L, et al: Hematologic changes following burns. J Surg Res 22:626–635, 1977
160.  Simon TL, Curreri PW, Harker LA: Kinetic characterization of hemostasis in thermal injury. J Lab Clin Med 89:702–711, 1977
161.  McManus WF, Eurenius K, Pruitt BA Jr: Disseminated intravascular coagulation in burned patients. J Trauma 13:416–422, 1973
162.  Ports TA, Deuel TF: Intravascular coagulation in fresh-water submersion. Report of three cases. Ann Intern Med 87:60–61, 1977
163.  Bleisch V: In Aach R, Kissane M: A sixty-five year old woman with heat stroke. Am J Med 43:113–124, 1967

164. Shibolet S, Fisher S, Gilat T, et al: Fibrinolysis and hemorrhages in fatal heat stroke. N Engl J Med 266:169–173, 1962

165. Sohal RS, Sun SC, Colcolough HL, et al: Heat stroke. An electron microscopic study of endothelial cell damage and disseminated intravascular coagulation. Arch Intern Med 122: 43–47, 1968

166. Weber MB, Blakely JA: The hemorrhagic diathesis of heat stroke. A consumption coagulopathy successfully treated with heparin. Lancet 1:1190–1192, 1969

167. Johansson BW, Nilsson IM: The effect of heparin and ∊-aminocaproic acid on the coagulation in hypothermic dogs. Acta Physiol Scand 60:267–277, 1964

168. Chadd MA, Gray OP: Hypothermia and coagulation defects in the newborn. Arch Dis Child 47:819–821, 1972

169. Cohen IJ: Cold injury in early infancy. Relationship between mortality and disseminated intravascular coagulation. Isr J Med Sci 13:405–409, 1977

170. Mahood JM, Evans A: Accidental hypothermia, disseminated intravascular coagulation and pancreatitis. NZ Med J 87:283–284, 1978

171. Mahajan SL, Myers TJ, Baldini MG: Disseminated intravascular coagulation during rewarming following hypothermia. JAMA 245:2517–2518, 1981

172. Thomas JE, Ayyar DR: Systemic fat embolism. A diagnostic profile in 24 patients. Arch Neurol 26:517–523, 1972

173. Dines DE, Burgher LW, Okazaki H: The clinical and pathologic correlation of fat embolism syndrome. Mayo Clin Proc 50:407–411, 1975

174. Horne RH, Horne JH: Fat embolization prophylaxis. Arch Intern Med 133:188–291, 1974

175. Riseborough EJ, Herndon JH: Alterations in pulmonary function, coagulation and fat metabolism in patients with fractures of the lower limbs. Clin Orthop 115:248–267, 1976

176. Bradford DS, Foster RR, Nossel HL: Coagulation alterations, hypoxemia and fat embolism in fracture patients. J Trauma 10:307–321, 1970

177. Saldeen T: The importance of intravascular coagulation and inhibition of the fibrinolytic system in experimental fat embolism. J Trauma 10:287–298, 1970

178. Gossling HR: The fat embolism syndrome. JAMA 241:2740–2742, 1979

179. Wilson JJ, Neame PB, Kelton JG: Infection-induced thrombocytopenia. Semin Thromb Hemostas 8:217–233, 1982

180. McGehee WG, Rapaport SI, Hjort PF: Intravascular coagulation in fulminant meningococcemia. Ann Intern Med 67:250–260, 1967

181. Ratnoff OD, Nebehay WG: Multiple coagulative defects in a patient with Waterhouse-Friderichsen syndrome. Ann Intern Med 56:627–632, 1962

182. Bisno AL, Freeman JC: The syndrome of asplenia, pneumococcal sepsis, and disseminated intravascular coagulation. Ann Intern Med 72:389–393, 1970

183. Gopal V, Bisno AL: Fulminant pneumococcal infections in normal 'asplenic' hosts. Arch Intern Med 137:1526–1530, 1977

184. Ammann AJ, Addiego J, Wara DW, et al: Polyvalent pneumococcal-polysaccharide immunization of patients with sickle-cell anemia and patients with splenectomy. N Engl J Med 297:897–900, 1977

185. Overturf GD, Field R, Edmonds R: Death from type 6 pneumococcal septicemia in a vaccinated child with sickle-cell disease. N Engl J Med 300:143, 1979 (letter)

186. Hjort PF, Rapaport SI, Jørgensen L: Purpura fulminans. Report of a case successfully treated with heparin and hydrocortisone. Review of 50 cases from the literature. Scand J Haematol 1:169–192, 1964

187. Chambers WN, Holyoke JB, Wilson RF: Purpura fulminans. Report of two cases following scarlet fever. N Engl J Med 297:933–935, 1952

188. Heal FC, Kent G: Purpura fulminans with afibrinogenaemia. Can Med Assoc J 69:367–370, 1953

189. Antley RM, McMillan C: Sequential coagulation studies in purpura fulminans. N Engl J Med 276:1287–1290, 1967
190. Spicer TE, Rau JM: Purpura fulminans. Am J Med 61:566–570, 1976
191. Little JR: Purpura fulminans treated successfully with anticoagulation. JAMA 169:36–40, 1959
192. Kasabach HH, Merritt KK: Capillary hemangioma with extensive purpura. Report of a case. Am J Dis Child 59:1063–1070, 1940
193. Verstraete M, Vermylen C, Vermylen J, et al: Excessive consumption of blood coagulation components as a cause of hemorrhagic diathesis. Am J Med 38:899–908, 1965
194. Bachman F, Vietti T, Kulapongs P: Consumption coagulopathy. Sequential studies in a patient with Kasabach-Merritt syndrome. Blood 28:1016–1017, 1966 (abstract)
195. Propp RP, Scharfman WB: Hemangioma-thrombocytopenia syndrome associated with microangiopathic hemolytic anemia. Blood 28:623–633, 1966
196. Inceman S, Tangün Y: Chronic defibrination syndrome due to a giant hemangioma associated with microangiopathic hemolytic anemia. Am J Med 46:997–1002, 1969
197. Beller FK, Ruhrmann G: Zur Pathogenese des Kasabach-Merritt syndroms (Riesenhämagiom, Blutung, Thrombopenie und Afibrinogenämie). Klin Wochenschr 37:1078–1082, 1959
198. Good TA, Carnazzo SF, Good RA: Thrombocytopenia and giant hemangioma in infants. AMA Am J Dis Child 90:260–274, 1955
199. D'Amico JA, Hoffman GC, Dyment PG: Klippel-Trénaunay syndrome associated with chronic disseminated intravascular coagulation and massive osteolysis. Cleve Clin Q 44:181–188, 1977
200. Shanberge JH, Tanaka K, Gruhl MC: Chronic consumption coagulopathy due to hemangiomatous transformation of the spleen. Am J Clin Pathol 56:723–729, 1971
201. Alpert LI, Benesch B: Hemangioendothelioma of the liver associated with microangiopathic hemolytic anemia. Am J Med 48:624–628, 1970
202. Blix S, Jacobsen CD: The defibrination syndrome in a patient with haemangio-endothelio-sarcoma. Acta Med Scand 173:377–383, 1963
203. Fine NL, Applebaum J, Elguezabal A, et al: Multiple coagulation defects in association with dissecting aneurysm. Arch Intern Med 119:522–526, 1967
204. Mulcare RD, Royster TS, Weiss HJ, et al: Disseminated intravascular coagulation as a complication of abdominal aortic aneurysm repair. Ann Surg 180:343–349, 1974
205. Straub PW, Kessler S: Umsatz und Lokalisation von $^{131}$I-Fibrinogen bei chronischer intravasale Gerinnung. Schweiz Med Wochenschr 100:2001–2003, 1970
206. Cate JW ten, Timmers H, Becker AE: Coagulopathy in ruptured or dissecting aneurysm. Am J Med 59:171–176, 1975
207. Moschcowitz E: An acute febrile pleiochromic anemia with hyaline thrombosis of the terminal arterioles and capillaries. An undescribed disease. Arch Intern Med 36:89–93, 1925
208. Pisciotta AV, Gottschall JL: Clinical features of thrombotic thrombocytopenic purpura. Semin Thromb Hemostas 6:330–340, 1980
209. Crain SM, Choudhury AM: Thrombotic thrombocytopenic purpura. A reappraisal. JAMA 246:1243–1246, 1981
210. Ridolfi RL, Bell WR: Thrombotic thrombocytopenic purpura. Report of 25 cases and review of the literature. Medicine 60:413–428, 1981
211. Kwann HC: Thrombotic thrombocytopenic purpura, in Kwann HC, Bowie EJW (eds): Thrombosis. Philadelphia, WB Saunders Co, 1982, pp 185–194
212. Orbison JL: Morphology of thrombotic thrombocytopenic purpura with demonstration of aneurysms. Am J Pathol 28:129–143, 1952
213. Jaffe EA, Nachman RL, Merskey C: Thrombotic thrombocytopenic purpura—Coagulation parameters in twelve patients. Blood 42:499–507, 1973
214. Lian ECY, Harkness DR, Byrnes JJ, et al: Presence of a platelet aggregating factor in the plasma of patients with thrombotic thrombocytopenic purpura (TTP) and its inhibition by normal plasma. Blood 53:333–338, 1979

215. Burns ER, Zucker-Franklin D: Pathologic effects of plasma from patients with thrombotic thrombocytopenic purpura on platelets and cultured endothelial cells. Blood 60:1030–1037, 1982

216. Remuzzi G, Rossi EC, Misiani R, et al: Prostacyclin and thrombotic microangiopathy. Semin Thromb Hemostas 6:391–394, 1980

217. Moake JL, Rudy CK, Troll JH, et al: Unusually large plasma factor VIII: von Willebrand factor multimers in chronic relapsing thrombotic thrombocytopenic purpura. N Engl Med 307:1432–1435, 1982

218. Rubenstein MA, Kagan BM, MacGillviray H, et al: Unusual remission in a case of thrombotic thrombocytopenic purpura syndrome following fresh blood exchange transfusion. Ann Intern Med 51:1409–1419, 1959

219. Bukowski RM, Hewlett JS, Reimer RR, et al: Therapy of thrombotic thrombocytopenic purpura: An overview. Semin Thromb Hemostas 7:1–8, 1981

220. Gasser von C, Gautier E, Steck A, et al: Hämolytisch-Urämische Syndrome: Bilaterale Nierenindennekrosen bei akute erworbenen hämolytischen Anämien. Schweiz Med Wochenschr 85:905–909, 1955

221. McQuiggan MC, Oliver WJ, Littler ER, et al: Hemolytic uremic syndrome. JAMA 191:787–792, 1965

222. Vitsky BH, Suzuki Y, Strauss L, et al: Hemolytic-uremic syndrome. A study of renal pathologic alterations. Am J Pathol 57:627–648, 1969

223. Kaplan BS, Drummond KN: The hemolytic-uremic syndrome is a syndrome. N Engl J Med 298:964–966, 1978

224. Brain MC: Hemolysis and renal disease, in Jepson JH (ed): Hematologic Problems in Renal Disease. Menlo Park, Calif, Addison-Wesley, 1979, pp 38–68

225. Katz J, Krawitz S, Sacks PV, et al: Platelet, erythrocyte, and fibrinogen kinetics in the hemolytic-uremic syndrome of infancy. J Pediatr 83:739–748, 1973

226. George CRP, Slichter SJ, Quadracci LJ, et al: A kinetic evaluation of hemostasis in renal disease. N Engl J Med 291:1111–1115, 1974

227. Ponticelli C, Rivolta E, Imbasciati E, et al: Hemolytic-uremic syndrome in adults. Arch Intern Med 140:353–357, 1980

228. Sorrenti LY, Lewy PR: The hemolytic-uremic syndrome. Experience at a center in the Midwest. Am J Dis Child 132:59–62, 1977

229. Longmore DB, Bennett JG, Hoyle PM, et al: Prostacyclin administration during cardiopulmonary bypass in man. Lancet 1:800–804, 1981

230. Harker LA, Malpass TW, Branson HE, et al: Mechanism of abnormal bleeding in patients undergoing cardiopulmonary bypass: Acquired transient platelet dysfunction associated with selective α-granule release. Blood 56:824–834, 1980

231. Ruckley CV, Das PC, Leitch AG, et al: Serum fibrin/fibrinogen degradation products associated with postoperative pulmonary embolus and venous thrombosis. Br Med J 4:395–398, 1970

232. Hedner U, Nilsson IM: Clinical experience with determination of fibrinogen degradation products. Acta Med Scand 189:471–477, 1971

233. Bick RL: The clinical significance of fibrinogen degradation products. Semin Thromb Hemostas 8:302–330, 1982

234. Klein HG, Bell WR: Disseminated intravascular coagulation during heparin therapy. Ann Intern Med 80:477–481, 1974

235. Clarkson AR, MacDonald MK, Petrie JJB, et al: Serum and urinary fibrin/fibrinogen degradation products in glomerulonephritis. Br Med J 3:447–451, 1971

236. Kanyerezi BR, Lwanga SK, Bloch KJ: Fibrinogen degradation products in serum and urine of patients with systemic lupus erythematosus. Relation to renal disease and pathogenetic mechanisms. Arthritis Rheum 14:267–275, 1971

237.  deGaetano G, Vermylen J, Donati MB, et al: Indomethacin and platelet aggregation in chronic glomerulonephritis: Existence of non-responders. Br Med J 2:301–303, 1974

238.  Robson AM, Cole BR, Kienstra RA, et al: Severe glomerulonephritis complicated by coagulopathy: Treatment with anticoagulant immunosuppressive drugs. J Pediatr 90:881–892, 1977

239.  Editorial: Anti-platelet agents in nephrology. Lancet 1:426–427, 1981

240.  Lichtman MA, Hoyer LW, Sears DA: Erythrocyte deformation and hemolytic anemia coincident with the microvacular disease of rejected renal homotransplants. Am J Med Sci 256:239–246, 1968

241.  Hutton MM, Prentice CRM, Allison MEM, et al: Renal homotransplantation rejection associated with microangiopathic haemolytic anemia. Br Med J 3:87–88, 1970

242.  Starzl TE, Boehmig HJ, Amemiya H, et al: Clotting changes, including disseminated intravascular coagulation, during rapid renal-homograft rejection. N Engl J Med 283:383–390, 1970

243.  Williams GM, Hume DM, Hudson RP Jr, et al: "Hyperacute" renal-homograft rejection in man. N Engl J Med 279:611–618, 1968

244.  Guttmann RD: Medical progress: Renal transplantation. N Engl J Med 301:1038–1048, 1979

Bruce Bennett
Derek Ogston

# 9

# Fibrinolytic Bleeding Syndromes

Fibrin deposits in the body are removed in healthy individuals. This is achieved by the action of the fibrinolytic enzyme system. Abnormally increased activity in this system results in hemorrhage, but bleeding due to overactive fibrinolysis is a rare event. When it does occur, however, it can be very severe and may be fatal. Fibrinolytic bleeding can be divided, broadly speaking, into two types, primary and secondary. Primary fibrinolysis, as its name implies, occurs without any other detected disorder of the hemostatic mechanism; it is thus a relatively clearly defined disorder, and specific inhibitors of fibrinolysis are useful in its control. Secondary fibrinolysis is the term used to describe overactivity of the system in patients whose primary hemostatic disorder is thought to be disseminated (or local) intravascular coagulation (DIC); here the enhanced fibrinolysis is sometimes regarded as representing a compensatory mechanism which may protect the organism by removing the widespread intravascular deposits of fibrin which occur in DIC. Both the intravascular clotting and the increased fibrinolytic activity will, however, contribute to the hemorrhagic disorder, the former by depleting or consuming plasma clotting factors during coagulation and the latter by digesting some of them and generating breakdown products of fibrin or fibrinogen which themselves have anticoagulant properties. If the belief that secondary fibrinolysis is a protective mechanism is correct, it is clearly irrational to attempt to inhibit it therapeutically, and animal experiments indicate that doing so in the presence of DIC may markedly increase organ damage by enhancing the persistence of deposited fibrin.

## THE FIBRINOLYTIC ENZYME SYSTEM

Fibrinolysis is the result of the action of the protease plasmin, which is not normally detectable in circulating blood. Its inert precursor, plasminogen, circulates in the plasma as a potential source of plasmin. Conversion of plasminogen to plasmin may be achieved by a number of agents known collectively as plasminogen activators *(PA)*, whose nature

Previously unreported studies reported here were supported by grants G978/718/S–G812/289/ISA from the Medical Research Council of Great Britain.

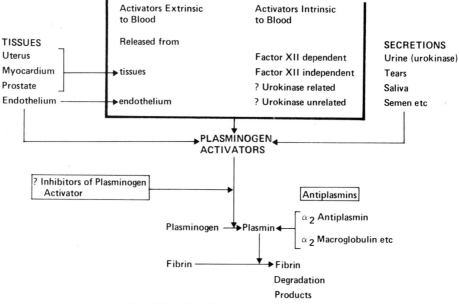

**Fig. 9-1.** The fibrinolytic enzyme system.

and interrelationships are only now being elucidated. The system itself is held rigorously in check in the circulating blood by several inhibitors, the principal one of which, $\alpha_2$-antiplasmin, very rapidly combines with and neutralizes any plasmin formed, thus protecting the plasma proteins from digestion by plasmin. An outline of the system appears in Figure 9-1.

## Plasminogen and Plasmin

The circulating proenzyme plasminogen has a molecular weight of approximately 80,000,[1] and is a single-chain molecule of established amino acid sequence.[2] It occupies a position in the fibrinolytic system analogous to that of prothrombin in coagulation and has other similarities to prothrombin in that it contains several internal disulfide bonds which produce a number of triple loop or "kringle" structures in the protein chain. The circulating form of the protein has glutamic acid at its $NH_2$-terminus (Glu-plasminogen),[3] but a second form with $NH_2$-terminal lysine (Lys-plasminogen) is produced by removal of a small peptide.[4] Lys-plasminogen is more readily converted to plasmin than the glu form and is adsorbed onto fibrin but its role in physiological fibrinolysis is not yet clear. Rupture of a specific bond (Arg 560-Val 561) converts the molecule to plasmin, a two-chain structure linked by internal disulfide bonds of the original plasminogen molecule. The active site of the enzyme is situated on the light (B) chain and contains serine and histidine.[5] The heavy chain contains sites with affinity for lysine[6] which participate in the linking of the molecule to fibrinogen and its interactions with its major inhibitor, $\alpha_2$-antiplasmin.

Plasmin is capable of digesting many proteins [e.g., fibrin, fibrinogen, factors V (proaccelerin) and VIII (antihemophilic factor), and casein], various esters, and amides. Assays of plasmin are based on one or another of these properties.[1] Plasminogen has no such activity, but it may be assayed after conversion to plasmin in similar systems.[1,7]

## Activators of Plasminogen

PAs which convert plasminogen to plasmin, are less well defined than plasminogen or plasmin. It is known that several such agents exist in the blood, vascular endothelium, solid tissues, and various secretions, but their interrelationships are only now being investigated in detail.[8] Figure 9-1 outlines the sources of PA, but which is of major physiological importance is not established.

Urokinase, the activator secreted in human urine, has been studied in detail. It has been purified, and two forms with a molecular size of approximately 30,000 and 50,000 are recognized.[9] It converts plasminogen to plasmin by digestion of the single bond mentioned above, is nonantigenic in man, and has been widely used to achieve therapeutic thrombolysis. It is not adsorbed strongly onto fibrin, which is a disadvantage in its use as a thrombolytic agent.

Blood vessel endothelium, particularly that of veins,[10] produces PA. Activator purified from the washouts of cadaveric leg veins presumably represents this endothelial activator. It has a molecular weight of approximately 65,000[11] in the purified form, has been reported to exist as a single-chain[12] molecule, and is adsorbed onto fibrin. Cultured endothelial cells produce activator which is released into the culture medium.[13]

Many tissues, including myocardium, uterus, and prostate, have been shown to contain PA. Activator purified from human myometrium also has a molecular weight of 65,000[14] and has been reported to exist in both single-chain and two-chain molecular forms. The significance of the difference between the two forms is unknown, as they appear to have similar fibrinolytic properties;[15] possibly the two-chain form is the result of proteolysis of the single-chain one.[16] Human myocardial PA has a molecular size similar to that of the uterus and appears to exist as a single-chain molecule.[8,17]

Circulating blood appears to contain several types of PA.[8,18] Activator levels in normal blood are very low, which has delayed their identification and characterization. Levels rise sharply after many stimuli such as exercise, injection of adrenalin, and venous occlusion. The activator present after prolonged venous occlusion has been partially purified.[19] On chromatography on Sephadex gels, it separates as molecules of large size in buffers containing high salt concentrations as if a complex had been disrupted. This activator is avidly adsorbed by fibrin.[19] It may represent activator released from the venous endothelium, as it has physical and immunological properties similar to those of the activators from cadaveric endothelium and some tissues but different from those of urokinase.[18,20] It is sometimes called the extrinsic activator of the blood on the assumption that it does arise from outside the blood itself.

Blood collected from resting individuals not stimulated by exercise, adrenalin, venous occlusion, etc. does contain very small amounts of PA. This material is thought to be different from that present after exercise on the basis of its sensitivity to C1 inactivator. This activator is sometimes termed intrinsic activator on the assumption that it arises from the blood itself. Whether this is true or not, it is clear that, although the PA present after exercise, occlusion, etc. is directly demonstrable in plasma, activator may also be generated from plasma by incubation with kaolin or other agents known to activate the contact phase of coagulation.[22] This generation is a time-dependent process, and such generated activators may be regarded as intrinsic to the blood. This pathway to the generation of PA is defective in Hageman trait, Fletcher trait, and Fitzgerald trait plasmas. The pathway therefore requires factor XII,[22] plasma prekallikrein,[23] and high molecular weight kininogen[24] to generate PA and other less clearly defined factors[22] as well. The agent generated by this pathway which actually activates plasminogen has not been identified. Kallikrein,[25] activated Hageman factor, and, to a lesser degree, Hageman factor fragments[26] activate plasminogen in pure systems, but the contact-dependent activator is probably separate from these[27]; it has some properties similar to those of postocclusion (extrinsic) activator and PA from vascular endothelium or human myocardium,[18] but has not been purified or examined by immunological methods. This pathway to activator formation is inhibited by $\bar{C1}$ inactivator[21] and by a separate inhibitor detected first by its ability to inhibit urokinose[28] both of these agents inhibit activated factor XII, and some of their inhibitory properties may reflect this action. As if this were not complex enough, it is now suggested that there are "intrinsic activators" independent of factor XII,[29,30] and that some intrinsic activators are related to urokinase whereas others[30,31] are not. So, just as there may be several different extrinsic activators derived from different tissues, so there may be more than one form of intrinsic activator of plasminogen. This problem should be clarified in the future.

## Inhibitors of Fibrinolysis

Plasma contains several protease inhibitors which are capable of neutralizing the action of plasmin in pure systems. For many years, the principal plasma inhibitors of plasmin (or antiplasmins) were thought to be $\alpha_2$-macroglobulin and $\alpha_1$-antitrypsin. Recently, however, it has been shown that a protein different from these agents is responsible for the major part of plasmin neutralization in plasma.[32] This protein is now known as $\alpha_2$-antiplasmin.[32a] It has a molecular weight of 60,000–70,000 and is a single-chain structure which has been partially sequenced. It forms a 1:1 molecular complex with plasmin exceedingly rapidly,[33] a fact which may account for the observation that free plasmin is only very rarely detectable in circulating blood. The rate of interaction of this protein with plasmin is influenced by the availability of the lysine-binding sites on the plasmin molecule, and its complexing with plasmin neutralizes the enzyme activity of the molecule completely and irreversibly. The observations illustrated in Figure 9-2 (p 331) indicate that the complexes, once formed, are rapidly cleared from the blood. This agent thus accounts for most of the immediate neutralization of plasmin formed within the body. If its ability to do this is overwhelmed, then plasmin inhibition may result from the action of $\alpha_2$-macroglobulin,[34] which thus acts as a reserve of antiplasmin activity. $\alpha_1$-Antitrypsin, antithrombin III, $\bar{C1}$ inactivator, and inter-$\alpha$-trypsin inhibitor are all proteins shown to have some antiplasmin activity in vitro.[35] Their role as physiological antiplasmins in vivo is probably minor. Isolated deficiency of $\alpha_2$-antiplasmin results in a severe bleeding disorder, whereas deficiencies of the other antiplasmins do not.[36]

Most of the work on inhibitors of fibrinolysis has centered on molecules with antiplasmin activity. As overall blood fibrinolytic activity or potential activity probably depends primarily upon PA levels, however, the possibility that inhibitors of activator exist is of major interest, as these inhibitors may represent a further mechanism for the regulation of in vivo fibrinolysis. Methodological problems, particularly the absence of specific substrates for PA other than plasminogen itself, have complicated these studies. (Because plasminogen has been used as the substrate, and is measurable only in plasmin assays, the distinction between inhibition of activator and that of plasmin has not been clearly made.) Some evidence has been obtained suggesting that inhibitors of urokinase exist in the blood, apart from antiplasmin,[8,28,32] but as many human activators are not related to urokinase, the significance of these inhibitors in vivo is unknown. One carefully studied protein, detected initially by virtue of its ability to inhibit urokinase-induced clot lysis, has since been shown to inhibit activated factor XII and factor XIIa-induced clot lysis and to be separate from known plasmin inhibitors[37]; it may thus have a role in control of intrinsic fibrinolytic mechanisms in the body. $C\bar{1}$ inactivator may have a similar function.[21] Information on inhibitors of tissue or endothelial (extrinsic) blood activators is meager. Such inhibitors have been described in endothelial cell cultures[38] and in plasma,[39] apparently separate from antiplasmins, but some workers doubt that they have an important physiological role and propose that activator levels are controlled in vivo by clearance via mechanisms other than neutralization by plasma inhibitors.[40]

An interesting observation, recently made, indicates that histidine-rich glycoprotein may slow the interaction between plasmin and $\alpha_2$-antiplasmin.[41] The potential importance of any agent which influences this interaction is clearly considerable, but the actual physiological role of this protein is still undefined.

## FIBRINOLYSIS AND ITS CONTROL IN THE BODY

Fibrin thrombi may lyse spontaneously, and fibrin that is deposited in tissues damaged by mechanical trauma or pathological processes such as pneumonia or nephritis is removed as tissues heal or scars form. As free plasmin is virtually never detected in the circulating blood, this process must occur as a local phenomenon by local activation of fibrinolysis; any plasmin formed locally and diffusing away from the site of activity must be neutralized so rapidly that it is not detectable on blood sampling. This must indicate a sophisticated mechanism ensuring local lysis of fibrin while protecting the organism from plasmin-induced digestion of proteins in the circulating blood. How is this achieved? It is currently believed that the balance which allows local fibrin lysis to occur while preventing systemic hyperplasminemia depends on two principal factors, namely, the avidity of formed fibrin for plasminogen and certain of the plasminogen activators, and the opposing avidity of plasma $\alpha_2$-antiplasmin for formed plasmin.[42]

Small quantities of plasminogen are adsorbed onto insoluble fibrin.[43] Such adsorption depends upon the availability of the lysine binding sites in the plasminogen chain and is impaired if these sites are blocked by lysine or fibrinolytic inhibitors such as epsilon aminocaproic acid or tranexamic acid. If its lysine binding sites are unoccupied, formed plasmin is also presumably adsorbed onto fibrin. Certain PAs, namely, the postocclusion,[19] endothelial,[44] and tissue[45] activators, have a marked affinity for fibrin and are adsorbed onto it; the activity of PAs may be enhanced in the presence of fibrin or fibrin monomer.[46] Plasminogen and activator thus are preferentially concentrated on solid fibrin strands, where conversion of plasminogen to plasmin may take place. Plasmin so formed will be protected from rapid inactivation by plasma antiplasmins, as its lysine binding sites are occupied by its adsorption to the fibrin molecule. Thus the combination of these plasmin molecules with $\alpha_2$-antiplasmin is impeded.[42,47] Should plasmin be detached from the fibrin clot and diffuse away, its lysine binding sites presumably become free and allow its rapid inactivation by virtue of its combination with $\alpha_2$-antiplasmin. Similarly, should any plasmin be formed in the circulation remote from fibrin, it will be rapidly neutralized by combination with $\alpha_2$-antiplasmin. The unique property of fibrin of adsorbing both plasminogen (by bonds involving sites which participate in the inhibition of any plasmin formed from these molecules) and PA thus accounts for the specificity of action of the fibrinolytic system for fibrin itself, whereas the rapidity with which $\alpha_2$-antiplasmin neutralizes any free plasmin in the circulation under normal circumstances protects the plasma proteins from digestion by plasmin. It should be noted that fibrinogen does not share with fibrin the property of attracting or complexing with plasminogen or activator. The nature of the sites of adsorption of plasminogen on the fibrin molecule remains to be defined, as does the nature of the activator-fibrin interaction.

To allow these mechanisms for control of fibrinolysis to function, it is necessary that adequate levels of plasminogen, PA, and $\alpha_2$-antiplasmin be maintained. The levels of plasminogen and activator necessary to secure lysis of thrombi in the body, and of $\alpha_2$-antiplasmin to prevent fibrinolytic bleeding, are not as yet clearly established.

## MEASUREMENT OF ENHANCED FIBRINOLYTIC ACTIVITY IN THE BODY

The presence of abnormally increased fibrinolytic activity in the circulating blood is easy to establish, and involves the detection of either plasmin or PA activity. Free plasmin is very rarely present, but may appear if an overwhelming and sudden episode of fibrinolytic activity occurs such as results from the injection of very large doses of urokinase or streptokinase or, perhaps, an acute clinical event such as amniotic fluid embolism. Under these circumstances, plasmin may be generated in quantities too great for immediate inhibition by $\alpha_2$-antiplasmin, and free plasmin will thus be detectable. More commonly, pathologically enhanced fibrinolysis is due to excessive quantities of PA in the blood which, without causing directly demonstrable systemic hyperplasminemia, may be associated with hemorrhage. Screening tests which, in the clinical context of severe hemorrhage, will indicate whether systemic hyperfibrinolysis is a causative factor are discussed next.

1. The whole blood clot lysis time (WBCLT) is the simplest test of pathologically increased fibrinolytic activity. If a nonanticoagulated blood sample obtained from a bleeding patient is seen to clot spontaneously in a test tube and the clot then lyses spontaneously at 37°C in 8 hours or less, there can be no doubt that excessive systemic fibrinolytic activity is present. This is a very simple, direct test of value in the acute situation. It does not distinguish between increased levels of PA and plasmin itself. Whole blood clots from normal individuals show no visible lysis within 48 hours although they may retract.

2. A minor refinement of the WBCLT is the plasma euglobulin clot lysis time (ELT). This involves precipitation of the euglobulin fraction of plasma (which contains a proportion of the plasma fibrinogen, plasminogen, and PA, but leaves most of the inhibitors of fibrinolysis in the supernatant), clotting of the precipitate after it is redissolved in buffer, with thrombin, and observation of the time it takes for clot lysis to occur. This test is clearly more time-consuming in preparation than the WBCLT, but exclusion of the bulk of plasma inhibitors from the system means that overall clot lysis times are much more rapid and the test result is available sooner. ELTs from resting normal individuals in our laboratory are usually over 80 minutes, whereas times of 20 minutes have been recorded in patients with excessive fibrinolysis that may possibly cause bleeding. It should be noted, however, that under extreme physiological conditions in normal individuals, namely, prolonged exercise, we have noted ELTs in this rapid range with no hemorrhagic phenomena and no change in plasma fibrinogen or plasminogen levels.[8]

3. Neither of the above tests distinguishes high activator levels from the presence of free plasmin, although the former is far more common. Additionally, both methods depend on plasma plasminogen for the expression of PA levels, and the very low levels of plasminogen sometimes encountered during therapeutic infusion of urokinase or streptokinase may result in a prolonged WBCLT or ELT even when activator levels are high. This

problem may be circumvented by the use of a method which observes the lysis of pre-formed fibrin which either does or does not contain plasminogen. Lysis of plasminogen-free fibrin indicates the presence of plasmin, whereas lysis of plasminogen-containing fibrin indicates the presence of plasmin *or* PA. The simplest such system is the fibrin plate assay, in which a film of fibrin (with or without plasminogen) is prepared in a Petri dish, a standard volume of plasma (e.g., 30λ) is placed on the film as a drop from a micropipette, and the area of lysis resulting after a fixed period at 37°C is measured. The concurrent use of plasminogen-containing and plasminogen-free fibrin plates will distinguish plasmin from PA in the applied sample, but for clinical purposes this is probably academic. In our labora-tory, plasma from resting normal individuals never produces lysis of such plasminogen-containing plates in 6 hours and rarely in 24 hours; in patients with fibrinolytic bleeding, significant lysis is detectable in 6 hours. More sophisticated assays involving lysis of pre-formed radiolabeled fibrin exist but are too complex for routine use in clinical laboratories.

These three simple tests therefore will, within a few hours, indicate the presence or absence of fibrinolytic activity increased to a degree likely to contribute to bleeding. No additional test is required for this assessment to be made. As the WBCLT can be set up by a totally untrained individual, provided there is reasonable access to a 37°C water bath, a decision as to whether increased systemic fibrinolysis is current and operative may reason-ably be made on the basis of this assay alone in extreme circumstances. The other two tests require preparedness in the laboratory but only very modest expertise. These tests are therefore sufficient to allow a conclusion as to the current involvement of fibrinolysis in a bleeding episode and a decision as to whether intervention might modify it. They do not indicate whether fibrinolysis is primary or secondary, that is, whether DIC is contributing to the disorder. This decision is a clinically important and sometimes difficult one, and is discussed later in this chapter and in Chapter 8.

Other measurements undertaken routinely in the investigation of bleeding disorders or more specialized studies accessible to most routine laboratories may reflect indirectly the activity of the fibrinolytic system at the moment of sampling or in the period prior to sampling. This distinction is important. Only tests that detect plasmin or PA activity indi-cate that fibrinolysis is systemically enhanced at the moment of blood sampling, and it is clearly fruitless to intervene in an attempt to control overactive fibrinolysis if this is a transient phenomenon which has passed.

Tests which may provide an indirect indication of current or recent fibrinolytic activ-ity are now described.

4. Routine screening tests of coagulation pathways such as the thrombin (TT), pro-thrombin (PT), and partial thromboplastin times (PTT) may be prolonged in severe sys-temic fibrinolytic episodes due to depletion of plasma fibrinogen or other procoagulants such as factors V or VIII. This may occur in episodes of primary fibrinolysis, although, as discussed later, it is easier to establish that fibrinolysis is primary if these tests are not severely abnormal. Marked prolongation of these screening tests is commonly encoun-tered in episodes of intravascular coagulation with secondary fibrinolysis. In this situation, the relative contribution to depletion of clotting factors by the coagulant component of the syndrome (by "consumption" during fibrin formation) as opposed to the fibrinolytic com-ponent (by digestion of clotting factors by plasmin) is impossible to quantify clearly. Although acute intravascular coagulation with secondary fibrinolysis is typically accompa-nied by severe prolongation of the TT, PT, and PTT, and although primary fibrinolysis is usually identified with certainty only when minor changes in these screening tests exist, there is no conceptual reason why primary fibrinolysis may not occasionally cause severe

prolongation of all three tests. Experience with the therapeutic use of PA confirms that this may occur.

A further reason for some prolongation of these tests exists in severe fibrinolytic episodes quite apart from the reduction in the levels of clotting factors. This is the anticoagulant effect of the breakdown products of fibrinogen, which may impede thrombin formation and the thrombin–fibrinogen interaction or impair fibrin polymerization and thus prolong the clotting time observed in any test.

It may thus be said that normality of these screening tests (or normality of the levels of individual clotting factors, if they are specifically measured) in a hemorrhagic patient who has evidence of pathologically enhanced fibrinolysis in the studies described above suggests that primary fibrinolytic bleeding is occurring. Abnormality of the coagulation studies may indicate intravascular coagulation with or without secondary fibrinolysis or severe primary fibrinolysis.

5. The detection in serum of agents believed to represent breakdown products of fibrinogen or fibrin is widely used to indicate that fibrinolysis is active in the body. Plasmin digests fibrinogen, producing a number of fragments known as fibrinogen breakdown products, which were originally designated A, B, C, D, and E according to their size and the order in which they were produced.[48] Other breakdown products have been separately identified, larger fragments now being known as X and Y.[49] Plasmin also digests fibrin, producing fibrin breakdown products. Lysis of fibrin which has not been cross-linked by the action of factor XIII (fibrin-stabilizing factor) produces breakdown products similar to those resulting from the digestion of fibrinogen itself.[50,51] Factor XIII-induced cross-linking of fibrin, however, renders it more resistant to the action of plasmin. Breakdown products of cross-linked fibrin are, not surprisingly, structurally different from those produced from fibrinogen or non-cross-linked fibrin, as they may contain the interchain bonds induced by factor XIII. The fragments of cross-linked fibrin which have received most study are the dimer of the D fragment (D: dimer), and the one formed when this dimer retains its link to fragment E (D: dimer-E). It has been suggested that these fragments, or aggregates of them, represent the agents most commonly resulting from in vivo lysis of cross-linked fibrin[52]; this is not undisputed, and other large fragments may be generated.[53,54]

Specific detection of these different breakdown products may thus theoretically allow the distinction of fibrinogenolysis from lysis of cross-linked fibrin in the body, that is, it may distinguish current or recent generalized hyperplasminemia with digestion of circulating fibrinogen (undesirable) from digestion of deposits of cross-linked fibrin (usually desirable). Rapid, convenient methods for making such distinctions are not yet generally available.

Early methods used for demonstrating the presence of degradation products of fibrinogen or fibrin in blood relied on the demonstration of antigenic material similar to fibrinogen in the serum after clotting of blood by thrombin had been induced. That is, they demonstrated the presence of noncoagulable agents in serum using antisera to fibrinogen itself; the methods employed included tanned red cell hemagglutination inhibition.[55] Although this was a major advance, the use of antisera to fibrinogen itself does not allow the distinction of fragments of fibrin from those of fibrinogen. The currently widely used latex agglutination technique for the detection of fibrin(ogen) degradation products (FDP) employs latex coated with antibodies raised to the D and E fragments of fibrinogen. This is an extremely convenient and rapid technique but, like the assay depending on antisera to fibrinogen itself, will not distinguish fibrin from fibrinogen lysis because of the marked immunological similarity of the breakdown products of fibrinogen and fibrin.

A further problem in interpretation of the results of such techniques came with the demonstration that, under some circumstances, fibrin monomer may complex with fibrinogen itself or with some of the larger breakdown products of fibrinogen[56-58] these complexes may not always be coagulable with thrombin, and on occasion may appear in the serum. It is thus possible that immunologically based methods for the demonstration of FDP may sometimes detect, at least in part, fibrin monomer, a molecule produced by the action of thrombin, not plasmin, and thus ineligible for the title FDP. The current widely available assays are therefore best regarded as detecting fibrinogen- or fibrin-related antigens, or FRA (a term which includes fibrin monomer complexes, and fibrin- or fibrinogen-degradation products) rather than FDP specifically, and the makers of latex agglutination assay kits recognize this fact. Clotting of blood with thrombin prior to the performance of these immunoassays probably excludes most fibrin monomer complexes, but whether it invariably does so is not clearly established. In the last analysis, of course, plasma and not serum circulates in the body, and it is the agents present in vivo which we wish to detect. As one of the pioneers of the study of these agents has stated:[59]

The amount of FR-antigen in the serum is helpful in the diagnosis . . . but the antigen is biochemically undefined and the per cent recovered is unpredictable; thus it is of little pathogenic significance. Moreover, in the process of obtaining serum much of the enzyme-degraded FR-antigen is incorporated in the clot and all the fibrinogen in the sample is exposed to the enzymic action of thrombin in vitro, masking the effects of thrombin on the structure of FR-antigen in vivo.

These admirably judicious remarks remind us that the use of antibodies will indicate that antigen is detected, but will reveal little about the nature of the antigen. As indicated above, many fibrin(ogen)-related (FR) antigens may exist. A huge literature describes attempts to define more clearly the various FR antigens. From the clinical point of view, they will be useful if they result in techniques which a clinical laboratory can employ

1. to detect fibrinogen degradation products;
2. to detect fibrin degradation products;
3. to detect fibrin monomer or complexes of this in circulating blood;

and to differentiate clearly among these agents. Techniques used in research laboratories aimed at achieving these goals include

1. examination of the physical properties of FRA such as molecular size or charge[53,54,60-64];
2. examination of the chain structure of FRA[53,62,63];
3. examination of the ability of the components of FRA to dissociate, and the nature of the cross-links between them[53,62,63,65];
4. N-terminal analysis of FRA[66];
5. detection and characterization of neoantigens revealed on formation of certain FRA[62,67-70]

Few of the techniques used in these studies are appropriate for use in a routine clinical laboratory. Methods for characterization of FRA in terms of molecular size or charge, chain structure, or N-terminal properties are too complex and time-consuming for routine use, and the neoantigens detected on formation of some FRA have not resulted in simple immunological techniques for their specific detection in investigation of hemorrhagic patients.

Currently, therefore, the detection of FRA in serum using antisera to fibrinogen or to its D or E fragments allows the conclusion that fibrinolysis has been active in the recent past but

1. does not indicate that it is active at the moment of sampling;
2. does not distinguish clearly between lysis of fibrin or fibrinogen;
3. does not indicate whether some of the FRA identified represent soluble fibrin monomer (generated via intravascular coagulation) complexed with other FRA in noncoagulable forms.

These qualifications indicate that detection of FRA in serum does not distinguish systemic fibrinolysis with fibrinogen digestion, which is likely to be associated with a hemorrhagic risk, from episodes of local lysis of fibrin which are likely to be of value to the organism with little risk of bleeding (large quantities of FRA are detectable in episodes of pulmonary embolism, for instance). Clearly, however, the absence of significant quantities of FRA establishes the fact that significant fibrin or fibrinogen lysis has not occured in the recent past and that systemic fibrinolysis cannot easily be invoked as a cause of bleeding.

6. A different approach may prove useful in the future for establishing that pathological bleeding is due to enhanced fibrinolysis where doubt exists. It is established that $\alpha_2$-antiplasmin is the principal inhibitor of plasmin, and that it complexes very rapidly with free plasmin formed in the circulating blood. It is now possible to demonstrate the presence of large quantities of these complexes in the blood by the simple and accessible technique of two-dimensional immunoelectrophoresis of plasma against antisera to $\alpha_2$-antiplasmin.[71] Migration of the enzyme–inhibitor complex is slower than that of the uncomplexed inhibitor alone, allowing its detection by this method. Figure 9-2 shows a series of such observations in a patient with placental abruption and DIC, and Table 9-1 demonstrates that, although at the time of the onset of hemorrhage excessive fibrinolysis was present, it disappeared very rapidly. In contrast, plasmin–$\alpha_2$-antiplasmin complexes persisted in the plasma a little longer, although they too were cleared from the circulation fairly rapidly. In the context of acute intravascular clotting in labor, the detection of enhanced fibrinolysis by any technique is probably only of academic interest, as the disorder is self-limiting. Figure 9-2 is included to illustrate the phenomenon and to indicate the rapidity with which the complexes are cleared when the acute stimulus to their formation is transient. Use of this technique has been found to be of value in the authors' laboratory in the definition and management of the rarer event of primary fibrinolytic bleeding. It allows the convincing demonstration that plasmin is being generated in the circulation, although it may not be detectable in functional assays because of the rapidity with which it is complexed with and neutralized by $\alpha_2$-antiplasmin. The technique of two-dimensional immunoelectrophoresis is probably fairly insensitive and capable of detecting only large quantities of these complexes in the blood. This is not necessarily a disadvantage in the demonstration that pathological fibrinolysis is responsible for a hemorrhagic episode, as it indicates that a positive finding using the technique is of major importance. More sensitive methods for detection of plasmin-$\alpha_2$-antiplasmin complexes are being developed[72]; the complexes may exhibit neoantigens which will allow their detection by antisera specific to them. Such antisera are not yet generally available, but if their specificity for the complexes is clearly established in practice, immunoassays based on such antisera are likely to be useful in the definition of episodes of fibrinolytic bleeding.

Comparable approaches may also allow the detection of complexes between antithrombin III (ATIII) and activated procoagulants.[25] Whether or not complexed ATIII or complexed $\alpha_2$-antiplasmin, or both, are detected, may allow the assessment of the relative

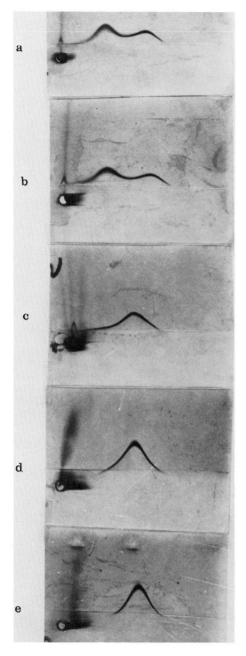

**Fig. 9-2.** Plasmin–$\alpha_2$-antiplasmin complexes in circulating blood demonstrated by two-dimensional immunoelectrophoresis of plasma against antiserum to $\alpha_2$-antiplasmin. Panels a, b, c, d, and e represent maternal blood findings during labor and 2, 18, 46, and 66 hours after delivery of a stillborn infant 3 hours after onset of placental abruption. (The routine hemostatic findings at these times are listed in Table 9-1.) The plasmin–$\alpha_2$-antiplasmin complex is clearly seen as the major slow-moving peak in panels a and b; panel c continues to show traces of complex 16 hours after the fibrin plate assay last showed significant systemic fibrinolytic activity. FRA disappeared later than did the plasmin–$\alpha_2$-antiplasmin complex. Panels d and e show a pattern identical to that seen in normal individuals. Vaginal bleeding was profuse for approximately 2–3 hours after delivery; the only treatment was transfusion of 7 U of whole blood.

**Table 9-1**

Findings on Routine Hemostatic Screening of the Patient, After an Episode of Placental Abruption, Whose Plasmin–$\alpha_2$-Antiplasmin Complexes are Illustrated in Figure 9-2

| Hours Post-partum | TT (sec) | PT (sec) | PTT (sec) | Serum FRA (μg/ml) | PA (fibrin plate) (mm²) | Plasmin–α-antiplasmin complex | Panel in Figure 9-2 |
|---|---|---|---|---|---|---|---|
| 0 | >120 | 20.5 | 73.2 | >40 | $12^2$ | +++ | a |
| 2 | >120 | 24.5 | 78.8 | >40 | $10^2$ | +++ | b |
| 5 | 14.5 | 14.5 | 38.0 | >40 | Trace | + | Not illustrated |
| 18 | 10.6 | 9.0 | 36.5 | >40 | 0 | Trace | c |
| 42 | 9.2 | 11.4 | 35.0 | >10 | 0 | 0 | d |
| 66 | 10.6 | 11.1 | 35.5 | <40 | | 0 | e |
| Control Values | 9.0–11.0 | 11.0–14.0 | 36.5–41.5 | 0 | 0 | 0 | — |

Key: TT, thrombin time; PT, prothrombin time; PTT, partial thromboplastin time; ELT, euglobulin clot-lysis time; PA, plasminogen activator (whole plasma applied to plasminogen-containing fibrin plate); FRA, fibrin/fibrinogen-related antigens; EACA, epsilon aminocaproic acid.

contributions of intravascular coagulation and fibrinolysis to bleeding episodes in a manner at least as useful as that hoped for by the specific detection of the different types of FRA.

7. Measurement of plasma plasminogen or plasma antiplasmin levels rarely contributes to the definition of a bleeding syndrome or to decisions on management. Plasminogen levels measured in functional assays are lowered during active systemic fibrinolytic episodes as plasminogen is converted to plasmin, which is neutralized by $\alpha_2$-antiplasmin; "fast" antiplasmin activity, the functional assay for $\alpha_2$-antiplasmin, may also be reduced as the inhibitor is utilized in the destruction of plasmin. These phenomena occur in both primary and secondary fibrinolysis and do not assist in their distinction. It should be noted that depletion of fast-acting antiplasmin activity, which occurred in the episodes of acute intravascular coagulation with secondary fibrinolysis we have studied, may not be accompanied by a similar reduction of the inhibitor measured by immunoassay (Table 9-3), whereas those patients with primary fibrinolysis had roughly equivalent reductions of antiplasmin in both the functional assays and immunoassays. After cessation of a fibrinolytic episode or of a stimulus such as the infusion of streptokinase and urokinase, levels of plasminogen return to normal over a period of about 48 hours and levels of fast-acting antiplasmin rise fairly rapidly.

With the exception, however, of the very rare hereditary deficiency of $\alpha_2$-antiplasmin, measurement of levels of the two proteins does not assist in defining acute bleeding disorders or in making decisions on their management. Technical descriptions of the assay techniques discussed in this section appear in detail in several publications.[7,73,74]

## HEREDITARY FIBRINOLYTIC BLEEDING

### $\alpha_2$-Antiplasmin Deficiency

Specific deficiency of this protein has now been described in two families.[75-77] In the first,[75] the affected individual had approximately 3 percent of the normal quantity of $\alpha_2$-antiplasmin in his blood, a severe bleeding tendency after injuries, and occasional spontaneous bleeding episodes. The levels of all clotting factors, including fibrinogen, were normal. Several of the individual's relatives had approximately 50 percent of normal $\alpha_2$-antiplasmin levels; he thus appeared to represent the homozygous form of the disorder. The heterozygotes had no bleeding problems, so that a value of 50 percent of normal appeared to be consistent with normal hemostasis. The other severely deficient patient[77] described had approximately 2 percent of normal levels of $\alpha_2$-antiplasmin and also had episodes of severe bleeding.

An interesting observation was the fact that serum FRA levels were not elevated, indicating that in spite of the absence of $\alpha_2$-antiplasmin, significant lysis of plasma fibrinogen presumably did not occur continuously. Clearly, the reserves of antiplasmin activity possessed by $\alpha_2$-macroglobulin and other inhibitors, or the forces preventing the amounts of activator normally circulating from activating plasma plasminogen, are considerable. The finding suggests that, although $\alpha_2$-antiplasmin may represent the principal defense against digestion of plasma proteins by plasmin once it has formed, other mechanisms, as yet undefined, are sufficient to prevent plasmin generation in the circulation in everyday life. This comment does not imply, however, that the concept of the central role of fibrin in securing local fibrin lysis is invalid.

## Plasminogen Activator Excess

A lifelong and ultimately fatal hemorrhagic disorder has been observed in our laboratory due to a different fibrinolytic disorder.[78,79] The patient had severe, prolonged bleeding after minor injuries and dental extractions, and ultimately developed a spontaneous cerebral hemorrhage at the age of 46. This individual had no deficiency of any known inhibitor of fibrinolysis. His blood invariably showed grossly elevated levels of a plasminogen activator that was physically and immunologically similar to tissue activator. This patient, however, showed signs of continuous fibrinolysis in his circulation. Whole blood clots invariably lysed within 6 hours; he had marginally low fibrinogen levels and consistently grossly raised levels of FRA. Although free plasmin was never detected in functional assays, plasmin–$\alpha_2$-antiplasmin complexes were always present in his blood. There was no deficiency of any procoagulant other than the minor deficiency of fibrinogen, and platelet function was normal. Inhibition of fibrinolysis with tranexamic acid was followed by a rapid, dramatic rise in fibrinogen levels, indicating that fibrinogen synthesis was normal or enhanced. The patient's mother and brother showed no clinical or laboratory abnormality of hemostasis, but no other family members were available for study. Thus, although this man's bleeding syndrome was lifelong, its hereditary basis could not be established.

## Hereditary Disorders of Fibrinolysis Predisposing to Thrombosis

Until recently, no hereditary disorder characterized by depressed fibrinolytic activity could be clearly identified as predisposing to thrombosis in spite of an extensive search. Now, however, several individuals have been described in whom the plasminogen molecules were physically abnormal in a number of ways, which hampered their conversion to plasmin by PA.[80–82] At least one of the disorders was shown to be hereditarily based.[80] Individuals with the abnormal forms of plasminogen appeared to have an increased incidence of thrombosis, although its severity varied. In the hereditary disorder, the propositus with thrombotic disease appeared to be a heterozygote. The family included an infant who apparently represented the homozygous form of the disorder, but at the time of this report it had not developed thrombotic symptoms.

## ACQUIRED FIBRINOLYTIC BLEEDING: PRIMARY

Hemorrhage due to excessive fibrinolysis alone, with no disorder of other hemostatic mechanisms, is rare, but when it does occur it may be very severe. The simplest and purest form of such primary fibrinolytic bleeding is a complication of the use of thrombolytic therapy and is thus iatrogenic.

## Thrombolytic Therapy

Past attempts at therapeutic lysis of intravascular clots have involved intravenous infusion of those PAs which were available in sufficient quantity in relatively pure form, namely, streptokinase and urokinase. Both of these agents suffer from disadvantages. Streptokinase is a foreign bacterial protein and, as such, produces allergic reactions which have been severe on occasion; in addition, the effectiveness of streptokinase is impaired by the

**Table 9-2**
Findings During Thrombolytic Therapy with the Currently Available
Agents Streptokinase and Urokinase

| | |
|---|---|
| WBCLT | Rapid ⎫ unless plasminogen levels are |
| ELT | Rapid ⎭ grossly depleted |
| Lysis of plasminogen-containing fibrin plates | Markedly enhanced |
| Plasma fibrinogen levels | Variably reduced |
| TT | ⎫ |
| PT | ⎬ Variably prolonged |
| PTT | ⎭ |
| Serum FRA levels | Increased |
| Plasmin–$\alpha_2$-antiplasmin complexes | Present |
| Plasma plasminogen levels | Reduced |
| Plasma antiplasmin levels | Reduced |

Key: TT, thrombin time; PT, prothrombin time; PTT, partial thromboplastin time; ELT, euglobulin clot-lysis time; FRA, fibrin/fibrinogen-related antigens.

variable quantities of antistreptococcal antibodies present in the plasma of most patients. Urokinase, a human protein, does not produce troublesome allergic reactions but is poorly adsorbed onto fibrin deposits. Attempts at thrombolytic therapy therefore require the production of a systemic fibrinolytic state to achieve lysis of fibrin localized in the thrombus under attack. Systemic fibrinolysis is thus an undesirable and costly side effect of therapy and may produce dangerous bleeding. Because of the clearly defined nature of the disorder, however, it provides a model against which spontaneous primary fibrinolytic bleeding episodes may be compared (Table 9-2). Typically, streptokinase or urokinase therapy is accompanied by evidence of active current fibrinolysis, with rapid whole blood or euglobulin clot lysis (unless plasma plasminogen levels are very severely depressed) and very active lysis of preformed plasminogen-containing fibrin plates. Progressive reduction of plasma fibrinogen and possibly other clotting factors occurs during therapy and may lead to prolongation of the TT, PT, and PTT. Levels of FRA may increase dramatically, representing breakdown products of either fibrin in the target thrombus or of plasma fibrinogen; the anticoagulant effect of some of these may contribute to prolongation of the TT, PT, and PTT. Plasmin–$\alpha_2$-antiplasmin complexes are demonstrable in the plasma.[83]

Although the derangement of hemostasis may be severe, bleeding does not necessarily result. It is far more likely to occur if a wound or raw surface is present, such as an operation scar, postpartum uterus, or arterial puncture site, and if it occurs bleeding may be severe. Management, however, is simple, as the disorder is iatrogenic and consists of cessation of the infusion. This is usually sufficient to reverse the bleeding tendency within hours. If bleeding is very severe, the use of an inhibitor of fibrinolysis such as epsilon aminocaproic acid or tranexamic acid orally or intravenously will control hemorrhage until natural recovery of hemostasis occurs. Replacement therapy with blood or red cells is given as necessary. Fresh blood or plasma will replace clotting factors rapidly if their levels are severely depressed, but this is rarely necessary.

In the future, thrombolytic regimens may be designed which are less likely to be complicated by undesirable systemic hyperfibrinolysis. Activators from human tissues are avidly adsorbed onto fibrin, which may localize their effect on formed fibrin and avoid plasminogen activation in the circulating plasma. "Tissue activators" are already being harvested in quantity from human melanoma cell lines in culture and have been used in both dogs and man,[84,85] securing local thrombolysis without inducing systemic fibrinogenolysis. If these or similar activators become available in quantity, thrombolytic therapy will be refined considerably and the likelihood of hemorrhagic complications reduced.

## Disease-Related Primary Fibrinolytic Bleeding

Only a small proportion of acquired bleeding disorders can be clearly shown to represent primary fibrinolytic states. There are numerous reports in the literature describing hemorrhage in association with evidence of grossly enhanced fibrinolysis in a variety of disorders, usually neoplastic. Examples include metastatic carcinoma of the prostate,[86] carcinoma of the pancreas,[87] leukemia of various types,[88,89] hepatic cirrhosis,[90,91] and disseminated lupus erythematosus.[92] Some of these conditions probably represent primary fibrinolytic episodes, but it is not always clear that intravascular coagulation may be excluded with certainty; the distinction between primary fibrinolysis and that secondary to intravascular coagulation is not always possible. Of the simple measurements thought to assist in making this distinction, the platelet count is often said to be crucial, and to be normal in the former but reduced in the latter. The discriminatory value of the platelet count is overemphasized. First, it may be influenced by factors unrelated to the hemostatic disorder; this is clearly the case in patients with leukemia, cirrhosis with hypersplenism, and metastatic malignant disease with marrow invasion. Second, unequivocal depression of the platelet count does not necessarily accompany syndromes currently regarded as classical prototypes of intravascular coagulation. We have recently seen two women, one with amniotic fluid embolism and one with premature separation of the placenta, both of whom had incoagulable blood and all the features regarded as diagnostic of massive intravascular coagulation; their platelet counts, however, were 240 and $220 \times 10^9$/liter. Similarly, reliance on screening tests of coagulation, or on fibrinogen levels, will not distinguish all episodes of primary from secondary fibrinolysis; as previously discussed, similar changes may occur in the TT, PT, and PTT and in fibrinogen levels in both syndromes, depending on the strength of the stimulus. Our preconceptions, based on analogies with animal experiments or previous experience with bleeding patients, lead us to conclude that gross fibrinogen depletion and gross prolongation of the coagulation screening tests are probably more likely to occur in episodes of intravascular coagulation; this is reasonable, but reflects probability rather than clear-cut proof when considering individual bleeding patients. Simple tests for the detection of fibrin monomers in the plasma would be invaluable in establishing whether intravascular coagulation was present; those tests that depend on the precipitability of these monomers, such as ethanol gelation,[93,94] protamine sulfate precipitation,[95,96] or ristocetin precipitation,[97] are promising but have proved somewhat variable in practice.[56,98–101] Perhaps in the future, the clearer characterization of fibrinopeptide A in plasma or FR-antigens in serum, or the detection of ATIII and $\alpha_2$-antiplasmin in complexed forms, will allow the better definition of bleeding episodes and firmer conclusions, based upon science rather than upon art or experience, that they are due to primary fibrinolysis or intravascular clotting.

In spite of these qualifications, however, some patients can be identified who have severe bleeding with grossly enhanced fibrinolysis in the absence of evidence of intravascular clotting. These patients do not have severe depletion of clotting factors and can be regarded as having primary fibrinolytic bleeding. They are thus likely to benefit from the use of fibrinolytic inhibitors. Table 9-3 summarizes the findings in several such patients with severe bleeding disorders recently studied in this laboratory. Their intrinsic and extrinsic pathways of thrombin generation were intact or only minimally disturbed, and their fibrinogen levels were normal or only slightly lowered; however, they had grossly enhanced fibrinolytic activity on clot lysis or fibrin plate assays and large amounts of circulating FR antigens. Additionally, although all showed clear evidence of plasmin–$\alpha_2$-antiplasmin complexes in their blood, none showed detectable complexed ATIII. Hemorrhage was controlled wholly or partly by the use of fibrinolytic inhibitors (2 patients had surgery without bleeding during such therapy), which reversed the abnormalities without resulting in the thrombosis which might have occurred had intravascular coagulation contributed to their bleeding but been undetected by the laboratory screening. Comparable results are included in Table 9-3 from a patient with amniotic fluid embolism and the clinical features of intravascular coagulation. This patient also showed evidence of pathologically enhanced fibrinolysis, but had severe depletion of clotting factors and evidence of complexed ATIII in the circulation as well. She did not, of course, receive fibrinolytic inhibitors.

Of the patients who had primary fibrinolysis, 3 presented with major hemorrhage into the gastrointestinal or urinary tract, with epistaxis and cutaneous hemorrhage sufficient to require recurrent transfusions at intervals of a few days. One presented with a history of severe bleeding at previous surgery or on trauma only. None presented with an acute torrential bleeding disorder such as that encountered in the patient with amniotic fluid embolism, but none, of course, had a site of potential hemorrhage in any way similar to that in the pregnant patient during labor.

## FIBRINOLYSIS SECONDARY TO INTRAVASCULAR CLOTTING

As emphasized earlier, the current belief is that fibrinolysis secondary to DIC assists in the rapid removal of fibrin deposited in the microcirculation, protecting the body from the tissue damage this would otherwise cause. In spite of this protective effect, the active fibrinolysis sometimes accompanying intravascular clotting will increase the tendency to bleed by digesting plasma fibrinogen, and possibly also factors V and VIII (already depleted by the coagulative process), and by generating fibrin or fibrinogen degradation products, some of which have anticoagulant properties. Two considerations indicate that suppression of the fibrinolytic component of such syndromes is unwise.

First, animal experiments indicate that the role of fibrinolysis in removing fibrin deposited in the course of experimentally induced intravascular clotting is of major benefit. Intravascular clotting induced by infusion of thrombin is not generally fatal, but if such infusions are accompanied by suppression of fibrinolysis by fibrinolytic inhibitors, renal cortical necrosis or other thrombotic tissue damage is common.[102,103]

Second, the acute episodes of intravascular clotting in which fatal hemorrhage is most likely and which are most frequently seen in clinical practice are those associated with complications of pregnancy and labor (with premature placental separation, amniotic fluid embolism, etc.). The period of active fibrinolysis is frequently very transient; it may well be over by the time blood sampling is undertaken. Thus, whereas generation of FRA and

**Table 9-3**

Findings in Patients with Primary Fibrinolysis, Normal Control Subjects,
and a Patient with DIC and Secondary Fibrinolysis Following
Amniotic Fluid Embolism

| Patient Presentation | Assays Reflecting Clotting Factor Levels* | | | | Assays Reflecting Intravascular Clotting | | Assays Reflecting Systemic Fibrinolytic Activity | | |
|---|---|---|---|---|---|---|---|---|---|
| | TT (sec) | PT (sec) | PTT (sec) | Fibrinogen (g/liter) | Thrombin–ATIII Complex | Ethanol Gelation | ELT (min) | PA (fibrin plate) ($mm^2$) | Plasminogen CU/ml |
| Massive intrapartum hemorrhage: amniotic fluid embolism | >120 | >120 | >120 | 0.40 | + + | + + | <30 | $18^2$ | — |
| Thrombolytic therapy (urokinase); no bleeding | Patient heparinized | | | 0.75 | 0 | 0 | 24 | $18^2$ | 1.6 |
| Severe multiple-site bleeding in: | | | | | | | | | |
| Metastatic breast carcinoma | 12.9 | 17.9 | 49.3 | 1.2 | 0 | 0 | <30 | $15^2$ | 1.2 |
| Lifelong disorder | 14.0 | 18.0 | 40.5 | 1.75 | 0 | 0 | 37 | $14^2$ | 4.5 |
| Metastatic prostatic carcinoma | 11.0 | 15.0 | 44.0 | 6.5 | 0 | 0 | 45 | $13^2$ | 2.5 |
| Acute myeloid leukemia | 10.0 | 17.0 | 38.2 | 4.9 | 0 | 0 | 40 | $9.5^2$ | 1.5 |
| Normal values | 9.5– 10.2 | 12.5– 15.0 | 41.0– 43.0 | 2.2– 3.0 | 0 | 0 | >80 | 0 | 3.6– 4.0 |

*Table 9-3 (continued)*

| Assays Reflecting Systemic Fibrinolytic Activity *(continued)* | | | Other Assays | | | | |
|---|---|---|---|---|---|---|---|
| $\alpha_2$-antiplasmin Activity (% normal) | $\alpha_2$-antiplasmin Antigen (% normal) | Plasmin–$\alpha_2$-anticomplex | Serum FRA (μg/ml) | Platelet Count ($10^9$/liter) | Clinical Response to EACA or tranexamic acid | Diagnosis |
| 0 | 83 | + + | >40 | 240 | Not given | DIC; secondary fibrinolysis |
| — | 40 | + | >40 | 280 | Not given | Primary fibrinolysis; iatrogenic |
| 35 | 31 | + + | >40 | 107 | moderate | Primary fibrinolysis; noniatrogenic |
| 60 | 76 | + | >40 | 100 | good | Primary fibrinolysis; noniatrogenic |
| 35 | 29 | + | >40 | 327 | good | Primary fibrinolysis; noniatrogenic |
| 29 | 40 | + | >40 | 44 | moderate | Primary fibrinolysis; noniatrogenic |
| 100 | 100 | 0 | <5 | >120 | — | Normal healthy subjects |

Key: TT, thrombin time; PT, prothrombin time; PTT, partial thromboplastin time; ELT, euglobulin clot-lysis time; PA, plasminogen activator (whole plasma applied to plasminogen-containing fibrin plate); FRA, fibrin/fibrinogen-related antigens; EACA, epsilon aminocaproic acid; 0; none; —; test not done.
*Note that depletion of clotting factors may reflect either plasmin or thrombin generation.

part of the depletion of clotting factors are attributable to the episode of fibrinolysis and may be demonstrated when the blood is studied, WBCLT, ELT, or fibrin plate assays may indicate that the systemic fibrinolytic phase has passed spontaneously; Table 9-1 shows that this occurs rapidly, although evidence of it persists for many hours longer. It is therefore clear that intervention in the attempt to suppress fibrinolysis may not only expose the patient to the risks mentioned above but will certainly not diminish the likelihood of hemorrhage, as active systemic fibrinolysis is no longer present. DIC is extensively discussed in Chapter 8 and will not be dealt with at length here. The acute episodes of the disorders that complicate pregnancy and labor are discussed here merely to illustrate the fruitlessness of attempts to suppress fibrinolysis which may occur secondary to such events. Use of inhibitors of fibrinolysis in these situations is not only potentially dangerous but almost always occurs too late to influence the phase of active fibrinolysis. Treatment should involve the maintenance of blood volume until the uterus is emptied; after this happens, the hemostatic derangement corrects itself spontaneously within a few hours. As discussed in chapters 8 and 12, DIC may complicate many disorders other than complications of pregnancy. In these situations, too, suppression of secondary fibrinolysis is not rational for reasons similar to those discussed above, and treatment is directed at the control or removal of the stimulus initiating intravascular clotting.

## TREATMENT

When inhibition of fibrinolysis is indicated, two principal agents are available. Their chemical nature and pharmacological properties have been described in detail elsewhere[104] and in Chapter 5 and are summarized here.

### Epsilon Aminocaproic Acid (EACA: 6-Aminohexanoic Acid)

EACA, at concentrations of $10^{-4}$ $M$ and above, will inhibit activation of plasminogen competitively, whereas at concentrations of over $5 \times 10^{-2} M$ it will act as a noncompetitive inhibitor of plasmin. Its in vivo action may reflect interference with the association of plasminogen with the fibrin surface.[43,45] It is rapidly absorbed from the gastrointestinal tract, is widely distributed throughout extracellular and intracellular fluid, and is excreted in the urine within a period of about 12 hours. Preparations for intravenous use are available. The conventional dosage is 3 g initially, followed by similar doses every 6 hours.

### Tranexamic Acid (AMCA: Trans-4-Aminomethyl Cyclohexane Carboxylic Acid)

This agent has properties similar to those of EACA but is more potent on a weight-for-weight basis. It is also absorbed from the gastrointestinal tract, although somewhat less completely than EACA, is widely distributed throughout body fluid compartments, and is excreted in the urine. Dosages of 10 mg/kg intravenously or 30–50 mg/kg orally every four hours have been recommended for control of systemically enhanced fibrinolysis.

The therapeutic use of inhibitors of fibrinolysis is indicated in systemic primary fibrinolysis sufficient to cause hemorrhage. Their use is contraindicated in fibrinolysis secondary to intravascular clotting. The following points may be of value in elaborating on these two basic statements.

1.  Primary fibrinolysis is rare.
2.  In general, primary fibrinolysis is a subacute rather than an overwhelming hemorrhagic syndrome. Several patients described in Table 9-3 with primary fibrinolysis had very severe bleeding, necessitating frequent transfusion; however, none was exsanguinating, as are some cases with acute DIC. The authors have not personally encountered a patient with primary fibrinolysis with torrential bleeding, but doubtless would have, had some of these patients undergone surgery unprotected by antifibrinolytic drugs. This does not, of course, mean that episodes of exsanguinating hemorrhage may never occur due to primary fibrinolysis.
3.  In general, primary fibrinolysis can most clearly be shown to exist when little or no depletion of clotting factors occurs. Gross reduction of these factors always raises the possibility of DIC, but experience with thrombolytic agents shows that such depletion may occur in primary fibrinolysis.
4.  If WBCLT, ELT, or lysis of preformed fibrin fails to show grossly enhanced current fibrinolytic activity, intervention with fibrinolytic inhibitors is never indicated in systemic bleeding syndromes under any circumstances. Occasionally, the clot lysis assays may be deceptive if plasminogen levels are very severely depleted, but this has been reported only during thrombolytic therapy; theoretically, it may occur in other situations. Lysis of a plasminogen-containing fibrin plate, however, will detect raised activator levels even in the absence of plasma plasminogen.
5.  Currently, widely available tests for FR antigens do not distinguish fibrinogen from FDP or from fibrin monomers. Detection of FR antigens in excessive quantities is never an indication for the use of fibrinolytic inhibitors unless the assays listed in (4) demonstrate enhanced fibrinolysis. The detection of fibrin monomer in plasma should indicate that intravascular coagulation is current and that fibrinolytic inhibitors are contraindicated. No test currently available to routine laboratories detects fibrin monomer with absolute certainty; ethanol gelation and protamine sulfate precipitation tests may be useful, but both false-positive and false-negative results have been reported. As FR antigens in plasma may represent the results of either coagulation (fibrin monomer) or fibrinolysis (fibrin or fibrinogen degradation products), the crucial distinction between primary fibrinolysis and that secondary to intravascular coagulation may perhaps be more readily achieved by demonstrating that thrombin has been generated. A test which does this readily and simply is not now widely available. The detection of ATIII complexed with activated clotting factors and $\alpha_2$-antiplasmin complexed with plasmin may, in the future, prove useful in the study of fibrinolysis and may show whether it is associated with intravascular clotting.

## BLEEDING DUE TO LOCAL FIBRINOLYSIS

Thus far, we have been concerned with generalized bleeding tendencies due to systemic activation of fibrinolysis detectable by the study of venous blood samples. Physiological fibrinolysis, as discussed earlier, depends on the activation of the enzyme system locally within deposits of fibrin without its activation in the circulating blood. The possibility therefore arises that excessive local enhancement of fibrinolysis may account for local bleeding. Clearly, such a process may be undetected by the study of peripheral blood specimens. In unusual cases, local bleeding may be clearly shown to reflect locally enhanced fibrinolysis with no abnormality in the individual's venous blood samples, and to respond to the use of fibrinolytic inhibitors[105]; however, this situation is excessively rare. Locally enhanced fibrinolysis has been invoked as causing or contributing to bleeding in a wide variety of disorders including bleeding after prostatectomy or adenotonsillectomy, gastrointestinal bleeding, subarachnoid hemorrhage, epistaxis, menorrhagia or bleeding complicating the use of intrauterine devices, and in hemophilic patients who have hematuria, dental extraction, or synovectomy.

Evidence suggests that locally enhanced fibrinolysis may occur in individuals who are bleeding from some of these sites,[106,107] but the difficulty of obtaining appropriate samples for testing indicates that such studies cannot be performed in routine laboratories in the study of single patients. Reduction of bleeding or rebleeding with the use of inhibitors of fibrinolysis has been claimed on the basis of double-blind trials in the following situations: in hemophilic patients after dental extraction,[108,109] in hemophilic patients with spontaneous hemarthroses,[110,111] in patients with menorrhagia,[112–115] in patients using intrauterine devices[116,117] or having certain gynecological operations,[118] in some forms of gastrointestinal bleeding,[119–121] after prostatectomy,[122–128] after subarachnoid hemorrhage,[129,130] after adenotonsillectomy,[131,132] and in patients with traumatic hyphema.[133–135]

The positive results quoted in some of these trials have not always been confirmed by others and, in some, the incidence of side effects has been unacceptably high or the possibility of deleterious side effects has been raised.[136–142] It is clear, for instance, that although bleeding from the kidney can be controlled in hemophilic patients by the use of fibrinolytic inhibitors,[124,143,144] the high incidence of urinary tract obstruction observed makes their use unjustifiable[145,146]; similarly, their systemic use for the control of postprostatectomy bleeding has been associated with the occurrence of large clots in the bladder.[122] Additionally, the systemic use of inhibitors of fibrinolysis may be complicated occasionally by thrombotic episodes remote from the sites of bleeding which they are administered to control,[147–151] although other side effects appear rare.[152] The positive trials quoted above indicate that a reduction in the use of blood or blood products, or occasionally, and more crucially, in the requirement for surgery in some of the groups studied has been achieved by the use of fibrinolytic inhibitors. It is evident, however, that in contrast to the systemic bleeding disorders described earlier in this chapter, demonstration of the benefits of fibrinolytic inhibitors in the local bleeding phenomena discussed in this section often depends on the statistical approach used and may be difficult to identify in an individual patient. This problem, which is more familiar to those concerned with the prevention of thrombosis than to those who desire to prevent hemorrhage, will not be confronted here.

## REFERENCES

1. Robbins KC: The biochemistry of plasminogen and plasmin, in Ogston D, Bennett B (eds): Hemostasis, Biochemistry, Physiology and Pathology. New York, Wiley, 1977, pp 208–220
2. Sottrup-Jensen L, Claeys H, Zajdel M, et al: The primary structure of human plasminogen, in Davidson JF, Rowan RM, Samama MM, et al (eds): Progress in Chemical Fibrinolysis and Thrombolysis, vol. 3. New York, Raven Press, 1978, pp 191–209
3. Wiman B, Wallen P: Activation of human plasminogen by an insoluble derivative of urokinase. Eur J Biochem 36:25–31, 1973
4. Robbins KC, Summaria L, Hsieh B, et al: The peptide chains of human plasmin. Mechanism of activation of human plasminogen to plasmin. J Biol Chem 242:2333–2342, 1967
5. Robbins KC, Bernabe P, Arzedon L, et al: The primary structure of human plasminogen II.

The histidine loop of human plasmin; light (B) chain active center histidine sequence. J Biol Chem 248:1631–1633, 1973

6. Rickli EE, Otavsky WI: A new method of isolation and some properties of the heavy chain of human plasmin. Eur J Biochem 59:441–447, 1975

7. Davidson JF, Samama MM, Desnoyers PC (eds): Progress in Chemical Fibrinolysis and Thrombolysis, vol. 2: Methodology. New York, Raven Press, 1976

8. Bennett B, Ogston D, Douglas AS: The fibrinolytic enzyme system, in Biggs R, Rizza CR (eds): Human Blood Coagulation, Hemostasis and Thrombosis. Oxford, Blackwell Scientific Publications, in press

9. White WF, Barlow GH, Mozen MM: The isolation and characterization of plasminogen activators (urokinase) from human urine. Biochemistry 5:2160–2169, 1966

10. Todd AS: The histological localisation of fibrinolysin activator. J Pathol Bacteriol 78:281–283, 1959

11. Aoki N, von Kaulla KN: The extraction of vascular plasminogen activator from human cadavers and a description of its properties. Am J Clin Pathol 55:171–179, 1971

12. Binder BR, Spragg J, Austen KF: Purification and characterization of human vascular plasminogen activator derived from blood vessel perfusate. J Biol Chem 254:1998–2003, 1979

13. Loskutoff DP, Edgington TS: Synthesis of a fibrinolytic activator and inhibitor by endothelial cells. Proc Natl Acad Sci USA 74:3903–3907, 1977

14. Rijken DC, Wijngaards G, Zaal de Jong M, et al: Purification and partial characterization of plasminogen activator from human uterine tissue. Biochem Biophys Acta 580:140–153, 1979

15. Rijken DC, Hoylaerts M, Collen D: On the fibrinolytic properties of single-chain and two-chain human tissue plasminogen activator. Thromb Haemost 46:12, 1981 (abstract)

16. Wallen P, Ranby M, Bergsdorf N, et al: Purification and characterization of tissue plasminogen activator: On the occurrence of two different forms and their enzymatic properties, in Davidson JF, Nilsson IM, Astedt P (eds): Progress in Chemical Fibrinolysis V. Edinburgh, Churchill Livingstone, 1981, pp 16–23

17. Rickli EE, Zaugg H: Isolation and purification of highly enriched tissue plasminogen activator from pig heart. Thromb Diath Haemorrh 23:64–76, 1970

18. Mackie M, Booth NA, Bennett B: Comparative studies on human activators of plasminogen. Br J Haematol 47:77–90, 1981

19. Ogston D, Bennett B, Mackie M: Properties of a partially purified preparation of a circulating plasminogen activator. Thromb Res 8:276–284, 1976

20. Rijken DC, Wijngaards G, Welbergen J: Immunological characterization of plasminogen activator activities in human tissues and body fluids. J Lab Clin Med 97:477–486, 1981

21. Kluft C: C1-inactivator resistant fibrinolytic activity in plasma euglobulin fractions. Its relationship to vascular activator in the blood and its role in euglobulin fibrinolysis. Thromb Res 13:135–151, 1978

22. Ogston D, Ogston CM, Ratnoff OD, et al: Studies on a complex mechanism for the activation of plasminogen by kaolin and by chloroform. The participation of Hageman factor and additional co-factors. J Clin Invest 48:1786–1801, 1969

23. Wuepper KD: Prekallikrein deficiency in man. J Exp Med 138:1345–1355, 1973

24. Saito H, Ratnoff OD, Waldmann R, et al: Fitzgerald trait: Deficiency of a hitherto unrecognized agent, Fitzgerald factor, participating in surface mediated reactions of clotting, fibrinolysis, generation of kinins and the property of diluted plasma enhancing vascular permeability (PF/Dil). J Clin Invest 55:1082–1089, 1975

25. Colman RW: Activation of plasminogen by human plasma kallikrein. Biochem Biophys Res Commun 35:273–279, 1969

26. Goldsmith GH Jr, Saito H, Ratnoff OD: The activation of plasminogen by Hageman factor (factor XII) and Hageman factor fragments. J Clin Invest 62:54–60, 1978

27. Binder BR, Beckman R, Jorg M: Plasminogen activator activity of urokinase, the vascular plasminogen activator, plasma kallikrein and Hageman factor in the presence and absence of fibrin. Thromb Haemost 46:12, 1981 (abstract)

28. Hedner U: Inhibitors of plasminogen activation distinct from the other plasma protein inhibitors, in Tilsner V, Lenau H (eds): Fibrinolysis and Urokinase, vol. 31. Proceedings of the Serono Symposia. New York, Academic Press, 1980, pp 19–25

29. Astrup T, Rosa AT: A plasminogen proactivator-activator system in human blood effective in absence of Hageman factor. Thromb Res 4:609–613, 1974

30. Kluft C, Wijngaards G, Jie AFH: The factor XII-independent plasminogen proactivator system of plasma includes urokinase-related activity. Thromb Haemost 46:343, 1981 (abstract)

31. Wijngaards G, Kluft C: Urokinase-related fibrinolytic activity in human plasma. Thromb Haemost 46:385, 1981 (abstract)

32. Mullertz S: Different molecular forms of plasminogen and plasmin produced by urokinase in human plasma and their relation to protease inhibitors and lysis of fibrinogen and fibrin. Biochem J 143:273–283, 1974

32a. Moroi M, Aoki N: Isolation and characterization of $\alpha_2$-plasmin inhibitor from human plasma. J Biol Chem 251:5956–5965, 1976

33. Collen D: Biochemical background of fibrinolytic therapy, in Tilsner V, Lenau H (eds): Fibrinolysis and Urokinase, vol. 31. Proceedings of the Serono Symposia. New York, Academic Press, 1980, pp 9–17

34. Harpel PC, Mosesson MW: Degradation of human fibrinogen by plasma $\alpha_2$-macroglobulin–enzyme complexes. J Clin Invest 52:2175–2184, 1973

35. Ogston D, Bennett B: Biochemistry of the naturally occurring inhibitors of the fibrinolytic enzyme system, in Ogston D, Bennett B (eds): Hemostasis: Biochemistry, Physiology and Pathology. New York, Wiley, 1977, pp 230–238

36. Bennett B, Ogston D: Role of complement, coagulation and fibrinolysis in normal haemostasis and disease, in Bloom AL, Thomas D (eds): Haemostasis and Thrombosis. Edinburgh, Churchill-Livingstone, 1981, pp 236–251

37. Hedner U, Martinsson G: Inhibition of activated Hageman factor (Factor XIIa) by an inhibitor of plasminogen activation (PA inhibitor). Thromb Res 12:1015–1023, 1978

38. Loskutoff DJ, Edgington TS: An inhibitor of plasminogen activator in rabbit endothelial cells. Thromb Haemost 46:82, 1981 (abstract)

39. Walker JE, Ogston D: The inhibition of tissue activators and urokinase by human plasma. Thromb Haemost 46:280, 1981 (abstract)

40. Collen D: Natural inhibitors of haemostasis with particular reference to fibrinolysis, in Bloom AL, Thomas D (eds): Haemostasis and Thrombosis. Edinburgh, Churchill Livingstone, 1981, pp 225–235

41. Lijnen HR, Hoylaerts M, Collen D: Isolation and characterization of a human plasma protein with affinity for lysine-binding sites in plasminogen. Role in regulation of fibrinolysis and identification as histidine-rich glycoprotein. J Biol Chem 255:10214–10222, 1980

42. Wiman B, Collen D: Molecular mechanism of physiological fibrinolysis. Nature 272:549–550, 1978

43. Thorsen S: Differences in the binding to fibrin of native plasminogen and plasminogen modified by proteolytic degradation. Influence of omega-amino carboxylic acids. Biochim Biophys Acta 393:55–65, 1975

44. Mackie M, Bennett B: Unpublished observations, 1978

45. Thorsen S, Glas-Greenwalt P, Astrup T: Differences in the binding to fibrin of urokinase and tissue plasminogen activator. Thromb Diath Haemorrh 28:65–74, 1972

46. Allen RA, Pepper DS: Isolation and properties of human vascular plasminogen activator. Thromb Haemost 45:43–50, 1981

47. Christensen U, Clemmensen I: Kinetic properties of the primary inhibitor of plasmin from human plasma. Biochem J 163:389–391, 1977

48. Nussenzweig V, Seligmann M, Pelmont J, et al: Les produits de degradation du fibrinogene humaine par la plasmine. Ann Institut Pasteur 100:377–387, 1961

49. Larrieu M-J, Mardar VJ, Inceman S: Effects of fibrinogen degradation products on platelets and coagulation. Thromb Diath Haemost Suppl 20:215–226, 1966

50. Gaffney PJ: Subunit relationships between fibrinogen and fibrin degradation products. Thromb Res 2:201–218, 1973

51. Pizzo SV, Taylor LM, Schwartz ML, et al: Subunit structure of fragment D from fibrinogen and cross-linked fibrin. J Biol Chem 248:4584–4590, 1973

52. Gaffney PJ, Joe F: The lysis of cross linked fibrin by plasmin yields initially a single molecular complex D dimer: E. Thromb Res 15:673–687, 1979

53. Francis CW, Mardar VJ, Barlow GW: Plasmic degradation of cross-linked fibrin. Characterization of new macromolecular soluble complexes and a model of their structure. J Clin Invest 66:1033–1043, 1980

54. Francis CW, Mardar VJ, Martin SE: Detection of circulating cross-linked fibrin by a heat extraction-SDS gradient gel electrophoresis technique. Blood 54:1282–1295, 1979

55. Merskey C, Kleiner GJ, Johnson AJ: Quantitative estimation of split products of fibrinogen in human serum, relation to diagnosis and treatment. Blood 28:1–18, 1966

56. Bang NV, Chang ML: Soluble fibrin complexes. Semin Thromb Haemost 1:91–128, 1973

57. Sasaki T, Page IH, Shainoff JR: Stable complex of fibrinogen and fibrin. Science 152:1069–1071, 1966

58. Shainoff JR, Page IH: Significance of cryoprofibrin in fibrinogen–fibrin conversion. J Exp Med 116:687–707, 1962

59. Merksey C, Johnson AJ, Harris JU, et al: Isolation of fibrinogen-fibrin related antigen from human plasma by immuno-affinity chromatography: Its characterization in normal subjects and in defibrinating patients with abruptio placentae and disseminated cancer. Br J Haematol 44:655–670, 1980

60. Alkjaersig N, Davies A, Fletcher AP: Fibrin and fibrinogen proteolysis products: Comparison between gel-filtration and SDS polyacrylamide electrophoresis analysis. Thromb Haemost 38:524–535, 1977

61. Fletcher AP, Alkjaersig N, O'Brien JR, et al: Fibrinogen catabolism in the surgically operated patient and in those with postoperative venous thrombosis. Correlation of plasma fibrinogen chromatographic findings with [125]I-labelled fibrinogen scan findings. J Lab Clin Med 89:1349–1364, 1977

62. Gaffney PJ: The fibrinolytic system, in Bloom AL, Thomas D (eds): Haemostasis and Thrombosis. New York, Churchill Livingstone, 1981, pp 198–224

63. Graeff H, Hafter R, Bachman L: Subunits and macromolecular structure of circulating fibrin in obstetric patients with intravascular coagulation. Thromb Res 16:313–328, 1979

64. Shainoff JR, Dardik BN: Role of fibrinogen in fibrin transport. Chromatographic studies. Thromb Res 17:491–500, 1980

65. Müller-Berghaus G, Mahn I, Krell W: Formation and dissociation of soluble fibrin complexes in plasma at 20°C and 37°C. Thromb Res 14:561–572, 1979

66. Kierulf P: Studies on soluble fibrin in plasma. II. N-terminal analysis of a modified fraction I (Cohn) from patient's plasmas. Scand J Clin Lab Invest 31:37–42, 1973

67. Budzynski A, Mardar VJ, Parker ME, et al: Antigenic markers on fragment DD, a unique plasmic derivative of human cross-linked fibrin. Blood 54:794–804, 1979

67a. Krohnke I, Mahn I, Krell W, et al: Studies on circulating soluble fibrin: Separation of [125]I-des AB fibrin and [131]I-fibrinogen by gel filtration. Br J Haematol 45:131–141, 1980

68. Lee-Own V, Gordon YB, Chard T: The detection of neoantigenic sites on the D dimer peptide isolated from plasmin-digested cross-linked fibrin. Thromb Res 14:77–84, 1979

69. Plow EF, Edgington TS: Immunobiology of fibrinogen: Emergence of neoantigenic expression during physiologic cleavage in vitro and in vivo. J Clin Invest 52:273–282, 1973

70. Plow EF, Edgington TS: A cleavage-associated neoantigenic marker for a $\gamma$ chain site in the $NH_2$ terminal aspect of the fibrinogen molecule. J Biol Chem 250:3368–3392, 1975

71. Booth NA, Bennett B: Plasmin-$\alpha_2$-antiplasmin complex as an indicator of in vivo fibrinolysis. Br J Haematol 50:537–541, 1982

72. Collen D: Thrombin–antithrombin III and plasmin–antiplasmin complex as indicators of in vivo activation of the coagulation and/or fibrinolytic systems. Acta Clin Belg 32:398–402, 1977

73. Biggs R, Rizza CR: Human Blood Coagulation, Haemostasis and Thrombosis (ed 3). Oxford, Blackwell Scientific Publications, in press
74. Holmberg L, Nilsson I-M: Assessment of blood coagulation and general haemostasis, in Bloom AL, Thomas D (eds): Haemostasis and Thrombosis. Edinburgh, Churchill Livingstone, 1981, pp 768–774
75. Aoki N, Saito H, Kamiya T, et al: Congenital deficiency of $\alpha_2$-plasmin inhibitor associated with severe hemorrhagic tendency. J Clin Invest 63:877–884, 1979
76. Aoki N, Sakata Y, Matsuda M, et al: Fibrinolytic states in a patient with congenital deficiency of $\alpha_2$-plasmin inhibitor. Blood 55:483–488, 1980
77. Kluft C, Vellenga E, Brommer EJP: Homozygous $\alpha_2$-antiplasmin deficiency. Lancet 2:206, 1979 (letter)
78. Booth NA, Cumming AM, Cook IA, et al: Hyperactive fibrinolysis in a patient with gross hyperlipidemia, in Davidson J, Nilsson IM, Astedt B (eds): Progress in Fibrinolysis V. Edinburgh, Churchill Livingstone, 1981, pp 342–344
79. Booth NA, Bennett B, Wijngaards G, et al: A new life-long hemorrhagic disorder due to excess of plasminogen activator. Blood 61:267–275, 1983
80. Aoki N, Moroi M, Sakata Y, et al: Abnormal plasminogen. A hereditary molecular abnormality found in a patient with recurrent thrombosis. J Clin Invest 61:1186–1195, 1978
81. Robbins KC: The regulation and control of the blood fibrinolytic system, in Davidson JF, Nilsson IM, Astedt B (eds): Progress in Fibrinolysis. Edinburgh, Churchill Livingstone, 1981, pp 3–13
82. Sakata Y, Aoki N: Molecular abnormality of plasminogen. J Biol Chem 255:5442–5447, 1980
82a. Wohl RC, Summaria L, Robbins KC: Physiological activation of the human fibrinolytic system. Isolation and characterization of human plasminogen variants Chicago I and Chicago II. J Biol Chem 254:9063–9069, 1979
83. Verstraete M, Vermylen J, Schetz J: Biochemical changes noted during intermittent administration of streptokinase. Thromb Haemost 39:61–68, 1978
84. Korninger C, Matsuo O, Suy R, et al: Thrombolytic properties of purified human tissue plasminogen activator in a dog femoral vein thrombosis model. Thromb Haemost 46:209, 1981 (abstract)
85. Weimar W, Stibbe J, van Seyen AJ, et al: Specific lysis of an iliofemoral thrombus by administration of extrinsic (tissue type) plasminogen activator. Lancet 2:1018–1020, 1981
86. Tagnon HJ, Whitmore WF, Schulman NR: Fibrinolysis in metastatic carcinoma of the prostate. Cancer 5:9–12, 1952
87. Ratnoff OD: Studies on a proteolytic enzyme in human plasma VII. A fatal hemorrhagic state associated with excessive plasma proteolytic activity in a patient undergoing surgery for carcinoma of the head of the pancreas. J Clin Invest 31:521–528, 1952
88. Mikata I, Hasegawa M, Igarashi T, et al: Variations of plasmin in hemorrhagic blood disease. Keio J Med 8:278–292, 1959
89. Pisciotta AV, Schultz EJ: Fibrinolytic purpura in acute leukemia. Am J Med 19:824–828, 1955
90. Fletcher AP, Biederman O, Moore D, et al: Abnormal plasminogen–plasmin system activity (fibrinolysis) in patients with hepatic cirrhosis: its cause and consequences. J Clin Invest 43:681–695, 1964
91. Grossi CE, Moreno AH, Rousselot LM: Studies on spontaneous fibrinolytic activity in patients with cirrhosis of the liver and its inhibition by epsilon aminocaproic acid. Ann Surg 153:383–393, 1961
92. Zywicka H, Kopec M, Latallo Z, et al: Anticoagulant circulant ressemblant a l'antithrombin IV au cours d'un lupus erythemateux dissemine. Thromb Diath Haemorrh 6:63–72, 1961
93. Breen FA, Tullis JL: Ethanol gelatin: A rapid screening test for intravascular coagulation. Ann Intern Med 69:1197–1206, 1968

94. Godal HC, Abildgaard U: Gelation of soluble fibrin by ethanol. Scand J Haematol 3:342–350, 1966

95. Lipinski B, Worowski K: Detection of soluble fibrin complexes in blood by means of protamine sulphate test. Thromb Diath Haemorrh 20:44–49, 1968

96. Niewiarowski S, Gurewich V: Laboratory identification of intravascular coagulation. The serial dilution protamine sulfate test for the detection of fibrin monomer and fibrin degradation products. J Lab Clin Med 77:665–676, 1971

97. Watanabe K, Tullis JL: Ristocetin precipitation: A new simple test for detection of fibrin monomer and fibrin degradation products. Am J Clin Pathol 70:691–696, 1978

98. Deykin D: The clinical challenge of disseminated intravascular coagulation. N Engl J Med 283:636–644, 1970

99. Gurewich V, Lipinski B, Lipinska I: A comparative study of precipitation and paracoagulation by protamine sulfate and ethanol gelation tests. Thromb Res 2:539–556, 1973

100. Kisker TC: Detection of fibrin monomer. Comparison of immune precipitation method with the serial dilution protamine sulfate test and the ethanol gelation test. Am J Clin Pathol 72:405–409, 1979

101. Margolis CZ: Ethanol gelation test. N Engl J Med 284:53–54, 1971

102. Margaretten W, Zunker HO, McKay DG: Production of the generalized Shwartzman reaction in rats by intravenous infusion of thrombin. Lab Invest 13:552–559, 1964

103. Margaretten W, Csavossy I, McKay DG: An electron microscope study of thrombin induced disseminated intravascular coagulation. Blood 29:169–181, 1967

104. Ogston D, Bennett B, Douglas AS: Thrombolytic therapy and fibrinolytic inhibitors, in Biggs R, Rizza CR (eds): Human Blood Coagulation. (in press)

105. Davidson JF, McNicol GP, Frank GL, et al: A plasminogen activator-producing tumor. Br Med J 1:88–91, 1969

106. Poller L: Fibrinolysis and gastrointestinal hemorrhage. J Clin Pathol 33(suppl 14):63–67, 1980

107. Rybo G: Plasminogen activators in the endometrium II. Clinical aspects. Acta Obstet Gynecol Scand 45:429–450, 1966

108. Forbes CD, Barr RD, Reid G, et al: Tranexamic acid in control of haemorrhage after dental extraction in haemophilia and Christmas Disease. Br Med J 2:311–313, 1972

109. Walsh PN, Rizza CR, Matthews JM, et al: Epsilon aminocaproic acid therapy for dental extractions in haemophilia and Christmas disease: A double blind controlled trial. Br J Haematol 20:463–475, 1971

110. Gordon AM, McNicol GP, Dubber AHC, et al: Clinical trial of epsilon aminocaproic acid in severe haemophilia. Br Med J 1:1632–1635, 1965

111. Rainsford SG, Jouhar AJ, Hall A: Tranexamic acid in the control of spontaneous bleeding in severe haemophilia. Thromb Diath Haemorrh 30:272–279, 1973

112. Calendar ST, Warner GT, Cope E: Treatment of menorrhagia with tranexamic acid. A double blind trial. Br Med J 4:214–216, 1970

113. Nilsson L, Rybo G: Treatment of menorrhagia with an antifibrinolytic agent tranexamic acid (AMCA). A double blind investigation. Acta Obstet Gynecol Scand 46:572–580, 1967

114. Nilsson L, Rybo G: Treatment of menorrhagia with epsilon aminocaproic acid. A double blind investigation. Acta Obstet Gynecol Scand 44:467–473, 1965

115. Vermylen J, Verhaegen-Declecq ML, Verstraete M, et al: A double blind study on the effect of tranexamic acid in essential menorrhagia. Thromb Diath Haemorrh 20:583–587, 1968

116. Kasonde JM, Bonnar J: Effect of ethamsylate and aminocaproic acid on menstrual blood loss in women using intrauterine devices. Br Med J 4:21–22, 1975

117. Westrom L, Bengtsson LP: Effect of tranexamic acid (AMCA) in menorrhagia with intrauterine contraceptive devices. A double blind study. J Reprod Med 5:154–161, 1970

118. Rybo G, Westerberg H: The effect of tranexamic acid (AMCA) on postoperative bleeding after conization. Acta Obstet Gynecol Scand 51:347–350, 1972

119. Biggs JC, Hugh TB, Dodds AJ: Tranexamic acid and upper gastrointestinal haemorrhage—a double-blind trial. Gut 17:729–734, 1976

120. Cormack F, Jouhar AJ, Chakrabarti RR, Fearnley GP: Tranexamic acid in upper gastrointestinal haemorrhage. Lancet 1:1207–1208, 1973

121. Engqvist A, Bostrom O, von Feilitzen F, et al: Tranexamic acid in massive hemorrhage from the upper gastrointestinal tract. A double blind study. Scand J Gastroenterol 14:839–844, 1980

122. Hedlund PO: Antifibrinolytic therapy with Cyclokapron in connection with prostatectomy. A double blind study. Scand J Urol Nephrol 3:177–182, 1969

123. Lawrence ACK, Ward-McQuaid JN, Holdom GL: The effect of epsilon aminocaproic acid on the blood loss after retropubic prostatectomy. Br J Urol 38:308–310, 1966

124. McNicol GP, Fletcher AP, Alkjaersig N, et al: The use of epsilon aminocaproic acid, a potent inhibitor of fibrinolytic activity in the management of postoperative hematuria. J Urol 86:829–837, 1961

125. Madsen PO, Strauch AE: The effect of aminocaproic acid on bleeding following transurethral prostatectomy. J Urol (Balt) 96:255–256, 1966

126. Smart CJ, Turnbull AR, Jenkins JD: The use of frusemide and epsilon-aminocaproic acid in transurethral prostatectomy. Br J Urol 46:521–525, 1974

127. Vinnicombe J, Shuttleworth KED: Aminocaproic acid in the control of hemorrhage after prostatectomy. Safety of aminocaproic acid. A controlled trial. Lancet 1:232–234, 1966

128. Warren JW Jr, Stanley KE Jr: A new anti-hemorrhagic agent. Epsilon aminocaproic acid for control of hemorrhage after transurethral prostate resection: A controlled study. J Kans Med Soc 20:173–176, 1969

129. Fodstad H, Liliequist B, Schannong M, et al: Use of tranexamic acid (AMCA) in the preoperative management of patients with ruptured intracranial aneurysms. Surg Neurol 9:9–15, 1978

130. Maurice-Williams RS: Prolonged antifibrinolysis: An effective non-surgical treatment for ruptured intracranial aneurysms? Br Med J 1:945–947, 1978

131. Verstraete M, Vermylen J, Tyberghein J: Double blind evaluation of the hemostatic effect of adrenochrome monosemicarbazone, conjugated estrogens and epsilon aminocaproic acid after adenotonsillectomy. Acta Haematol 40:154–161, 1968

132. Verstraete M, Tyberghein J, Degreef Y, et al: Double blind trials with ethamsylate, batroxobin or tranexamic acid on blood loss after adenotonsillectomy. Acta Clin Belg 32:136–141, 1977

133. Bramsen T: Traumatic hyphaema treated with the antifibrinolytic drug tranexamic acid. Acta Ophthalmol 54:250–256, 1976

134. Jerndal T, Frisen M: Tranexamic acid (AMCA) and late hyphema—a double blind study in cataract surgery. Acta Ophthalmol 54:417–429, 1976

135. Mortensen KK, Sjølie AK: Secondary haemorrhage following traumatic hyphaema. A comparative study of conservative and tranexamic acid treatment. Acta Ophthalmol 56:763–768, 1978

136. Bennett AE, Ingram GIC, Inglish PJ: Antifibrinolytic treatment in haemophilia: A controlled trial of prophylaxis with tranexamic acid. Br J Haematol 24:83–88, 1973

137. Fodstad H: Tranexamic acid (AMCA) in aneurysmal subarachnoid hemorrhage. J Clin Pathol 33(suppl 14):68–73, 1980

138. Kaste M, Ramsey M: Effect of tranexamic acid on fatal rebleeds after subarachnoid hemorrhage. Double blind study. Acta Neurol Scand Suppl 67:254, 1978 (abstract)

139. Post KD, Flamm ES, Goodgold A, et al: Ruptured intracranial aneurysms: Case morbidity and mortality. J Neurosurg 46:290–295, 1977

140. Strauss HS, Kevy SV, Diamond LK: Ineffectiveness of prophylactic epsilon aminocaproic acid in severe hemophilia. N Engl J Med 273:301–304, 1965

141. Sundt TM, Whisnant JP: Subarachnoid hemorrhage from intracranial aneurysms. Surgical management and natural history of disease. N Engl J Med 229:116–122, 1978

142. Van Rossum J, Wintzen AR, Endtz LJ, et al: Effect of tranexamic acid on rebleeding after subarachnoid hemorrhage: A double blind controlled trial. Ann Neurol 2:242–245, 1977
143. Barkhan P: Hematuria in a hemophiliac treated with ε-aminocaproic acid. Lancet 2:1061, 1964
144. Tsevrenis H, Mandalaki T: Haematuria in a haemophiliac treated with ε-aminocaproic acid. Lancet 1:610, 1965
145. Itterbeck H van, Vermylen J, Verstraete M: High obstruction of urine flow as a complication of treatment with fibrinolysis inhibitors of haematuria in haemophiliacs. Acta Haematol 39: 237–242, 1968
146. Stark SN, White JG, Langer L, et al: Epsilon-aminocaproic acid as a cause of intrarenal obstruction in haematuria of haemophiliacs. Scand J Haematol 2:99–107, 1965
147. Davies D, Howell DA: Tranexamic acid and arterial thrombosis. Lancet 1:49, 1977
148. Fletcher AP, Alkjaersig N, Sherry S: Fibrinolytic mechanisms and the development of thrombolytic therapy. Am J Med 33:738–752, 1962
149. Hoffman EP, Koo AH: Cerebral thrombosis associated with Amicar. Radiology 131:687–689, 1979
150. McNicol GP: Disordered fibrinolytic activity and its control. Scott Med J 7:266–276, 1962
151. Naeye RI: Thrombotic state after hemorrhagic diathesis, a possible complication of therapy with epsilon-aminocaproic acid. Blood 19:694–701, 1962
152. Lane RJM, Martin AM, McLelland NJ, et al: Epsilon aminocaproic acid (EACA) myopathy. Postgraduate Medical Journal 55:282–285, 1979

George H. Goldsmith, Jr.

# 10
# Hemostatic Disorders Associated with Neoplasia

Every known component of the normal hemostatic mechanism may be adversely affected by neoplastic growths (Table 10-1). The clinical syndromes resulting from these interactions include both hemorrhagic states, reflecting impaired platelet and/or plasma coagulation, and vasooclusive events in both the venous and arterial circulations.

Investigations stimulated by the diverse hemostatic alterations occurring in patients with a wide variety of neoplasms have, in recent years, indicated that the entire sequence of cancer cell growth and metastasis seems intimately entwined with, and perhaps influenced by, the hemostatic system. Local tumor growth and extension appears to be influenced by the fibrin deposits commonly found at the tumor periphery; in different tumor models, evidence that these deposits may function to retard escape of cells from the primary lesion or that they impair attack by the host upon the malignant cells has been put forward.[1,2] Extension of focal malignant deposits may also reflect impaired production or utilization[3] of fibronectin; this cell surface protein mediates cellular adhesion to collagen and is cross-linked to fibrinogen or fibrin by factor XIII. Current data suggest that this impaired fibronectin-mediated adhesion to collagen and/or fibrin, enhancing the ability of the malignant cell to migrate along fibrin deposits, may provide a biochemical basis for extension and growth of malignant cell populations. Plasminogen activators, proteases commonly produced by transformed or malignant cell lines,[4] produce proteolytic products of plasminogen and fibrinogen that are mitogenic and enhance local vascular permeability. Platelet-derived prostaglandins[5] and growth factors[6] may also influence tumor cell proliferation. Metastatic tumor dissemination may be mediated by the interaction of tumor–platelet–emboli with normal or damaged endothelium at specific microvascular sites.[7]

These and a rapidly growing body of similar data derived from animal tumor models and cell culture systems can, at present, be only conjecturally applied to the more complex in vivo situation of naturally arising malignancy. There seems little question, however, that both local and systemic changes in the hemostatic system are intimately related to the processes of local tumor growth and metastasis. The pertinent details of this interaction may well differ according to individual tumor and host characteristics, and with the stage of disease.

In view of our limited understanding of the complex and variable network of interac-

**Table 10-1**

Hemostatic Disorders in Neoplasia

Intravascular coagulation and fibrinolysis (DIC)
Impaired plasma coagulation
    Pathological inhibitors
    Isolated factor deficiencies
    Hepatic or renal damage
    Iatrogenic defects
Platelet abnormalities
    Thrombocytopenia
    Thrombocytosis
    Platelet dysfunction
Vascular disorders

tions between malignant cells and the coagulation system, it is not surprising that attempts to influence tumor progression by pharmacologic manipulation of the hemostatic mechanism have given mixed results to date. Recently, adjuvant treatment with warfarin in patients with small-cell carcinoma also receiving systemic chemotherapy resulted in a longer survival time of warfarin-treated patients responding to chemotherapy as compared to a control group of responders.[8] In a wide variety of other solid tumors receiving similar warfarin treatment, improved survival has also been reported with some lymphomas, breast cancer, ovarian carcinoma, and osteogenic sarcoma.[9] Other studies employing warfarin therapy have shown no benefit, however. Adjunctive heparin and platelet-inhibiting agents have been less extensively studied and have yielded equivocal results to date.

## INTRAVASCULAR COAGULATION AND FIBRINOLYSIS

The particular predisposition of patients with neoplasms to develop apparently spontaneous thromboembolic and hemorrhagic lesions has become well established since Trousseau's linkage of vascular thrombosis with visceral cancer in 1865,[10] and the association of these complications with laboratory evidence of disseminated intravascular coagulation (DIC) and fibrinolysis is also long-standing.[11]

In different studies of patients with cancer, the incidence of laboratory abnormalities suggestive of DIC has varied widely, reflecting differences in the sensitivity of the assays employed, in the distribution of tumor types, and in the incidence and severity of metastatic disease. Surveys employing tests such as the whole blood clotting time, prothrombin time (PT), partial thromboplastin time (PTT), thrombin time (TT), fibrinogen level, platelet count, and measurements of fibrin/fibrinogen degradation products have typically shown abnormalities in one or more of these tests in over 50 percent of patients with cancer and in over 90 percent of patients with extensive metastatic disease.[12,13] The patterns of abnormalities, which include shortening as well as prolongation of clotting times and abnormal elevation of platelet counts and coagulation factor levels, vary markedly among affected patients. Increased platelet and fibrinogen turnover has been described in patients with both abnormal and normal coagulation parameters, and in some studies was found to correlate with both the extent and type of malignancy.[14] Increased plasma levels of fibrinopeptide A, indicative of ongoing in vivo thrombin generation, appear to be the single most sensitive index of deranged hemostasis in patients with cancer; recent studies have found this abnormality in over 90 percent of patients with metastatic cancer.[15]

Even allowing for disparities in the types and extent of cancer in published series, it is clear that the incidence of laboratory abnormalities of hemostasis greatly exceeds the incidence of clinically apparent thrombotic or hemorrhagic complications in cancer patients. Although several postmortem studies have found thrombi in 20–50 percent of patients with metastatic carcinoma, clinically evident thromboembolic and hemorrhagic disease in series reflecting different tumor types and varying tumor burdens has ranged from 0 to 15 percent.[14,16]

This coupling of frequent, but variable, laboratory abnormalities of coagulation with an increased, but less frequent, incidence of clinical hemostatic abnormalities is currently interpreted as evidence for a high incidence of ongoing or intermittent intravascular coagulation and fibrinolysis or DIC (see Chapter 8) in patients with cancer. In this patient population, it is both conceptually and clinically useful to separate the diverse forms of DIC into an acute syndrome, characterized by marked consumption and depletion of coagulation factors and platelets in association with diffuse thrombotic and/or hemorrhagic lesions, and a chronic syndrome, in which a presumably lower rate of thrombin formation produces less marked laboratory abnormalities and may or may not be accompanied by clinically apparent thrombosis or hemorrhage. Affected patients with solid tumors, for example, most commonly have persistent laboratory and clinical profiles that correspond more closely to that of "chronic" DIC. The fluctuating clinical and laboratory manifestations of DIC that are common in patients with large tumor burdens may also be characterized according to the ability of the patient's hemostatic mechanism to compensate for the aberrant procoagulant stimulus. That is, "decompensated" DIC, with decreased levels of platelets, fibrinogen, and other coagulation factors, reflects consumption in excess of production. "Compensated" DIC, reflecting balanced consumption and production, is characterized by largely normal levels of coagulation factors in conjunction with other evidence of thrombin formation, such as elevated plasma levels of fibrinogen-related antigens (FDP or FRA) or of fibrinopeptide A. In "overcompensated" DIC, platelets and/or coagulation factors are present at above-normal levels, reflecting production in excess of the current rate of consumption.

Many etiologic mechanisms for DIC due to cancer have been proposed. Granulocytic proteases from leukemic cells may directly activate the coagulation mechanism.[17] Carcinoma cells may produce both tissue thromboplastin and enzymes capable of direct activation of plasma factor X (Stuart factor).[18,19] Necrosis of rapidly growing tumors may potentiate thrombin generation by chronic release of thromboplastin to the circulation. Tumor cell-induced platelet aggregation[20] may also activate coagulation. In addition, procoagulant activities may be induced in normal circulating leukocytes of patients with cancer, perhaps by immune responses of the host to tumor tissue.[21]

In clinical situations, precise definition of either the etiology or the site of cancer-related activation of the hemostatic system is usually not possible. Assays ordinarily employed for evaluation of DIC do not distinguish between activation and consumption of clotting factors at local sites and the actual circulation of released procoagulant material that induces a truly disseminated coagulopathy. Recent data suggest that both mechanisms may be operative, even in the absence of clinical complications of DIC. In a group of cancer patients lacking clinical evidence of thromboembolism or hemorrhage, a subgroup of patients was identified whose plasmas possessed both increased levels of fibrinopeptide A, and increased in vitro production of fibrinopeptide A, indicating the presence of a circulating thrombinlike or thrombin-generating activity. Heparin treatment abolished in vitro production of fibrinopeptide A without reducing it to normal levels.[15] This suggests that concomitant localized thrombinlike activity, not susceptible to systemic heparin-antithrombin inhibition, and release of procoagulant species susceptible to such inhibition to the circulation may both occur in at least some patients with disseminated carcinoma.

## Clinical Features

The clinical manifestations of this abnormal activation of the coagulation mechanism in patients with cancer are as protean as the associated laboratory abnormalities. In patients with solid tumors, thromboembolic events are the most common complications. Venous thrombosis, either localized or recurrent and migratory, occurs in over one-half of clinically affected patients, and may coincide with or precede diagnosis of the underlying malignancy.[11] As many as 25 percent of affected patients sustain arterial embolic complications, usually in conjunction with nonbacterial thrombotic endocarditis; the predominantly fibrin-platelet valvuler lesions found at autopsy most commonly involve the aortic and mitral valves, but tricuspid involvement may also occur.[11] Common sites of embolization include large and small cerebral vessels, spleen, kidneys, and peripheral arteries. Myocardial infarction due to coronary artery occlusion has also been observed. It should be noted that the neurologic manifestations of cerebral involvement are not limited to the sudden onset of focal neurologic deficits. Multifocal small ischemic or hemorrhagic infarctions associated with fibrin thromboemboli may be manifested as confusion, disorientation, or other disorders of consciousness that are initially confused with metabolic encephalopathy or diffuse central nervous system infection.[22]

Hemorrhagic complications in affected patients with solid tumors may range from minor mucocutaneous bleeding to massive gastrointestinal, pulmonary, or intracerebral hemorrhage; the incidence in different series has ranged by 6 to 40 percent.[11] Notably, manifestations of two or all three of these clinical syndromes may develop in the same patient either concomitantly or in sequence.

Recognition of these syndromes as manifestations of abnormal activation of the coagulation mechanism is usually not difficult, if the predisposition of patients with carcinoma to undergo the sequences described above is kept in mind. The likelihood of a patient's being affected is also roughly proportional to the tumor burden, in that extensive metastatic disease is much more frequently complicated by these syndromes than is localized carcinoma. Anticipation of predisposition by type of tumor is clinically less useful. Although pancreatic and other mucinous adenocarcinomas have been particularly associated with thromboembolic events, and prostate carcinoma with hemorrhagic ones, it should be recognized that solid tumors of a wide variety of anatomic sites and histologic types[11] have been complicated by each form of hemostatic disorder described. Typical manifestations of an underlying disordered hemostatic mechanism such as migratory thrombophlebitis; coincident or sequential occurrence of the venous occlusive, arterial embolic, and hemorrhagic syndromes previously described; or multifocal sites of simultaneous hemorrhage should all immediately suggest the clinical likelihood of DIC.

Awareness of the possibility of a low-grade, compensated process of intravascular coagulation also prepares the clinician for the increased frequency of thromboembolic and hemorrhagic complications that may follow any additional insult to the affected patient's hemostatic mechanism. Thromboembolism or bleeding following even minor surgery may result from disruption of this delicate balance; deep venous thrombosis has occurred 3–4 times more frequently in patients with cancer than in patients without cancer undergoing comparable procedures.[18] Similarly, severe intercurrent infections, venous stasis with immobility, or initiation of cytotoxic chemotherapy or radiation therapy may produce decompensation of an already stressed hemostatic mechanism and thrombosis or hemorrhage.

In contrast to the solid tumors, hemorrhage is the most common hemostatic complication encountered in the acute leukemias. Since thrombocytopenia consequent to impaired bone marrow function is common with these disorders, intravascular coagulation itself may not be the dominant etiology. In acute promyelocytic leukemia[23] and, to a lesser extent, acute myelocytic leukemia, however, laboratory manifestations of DIC are quite common. In the former disorder, administration of heparin during initial cytotoxic chemotherapy has reduced the frequency of complicating hemorrhage.[24]

Hemorrhage is less common in the chronic leukemias until late in the course of the disease, but chronic lymphocytic leukemia appears to be complicated by a greater than expected frequency of thrombophlebitis,[25] and the increased frequency of both thromboembolism and hemorrhage in the myeloproliferative disorders may be due, in part, to the induction of a chronic intravascular coagulation by abnormally functioning platelets.

As noted previously, the laboratory abnormalities associated with diverse clinical DIC syndromes are quite variable. Patients with acute, decompensated DIC will commonly have thrombocytopenia, hypofibrinogenemia, prolonged TT, PT, and PTT and elevated levels of circulating FDP; antithrombin III levels are often also reduced. Less commonly, peripheral blood smears will show microangiopathic evidence of red blood cell fragmentation. Patients with less fulminant forms of DIC usually show less severe abnormalities. The demonstration of consistent laboratory abnormalities assists in confirming the diagnosis of DIC. However, there is such great variation in the number, type, and severity of hemostatic abnormalities in this group of patients that virtually all combinations of normal and abnormal test parameters of hemostasis may be present at a given time in a given patient; even a completely normal PT, PTT, fibrinogen level, platelet count, and FDP titer may not exclude the presence of some degree of abnormal activation of coagulation. Although increased levels of fibrinopeptide A seem to be the most sensitive index of ongoing thrombin generation currently available to the clinician, assay results are usually not rapidly available.

Despite the somewhat loose correlation between individual assay results and clinical severity of the syndrome in different patients, sequential determination of coagulation assays is often useful in patient management. Acute vascular events are commonly associated with changes in platelet count and fibrinogen level, so that individual patterns of change in such assays as the PT, PTT, TT, platelet count, and fibrinogen level can often be used both for correlation with clinical events and as an aid in judging the response to therapy. Sequential laboratory determinations can also aid in detection of coincident defects of hemostasis distinct from the DIC syndrome. A patient whose DIC was manifested, in part, by hypofibrinogenemia and thrombocytopenia, for example, and who had responded to therapy with a return of these values to normal levels but who now also shows a new prolongation of his PT and PTT, may have a superimposed vitamin K deficiency resulting from malnutrition and antibiotic therapy.

## Therapy

As with DIC in other settings (Chapter 8), success in controlling the coagulopathy in patients with cancer ultimately requires successful control of the underlying disease process; treatment directed solely at the coagulopathy is of limited long-term value. When laboratory abnormalities are found in the absence of clinical complications, treatment of the coagulopathy is ordinarily not indicated. One apparent exception to this guideline is subclinical DIC complicating acute promyelocytic leukemia, in which the incidence of overt and fulminant DIC during treatment with cytotoxic agents is so common that heparin therapy is often used as part of the initial chemotherapy regimen.[24,26] Most authorities agree that laboratory evidence of DIC in this disease, even in the absence of clinical mani-festations, is sufficient indication for heparin therapy. The usual initial heparin dosage is 50 U/kg intravenously every six hours, or the equivalent administered as a continuous intravenous infusion.[27] Concomitantly, platelets are administered as required to maintain a platelet count equal to or greater than 20,000/μl. some authorities recommend doubling the dosage of heparin if there is no improvement within 24 hours, or if hypofibrinogenemia and circulating FDP become more abnormal. Others believe that heparin in excess of the initial dosage is accompanied by an unacceptable risk of bleeding in the presence of severe thrombocytopenia.

For other neoplastic disorders complicated by acute and chronic DIC syndromes, there is considerable disagreement over indications for treatment and specific treatment programs; no published data clearly demonstrate the superiority of one specific treatment approach over another. Anticoagulant therapy appears to exert a more clearly beneficial effect upon chronic rather than acute DIC syndromes;[11,28,29] Heparin has been demonstrably superior to warfarin in controlling chronic DIC.[11] Although antiplatelet drugs have been recom-mended for initial treatment of chronic DIC syndromes,[30] the equivalence or superiority of this approach has not been demonstrated. Concern over exacerbating the coagulopathy (''feeding the fire'') with transfused platelets and coagulation factors has largely abated in recent years. Replacement therapy with platelets and plasma components is now com-monly recommended in conjunction with anticoagulant therapy, but only limited data are available to support their efficacy[31] in DIC.

Acute DIC, with severe clinical complications and pronounced decompensation of the hemostatic system, often occurs in conjunction with catastrophic dysfunction of other organ systems that is the major threat to life, such as the adult respiratory distress syndrome, sepsis with acute renal failure, diffuse pulmonary hemorrhage with respiratory insufficiency, and extensive peripheral cutaneous infarction.[29] This may account for the apparently mar-ginal benefits of treatment directed at the coagulopathy itself. Nonetheless, it would ap-pear that vascular thrombosis and pathological bleeding into the gastrointestinal tract, central nervous system, and lungs are major contributions of the coagulopathy to the high mortal-ity of this patient population,[11,29] and treatment decisions should include this consideration.

Heparin therapy should be considered in acute DIC syndromes other than those asso-ciated with an acute treatable event such as sepsis, or when bleeding or other complica-tions of the coagulopathy appear to be a dominant feature of the clinical picture in a patient with a treatable malignancy. Serial determinations of laboratory tests of hemostasis often help in making this assessment. Although a variety of dosages have been recommended, most often standard doses of 15–20 U/kg/hr by continuous infusion or 70–140 U/kg intra-venously every 4 hours are used. When significant (less than or equal to 50,000/μl) thrombocytopenia is present, reduced doses of 10–12 U/kg/hr are used initially. Concomi-tant replacement therapy with platelets may require repeated transfusion of 10–20 U of platelet concentrates. Severe hypofibrinogenemia may be treated with cryoprecipitate as required to obtain fibrinogen levels equal to or greater than 150 mg/dl; 15 U of cryoprecip-itate, containing about 3 g of fibrinogen, will contribute about 100 mg/dl to the circulation of a 70-kg adult. Heparin should be used cautiously, if at all, in the setting of severe renal or hepatic failure, when extensive vascular damage is present, or when very severe thrombocytopenia and hypofibrinogenemia are found. If DIC appears to be arrested, but very high levels of FDP persist, continued heparin treatment may produce hemorrhagic complications of a predominantly fibrin(ogen)olytic process.[28]

Heparin therapy offers clearer benefits for control of the thrombotic and hemorrhagic manifestations of the chronic DIC syndromes in cancer patients. Most patients will respond to treatment with standard doses of heparin,[11] and lower doses (5–10 U/kg/hr intravenously or 5000–10,000 U subcutaneously for 8–12 hours have also been used successfully. Recurrent thrombosis, however, commonly follows cessation of heparin or conversion to oral anticoagulant therapy. In general, heparin therapy for significant thrombotic or thromboembolic complications of DIC in patients without severe thrombocytopenia (greater than or equal to 50,000/μl) or hypofibrinogenemia (greater than or equal to 100 mg/dl) should continue until both resolution of thrombophlebitis or other clinical manifestations of the coagulopathy and improvement in laboratory abnormalities have occurred. Subsequently, in patients who have had a single episode of venous thrombosis or coincident significant reduction in tumor burden, heparin may be discontinued, with careful observation of clinical and laboratory parameters for signs of relapse. In patients with stable tumor burdens, continued therapy with oral anticoagulants sometimes seems beneficial, but warfarin treatment, as noted previously, often fails to prevent recurrence; this is especially true in cases with tumor progression. Recurrent thromboembolic disease, especially in the setting of stable or increasing tumor burden, usually requires continued heparin therapy for a prolonged period. Once control of acute symptoms is achieved, outpatient management with subcutaneous heparin is often successful. The dosage required varies in individual cases, but an average initial regimen of 5000 U subcutaneously three times a day, followed by reduction to 5000 U two times a day, is often adequate. Spontaneous bleeding complications with this regimen seem to be infrequent, and recurrent hemorrhage is usually accompanied by hypofibrinogenemia and thrombocytopenia, indicative of worsening DIC or heparin toxicity.[32] Patients for whom effective treatment of the underlying tumor is not available do not ordinarily survive long enough to develop such complications of chronic heparin therapy as neurotoxicity, osteoporosis, and alopecia. Patients who do not respond to heparin therapy initially may be treated with antiplatelet agents, such as aspirin, 300 mg twice a day, and dipyridamole, 50 mg four times a day.[30]

For control of minor hemorrhagic complications such as recurrent epistaxis and gingival bleeding not associated with severe thrombocytopenia, the author prefers an initial trial of low-dose heparin (2500–5000 U subcutaneously 2–3 times a day) but has also observed responses to antiplatelet agents as described above.

Replacement therapy with platelets and plasma fractions is less commonly needed in the chronic DIC syndromes, but may be administered as needed according to the guidelines discussed previously.

## FIBRIN(OGEN)OLYSIS

So-called primary fibrin(ogen)olysis, in which the dominant detectable disorder of coagulation is uncontrolled plasmin-mediated digestion of fibrin and fibrinogen, appears to be rare in disorders other than prostatic-carcinoma.[30,33] Distinction from a coexisting DIC syndrome may be difficult, but must be made before treatment with inhibitors of plasminogen activation, such as epsilon aminocaproic acid, is considered. Hypofibrinogenemia, high circulating levels of FDP, relatively normal levels of platelets, and a shortened whole blood or euglobulin clot-lysis time should be present. Although coagulation factors other than fibrinogen, factor V (proaccelerin) and factor VIII (antihemophilic factor) are not reduced by circulating plasmin, the TT, PT, and PTT are commonly prolonged due to the anticoagulant effect of circulating FDP. The appropriate clinical setting and

**Table 10-2**
Selective Impairment of Plasma Coagulation in Cancer

Pathological inhibitors
    Paraproteins in plasma cell dyscrasias
    Lupuslike: Hodgkin's disease, non-Hodgkin's lymphoma, myelofibrosis, carcinoma
    Factor XI inhibitors: carcinomas of the colon, prostate
    Factor VII inhibitor: bronchogenic carcinoma
    Heparinoid: plasma cell dyscrasia, lung cancer
Isolated factor deficienceis
    XIII: Acute leukemias, chronic myelocytic leukemia (CML)
    XII: CML
    XI: Malignant melanoma
    X: Multiple myeloma with amyloidosis, mycoplasma pneumonia
    VIIR:RC and/or VIIIR:Ag: Macroglobulinemia, chronic lymphocytic leukemia, Wilms' tumor
    V: CML, polycythemia vera

laboratory profile must be confirmed before administration of epsilon aminocapoic acid, since severe thrombotic complications may follow its administration in DIC.[34]

## OTHER DIRECT EFFECTS OF NEOPLASTIC TISSUE ON PLASMA COAGULATION

Neoplasms may also form products that directly impair one or more components of the plasma coagulation mechanism (Table 10-2). This is particularly true in multiple myeloma and other malignant paraprotein disorders as a result of inhibition of coagulation by paraprotein. Although anticoagulant activity directed against the surface-mediated system and the individual coagulation factors prothrombin, V, VII, VIII, and X has been described, the most common inhibitory activity is directed against the thrombin–fibrinogen interaction and fibrin monomer polymerization.[35–38] Other anticoagulant paraproteins have been shown to inhibit coagulation through impairment of phospholipid function (lupus-type inhibitor, Chapter 7)[39–41] and by abnormal calcium binding.[42] One unusual paraprotein inhibitor of factor VIII appeared to function as a lymphocyte-associated immunoabsorbent that depleted the patient's plasma of factor VIII.[43] The clinical significance of such coagulation abnormalities in malignant paraprotein diseases is conjectural. From 15 to 60 percent of patient with multiple myeloma, Waldenström's macroglobulinemia, and other lymphoproliferative diseases associated with paraproteinemias have some hemorrhagic complication.[35] Defective platelet function, thrombocytopenia, and abnormalities of liver function are also commonly present at the time of bleeding episodes, and there is usually poor correlation between laboratory abnormalities of plasma coagulation and hemorrhagic symptoms.

Lupuslike inhibitors have also been identified in a few patients with Hodgkin's disease, non-Hodgkin's lymphoma, myelofibrosis, and carcinoma.[40,44,45] When present as isolated abnormalities, these are not associated with a bleeding disorder; in contrast, some data suggest an increased risk of thrombosis in patients with these anticoagulants.[46]

Inhibitors of factor XI (plasma thromboplastin antecedent, PTA) have been detected in patients with carcinoma of the colon[47] and prostate.[48] An inhibitor of factor VII in a patient with bronchogenic carcinoma[49] and heparinlike anticoagulants in isolated cases of plasma cell dyscrasia and lung cancer[50,51] have been reported. Several other cases of heparinemia or antithrombinlike anticoagulants reported in the older literature may have been manifestations of circulating FDP due to DIC.

Isolated deficiencies of individual coagulation factors in patients with malignant disorders are rare, and for the most part, the etiology of the acquired deficiency state is unknown. Individual cases of chronic myelocytic leukemia have been associated with deficiencies of Factor XII (Hageman factor),[52] factor XIII (fibrin-stabilizing factor),[53] and factor V.[54] Factor XIII deficiency has also been identified in several cases of acute leukemia, especially acute promyelocytic leukemia.[53] Factor V deficiency has also been detected in polycythemia vera, along with a variety of less well-characterized abnormalities of coagulation and fibrinolysis.[55] Factor XI (PTA) deficiency and another uncharacterized abnormality of the surface-activated components of coagulation were found in one case of malignant melanoma.[56]

Hemorrhage of varying severity in conjunction with reduced levels of factor VIIIR:RC and/or factor VIIIR:Ag has been reported in patients with chronic lymphocytic leukemia and Wilms' tumor,[57,58] as well as in Waldenström's macroglobulinemia.[59,43] Amyloidosis, either primary or as a complication of multiple myeloma, has been associated with an acquired, selective deficiency of factor X (Stuart factor).[59a,60-62] Affected patients may sustain ecchymoses or intramuscular, mucosal, gastrointestinal or genitourinary tract bleeding. Surprisingly, some may have no clinical evidence of a hemorrhagic disorder. The titer of factor X has ranged from 1 to 20 percent of normal. In some patients, too, deficiencies of factor IX, factor VII, or prothrombin have also been detected, and the thrombin time has been greatly prolonged. The deficiency of factor X is corrected poorly, if at all, by transfusion of plasma or concentrates of the vitamin K-dependent clotting factors. This poor response is readily understandable since considerable evidence has accrued that amyloid fibrils bind factor X, extracting it from the circulation.[63] In several reported cases, bleeding decreased after splenectomy and the titer of factor X rose to near-normal levels.[63a] Isolated deficiency of factor X is not pathognomonic for amyloidosis, as it has also been detected in association with mycoplasmal pneumonia, and other situations.

Other abnormalities of plasma coagulation[64] and of the plasma fibrinolytic system[65] in patients with hematologic malignancies have not been clearly linked with abnormalities in the individual components of these mechanisms. These abnormalities, manifested by changes in the TT and euglobulin lysis time, appear to be of little clinical significance compared to other coexistent abnormalities of platelets and plasma coagulation in this patient population.

## COAGULATION DEFECTS RESULTING FROM ORGAN DAMAGE AND THERAPY

Hepatic dysfunction, due to neoplastic parenchymal damage or to obstruction of the hepatobiliary system, may produce a wide variety of coagulation defects reflecting reduced synthesis of coagulation factors, production of abnormal fibrinogens, decreased absorption of vitamin K, and other coagulation abnormalities that also result from liver disease of other etiologies (see Chapter 14). Similarly, malabsorption syndromes resulting from pancreatic or small bowel invasion may cause deficiency of vitamin K-dependent factors, as may the combination of the malnutrition that is common in advanced malignancy with broad-spectrum antibiotic treatment for intercurrent infection. In these situations, a therapeutic trial of vitamin $K_1$, 25 mg/day parenterally, for three days, is worthwhile since some improvement may occur even in the presence of hepatic parenchymal damage.

Renal damage resulting from anatomic or metabolic complications of malignancy usually affects hemostasis primarily through the platelet functional defects associated with uremia. Occasionally, the paraneoplastic nephrotic syndrome that may accompany Hodgkin's disease will cause an abnormal prolongation of the PTT due to urinary losses of Hageman factor and/or PTA.

Coagulation abnormalities may also result from cytotoxic agents used to treat the underlying disorder. L-Asparaginase therapy commonly produces hypofibrinogenemia and a functionally abnormal fibrinogen; reduced hepatic synthesis of other coagulation factors (II, V, VII, IX, and X) has also been noted.[66-68] Despite reduced fibrinogen levels in up to 70 percent of treated patients, very little clinically significant hemorrhage occurs as a direct result of impaired coagulation factor production. Mithramycin treatment programs are routinely accompanied by thrombocytopenia, platelet dysfunction, and variable reductions in the coagulation factors prothrombin, V, VII, and X, perhaps reflecting the induction of a DIC syndrome.[69] Hemorrhage after use of actinomycin D has been attributed to vitamin K antagonism by this agent, with impaired production of vitamin K-dependent factors.[70] Other abnormalities of coagulation, such as enhanced in vitro fibrinolysis in the presence of adriamycin and daunorubicin,[30] have also been described, but their clinical significance is not established.

## PLATELET ABNORMALITIES

Abnormal platelet production, survival, and function may stem from direct effects of the tumor or from alterations in the host induced by the tumor.

### Thrombocytopenia

Thrombocytopenia is the single most common cause of bleeding in patients with cancer. Bone marrow suppression from systemic chemotherapy or radiation therapy is probably the most common current cause of thrombocytopenia in this patient population. Decreased platelet production may also result from bone marrow dysfunction due to tumor invasion. Significant thrombocytopenia due to metastatic carcinoma usually reflects extensive marrow metastases that are heralded by a myelophthisic peripheral blood picture and are confirmed by closed needle biopsy of the bone marrow. Nutritional (folate) deficiency and/or intercurrent infection may also contribute to bone marrow hypoplasia in these patients. Replacement therapy with platelet concentrates will improve hemostasis temporarily under these conditions. No strict guidelines for their administration in this setting can be provided. Clinically significant bleeding is common with platelet counts of less than 20,000/μl due to marrow hypoplasia and is uncommon when the only hemostatic defect is moderate thrombocytopenia (greater than or equal to 40,000/μl).[71] Patients with neoplastic disorders, however, commonly have combined defects in platelets and plasma coagulation, and decisions regarding replacement therapy must reflect an assessment of the contribution of thrombocytopenia to the clinical problem at hand.

Thrombocytopenia due to increased peripheral destruction of platelets most commonly indicates the presence of intravascular coagulation, as discussed previously, and is ordinarily accompanied by other evidence of DIC. In lymphoproliferative malignancies and Hodgkin's disease, increased platelet destruction due to an apparently immunoglobulin-mediated (idiopathic thrombocytopenic purpuralike) process has been repeatedly observed, although the exact frequency is not well documented.[72,75] Rarely, a similar platelet-destructive process occurs in carcinomas.[76]

Distinction of antibody-mediated thrombocytopenia from hypoplastic thrombocytopenia is aided by detection in the former of increased platelet size on peripheral blood smear and adequate to increased numbers of megakaryocytes within the bone marrow. The risk of hemorrhage due to thrombocytopenia at platelet counts greater than or equal to $10,000/\mu l$ is greatly reduced in this situation compared to hypoplastic thrombocytopenia with an equivalent platelet count, and treatment with corticosteroids without platelet transfusion is ordinarily satisfactory. Rarely, severe thrombocytopenia and acute hemorrhage may require initial treatment with large quantities (greater than or equal to 10 U) of platelets to achieve initial control of life-threatening bleeding.

Drugs commonly required for treatment of complications of the malignant process, such as penicillin or carbenicillin, may also induce an immune-mediated thrombocytopenia. Withdrawal of the responsible drug is sufficient treatment in these situations unless life-threatening hemorrhage requires initial treatment with platelet transfusions. Heparin therapy may also be complicated by thrombocytopenia.[32] Suggested mechanisms to explain heparin-induced thrombocytopenia include immune-mediated destruction, direct heparin-induced platelet aggregation, and heparin-induced DIC. Since heparin therapy in patients with malignant disorders is usually initiated for treatment of a complication of DIC, it may be difficult to differentiate this side effect from the underlying process being treated. A pragmatic approach to this problem is to entertain seriously the diagnosis of heparin-induced thrombocytopenia when significantly worsened thrombocytopenia occurs within 10 days of initiating heparin therapy[32] despite improvement in other clinical and laboratory manifestions of the initial coagulopathy. Given this sequence, the severity of the thrombocytopenia and the need for continued anticoagulant therapy in the case at hand will dictate whether or not to discontinue heparin for the 2–4 days ordinarily required for improvement in this drug-induced thrombocytopenia.

Very rarely, increased platelet destruction due to a thrombotic thrombocytopenic purpuralike syndrome may occur with malignancy.[77] Diagnosis and treatment are as discussed in Chapters 4 and 8.

Finally, thrombocytopenia may reflect abnormal sequestration of the circulating platelet mass in an enlarged spleen or in the extensive and abnormal vascular channels of hemangiomas. In the latter situation, there is ordinarily concurrent DIC and microangiopathic hemolysis.[78]

## Thrombocytosis

Thrombocytosis, often with a platelet count of more than $10^6/\mu l$ and accompanied by qualitatively abnormal platelet function and abnormal morphology, is common in myeloproliferative disorders such as essential thrombocythemia and polycythemia vera.[79,80] Hemorrhagic and/or thrombotic complications are often associated with this increased platelet mass. In contrast, the increased number of circulating platelets ordinarily found in conjunction with neoplasms of many other types is usually modest ($400,000–600,000/\mu l$), although occasionally marked (exceeding $10^6/\mu l$),[81] associated with morphologically normal platelets, and not associated, in itself, with a bleeding disorder. The basis for this association is not known. Iron deficiency anemia also commonly contributes to modest elevations of the platelet count in patients with cancer.

Treatment of thrombocytosis is ordinarily required only in the myeloproliferative disorders. The choice between acute therapy with plateletpheresis or an intravenous alkylating agent, or more gradual control of the process with such agents as hydroxyurea, will depend upon the urgency of the clinical picture. Although antiplatelet agents such as aspirin have been utilized in the treatment of thromboembolic complications of thrombocytosis, their utility in this situation is not established.

## Qualitative Platelet Disorders

Abnormal platelet function is common in both solid tumors and hematologic malignancies. In the myeloproliferative disorders, increased or reduced platelet responsiveness to aggregating agents, impaired prostaglandin metabolism, reduced platelet factor 3 release, and impaired adhesion to glass beads are associated with abnormal platelet ultrastructure by electron microscopy. Some investigators have found that these functional abnormalities correlate better with hemorrhagic complications than does the platelet count, and, similarly, that platelet hyperreactivity in these assays corresponds to vasoocclusive complications.[79,82]

In the paraproteinemias, impaired in vitro platelet function is attributed to coating of the platelet canalicular system with paraprotein;[83] normal platelets incubated in affected patients' plasmas acquire the same defects. In contrast to the myeloproliferative disorders, however, there appears to be poor correlation between in vitro platelet functional defects and clinical hemorrhage. In solid tumors, the most common correlate with defective platelet function is the presence of FDP resulting from DIC. Other disease complications, including hepatic destruction and uremia, may also contribute to platelet dysfunction. Chemotherapeutic agents (melphalan, cytosine arabinoside, duanomycin) and antibiotics (carbenicillin) may also produce abnormalities in in vitro tests of platelet function. Mithramycin appears to induce a functional platelet disorder characterized by reduced platelet adenosine diphosphate (ADP) stores, prolonged bleeding time, and mucocutaneous hemorrhage which is independent of the previously described plasma coagulation defects.[84]

Except in the myeloproliferative disorders, the clinical significance of these platelet functional abnormalities is not established. It is reasonable to regard them as potential aggravators of hemorrhage due to other coagulopathies or thrombocytopenia. But it would appear unlikely that they present a major hemostatic problem in most bleeding patients with cancer. Dialysis to prevent or ameliorate bleeding due to uremia, or plasmapheresis for removal of paraproteins may be useful on rare occasions, but in general, the only therapy required is avoidance of additional contributions to platelet dysfunction by aspirin or other nonsteroidal anti-inflammatory agents. In the myeloproliferative disorders, these platelet-inhibiting agents have been used to prevent vasoocclusive complications attributed to platelet hyperfunction, but evidence supporting their efficacy for this purpose is not yet available.

## VASCULAR DISORDERS

Kaposi's sarcoma characteristically produces brown to violaceous cutaneous lesions with vascular disruption.[85] Cutaneous metastases of other tumors may occasionally be associated with local hemorrhage.

Generalized amyloidosis may produce purpuric skin lesions due to vascular infiltration and, in some cases, the abnormal protein may adsorb factor X from circulating blood.[63] Vascular purpura and mucocutaneous hemorrhage associated with malignant paraproteinemias, especially Waldenström's macroglobulinemia, are commonly attributed to direct vascular damage from sludging of red blood cells or cryoprecipitates; it is, however, difficult in these cases to distinguish the significance of direct paraprotein-induced vascular injury from the plasma coagulation and platelet functional defects described previously. Similarly, purpuric lesions attributed in the older literature to small-vessel injury by hematogenous tumor embolization[86] may also have been associated with other undiagnosed defects of hemostasis.

Corticosteroid excess, either iatrogenic or as part of a paraneoplastic syndrome, commonly produces purpuric cutaneous lesions; these most probably result from degenerative changes in vascular supporting tissue, with consequent loss of small-vessel protection against minor shearing insults, much as occurs in so-called senile purpura.[87]

With the exception of mucocutaneous hemorrhage in some paraproteinemias, these vascular lesions are of only cosmetic significance and require no specific therapy.

## REFERENCES

1. Dvorak HF, Dvorak AM, Manseau EJ, et al: Fibrin gel investment associated with line 1 and line 10 solid tumor growth angiogenesis, and fibroplasia in guinea pigs. Role of cellular immunity, myofibroblasts, microvascular damage and infarction in line 1 tumor regression. J Natl Can Inst 62:1459–1472, 1979
2. Dvorak HF, Orenstein NS, Carvalho AC, et al: Induction of a fibrin-gel investment: An early event in line 10 hepatocarcinoma growth mediated by tumor-secreted products. J Immunol 122:166–174, 1979
3. Chen LB, Gallimore PH, McDougall JK: Correlation between tumor induction and the large external transformation sensitive protein on the cell surface. Proc Natl Acad Sci USA 73:3570–3574, 1976
4. Peterson H-I: Fibrinolysis and antifibrinolytic drugs in the growth and spread of tumors. Cancer Treat Rev 1:213–217, 1977
5. Santoro MG, Philpott GW, Jaffe BM: Inhibition of tumor growth in vivo and in vitro by prostaglandin E. Nature 263:777–779, 1976
6. Ross R, Voge A: The platelet derived growth factor: Review. Cell 14:203–210, 1978
7. Warren BA: Cancer cell endothelial reactions: The microinjury hypothesis and localized thromboses in the formation of micrometastases, in Donati MG, Davidson JF, Garattini S (eds): Malignancy and the Hemostatic System. New York, Raven Press, 1981, pp 5–26.
8. Zacharski LR, Henderson WG, Rickles FJ, et al: Effect of warfarin on survival in small cell carcinoma of the lung. JAMA 245:831–835, 1981
9. Thornes RD: Oral anticoagulant therapy of human cancer. J Med 5:83–91, 1974
10. Trousseau A: Phlegmassia alba dolens. Clinique médicale de l'Hotel-Dieu de Paris, Vol. 3. London, New Sydenham Society, 1865, p 94
11. Sack GH, Levin J, Bell WR: Trousseau's syndrome and other manifestations of chronic disseminiated coagulopathy in patients with neoplasms: Clinical, pathophysiologic, and therapeutic features. Medicine (Balt) 56:1–37, 1977
12. Miller SP, Sanchez-Avalos J, Stefanski T, et al: Coagulation disorders in cancer. I. Clinical and laboratory studies. Cancer 20:1452–1465, 1967
13. Hagedorn AB, Bowie EJW, Eleback LR, et al: Coagulation abnormalities in patients with inoperable lung cancer. Mayo Clin Proc 49:647–653, 1974

14. Slichter SJ, Harker LA: Hemostasis in malignancy. Ann NY Acad Sci 230:252–261, 1974
15. Peuscher FW, Cleton FJ, Armstrong L, et al: Significance of plasma fibrinopeptide A (fpA) in patients with malignancy. J Lab Clin Med 96:5–14, 1980
16. Sun NCJ, McAfee WM, Hum GJ, et al: Hemostatic abnormalities in malignancy, a prospective study of one hundred eight patients. Am J Clin Pathol 71:10–16, 1979
17. Egbring, R, Schmidt W, Fuchs G, et al: Demonstration of granulocytic protease in plasma of patients with acute leukemia and septicemia with coagulation defects. Blood 49:219–231, 1977
18. Pineo GF, Brain MC, Gallus AS, et al: Tumors, mucus production, and hypercoaguability. Ann NY Acad Sci 230:262–270, 1974
19. Svanberg L: Thromboplastic activity of human ovarian tumors. Thromb Res 6:307–313, 1975
20. Gasic GJ, Catalfamo JL, Gasic TB, et al: In vitro mechanism of platelet aggregation by purified plasma membrane vesicles shed by mouse 15091A tumor. Thromb Res 6:27–36, 1981
21. Edgington TS: Activation of the coagulation system in association with neoplasia. J Lab Clin Med 96:1–4, 1980
22. Collins RC, Al-Mondhiry H, Chernik NL, et al: Neurologic manifestations of intravascular coagulation in cancer: A clinicopathologic analysis of 12 cases. Neurology 25:795–806, 1975
23. Gralnick HR, Bagley J, Abrell E: Heparin treatment for the hemorrhagic diathesis of acute promyelocytic leukemia. Am J Med 52:167–174, 1972
24. Drapkin RL, Gees TS, Dowling MD, et al: Prophylactic heparin therapy in acute promyelocytic leukemia. Cancer 41:2484–2490, 1978
25. Lisiewicz J: Mechanisms of hemorrhage in leukemias. Semin Thromb Hemostas 4:241–267, 1978
26. Daly PA, Schiffer CA, Wiernik PH: Acute promyelocytic leukemia—clinical management of 15 patients. Am J Hematol 8:347–359, 1980
27. Acquired coagulation disorders, in Wintrobe MW, Lee GR, Boggs DR, et al (eds): Clinical Hematology, Philadelphia, Lea & Febiger, 1981, pp 1206–1246
28. Green D, Seeler RA, Allen NA, et al: The role of heparin in the management of consumption coagulopathy. Med Clin North Am 56:193–200, 1972
29. Colman RW, Robboy SJ, Minna JD: Disseminated intravascular coagulation. A reappraisal. Ann Rev Med 30:359–374, 1979
30. Bick RL: Alterations of hemostasis associated with malignancy: Etiology, pathophysiology, diagnosis and management. Semin Throm Hemostas 5:1–26, 1978
31. Bick RL, Schmalhorst WR, Fekete L: Disseminated intravascular coagulation and blood component therapy. Transfusion 16:361–365, 1976
32. Babcock RB, Dumper CW, Sharfman WB: Heparin-induced immune thrombocytopenia. N Eng J Med 295:237–241, 1976
33. Soong BC-F, Miller SP: Coagulation disorders in cancer: Fibrinolysis and inhibitors. Cancer 25:867–74, 1970
34. Ratnoff OD: The haemostatic defects of liver disease, in Ogston D, Bennett B (eds): Haemostasis: Biochemistry, Pathology, Physiology. New York, Wiley, 1977, p 446
35. Perkins HA, MacKenzie MR, Fudenburg HA: Hemostatic defects in dysproteinemias. Blood 35:659–707, 1970
36. Lackner H: Hemostatic abnormalities associated with dysproteinemias. Semin Hematol 10:125–133, 1973
37. Valentin IR, Rimon A, Lahav M: Inhibition of blood coagulation factor XI-XII by monoclonal IgM. Isr J Med Sci 11:1392–1396, 1975
38. Niléhn J-E, Nilsson IM: Coagulation studies in different types of myeloma. Acta Med Scand Suppl 445:194–199, 1966
39. Cooper MR, Cohen HJ, Huntley CC, et al: A monoclonal IgM with antibody-like specificities for phospholipids in a patient with lymphoma. Blood 43:493–504, 1974
40. Goldsmith GH, Saito H, Muir WA: Labile anticoagulant in a patient with lymphoma. Am J Hematol 10:305–311, 1981

41. Thiagarajan P, DeMarioh M, Shapiro SS: A monoclonal IgM coagulation inhibitor with immunologic specificity toward phospholipid. Blood 54:306a, 1979 (abstract)

42. Glueck HI, Wayne L, goldsmith R: Abnormal calcium binding association with hyperglobulinemia, clotting defects, and osteoporosis. J Lab Clin Med 59:40–64, 1962

43. Brady JI, Haidar AB, Rossman RE: A hemorrhagic syndrome in Waldenström's macroglobulinemia secondary to immunoadsorption of Factor VIII. N Engl J Med 300:408–410, 1979

44. Schleider MA, Nachman RL, Jaffe EA, et al: A clinical study of the lupus anticoagulant. Blood 48:499–509, 1976

45. Yang HC, Kuzur M: Procoagulant specificity of factor VIII inhibitor. Br J Haematol 37:429–433, 1977

46. Mueh JR, Herbst KD, Rapaport SI: Thrombosis in patients with the lupus anticoagulant. Ann Intern Med 92:156–159, 1980

47. Criel A, Collen D, Masson PL: A case of IgM antibodies which inhibit the contact activation of blood coagulation. Thromb Res 12:883–892, 1978

48. Ratnoff OD: Personal communication

49. Campbell EB, Sanal S, Mattson J, et al: Factor VII inhibitor. Am J Med 68:962–964, 1980

50. Khoory MS, Nesheim ME, Bowie EJW, et al: Circulating heparan sulfate proteoglycan anticoagulant from a patient with a plasma cell disorder. J Clin Invest 65:666–674, 1980

51. Margolius A, Jackson DP, Ratnoff OD: Circulating anticoagulants: A study of 40 cases and a review of the literature. Medicine (Balt) 40:145–202, 1961

52. McGrath K, Koutts J: A case of Hageman factor deficiency with myeloid leukemia. Aust NZ J Med 5:155–157, 1975

53. Rasche H, Dietrich M, Gaus W, et al: Factor XIII-activity and fibrin subunit structure in acute leukemia. Biomed 21:61–66, 1974

54. Hasegawa DK, Bennett AJ, Coccia PF, et al: Factor V deficiency in Philadelphia-positive chronic myelogenous leukemia. Blood 56:585–595, 1980

55. Wasserman LR, Gilbert HS: Surgical bleeding in polycythemia vera. Ann NY Acad Sci 115:122–138, 1964

56. Phillips JD, O'Shea MJ: A new coagulation defect associated with a case of melanomatosis. J Clin Pathol 30:547–550, 1977

57. Wautier JL, Levy-Toledano S, Caen JP: Acquired von Willebrand's syndrome and thrombopathy in a patient with chronic lymphocytic leukemia. Scand J Haematol 16:128–134, 1976

58. Noronha PA, Hruby MA, Maurer HS: Acquired von Willebrand's disease in a patient with Wilms' tumor. J Pediatr 95:997–999, 1979

59. Joist JH, Cowan JF, Zimmerman TS: Acquired von Willebrand's disease. Evidence for a qualitative and quantitative disorder. N Engl J Med 298:988–991, 1978

59a. Greipp PR, Kyle RA, Bowie EJW: Factor X deficiency in amyloidosis: a critical review. Am J Hematol 11:443–450, 1981

60. Sugai S: Iga pyroglobulin, hyperviscosity syndrome, and coagulation abnormality in a patient with multiple myeloma. Blood 39:224–237, 1972

61. Howell M: Acquired factor X deficiency associated with systematized amyloidosis—a report of a case. Blood 21:739–744, 1963

62. McPherson RA, Onstad JW, Ugorets RJ, et al: Coagulopathy in amyloidosis: Combined deficiency of factors IX and X. Am J Hematol 3:225–235, 1977

63. Furie B, Voo L, McAdam KPWJ, et al: Mechanism of factor X deficiency in systemic amyloidosis. N Engl J Med 304:827–830, 1981

63a. Greipp PR, Kyle RA, Bowie EJW: Factor X deficiency in primary amyloidosis. Resolution after splenectomy. N Engl J Med 301:1050–1051, 1979

64. Gilbert HS, Wasserman LR: Hemorrhage in surgery in myelofibrosis, multiple myeloma, leukemia, and lymphomas. Ann NY Acad Sci 115:169–178, 1964

65. Ogston D, Dawson AA: The fibrinolytic enzyme system in malignant lymphomas. Acta Haematol 49:89–95, 1973

66. Brodsky I, Kahn SB, Vash G, et al: Fibrinogen survival with ($^{75}$Se) selenomethionine during L-asparaginase therapy. Br J Haematol 20:477–487, 1971

67. Capizzi RL, Bertino JR, Skeel RT: L-Asparaginase: Clinical, biochemical, pharmacological, and immunological studies. Ann Intern Med 74:893–901, 1971

68. Ramsay NKC, Coccia PF, Krivit W, et al: The effect of L-asparaginase on plasma coagulation factors in acute lymphoblastic leukemia. Cancer 40:1398–1401, 1977

69. Monto RW, Talley RW, Caldwell MJ, et al: Observations on the mechanisms of hemorrhagic toxicity in mithramycin therapy. Cancer Res 29:697–704, 1969

70. Olson RE: Vitamin K-induced prothrombin formation: Antagonism by actinomycin D. Science 145:926–928, 1964

71. Gardner FH: Platelet transfusion, in Baldini MG, Elbe S, (eds): Platelets: Production, Function, Transfusion and Storage. New York, Grune & Stratton, 1974, pp 393–405

72. Ebbe S, Wittels B, Dameshak W: Autoimmune thrombocytopenic purpura with chronic lymphocytic leukemia. Blood 19:23–37, 1962

73. Hassidim K, McMillan R, Conjalka MS, et al: Immune thrombocytopenic purpura in Hodgkin disease. Am J Hematol 6:149–153, 1979

74. Waddell CC, Cimo PL: Idiopathic thrombocytopenic purpura occurring in Hodgkin disease after splenectomy: Report of two cases and review of the literature. Am J Hematol 7:381–387, 1979

75. Doan CA, Bouroncle BA, Wiseman BK: Idiopathic and secondary thrombocytopenic purpura: Clinical study and evaluation of 381 cases over a period of 28 years. Ann Intern Med 53:861–876, 1960

76. Kim HD, Boggs DR: A syndrome resembling idiopathic thrombocytopenic purpura in 10 patients with diverse forms of cancer. Am J Med 67:371–377, 1979

77. Brook J, Konwaler BE: Thrombotic thrombocytopenic purpura. Association with metastatic gastric carcinoma and a possible autoimmune disorder. Calif Med 102:222–227, 1965

78. Rodríguez-Erdmann F, Button L, Murray JE, et al: Kasabach-Merritt syndrome: Coaguloanalytical observations. Am J Med Sci 261:9–15, 1971

79. McClure PD, Ingram GIC, Stacey RS, et al: Platelet function tests in thrombocythemia and thrombocytosis. Br J Haematol 12:478–498, 1966

80. Kaywin P, McDonough M, Insel PA, et al: Platelet function in essential thrombocythemia. N Engl J Med 299:505–509, 1978

81. Levin J, Conley CL: Thrombocytosis associated with malignant disease. Arch Intern Med 114:497–500, 1964

82. Cortellazzo S, Colucci M, Barbui T, et al: Reduced platelet factor X activating activity: A possible contribution to bleeding complications in polycythemia vera and essential thrombocythemia. Haemostasis 10:37–50, 1981

83. Pachter MR, Johnson SA, Neblett TR, et al: Bleeding, platelets and macroglobulinemia. Am J Clin Pathol 31:467–482, 1959

84. Ahr DJ, Scialla SJ, Kimball DB Jr: Acquired platelet dysfunction following mithramycin therapy. Cancer 41:448–454, 1978

85. Reynolds WA, Winkelmann RK, Soule EH: Kaposi's sarcoma. A clinicopathologic study with particular reference to its relationship to the reticuloendothelial system. Medicine 44:419–443, 1965

86. Smith WT, Whitefield AGN: Intravascular micro-embolic carcinomatosis as a cause of purpura. Report of a case associated with focal histologic lesions in the nervous system. Br J Cancer 8:97–106, 1954

87. Schuster S, Scarborough H: Senile purpura. Q J Med 30:33–40, 1961

Jack Levin

# 11

## Bleeding with Infectious Diseases

Hemorrhage can occur whenever any of the components that contribute to normal hemostasis are sufficiently compromised. Accordingly, deficient or defective platelets, abnormalities of blood vessels, or defective blood coagulation can result in inadequate hemostasis. Whether clinically significant bleeding then occurs depends upon a variety of factors, including the general status of the patient, the presence and nature of underlying diseases, administration of certain drugs, and localized anatomic conditions. Since many infectious disorders produce or are associated with abnormalities of the hemostatic mechanism(s), patients with infections have an increased susceptibility to experience abnormal bleeding.

### THROMBOCYTOPENIA

In almost all studies, thrombocytopenia has been defined as a platelet count of less than 150,000/μl (150 × 10$^9$/liter). An analysis of 11 studies (which included 1074 patients) in which data were available indicates that approximately 62 percent of patients with severe bacterial infections (most of whom had documented septicemia) were thrombocytopenic[1-11] (Table 11-1). Some of the thrombocytopenic patients had other laboratory data suggestive of disseminated intravascular coagulopathy (DIC), which will be discussed later in this chapter. Although, for obvious reasons, thrombocytopenia has received more attention, it is important to realize that infection may also cause thrombocytosis.[8,12-14] Thrombocytosis is common during pulmonary infections caused by bacteria, and usually does not disappear until the infectious process has resolved.

Thrombocytopenia associated with infections has some important clinical features. Both gram-negative and gram-positive infections are associated with thrombocytopenia (Table 11-2).[1,3,6,8,15] In most instances, the degree of thrombocytopenia is not severe. Corrigan[3] and Riedler et al.[6] reported that approximately 60–65 percent of patients who had thrombocytopenia secondary to infection had platelet counts of greater than 50,000/μl. Since this level of circulating platelets is almost always sufficient to provide adequate hemostasis in the absence of other abnormalities, this accounts for the relative rarity of hemorrhage in patients who become thrombocytopenic as the result of infection. Oppenheimer et al.[4] and Goldenfarb et al.[8] have stressed the absence of generalized bleeding in their

The preparation of this chapter was supported in part by the Veterans Administration.

**Table 11-1**

Frequency of Thrombocytopenia Associated
with Severe Bacterial Infection

| Reference | Total No. of Cases | Thrombocytopenia (%) |
|---|---|---|
| Emerson et al.[1] | 61 | 33 |
| Neame et al.[2] | 31 | 74 |
| Corrigan[3] | 46 | 65 |
| Oppenheimer et al.[4] | 28 | 93 |
| Corrigan et al.[5] | 36 | 61 |
| Riedler et al.[6] | 141 | 77 |
| Kelton et al.[7] | 44 | 46 |
| Goldenfarb et al.[8] | 34 | 35 |
| Milligan et al.[9] | 21 | 86 |
| Kreger et al.[10] | 612 | 56 |
| Cohen and Gardner[11] | 20 | 55 |

patients, even in association with surgery. In the report of Emerson et al, only four of 20 patients bled, and all had underlying diseases that had produced thrombocytopenia prior to the development of sepsis.[1] Only 10 percent of 21 patients who had thrombocytopenia in association with sepsis and hypotension died secondary to hemorrhage.[9] In the large series of patients with gram-negative sepsis studied by Kreger et al, only 16 of the 222 patients in whom tests of platelets and blood coagulation were performed had clinical indications for evaluation of hemostasis.[10] Overall, only 3 percent of their total group of 612 patients bled. A survey of over 7000 hospitalized patients revealed that 393 had platelet counts of less than 150,000/μl. Approximately 15 percent of patients with thrombocytopenia had infectious disorders.[15]

Since thrombocytopenia is apparently the most common effect of infection on hemostasis, a more detailed consideration of some of the mechanisms by which this occurs is warranted. Thrombocytopenia associated with bacteremia or viremia may be produced by a variety of potential mechanisms (Table 11-3). Infection may result in suppression of thrombopoiesis. Increased platelet destruction can occur during DIC or as the result of altered reticuloendothelial function. Splenomegaly may be associated with increased sequestration and decreased platelet viability. Bacterial or viral particles may damage endothelium, with resultant adhesion of platelets. Infectious particles or their components

**Table 11-2**

Some Infectious Diseases Associated with Thrombocytopenia

| | |
|---|---|
| Viral | Rubella, infectious mononucleosis, mumps, rubeola, cytomegalovirus infection, dengue, epidemic hemorrhagic fevers, hepatitis, herpes simplex, influenza, cat scratch fever,* Colorado tick fever, vaccinia, measles vaccine |
| Chlamydial | Psittacosis |
| Rickettsial | Rocky Mountain spotted fever, typhus |
| Bacterial | Sepsis due to gram-negative or gram-positive organisms, brucellosis, typhoid fever, diphtheria, scarlet fever, tuberculosis, subacute bacterial endocarditis |
| Spirochetal | Congenital syphilis |
| Mycotic | Histoplasmosis |
| Protozoan | Malaria, trypanosomiasis, kala-azar |

*Etiology disputed.

**Table 11-3**
Potential Mechanisms That Produce
Thrombocytopenia During Infection*

Bone marrow suppression
Increased platelet destruction
Endothelial damage
Direct bacterial (or viral) damage
Immune mechanisms

*Thrombocytopenia produced by infection has been re-
viewed recently.[16]

(i.e., bacterial endotoxins) may directly damage platelets, with a secondary decrease in viability and a more rapid loss from the circulation. Phagocytosis of bacteria by platelets may also potentially result in rapid disappearance of platelets from the circulation.

It is likely that in some instances, thrombocytopenia is produced by suppression of hematopoietic function, since it has been shown that infection can suppress erythropoiesis. However, few clinical data are available to document this effect. Megakaryocytes remain present in the bone marrow of infected patients, but careful quantification and evaluation of platelet production by megakaryocytes have not been adequately performed. Oski and Naiman have reported that following the administration of live measles vaccine, 86 percent of recipients developed modest thrombocytopenia, and the nadir occurred approximately 4–6 days after administration of the vaccine.[17] In three patients, the number of recognizable megakaryocytes was apparently reduced. Platelet counts returned to normal by the 21st day.

Studies of Newcastle disease virus (NDV) have indicated that the virus can become adsorbed to bone marrow cells, including megakaryocytes, and immunologic studies have indicated that viral particles subsequently appear in the cytoplasm of megakaryocytes.[18] The authors claimed that the presence of viral particles in megakaryocytes was associated with decreased maturation and thrombopoietic activity of the infected cells. Murine cytomegalovirus infection has been shown to produce gradual development of thrombocytopenia, with evidence of histologic changes and vacuolization of megakaryocytes.[19] These reports suggest that some types of viral infection can produce thrombocytopenia, at least in part, as the result of direct suppressive effects on megakaryocytes. However, much more information is required to establish that bacterial infections produce significant thrombocytopenia as the result of suppression of platelet production.

At least some episodes of thrombocytopenia caused by infection are associated with laboratory, if not clinical, evidence of DIC. In some studies, patients with reduced platelet counts also had abnormal tests of blood coagulation, such as prolonged prothrombin and partial thromboplastin times, reduced plasma fibrinogen, and elevated fibrinogen-fibrin degradation products (FDP-fdp).[2,3,4,5,8–10] The complexity of the relationship between DIC and thrombocytopenia is indicated by the lack of agreement as to whether DIC is[2,9] or is not[6,8] correlated with the degree of thrombocytopenia. The absence of hypofibrinogenemia in some patients suspected of having DIC is probably due to the stimulation of fibrinogen production that occurs as the result of infection or inflammation. Harker and Slichter have reported an increase in turnover of both platelets and fibrinogen in bacteremic patients who were thrombocytopenic but not hypofibrinogenemic.[20] In any case, there is agreement that in patients with infectious disease, significant clinical bleeding due to DIC is rare, even in the presence of thrombocytopenia.[1,8–10]

Increased platelet destruction can occur in the absence of DIC or immunologic mechanisms. Alteration of the status of thé reticuloendothelial system by infection may result in more rapid clearance of platelets that normally would continue to circulate. Splenomegaly may lead to sequestration and thrombocytopenia, even in the presence of increased platelet production. Direct interactions between bacteria or viruses and platelets can alter and damage platelets, with resultant increased rates of disappearance of platelets from the circulation. Following interaction of human platelets with bacteria, polymorphonuclear leukocytes have been shown to attach to aggregates of platelets, and to phagocytize the bacteria and occasionally also platelets.[21] Human blood platelets are capable of phagocytizing influenza virus[22] and perhaps under certain circumstances can phagocytize bacteria[23] as well. Clawson et al. have shown that *Staphylococcus* can stimulate human platelets to undergo the release reaction.[24] Recent studies by Hawiger et al. have demonstrated that staphylococci possess a receptor for the Fc fragment of immunoglobulin G (IgG), which provides a mechanism for the aggregation of human platelets by forming a complex composed of bacteria, IgG, and platelets.[25] Complement is not required.

Purified vaccinia virus is capable of binding to human platelets and causing release of serotonin.[26] Furthermore, the virus inhibits platelet aggregation, demonstrating that this virus alters platelet function. In contrast to vaccinia, which lacks neuraminidase, NDV, which contains neuraminidase activity, causes platelets to lose sialic acid.[27] Following exposure to NDV, platelet survival and responsiveness to thrombin and other aggregating agents were reduced.[27]

Collectively, these and other observations indicate that both bacteria and viruses are capable of interacting with platelets. Depending upon the nature of the infectious particles and other poorly understood variables, this interaction can produce platelet aggregation, release of platelet constituents, phagocytosis of the infectious agent, and ultimately a shortened platelet life span. However, the release reaction is not necessarily associated with loss of platelet viability. Under certain circumstances, it is possible that qualitatively altered platelets will continue to circulate. These possible effects and the predominance of a particular response that may result from the characteristics of a specific infectious particle provide a series of mechanisms by which infection can produce thrombocytopenia, bleeding due to qualitative platelet deficiencies, or platelet thrombi. Interactions between platelets and viruses or bacteria may provide a basis for the removal of infectious agents from the circulation.

## Bacterial Endotoxin

Gram-negative sepsis is commonly associated with thrombocytopenia. A unique characteristic of gram-negative bacteria is the presence of bacterial endotoxin (bacterial lipopolysaccharide, LPS) in their cell walls. Furthermore, LPS has been shown to have a wide variety of biological effects, including pyrogenicity, lethality, hypotension, and activation of the blood coagulation, kallikrein, and complement systems. Therefore, the effects of LPS on platelets have been of considerable interest. Human platelets have high-affinity binding sites for LPS.[28] The receptors appear to be phospholipids. MacIntyre et al. have shown that LPS aggregates rabbit and rat, but not pig or human platelets. Concentrations as high as 1 mg/ml were ineffective in causing aggregation of human platelets.[29] Complement was required for the aggregation of rat and rabbit platelets. Additional studies with rabbit platelets revealed that binding of LPS altered platelet surface proteins and increased the accessibility of possibly 3 surface proteins.[30]

These investigations and other studies which have demonstrated that the administration of LPS can produce thrombocytopenia suggest mechanisms by which gram-negative bacteria produce thrombocytopenia and trigger DIC in humans. In particular, alteration of platelet membranes might increase the availability of platelet factor 3 (PF3) and trigger the activation of intravascular coagulation. However, this hypothesis has not been fully established. Experimental in vitro models have demonstrated that human platelets are relatively resistant to the effects of LPS. Furthermore, concentrations required in vitro for human platelet activation have been 5–10 times greater than those required to produce pathophysiologic effects in vivo. The latter is particularly important since preparations of LPS are actually particulate suspensions,[29,31] and some of the results may be nonspecific. Finally, gram-positive organisms, which lack bacterial endotoxin, are also capable of producing thrombocytopenia and DIC. Accordingly, there must be mechanisms independent of bacterial LPS.

## Immunologic Mechanisms

Immunologic mechanisms are likely to play a role in the production of thrombocytopenia in at least some bacterial and viral infections. Antibodies directed against bacteria or viruses that have adhered to platelets may indirectly result in platelet destruction. Alteration of the surface characteristics of platelets by infectious particles may provide the basis for the production of autoantibodies. However, circulating immune complexes (CIC) have received much attention as a cause of thrombocytopenia in infectious diseases. Human platelets have been shown to possess an Fc receptor which can bind the Fc portion of CIC.[32] Complement is not required for this interaction. Human platelets have been shown, in vitro, to bind either DNA or DNA–anti-DNA complexes.[33]

Myllyla et al. apparently demonstrated that following the period of viremia, sera from patients recovering from rubella contained an immunoglobulin that, in combination with small, soluble antigens prepared from the virus, produced platelet aggregation.[34] Antibody titers were higher in patients with thrombocytopenia. Not only do the data confirm those of Hawiger et al.,[25] but complexes do not have to be immunologically related to platelets in order to bind.

Of newborns, 82 percent with severe viral or bacterial infections had increased levels of platelet-associated IgG.[35] DIC was not present. In another study, 73 percent of 44 patients with gram-negative or gram-positive sepsis and thrombocytopenia had elevated levels of platelet IgG.[7] Importantly, platelet IgG was increased only rarely in nonthrombocytopenic patients with sepsis.[7] Pertinently, some thrombocytopenic patients had CIC. Some studies, however, cast doubt on the significance of elevated platelet IgG in the pathogenesis of thrombocytopenia.[36] Thrombocytopenic purpura during infectious mononucleosis may be due to any of the mechanisms by which viruses produce thrombocytopenia, but an immunologic mechanism seems likely.[37]

Immunologic thrombocytopenic purpura (ITP) is often described an an autoimmune disease. However, many studies have demonstrated the presence of CIC in the blood of patients with ITP. Wautier et al. detected CIC in the plasma of approximately 40 percent of 36 patients with ITP using two different techniques.[38] In another study, over 80 percent of 72 patients with ITP were demonstrated to have circulating CIC.[39] Importantly, 74 percent of the CIC contained viral antigens, although there had been no history indicative of a preceding viral illness. Therefore, many cases of ITP may not represent autoimmune disease, but rather a prolonged sequela of subclinical (or clinical) viral infection. It has long been recognized that viral disease in children may be followed by a period of thrombocytopenic purpura. Trent et al. have detected CIC in the sera of 43 patients with chronic ITP, and the titer was inversely related to the platelet count.[40] Those workers suggested the possibility that platelets clear CIC. Unexplained was the presence of CIC in the sera of patients with nonimmune disorders. These data, in conjunction with the studies of Kelton et al., which demonstrated increased levels of platelet-associated IgG in patients with presumably non-immune disorders,[36] indicate that the signifance of elevated levels of platelet-associated IgG remains unclear, but that CIC may be an important cause of chronic thrombocytopenia. The relative and absolute concentrations of circulating antigens and antibodies and the physical characteristics of the circulating antigens may determine whether patients develop thrombocytopenia or vasculitis in many infectious diseases of bacterial, viral, or parasitic origin.[41,42]

## Rubella

An epidemic of rubella in the United States in 1964 provided an opportunity to evaluate the relationship between an acute viral infection and subsequent thrombocytopenia (which, in the absence of a recognized preceding viral illness, would have been designated as ITP). Examination of the bone marrow demonstrated that megakaryocytes were present.[43] The interval between onset of the rubella rash and acute purpura was approximately 4 days, and thrombocytopenia persisted for approximately 12 days.[43] Responses to platelet trans-fusions were compatible with increased peripheral destruction of circulating platelets. In other studies, approximately 45 percent of 38 cases of congenital rubella syndrome were thrombocytopenic.[44,45] Thrombocytopenia, which was present at birth, disappeared in 2 weeks, and platelet levels usually returned to normal within one month.[45] Interestingly, the patients were not anemic or leukopenic, and clinically significant bleeding did not occur in one series.[45] Megakaryocytes were markedly reduced or absent in this syndrome, suggesting that in contrast to the cause of thrombocytopenia in children with rubella, the congenital rubella syndrome was associated with decreased production of platelets. However, the study of Bayer et al. failed to detect thrombocytopenia in 11 purpuric newborn infants with congenital rubella.[46] The reason for this disparate finding is unclear, particularly since bleeding times were described as normal in these purpuric neonates. The authors suggested that purpura was due to viral-induced vascular damage.[46]

## DISSEMINATED INTRAVASCULAR COAGULOPATHY

As indicated above, laboratory evidence of DIC is much less common than thrombo-cytopenia in patients with severe infections. DIC has been fully discussed in Chapter 8, and therefore no attempt will be made to consider critically the basis for the laboratory diagnosis here. Infectious disorders associated with DIC have been reviewed.[47] A wide variety of viral diseases have been suggested to produce DIC and hemorrhagic manifesta-tions.[48] In addition to the many bacterial and viral disorders that have been associated with DIC, many parasitic infections have also been reported to produce this condition. Table 11-4 provides selected examples of parasitic, rickettsial, and viral diseases which apparently have caused DIC. However, it is important to emphasize that other studies have failed to detect DIC in patients with these infections.[56–59] Furthermore, in many instances, evidence of DIC has been limited to laboratory abnormalities and has not been associated with clinically significant bleeding. Vascular injury produced by sepsis may provide a mechanism for initiation of DIC by activation of factor XII (Hageman factor), and DIC,

**Table 11-4**
Examples of Viral, Rickettsial, and
Parasitic Diseases Reported to Produce
Disseminated Intravascular Coagulopathy

Dengue hemorrhagic fever [49-50]
Scrub typhus [51]
Malaria [52,53]
Influenza [54]
Trypanosomiasis [55]

once initiated, may be potentiated by the failure of a defective reticuloendothelial system to remove activated blood coagulation factors.[60] Bacterial endotoxin is also capable of directly activating factor XII. However, it is important to note that septic patients may have conditions other than DIC which are responsible for prolongation of the prothrombin and partial thromboplastin times and elevation of fibrinogen-related antigens, including FDP-fdp. For example, Goldenfarb et al. observed that 75 percent of patients with bacterial sepsis and elevated FDP-fdp did not have either hypofibrinogenemia or thrombocytopenia.[8] It does not appear that the severity of thrombocytopenia can be used as an indicator of DIC when sepsis is present, since there is disagreement about whether patients with DIC have lower platelet levels than those who do not.[2,6,8,9]

Regardless of the criteria utilized for the laboratory diagnosis of DIC in infected patients, and despite factors which may mask detection of abnormalities of blood coagulation, an analysis of studies with available data indicates that regardless of the presence of DIC in patients who have thrombocytopenia in association with sepsis, clinically significant hemorrhage (i.e., generalized bleeding in addition to cutaneous purpura) is rare. Only 7–10 percent of patients with sepsis and thrombocytopenia (with or without DIC) were described as having generalized hemorrhage,[1,8-10] and one study of 28 patients reported that none of the patients bled, although 30 percent had abnormalities in tests of blood coagulation and 93 percent were thrombocytopenic.[4] The only patients in the series of Emerson et al. who bled had thrombocytopenia which preceded the episodes of sepsis.[1] In a group of 612 patients with gram-negative sepsis, only 4 patients with DIC bled.[10] Overall, in that study there was no correlation between laboratory data compatible with DIC and clinical outcome. These authors' observations confirm the data of Corrigan and Jordan, which indicate that although heparin therapy can improve laboratory abnormalities in patients with DIC, there is no effect on the clinical outcome or mortality.[61]

Another view of the frequency and clinical significance of DIC in patients with sepsis can be gained from reports of collected series of patients with DIC. However, the data are obviously influenced by the manner in which patients were identified and the nature of the population in which the episodes of DIC occurred. In a series from Israel, 40 percent of patients with DIC were infected with gram-negative or gram-positive organisms.[62] Although clinically significant bleeding was described as occurring in 72 percent of patients with DIC and infection, it was unclear what proportion of the group had only cutaneous bleeding. Pertinently, liver and renal dysfunction were particularly common in infected patients and could have contributed to any hemorrhagic diathesis.

In another study, 346 persons were diagnosed as having DIC on the basis of at least 3 abnormal tests[63]; 26 percent had infections, and 54 percent of this group had sepsis. Overall, 77 percent had hemorrhagic manifestations, but the exact frequency of clinically significant hemorrhage in infected patients was not provided. Mortality was not significantly increased by the presence of clinical bleeding.[63] Although hemostasis was described as abnormal in a study of 56 cases of typhoid fever, 61 percent of patients with hemorrhage had gastrointestinal bleeding, which may have been directly due to the anatomic lesions produced by this infection.[64] Furthermore, laboratory abnormalities were minimal and unlikely to account for bleeding.

### Purpura Fulminans

Purpura fulminans is characterized by hemorrhagic ischemic necrosis, with marked cutaneous manifestations and often peripheral gangrene (Chapter 8). The lesions are usually symmetrical. Vascular occlusions may also occur in other organs. Historically, streptococcal infection has been associated with this severe thrombohemorrhagic complication of infection,[47] but it has also been reported in association with varicella.[47,48] It is considered to be an extreme form of DIC.

### White Blood Cells and DIC

Another mechanism by which DIC may be triggered by infection involves the generation of procoagulant activity by leukocytes. Bacterial endotoxins have been demonstrated to stimulate human mononuclear cells to generate procoagulant activity, designated tissue factor, both in vivo[65,66] and in vitro.[67,68] Furthermore, it appears that the lipid A portion of the bacterial endotoxin molecule is responsible for this effect of LPS.[69,70] This is an important observation because it has been demonstrated that lipid A is responsible for other biological effects of LPS. Interestingly, the generation of leukocyte procoagulant activity by endotoxin is enhanced in the presence of platelets, which are believed to provide a membrane lipoprotein surface for the interaction between lipid A and leukocytes.[71] The potential importance of this mechanism is suggested by observations that DIC can be produced in rabbits by the infusion of leukocyte procoagulant activity[72] and that the generalized Shwartzman reaction (an experimental model for intravascular coagulation) is inhibited by the prior production of leukopenia. The demonstration by Egbring et al. that the plasma of patients with sepsis and coagulation abnormalities contains granulocytic proteases provides another indication that white blood cells may play a role in the development of the altered coagulation that is observed in septic patients.[73]

## NONTHROMBOCYTOPENIC PURPURA

This form of vascular damage is due to the production of an aseptic vasculitis and occurs rarely during an infectious process or after administration of a drug. Nonthrombocytopenic purpura, in association with infection or drugs, appears to be mediated by deposition of immune complexes in the walls of the affected blood vessels.[74] It is characterized by often palpable, purpuric lesions of the extremities, with a remarkably symmetrical distribution. In contrast to the lesions of thrombocytopenic purpura, the cutaneous lesions of nonthrombocytopenic purpura often cause a feeling of vague discomfort or itching. In some instances, the gastrointestinal tract has been involved (Henoch-Schönlein purpura). This form is more common in children than adults.[75] A causal relationship between the Henoch-Schönlein syndrome and streptococcal infection has not been established. Nonthrombocytopenic purpura is easily distinguished from thrombocytopenic purpura by the nature of the cutaneous lesions and the presence of normal levels of circulating platelets.

## THERAPEUTIC CONSIDERATIONS

As the literature indicates, resolution of the various hemorrhagic complications of infectious disorders depends primarily on effective therapy and control of the underlying infection. Fortunately, even in the presence of deranged laboratory tests of hemostasis, bleeding in these patients is relatively rare. Thrombocytopenia should be treated as conservatively as possible, since recovery will take place with appropriate treatment of the infection. Platelets should be administered only if there is a specific clinical indication, and not solely because of severe thrombocytopenia in the absence of bleeding. Careful observation of patients with thrombocytopenic purpura is feasible because intracranial bleeding, the major cause of death in thrombocytopenia, usually does not take place until after petechial lesions of both the skin and mucous membranes have developed. Patients without the latter manifestations are unlikely to develop sudden intracranial hemorrhage. Furthermore, since it appears that most episodes of purpura in association with infection are due to peripheral destruction of platelets, platelet transfusions are unlikely to result in prolonged increases in platelet levels.

Most patients with laboratory tests consistent with DIC do not have evidence of significant clinical hemorrhage. Many of the laboratory abnormalities compatible with DIC may be due to other factors in these patients, and some reports indicate little correlation between DIC and outcome. In addition, bleeding, when it occurs, may be due to local factors. Interestingly, intracranial bleeding is a rare complication of DIC. Therefore, since no controlled studies have demonstrated the efficacy of heparin for the treatment of most forms of DIC (purpura fulminans apparently justifies the use of anticoagulants), heparin should be utilized only under rare circumstances, particularly since it may worsen ongoing bleeding without altering the outcome.[63,76]

## REFERENCES

1. Emerson WA, Zieve PD, Krevans JR: Hematologic changes in septicemia. Johns Hopkins Med J 126:69–76, 1970
2. Neame PB, Kelton JG, Walker IR, et al: Thrombocytopenia in septicemia: The role of disseminated intravascular coagulation. Blood 56:88–92, 1980
3. Corrigan JJ: Thrombocytopenia: A laboratory sign of septicemia in infants and children. J Pediatr 85:219–221, 1974
4. Oppenheimer L, Hryniuk WM, Bishop AJ: Thrombocytopenia in severe bacterial infections. J Surg Res 20:211–214, 1976
5. Corrigan JJ, Walker LR, May N: Changes in the blood coagulation system associated with septicemia. N Engl J Med 379:851–856, 1968
6. Riedler GF, Straub PW, Frick PG: Thrombocytopenia in septicemia. A clinical study for the evaluation of its incidence and diagnostic value. Helv Med Acta 36:23–38, 1971
7. Kelton JG, Neame PB, Gauldie J, et al: Elevated platelet-associated IgG in the thrombocytopenia of septicemia. N Engl J Med 300:760–764, 1979
8. Goldenfarb PB, Zucker S, Corrigan JJ Jr, et al: The coagulation mechanism in acute bacterial infection. Br J Haematol 18:643–652, 1970
9. Milligan GF, MacDonald JAE, Mellon A, et al: Pulmonary and hematologic disturbances during septic shock. Surg Gynecol Obstet 138:43–49, 1974
10. Kreger BE, Craven DE, McCabe WR: Gram-negative bacteremia. IV. Reevaluation of clinical features and treatment in 612 patients. Am J Med 68:344–355, 1980

11. Cohen P, Gardner FH: Thrombocytopenia as a laboratory sign and complication of gram-negative bacteremic infection. Arch Intern Med 117:113–124, 1966

12. Levin J, Conley CL: Thrombocytosis associated with malignant disease. Arch Intern Med 114:497–500, 1964

13. Marchasin S, Wallerstein RO, Aggeler PM: Variations of the platelet count in disease. Calif Med 101:95–100, 1964

14. Davis WM, Mendez Ross AO: Thrombocytosis and thrombocythemia: The laboratory and clinical significance of an elevated platelet count. Am J Clin Pathol 59:243–247, 1973

15. Pembrey RG, Handley DA, Kimber RJ: Causes of thrombocytopenia in a hospital population. A six-months survey of 7,750 patients. Med J Aust 1:583–588, 1971

16. Wilson JJ, Neame PB, Kelton JG: Infection-induced thrombocytopenia. Semin Thromb Hemostas 8:217–233, 1982

17. Oski FA, Naiman JL: Effect of live measles vaccine on the platelet count. N Engl J Med 275:352–356, 1966

18. Jerushalmy Z, Kaminski E, Kohn A, et al: Interaction of Newcastle disease virus with megakaryocytes in cell cultures of guinea pig bone marrow. Proc Soc Exp Biol Med 114:687–690, 1963

19. Osborn JE, Shahidi NT: Thrombocytopenia in murine cytomegalovirus infection. J Lab Clin Med 81:53–63, 1973

20. Harker LA, Slichter SJ: Platelet and fibrinogen consumption in man. N Engl J Med 287:999–1005, 1972

21. Smith SB: Platelets in host resistance: In vitro interaction of platelets, bacteria and polymorphonuclear leukocytes. Blut 25:104–107, 1972

22. Danon D, Jerushalmy Z, de Vries A: Incorporation of influenza virus in human blood platelets in vitro. Electron microscopical observation. Virology 9:719–722, 1959

23. Clawson CC: Platelet interaction with bacteria. III. Ultrastructure. Am J Pathol 70:449–471, 1973

24. Clawson CC, Rao GHR, White JG: Platelet interaction with bacteria. IV. Stimulation of the release reaction. Am J Pathol 81:411–419, 1975

25. Hawiger J, Steckley S, Hammond D, et al: Staphylococci-induced human platelet injury mediated by protein A and immunoglobulin G Fc fragment receptor. J Clin Invest 64:931–937, 1979

26. Bik T, Sarov I, Livne A: Interaction between vaccinia virus and human blood platelets. Blood 59:482–487, 1982

27. Scott S, Reimers H-J, Chernesky MA, et al: Effect of viruses on platelet aggregation and platelet survival in rabbits. Blood 52:47–55, 1978

28. Springer GF, Adye JC: Endotoxin-binding substances from human leukocytes and platelets. Infect Immun 12:978–986, 1975

29. MacIntyre DE, Allen AP, Thorne KJI, et al: Endotoxin-induced platelet aggregation and secretion. I. Morphological changes and pharmacological effects. J Cell Sci 28:211–223, 1977

30. Thorne KJI, Oliver RC, MacIntyre DE, et al: Endotoxin-induced platelet aggregation and secretion. II. Changes in plasma membrane proteins. J Cell Sci 28:225–236, 1977

31. Ausprunk DH, Das J: Endotoxin-induced changes in human platelet membranes: Morphologic evidence. Blood 51:487–495, 1978

32. Israels ED, Nisli G, Paraskevas F, et al: Platelet Fc receptor as a mechanism for Ag–Ab complex-induced platelet injury. Thromb Diathes Haemorrh 29:434–444, 1973

33. Clejan L, Menahem H: Binding of deoxyribonucleic acid to the surface of human platelets. Acta Haematol 58:84–88, 1977

34. Myllyla G, Vaheri A, Vesikari T, et al: Interaction between human blood platelets, viruses and antibodies. IV. Post-rubella thrombocytopenic purpura and platelet aggregation by rubella antigen-antibody interaction. Clin Exp Immunol 4:323–332, 1969

35. Tate DY, Carlton GT, Johnson D, et al: Immune thrombocytopenia in severe neonatal infections. J Pediatr 98:449–453, 1981

36. Kelton JG, Powers PJ, Carter CJ: A prospective study of the usefulness of the measurement of platelet-associated IgG for the diagnosis of idiopathic thrombocytopenic purpura. Blood 60:1050–1053, 1982

37. Clarke BF, Davies SH: Severe thrombocytopenia in infectious mononucleosis. Am J Med Sci 248:703–708, 1964

38. Wautier JL, Boizard B, Wautier MP, et al: Platelet-associated IgG and circulating immune complexes in thrombocytopenic purpura. Nouv Rev Fr Hematol 22:29–36, 1980

39. Lurhuma AZ, Riccomi H, Masson PL: The occurrence of circulating immune complexes and viral antigens in idiopathic thrombocytopenic purpura. Clin Exp Immunol 28:49–55, 1977

40. Trent RJ, Clancy RL, Danis V, et al: Immune complexes in thrombocytopenic patients: Cause or effect? Br J Haematol 44:645–654, 1980

41. Christian CL, Sergent JS: Vasculitis syndromes: Clinical and experimental models. Am J Med 61:385–392, 1976

42. Barnett EV, Knutson DW, Abrass CK, et al: Circulating immune complexes: Their immunochemistry, detection, and importance. Ann Intern Med 91:430–440, 1979

43. Morse EE, Zinkham WH, Jackson DP: Thrombocytopenic purpura following rubella infection in children and adults. Arch Intern Med 117:573–579, 1966

44. Plotkin SA, Oski FA, Hartnett EM, et al: Some recently recognized manifestations of the rubella syndrome. J Pediatr 67:182–191, 1965

45. Korones SB, Ainger LE, Monif GRG, et al: Congenital rubella syndrome: New clinical aspects with recovery of virus from affected infants. J Pediatr 67:166–181, 1965

46. Bayer WL, Sherman FE, Michaels RH, et al: Purpura in congenital and acquired rubella. N Engl J Med 273:1362–1366, 1965

47. Yoshikawa T, Tanaka KR, Guze LB: Infection and disseminated intravascular coagulation. Medicine 50:237–258, 1971

48. McKay DG, Margaretten W: Disseminated intravascular coagulation in virus diseases. Arch Intern Med 120:129–152, 1967

49. Srichaikul T, Nimmanitaya S, Artchararit N, et al: Fibrinogen metabolism and disseminated intravascular coagulation in dengue hemorrhagic fever. Am J Trop Med Hyg 26:525–532, 1977

50. Mitrakul C, Poshyachinda M, Futrakul P, et al: Hemostatic and platelet kinetic studies in dengue hemorrhagic fever. Am J Trop Med Hyg 26:975–984, 1977

51. Ognibene AJ, O'Leary DS, Czarnecki SW, et al: Myocarditis and disseminated intravascular coagulation in scrub typhus. Am J Med Sci 262:233–239, 1971

52. Dennis LH, Eichelberger JW, Inman MM, et al: Depletion of coagulaiton factors in drug-resistant Plasmodium falciparum malaria. Blood 29:713–721, 1967

53. Punyagupta S, Srichaikul T, Nitiyanant P, et al: Acute pulmonary insufficiency in falciparum malaria: Summary of 12 cases with evidence of disseminated intravascular coagulation. Am J Trop Med Hyg 23:551–559, 1974

54. Davison AM, Thomson D, Robson JS: Intravascular coagulation complicating influenza A virus infection. Br Med J 1:654–655, 1973

55. Barrett-Connor E, Ugoretz RJ, Braude AI: Disseminated intravascular coagulation in trypanosomiasis. Arch Intern Med 131:574–577, 1973

56. Neva FA, Sheagren JN, Shulman NR, et al: Malaria: Host-defense mechanisms and complications. Ann Intern Med 73:295–306, 1970

57. Nelson ER, Bierman HR, Chulajata R: Hematologic findings in the 1960 hemorrhagic fever epidemic (dengue) in Thailand. Am J Trop Med Hyg 13:642–649, 1964

58. Butler T, Tong MJ, Fletcher JR, et al: Blood coagulation studies in Plasmodium falciparum malaria. Am J Med Sci 265:63–67, 1973

59. Halstead SB: Dengue: Hematologic aspects. Semin Haematol 19:116–131, 1982

60. Colman RW, Robboy SJ, Minna JD: Disseminated intravascular coagulation (DIC): An approach. Am J Med 52:679–689, 1972

61. Corrigan JJ, Jordan CM: Heparin therapy in septicemia with disseminated intravascular

coagulation. Effect on mortality and on correction of hemostatic defects. N Engl J Med 283:778–782, 1970

62. Siegal T, Seligsohn U, Aghai E, et al: Clinical and laboratory aspects of disseminated intravascular coagulation (DIC): A study of 118 cases. Thromb Haemost 39:122–134, 1978

63. Spero JA, Lewis JH, Hasiba U: Disseminated intravascular coagulation. Findings in 346 patients. Thromb Haemost 43:28–33, 1980

64. Miro-Quesada M, Crosby E, Gotuzzo E, et al: Hemostasis in typhoid fever. Johns Hopkins Med J 148:73–77, 1981

65. Niemetz J: Coagulant activity in leukocytes. Tissue factor activity. J Clin Invest 51:307–313, 1972

66. Thiagarajan P, Niemetz J: Procoagulant-tissue factor activity of circulating peripheral blood leukocytes. Results of in vivo studies. Thromb Res 17:891–896, 1980

67. Edwards RL, Rickles FR, Bobrove AM: Mononuclear cell tissue factor: Cell of origin and requirements for activation. Blood 54:359–370, 1979

68. Muhlfelder TW, Khan I, Niemetz J: Factors influencing the release of procoagulant-tissue factor activity from leukocytes. J Lab Clin Med 92:65–72, 1978

69. Rickles FR, Rick PD, Van Why M: Structural features of *Salmonella typhimurium* lipopolysaccharide required for activation of tissue factor in human mononuclear cells. J Clin Invest 59:1188–1195, 1977

70. Niemetz J, Morrison DC: Lipid A as the biologically active moiety in bacterial endotoxin (LPS) -initiated generation of procoagulant activity by peripheral blood leukocytes. Blood 49:947–956, 1977

71. Niemetz J, Marcus AJ: The stimulatory effect of platelets and platelet membranes on the procoagulant activity of leukocytes. J Clin Invest 54:1437–1443, 1974

72. Kociba GJ, Griesemer RA: Disseminated intravascular coagulation induced with leukocyte procoagulant. Am J Pathol 69:407–416, 1972

73. Egbring R, Schmidt W, Fuchs G, et al: Demonstration of granulocytic proteases in plasma of patients with acute leukemia and septicemia with coagulation defects. Blood 49:219–231, 1977

74. Fauci AS, Haynes BF, Katz P: The spectrum of vasculitis. Clinical, pathologic, immunologic, and therapeutic considerations. Ann Intern Med 89:660–676, 1978

75. Meadow SR, Glasgow EF, White RHR, et al: Schonlein-Henoch nephritis. Q J Med 41:241–258, 1972

76. Mant MJ, King EG: Severe, acute disseminated intravascular coagulation. A reappraisal of its pathophysiology, clinical significance and therapy based on 47 patients. Am J Med 67:557–563, 1979

Rodger L. Bick

# 12

# Alterations of Hemostasis Associated with Surgery, Cardiopulmonary Bypass Surgery, and Prosthetic Devices

Surgery and cardiopulmonary bypass (CPB) surgery are procedures with which catastrophic intraoperative or postoperative hemorrhage may be associated. Surgical or CPB hemorrhage is of more than passing concern, as it not only places undue demands on local blood bank facilities but can also lead to prolonged hospitalization and significantly altered morbidity and mortality. Many instances of surgical and CPB hemorrhage are clearly due to inadequate surgical technique: an "acquired silk deficiency." However, many other instances are due to alterations in hemostasis. Often, a defect in hemostasis is present prior to the surgical procedure and is simply not detected. However, severe alterations in hemostasis are also created by CPB procedures. When managing a postsurgical patient with hemorrhage, it is obviously important to distinguish quickly between surgical and nonsurgical bleeding. This key question must be answered before a reasonable decision can be reached regarding surgical versus medical control of hemostasis. Perhaps the most important function of the hematologist in these instances is to be able to inform a surgeon or cardiac surgeon quickly if hemostasis is intact or potentially contributing to surgical or CPB hemorrhage. When surgical hemorrhage occurs, it is often fulminant and life-threatening; thus, effective management of patients and reasonable decisions regarding reexploration versus medical management require close teamwork between the hematologist, surgeon, cardiac surgeon, and pathologist. Only with this approach can optimal care be given to these critically ill patients, who in many instances have undergone an elective procedure.

## PREVENTION OF SURGICAL AND CARDIOVASCULAR SURGICAL BLEEDING

Since hemorrhage associated with surgery is usually catastrophic and often life-threatening, overcautiousness must be emphasized in regard to prevention, differential diagnosis, and rapid, efficacious therapy. Much attention must be given to preventing surgical hemorrhage by uncovering hereditary, acquired, or drug-induced bleeding diatheses before subjecting a patient to a general surgical procedure or CPB. An already existing bleeding diathesis, even though mild, when coupled with surgery or the alterations of hemostasis induced by CPB, can obviously lead to disastrous results.

## History Taking

Many cases of surgical or CPB hemorrhage could be averted by simply obtaining an adequate hemostasis history. Ideally, this should be obtained before hospital admission in order to allow time for appropriate evaluation if a potential problem with hemostasis is uncovered. Most historical information needed for detecting overt or covert bleeding tendencies is well known and covered in other areas of this textbook; however, for the surgeon or cardiovascular reader who is not often confronted with this aspect of medicine, the salient features of a bleeding history are outlined.[1] Key questions which often suggest a bleeding diathesis are: Does the patient suffer significant gingival bleeding with tooth brushing? Is there easy or, more significantly, spontaneous bruising? Has the patient experienced undue bleeding following dental extractions or prior surgical procedures? Is there a childhood history of epistaxis? Is menstrual flow normal or excessive? These simple questions certainly do not constitute a complete historical search for disorders of hemostasis, but a positive response is a good clue to the possibility of an underlying bleeding diathesis. Obviously, all patients considered for surgery or CPB should also be questioned regarding epistaxis, hemoptysis, hematemesis, melena, hematochezia, and hematuria.

The family history should always include inquiries about bleeding tendencies in parents, siblings, and children; this may uncover a hereditary bleeding tendency which has remained silent in the operative candidate because the hemostatic system has never been stressed by surgery or trauma. Of paramount importance and often neglected is a detailed drug history. In this author's experience, many instances of surgical and CPB hemorrhage could be explained in retrospect by noting the ingestion of drugs known to interfere with hemostasis, primarily platelet or, less commonly, vascular function.[2] Many drugs interfere with hemostasis. Often, the bleeding is mild and classified as bothersome. However, when drug-induced defects are combined with surgery or CPB surgery, hemorrhage may reach alarming proportions. Drugs may interfere with hemostasis by many mechanisms, most commonly platelet function. Significant drugs will be covered in specific sections of this chapter. If the drug history is positive and surgery or CPB is elective rather than emergent, surgery should be canceled for a full 14 days. Most drugs interfering with platelet function are generally effective for as long as 14 days, and this time period may be required for platelet function to return to normal and the surgical procedure to be performed safely. If the drug history is positive for antiplatelet agents and the drug has been ingested within 14 days, and surgery or CPB is emergent rather than elective, the patient should be given an appropriate dose of platelet concentrates (6–8 U for an adult) just prior to surgery. In addition, for CPB the patient should receive a similar dose of platelet concentrates just before leaving the operating room and then each morning for two postoperative days. This approach is somewhat vigorous, but is important if life-threatening CPB hemorrhage is to be avoided. For general surgical procedures, platelets are given preoperatively if the template bleeding time is greater than 15 minutes. They are then kept on hold for 2 days postoperatively and given only if bleeding occurs. Obviously, the presurgical patient should be questioned about the past use of warfarin or heparin anticoagulants.

## Physical Findings

For the benefit of surgical or cardiac surgical readers, the less obvious physical findings which provide clues to potential bleeding problems will be presented, since the more overt physical findings of a potential bleeding diathesis, such as hemarthroses, hematomegaly, and splenomegaly, are well known and covered in detail in appropriate chapters of this textbook. The patient's general appearance often provides hints of a bleeding tendency. All the hereditary and acquired connective tissue disorders are often associated with a significant vascular defect and the potential for surgical or CPB hemorrhage. In addition, most of the hereditary collagen vascular disorders are accompanied by poorly defined platelet functional defects. Clinical clues heralding the presence of a collagen disorder are well known to most clinicians and include the body habitus of Marfan's syndrome, blue sclerae, skeletal deformities, hyperextensible joints and skin, and nodular, spider, or pinpoint telangiectasia. These suggestive signs should promote a more complete investigation for the presence of a collagen vascular disorder before surgery is undertaken. The hereditary and acquired collagen vascular disorders which are most likely to be associated with general surgical bleeding will be discussed in appropriate sections. Other disorders which may be associated with a vascular defect and surgical bleeding include Cushing's syndrome, malignant paraproteinemias, the allergic purpuras, and hereditary hemorrhagic telangiectasia.

Other subtle hints of an occult bleeding tendency are uncovered by careful observation of the mucous membranes and the skin. Mucosal petechiae, purpura, or significant telangiectasia should be searched for and explained, if present. Likewise, petechiae, significant ecchymoses (large bruises greater than 2 cm in diameter), or telangiectasia of the skin or nail beds must be looked for; these findings are often suggestive of a vascular defect, platelet functional defect, or significant thrombocytopenia. If any of these findings are present, they should be investigated and thoroughly explained before surgery is performed. The usual physical findings of the more common clinical disorders associated with a significant hemorrhagic tendency, such as chronic liver disease, hypersplenism, chronic renal disease, rheumatoid arthritis, and systemic lupus erythematosus, are well known and will not be delineated here. In addition, prior laboratory screening will usually suggest the presence of any of these disorders if characteristic physical findings are absent. If the personal, family, or drug history or physical examination is suggestive of a potential or real bleeding tendency, surgery, especially cardiac, should be postponed until the defect is ruled out, or until it is fully delineated and a therapeutic plan for surgical hemostasis has been carefully designed. In this regard, it should be emphasized that a bleeding disorder of any type is rarely, if ever, a contraindication to performing general surgical procedures or CPB, provided the defect is delineated and a sound approach to correcting hemostasis during surgery and the postoperative period is designed.

## Presurgical Laboratory Screening

Any preoperative laboratory and hemostasis screen should generally be simple and involve a minimum of expense to the patient, while providing adequate information; usually however, presurgical or pre-bypass hemostasis screens are oversimplified.[1,2] As with an adequate history and physical examination, one cannot be too cautious in screening for defects in hemostasis when a surgical procedure is contemplated. When preexisting hemostatic defects are combined with general surgical procedures (vascular disruption) or the defects in hemostasis created by CPB, the resultant hemorrhage is often catastrophic but in many instances can be averted by wise screening of patients. The usually ordered SMA 12/60 biochemistry screening survey, electrolytes, complete blood count (CBC), and platelet count will detect the common acquired disorders often associated with a bleeding tendency, such as chronic liver disease, renal disease, and instances of "hypersplenism" or bone marrow failure of any etiology. Most commonly, a presurgical screen consists only of a prothrombin time, an activated partial thromboplastin time, and a platelet count. Although these simple tests will detect the majority of coagulation protein problems and thrombocytopenia, they provide absolutely no information about vascular or platelet function and ignore the possibility of fibrinolysis. In this author's experience, the vast majority of nontechnical hemorrhage associated with general surgical procedures or CPB hemorrhage are due to platelet functional defects and vascular defects; these are much more common in surgical bleeding than coagulation protein problems. Accordingly, we add 1 simple procedure to the routine preoperative surgical screen and would strongly advise all surgeons to consider the same. This test is a standardized template bleeding time as described by Mielke and co-workers,[3] and is performed on all patients prior to a general surgical procedure; it provides a reasonable surgical screen for adequate vascular and platelet function.[4] It should be recalled that the template bleeding time should not be performed until adequate platelet numbers are documented by count or smear evaluation. We use the Simplate-II.* For bypass surgery patients, we add a thrombin time or Fibrindex† to the pre-CPB screen.[5] In addition, the resultant clot is observed for 5 minutes after the test is performed. A normal thrombin time assures the absence of significant hypofibrinogenemia, dysfibrinogenemia, fibrinolysis, or fibrin(ogen) degradation product (FDP) elevation. The use of one or both of these tests in the routine presurgical screen adds only minimal cost and laboratory time, while providing valuable information not given by a simple prothrombin time, activated partial thromboplastin time, or platelet count. With respect to cardiovascular surgery, if hypothermic perfusion is to be done, cryoglobulins should also be measured prior to bypass. The preoperative hemostasis screen is summarized in Table 12-1.[3,6-9]

## HEMORRHAGE ASSOCIATED WITH NONCARDIAC SURGERY

### Vascular Defects

Although most vascular defects are not strictly hematological diseases, many are characterized or accompanied by a significant hemorrhagic diathesis and are often present in this form.[10] In addition, most, if not all, of these disorders can be accompanied by significant surgical hemorrhage; thus, the surgeon should be aware of the more common of these disorders, especially those which may lead to vascular hemorrhage with surgery. Vascular disorders are characteristically manifested by petechiae, ecchymoses, or telangiectasia.[11] Although these are the most common manifestations, mucous membrane bleeding (epistaxis, genitourinary, and gastrointestinal bleeding) may also occur. Commonly found in vascular disorders is a history of gingival bleeding with tooth brushing, bleeding after dental extraction, and a history of easy and spontaneous bruising.[11] The vast ma-

---

*General Diagnostics.
†Ortho Diagnostics (a standardized thrombin time).

**Table 12-1**
Presurgical Hemostasis Screen

Platelet count or blood smear
Prothrombin time
Activated partial thromboplastin time
Template bleeding time
Thrombin time (CPB surgery): observe clot for 5 minutes
Cryoglobulins (hypothermic CPB)

jority of vascular disorders and their propensity toward surgical hemorrhage will be detected by noting an abnormal template bleeding time and (usually) a normal platelet function test. The vascular disorders which most commonly lead to hemorrhage with a surgical procedure are depicted in Table 12-2 and include hereditary hemorrhagic telangiectasia (HHT), collagen vascular disorders with a microvascular component, Cushing's syndrome, malignant paraprotein disorders, amyloidosis, allergic purpuras, and aspirin ingestion.[12] In the face of a known vascular disorder, little can be done to prevent hemorrhage other than use of careful surgical technique. However, if the patient with a vascular disorder and a propensity to surgical hemorrhage has not taken antiplatelet agents prior to surgery, and careful surgical hemostasis is strictly adhered to, significant intra- or postoperative bleeding rarely occurs. It should be emphasized, however, that the surgeon is well advised to know that one of these disorders, and the possibility of surgical hemorrhage exist prior to subjecting a patient to a surgical procedure. It should be recalled that the template bleeding time is commonly normal in HHT and the allergic purpuras; thus, an adequate history and physical examination are imperative.

## Platelet Defects

Thrombocytopenia is not commonly encountered in a general surgical practice, and its causes most commonly seen by the surgeon are depicted in Table 12-3. These are almost always, if not always, detected by the presurgical platelet count or careful evaluation of the peripheral blood smear. However, in the busy laboratory, even severe thrombocytopenia may be missed on a smear evaluation, and the presurgical patient should always have a platelet count. When thrombocytopenia is noted, the etiology should be delineated before surgery is undertaken; the most common etiological mechanisms are listed in Table 12-3. In addition, the common drugs causing thrombocytopenia are listed in Table 12-4, and the patient should be questioned about their use when encountering presurgical

**Table 12-2**
Vascular Disorders Most
Commonly Associated with
Surgical Hemorrhage

Hereditary hemorrhagic telangiectasia
    (Osler-Weber-Rendu)
Cushing's syndrome
Collagen vascular disorders
Diabetes mellitus
Myeloma and amyloidosis
Aspirin-induced

Table 12-3
Causes of Thrombocytopenia
Commonly Seen in a
Surgical Practice
_____

ITP
Metastatic carcinoma
Myeloproliferative syndromes
Aplastic anemia
Severe iron deficiency
Splenomegaly and hypersplenism
Infection
Hemolytic-uremic syndrome
Multiple blood transfusions
Cirrhosis
DIC—usually low-grade
Drug-induced
_____

thrombocytopenia. Surgical bleeding commonly does not occur with a platelet count greater than 100,000/$\mu$l. However, if a patient has a platelet count below 100,000/$\mu$l and does not have idiopathic thrombocytopenic purpura (ITP), appropriate numbers of platelet concentrates are usually given prior to surgery and 6–8 U are kept on hold for the possibility of postsurgical hemorrhage. If the platelet count is greater than 100,000/$\mu$l, the patient is subjected to the surgical procedure with platelets on hold, which are given only if significant bleeding occurs intra- or postoperatively. In our experience, the most common causes of presurgical thrombocytopenia are malignancy and attendant chemotherapy, radiation therapy, marrow metastases, or drug-induced thrombocytopenia.[1,2,13]

## Platelet Functional Defects

Platelet functional defects clearly account for more than 50 percent of nontechnical surgical hemorrhage, and the surgical reader should be thoroughly familiar with this possibility.[1,2] Platelet functional defects that most commonly cause a surgical bleeding

Table 12-4
Most Common Drugs Causing
Thrombocytopenia in
Surgical Patients
_____

Acetaminophen
Aspirin
Cephalothins
Chlorothiazide
Chlorpropamide
Digitalis
Phenytoin
Meprobamate
Penicillin
Phenobarbital
Quinidine
Streptomycin
_____

**Table 12-5**
Platelet Functional Defects
Most Commonly Causing
Surgical Bleeding

Drug-induced
Hereditary storage pool defects
Uremia
Myeloproliferative syndromes
Myeloma
Cirrhosis
DIC
Presence of FDP

problem are depicted in Table 12-5. Most of the hereditary platelet functional defects are clinical oddities and extremely rare; the one most commonly seen and leading to surgical hemorrhage in our experience has been a hereditary storage pool defect, typically manifested by absent second wave aggregation to adenosine triphosphate (ADP) and epinephrine and totally absent aggregation to collagen in conjunction with normal ristocetin-induced agglutination. In addition, the possibility of a storage pool defect should be considered when noting normal platelet numbers and a prolonged template bleeding time. Much more commonly, however, the surgeon will be confronted with acquired or drug-induced platelet functional defects. Those common clinical disorders that induce abnormal platelet function are depicted in Table 12-5, and the common drugs which interfere with platelet function and lead to surgical hemorrhage are depicted in Table 12-6. It should be emphasized that these are only the common drugs inducing postsurgical hemorrhage; for more extensive lists, the reader is referred to several excellent reviews.[14–17] If presurgical template bleed-

**Table 12-6**
Common Drugs Inhibiting
Platelet Function and Leading
to Surgical Hemorrhage

Aspirin
Sulfinpyrazone
Dipyridamole
Motrin
Indocin
Benadryl
Papaverine
Phenothiazines
Tricyclic amines
Clofibrate
Furosamide
Nitrofurantoin
Propanolol
Glyceryl Guaiacolate (cough suppressant)
Penicillin
Carbenicillin
Ampicillin
Gentamycin

ing times are not performed, these disorders will not be detected by the routine presurgical screening of a prothrombin time, activated partial thromboplastin time, and platelet count.

When surgical bleeding thought to be potentially due to a platelet functional defect is suspected, a template bleeding time should be performed immediately; if it is prolonged, platelet aggregation should be measured and a careful drug and bleeding history taken from the patient immediately. Platelet functional defects are treated in essentially the same manner as for thrombocytopenia. If a patient has a platelet functional defect which has been uncovered preoperatively and has a template bleeding time of more than 15 minutes, he is infused with 6–8 U of platelet concentrates prior to the surgical procedure. If the template bleeding time is less than 15 minutes (normal, 4–9 minutes), then platelets are kept on hold and infused only if significant intraoperative or postoperative hemorrhage occurs. Alternatively, if the defect is not uncovered prior to surgery and postsurgical bleeding occurs, if the template bleeding time is prolonged and platelet aggregation abnormalities are noted, appropriate numbers of platelet concentrates are given immediately to abort hemorrhage: usually 6–8 U in the adult, given twice a day or every morning, depending upon the site and severity of bleeding. Our practice is to give platelets until significant hemorrhage stops.

## Isolated Coagulation Factor Deficiencies

Isolated coagulation factor deficiencies are rarely a surgical problem, except in centers specializing in hemophilia and congenital coagulation protein problems, and are discussed in appropriate sections of this text. However, far more commonly, the general and subspecialty surgeon will be faced with multiple compartment defects. The most common of these defects are disseminated intravascular coagulation (DIC) and hypoprothrombinemic-chronic liver disease-type problems. The bleeding diathesis associated with chronic liver disease is multifaceted and covered in detail in appropriate chapters of this text. It consists not only of coagulation factor problems, including deficiencies of the vitamin K-dependent clotting factors, but also of vascular and platelet defects.[18] The platelet defect (s) may be quantitative or qualitative. Hypoprothrombinemic bleeding may be seen in the warfarin-treated patient; in the patient with acute liver insults, including hepatitis; and in the individual with hepatic cirrhosis. However, most of these types of defects will be detected by a careful history and adequate presurgical laboratory screening. It should be noted that even though a patient who has been on warfarin prior to surgery has a prothrombin time which has returned to normal, he still has an increased bleeding risk with a surgical procedure.[19] When vitamin K-dependent clotting factor deficiency-type bleeding occurs, whether due to liver disease or to presurgical use of warfarin, it is best managed by the use of Aquamephyton, 20 mg intravenously (at 1 mg/min) or intramuscularly, and the use of fresh frozen plasma, 2–4 U as necessary, as the site and severity of bleeding dictate. If bleeding is truly emergent and life-threatening, we have resorted, on occasion, to the use of prothrombin complex concentrates to correct the hemostatic defect quickly.[20]

DIC-type syndromes not uncommonly lead to significant surgical hemorrhage. Typically, a patient with a disorder associated with a chronic "low-grade" underlying DIC is subjected to a surgical procedure, which then precipitates an acute, fulminant-type DIC process.[21] Those conditions most commonly associated with a chronic or subacute underlying DIC process in patients who are surgical candidates are depicted in Table 12-7 and include septicemia, disseminated solid malignancy, crush injuries, tissue necrosis, burns, and obstetric accidents including amniotic fluid embolism, placental abruption,

**Table 12-7**
DIC Syndromes in Surgical
Patients

Disseminated malignancy
Infection, sepsis
Hemolysis
Transfusion reactions
Acidosis/shock
Obstetrical accidents
Burns (extensive)
Crush injuries
Collagen vascular disorders
Ulcerative colitis

toxemia, and the retained fetus syndrome.[22,23] A detailed description of the etiology, pathophysiology, diagnosis, and management of DIC, when fulminant, is given in appropriate chapters of this text. It should be emphasized, however, that the surgeon should be aware of the disorders that may be associated with a chronic low-grade DIC process that may not be detected by the use of routine presurgical screening. Primary fibrin(ogen)olysis has been commonly blamed for many instances of posttransurethral prostatectomy (TURP) hemorrhage; however, in our experience, even though primary fibrin(ogen)olysis is occasionally seen and may account for massive post-TURP hematuria, far more common causes of post-TURP bleeding are drug-induced platelet functional defects and a chronic underlying DIC-type syndrome.[24] It has been suggested that a minimal DIC evaluation be performed on all patients undergoing TURP, as this may identify the patients who are predisposed to post-TURP hemorrhage.[25]

## ALTERATIONS OF HEMOSTASIS ASSOCIATED WITH CARDIOPULMONARY BYPASS

Cardiac surgery using CPB is now a common procedure and, with popularization of coronary artery bypass grafting, is no longer limited to large centers but is now performed in most community hospitals. Widespread use of CPB has brought renewed awareness of the catastrophic intraoperative or postoperative hemorrhage that may be associated with this procedure. Hemorrhage during or after bypass is of more than passing concern, as it can lead to significant morbidity and mortality from an elective procedure, places marked demands on blood bank facilities, and can lead to prolonged hospitalization.[26,27] The actual incidence of life-threatening hemorrhage associated with CPB appears to vary from 5 to 25 percent.[27-29]

Until recently, the pathophysiology of altered hemostasis created by CPB was poorly understood. Past failures to delineate the pathophysiology of altered hemostasis during CPB have, quite understandably, precluded development of uniform concepts of successful prevention, adequate and rapid diagnosis, and effective control of CPB hemorrhage. Lack of understanding of CPB hemorrhagic syndromes has derived from several factors: (1) Many past studies of hemostasis during CPB examined only isolated aspects of blood coagulation and ignored the complexities and interrelationships of the hemostasis system. (2) Many previous studies failed to utilize coagulationists or hematologists. In some instances, this led to the inappropriate choice of test systems and unclear interpretation of results. (3)

In spite of available and sophisticated advances in modalities to assess the hemostatic system, many previous studies utilized insensitive, inaccurate, or inappropriate test systems. For example, the euglobulin lysis time has been the most commonly utilized modality for studying CPB fibrinolysis, even though this test system has been questioned for the evaluation of clinical fibrinolysis.[30,31]

Various investigators have ascribed the hemorrhagic syndrome of CPB to a wide variety of defects; each investigator has likewise placed varying degrees of importance on each defect, depending upon which particular hemostatic parameters were monitored. In the past, the abnormalities most frequently cited to account for CPB hemorrhage have included (1) inadequate heparin neutralization, (2) protamine excess, (3) heparin rebound, (4) thrombocytopenia, (5) hypofibrinogenemia, (6) primary hyperfibrin(ogen)olysis, (7) DIC, (8) isolated coagulation factor deficiencies, (9) transfusion reactions, and (10) hypocalcemia. The suggestion that all of these defects may contribute to CPB hemorrhage clearly demonstrates that despite the finding of multiple defects, the basic pathophysiology of hemostasis during CPB remains confusing to many. It is equally clear that basic mechanisms of altered hemostasis associated with CPB must be completely understood and appreciated before an appropriate approach to rapid diagnosis and effective therapy can be designed.

## Thrombocytopenia

Early studies of hemostasis during CPB noted significant thrombocytopenia, about 50,000/$\mu$l, in patients undergoing bypass surgery; many authors thought this responsible for bypass hemorrhage. In addition, Kevy et al.[32] noted that the degree of thrombocytopenia was related to the time on bypass, and was much more pronounced with perfusions lasting longer than 60 minutes. A relationship between degree of thrombocytopenia and time on bypass was also reported by Signori et al.[33] Later studies noted similar findings,[34,35] and Porter and Silver[39] found that in the majority of patients undergoing CPB, the platelet count fell to one-third of the preoperative level; in addition, it was noted that thrombocytopenia did not abate until several days after CPB. Earlier studies by Wright and co-workers[36] and von Kaulla and Swan[37] also recognized thrombocytopenia in association with CPB, but these investigators concluded that thrombocytopenia bore little, if any, relationship to actual bypass hemorrhage. Some studies that found thrombocytopenia during CPB concluded that this represented thrombocytopenia of DIC.[38-41] We,[42-45] as well as others,[46-48] have failed to find significant thrombocytopenia during CPB. This wide variability in experience most likely represents different surgical and pumping techniques such as flow rates, normothermic perfusion, the oxygenation mechanism used, time on bypass, and the priming solution. In our experience, a flow rate of 40 ml/kg/min and a pump prime of 20 ml/kg of 5 percent dextrose in Ringer's lactate plus 5 percent dextrose in water in a ratio of 2:1 produces only minimal thrombocytopenia.[44] Figure 12-1 demonstrates changes in platelet number with this pumping technique. The dotted line represents the mean platelet counts in membrane-pumped patients and the solid line in bubble oxygenation patients.[18] A total of 300 consecutive patients are depicted. In our experience, the type of oxygenation mechanism used appears to play little role, if any, in causing thrombocytopenia. Thrombocytopenia with bubble oxygenators is slightly greater than that seen with membrane oxygenators, but does not reach clinical significance. The most commonly cited mechanisms in the development of CPB thrombocytopenia are (1) hemodilution, (2) formation of intravascular platelet thrombi, (3) platelet utilization in the pump and/or oxygena-

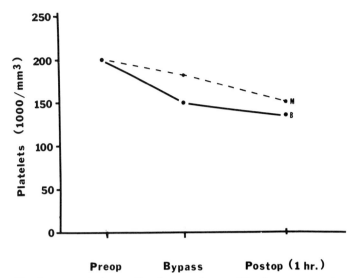

**Fig. 12-1.** Platelet counts during cardiopulmonary bypass. Membrane oxygenator: - - - -. Bubble oxygenator: ———.

tion system, and (4) peripheral utilization due to DIC. We have failed to find a correlation between CPB, hematocrit, and platelet count, suggesting that hemodilution is not a major factor.[45] Indeed, the role, if any, of these mechanisms in producing CPB thrombocytopenia remains totally unclear.

## Platelet Functional Defects

In contrast to the numerous investigations regarding platelet number during CPB, there has been a surprising lack of interest in assessing platelet function during this procedure. Early investigators[33] suspected that abnormalities of platelet function might occur when they noted faulty clot retraction. These results were of unclear significance, however, since other changes known to affect clot retraction, such as hypofibrinogenemia and thrombocytopenia, were also present. Another early study[49] assessed platelet function before placing patients on CPB but failed to evaluate platelet function during or after bypass. In this study, abnormal preoperative platelet adhesion in glass bead columns was associated with increased postoperative bleeding. Salzman[50] studied platelet adhesion before, during, and after bypass and noted decreased adhesion to glass bead columns in all patients during bypass; however, the significance of this defect was difficult to evalute since all patients had marked thrombocytopenia, which is definitely known to alter adhesion studies.[51–53] Further information from this study was that heparin, in doses using during CPB, did not alter platelet adhesion. This study concluded that a circulating anticoagulant might be responsible for this platelet functional defect, as plasma from CPB patients altered adhesion when added to normal platelets. This circulating anticoagulant most likely represented FDP. Salzman's study also noted that perfusion temperature and the type of priming solution did not correlate with the development of abnormal platelet function. More recently, platelet adhesion studies have been performed in patients undergoing CPB without significant thrombocytopenia.[42,44,45] In these studies, platelet function, as assessed by adhesion, decreased profoundly in all patients at the initiation of bypass; most patients demonstrated

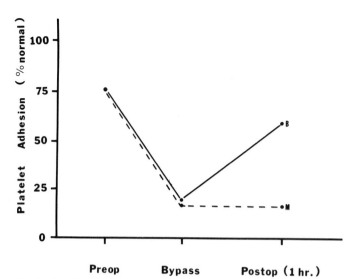

**Fig. 12-2.** Platelet function during cardiopulmonary bypass. Membrane oxygenator: - - - -. Bubble oxygenator: _____.

adhesion, which decreased to 17 percent of preoperative levels. In one study little correlation was noted between hematocrit, fibrinogen level, or FDP titer and abnormal platelet adhesion. In addition, poor correlation was noted between chest tube blood loss and abnormal platelet function, as assessed by adhesion. Figure 12-2 depicts platelet adhesion changes during CPB. This degree of abnormal platelet function would certainly be expected to compromise hemostasis severely. Membrane oxygenation patients are depicted by a dashed line, and bubble oxygenation patients are depicted by a solid line.[18] It appears that the platelet functional defect is slightly more severe and tends to correct much more slowly when a membrane oxygenator is used compared to a bubble oxygenator.

Platelet adhesion has been found to be abnormal in patients with qualitative platelet abnormalities,[53] von Willebrand's disease,[52] and myeloproliferative disorders.[54] Many factors, some possibly altered by CPB, affect platelet function as assessed by adhesion; these include (1) pH,[55] (2) absolute platelet count,[56] (3) hematocrit,[54] (4) drugs,[15] and (5) the presence of FDP.[57,58] Although most studies do not clearly define the reasons for abnormal platelet function during CPB, they do suggest that several of the above-mentioned mechanisms are most likely not involved. The finding of platelet counts greater than 100,000/$\mu$l and hematocrits greater than 30 percent in most patients with marked platelet functional defects 1 hour after CPB suggests that the absolute platelet count and the hematocrit do not account for altered platelet function. In addition, most patients have a normal or near-normal pH 1 hour after CPB; thus, a change in pH is unlikely to account for abnormal platelet function during bypass surgery. Heparin, at levels higher than those attained in patients undergoing CPB, has not been shown to alter platelet function.[50,53] Circulating FDP are known to interfere with platelet function, and these are present in approximately 85 percent of patients undergoing CPB. However, there is poor correlation between levels of circulating FDP and the degree of abnormal platelet function during bypass surgery. In addition, defective platelet function occurs in virtually 100 percent of patients undergoing CPB; thus, circulating FDP cannot account for altered platelet function in many instances. Other possible mechanisms of altered platelet function during CPB include platelet membrane damage by shearing force or contact with foreign material, resulting in partial release of platelet contents, platelet membrane coating with nonspecific proteins or protein degradation products, or incomplete platelet release or nonspecific platelet damage induced by fast flow rates. Recent studies have shown clear-cut platelet degranulation occurring during bypass surgery.[59] However, no studies reported thus far allow conclusions to be drawn regarding the contribution of any of these mechanisms to altered platelet function during CPB. Only 1 preliminary study has reported platelet aggregation studies during CPB.[60] In this series of 29 patients, only 20 percent developed aggregation abnormalities during CPB; however, after heparin reversal with protamine sulfate, 90 percent of patients developed aggregation abnormalities. These were thought to be due to a protamine–platelet interaction and not due to the bypass itself. Regardless of the mechanism(s) involved, studies to date clearly reveal that a significant platelet function defect is induced in all patients undergoing CPB. The magnitude of this defect would certainly be expected to have potentially serious consequences for hemostasis during and after bypass. In addition, patients who have ingested drugs known to interfere with platelet function would be expected to have more blood loss than those not ingesting such agents. In such patients, this would be expected to compound the defects already induced by CPB and potentiate the chance for hemorrhage. One small study has provided evidence for this conclusion.[56] Although diagnosis and management of hemorrhage associated with CPB will be discussed subsequently, it should be pointed out that this platelet function defect appears to be of major significance in post-CPB hemorrhage. In this author's experience, the use of platelet concentrates in the face of a normal platelet count will usually promptly correct or significantly reduce most episodes of CPB or post-CPB hemorrhage.

## Vascular Defects

Few studies of vascular defects during CPB have been reported. Recently, a syndrome of mild to moderate nonthrombocytopenic purpura accompanied by splenomegaly and atypical lymphocytosis following CPB has been reported by Behrendt and co-workers.[61] In this series, the purpura was benign, self-limited, and frequently manifested only after discharge from the hospital. Only 1 patient out of 7 suffered a complication following the development of this syndrome; this was glomerulonephritis of the type often seen in Henoch-Schönlein purpura. In addition, a case of fatal purpura fulminans was reported following extracorporeal circulation for coronary artery bypass grafting.[62] Massive purpura developed on the third postoperative day, followed by progressive renal failure. High doses of steroids and low molecular weight dextran produced no improvement, and the patient died of renal failure on the 18th postoperative day. No abnormalities in hemostasis were detected by extensive laboratory testing. These 2 reports suggest that an inflammatory vasculitis may be associated with CPB; the most benign forms represented by purpura simplex and, rarely, purpura fulminans (without DIC) may be expected to occur. Cardiac surgeons should be aware of this potential complication of bypass surgery. Aside from these 2 reports, no mention has been made of vascular defects associated with CPB.

## Isolated Coagulation Factor Defects

Numerous studies have examined and reported coagulation factor deficiencies during CPB. A wide variety of findings have been observed and, like the finding of thrombocytopenia, may only reflect differences in surgical or pumping techniques, such as flow rate,

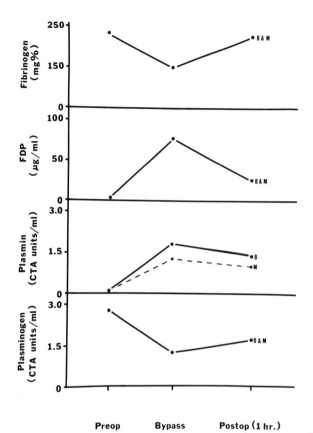

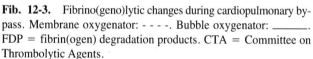

**Fig. 12-3.** Fibrino(geno)lytic changes during cardiopulmonary by-
pass. Membrane oxygenator: - - - -. Bubble oxygenator: _____.
FDP = fibrin(ogen) degradation products. CTA = Committee on
Thrombolytic Agents.

priming solution, etc. Most studies have noted significant hypofibrinogenemia[28,35,36,44,45]
which does not seem to be correlated with perfusion time. We,[44,45] and others,[28,35] have
found fibrinogen levels to be closely correlated with degree of CPB fibrinolysis; however,
other investigators[32,63] report little correlation between hypofibrinogenemia and degree of
CPB fibrin(ogen)olysis. Figure 12-3 depicts correlations noted between fibrinogen,
plasminogen, circulating plasmin, and FDP during CPB. The dashed line represents
membrane-pumped patients and the solid lines bubble oxygenator-pumped patients.[18] Some
studies have concluded that hypofibrinogenemia occurs primarily as a consequence of DIC
during pump surgery;[38,40,41] however, others have failed to find hypofibrinogenemia during CPB.[64,65] It seems reasonable to conclude from the studies reported that hypofibrinogenemia secondary to hyperfibrinolysis may be a frequent occurrence during CPB. This
appears to be a rather consistent finding in the carefully studied series noted above and is most
likely a major cause of hypofibrinogenemia associated with CPB. Hyperfibrin(ogen)olysis
occurs in approximately 85 percent of patients undergoing bypass surgery. Most studies
have also noted other coagulation deficiencies in association with CPB; those most
commonly found to be decreased and reported to play a role in CPB hemorrhage are
factor II (prothrombin), factor V (proaccelerin), and factor VIII:C (antihemophilic fac-

tor).[28,32,35,36,38,41] Some conclude that these changes are secondary to DIC,[38,48] whereas others ascribe these decreases to a primary hyperfibrin(ogen)olytic syndrome and plasmin-induced degradation of coagulation proteins.[28,44,45] Still others have failed to find a significant decrease in most coagulation factors during bypass surgery,[32,64,65] and 2 authors have reported increased factor VIII:C levels during perfusion.[64,66]

## Disseminated Intravascular Coagulation

The pathophysiology of DIC is depicted in detail in appropriate chapters. The question of whether it develops during bypass surgery has caused much confusion regarding altered hemostasis during and after bypass. Numerous early studies of hemostasis during CPB concluded that DIC took place.[38,40,41,67,68] However, many such studies monitored only isolated coagulation factors; and the measured decreases were empirically ascribed to presumed DIC, as no other explanation was evident. In particular, the findings of isolated fibrinogen, factor VIII:C,[36,40] or prothrombin complex factor[47] deficiencies were often assumed, perhaps erroneously, to be secondary to DIC, without appropriate confirmatory laboratory testing. In addition, 2 recent reports have concluded that DIC accounts for alterations of hemostasis during CPB.[48,69] In these reports of 9 patients, the authors concluded that DIC was present after noting that several measures of hemostasis worsened following heparin reversal with protamine. In particular, FDP elevation, hypofibrinogenemia, and hypoplasminogenemia appeared to become accentuated following the infusion of protamine. However, our experience,[44,45] as well as that of others,[28,33,34,37,65,70] has been the opposite; hypofibrinogenemia, hypoplasminogenemia, and FDP elevation are usually noted to correct rather rapidly and uniformly after the administration of protamine sulfate. These findings would suggest that DIC is not associated with CPB. DIC during CPB also seems unlikely in view of massive heparinization and the absence of significant or uniform thrombocytopenia reported in many studies in which hemostasis appears to be normal. Another finding which would certainly suggest that DIC is not present during CPB is the presence of normal or near-normal antithrombin III (ATIII) levels during CPB;[19,28] current evidence suggests that decreased ATIII levels are a reasonably good indicator of the development of acute or chronic DIC.[71] Only 1 study[48] has shown decreased levels of ATIII during CPB; however, in the 9 patients described, all had low levels of ATIII before bypass was initiated. In addition, the method used was quite old, and possibly influenced by the presence of FDP and/or heparin, rendering interpretation of these results unclear. Another consideration negating the probability that DIC occurs during CPB is the following: If DIC were present in patients undergoing CPB, the infusion of intravenous protamine sulfate would be expected to cause massive precipitation of soluble fibrin monomer, with resultant extensive micro- and/or macrovascular occlusion. In this author's experience, only 2 patients out of several thousand had DIC in association with CPB. Both patients developed DIC prior to CPB, one from cardiac arrest and the other from septicemia. In these 2 instances, bypass surgery was accomplished without incidence; however, when protamine sulfate was infused, massive vascular occlusion including carotid and renal artery thrombosis suddenly occurred.

To summarize, even though most early and several recent studies have detected primary fibrin(ogen)olysis in association with CPB, only a few have concluded that DIC occurs. These conclusions most likely derive from the marked superficial similarities between primary hyperfibrin(ogen)olysis and DIC, with the usual secondary fibrinolytic response, and from the difficulty in making a clear-cut differential diagnosis between these 2 states in the absence of sophisticated and complete coagulation studies.

## Primary Hyperfibrino(geno)lysis

Fibrinolytic activity is generally decreased or inhibited during and following most general surgical procedures.[72-75] However, most studies, utilizing a variety of laboratory modalities, have found increased fibrinolysis during and after cardiopulmonary bypass surgery.[28,32-35,44,45,63,65,70,76] Many earlier studies of hemostasis during CPB assessed fibrinolysis with the euglobulin lysis time; thus, the finding of fibrinolysis remained of unclear significance for a long period of time.[30,31] More recent studies of CPB hemostasis[34,44,45] which have utilized more specific methods for assessing fibrinolysis, primarily synthetic substrate assays,[77-81] have confirmed earlier reports of a primary hyperfibrin-(ogen)olytic syndrome in the majority of patients undergoing CPB. Figure 12-3 depicts changes in the fibrinolytic system in patients undergoing CPB. Because of early reports detecting primary hyperfibrin(ogen)olysis during CPB, the empirical use of antifibrinolytics, usually epsilon aminocaproic acid (EACA), has become commonplace. In spite of the attendant hazards of this agent, which include hypokalemia, hypotension, ventricular arrhythmias, local or disseminated thrombosis, and DIC syndromes,[82] many cardiovascular surgeons have frequently used this drug. Controlled studies with and without antifibrinolytics have failed to reveal any clear-cut differences in CPB hemorrhage,[28,29,35,63,83] and Gomes and McGoon,[70] and Tsuji and coworkers[65] have shown a clear-cut increase in post-CPB hemorrhage with the empirical use of antifibrinolytics. In our experience, the need to use EACA to control CPB hemorrhage is extremely rare; this agent should be used only when concrete laboratory evidence of primary hyperfibrin(ogen)olysis is noted in the severely hemorrhaging CPB patient. Several investigators finding primary fibrin(ogen)olysis during CPB have concluded this to be inconsequential as a cause of postperfusion hemorrhage,[33,35] whereas others have thought that this syndrome is triggered only by specific events such as pyrogenecity of equipment,[84] the use of Rheomacrodex,[85] or induction of anesthesia.[37] Since primary hyperfibrin(ogen)olysis occurs in the majority of patients subjected to CPB, it seems more likely that activation of the fibrinolytic system may be occurring in the oxygenation mechanism, or alternatively, that pump-induced acclerated flow rates may activate the plasminogen-plasmin system, or may alter endothelial plasminogen activator activity. In fact, the pathogenesis of fibrinolytic activation during CPB remains totally unclear. Although many investigators have noted enhanced fibrinolysis during CPB, a few studies have found only elevated fibrinolytic activator activity, with no systemically circulating plasmin.[32,63,67] Also, a few studies have failed to find any evidence of primary hyperfibrin(ogen)olysis in association with cardiopulmonary bypass.[29,35,36,67]

The pathophysiology of primary hyperfibrin(ogen)olysis is familiar to many readers; a comprehensive review is beyond the scope of this chapter. However, the salient features of this syndrome will be presented so that the cardiovascular reader can gain a complete understanding of the defects of hemostasis during CPB. The pathophysiology of primary hyperfibrin(ogen)olysis is depicted and summarized in Figure 12-4. Hemostasis is significantly altered when plasmin circulates systemically; the attendant systemic hypofibrinogenemia and plasmin degradation of factors V, VIII, and IX (Christmas factor)[86-88] may severely compromise the hemostatic system. In addition, the resultant FDP further derange hemostasis by interfering with thrombin activity,[89] interfering with fibrin monomer polymerization[90,91] and radically altering platelet function.[57,58,89]

These changes in hemostasis would certainly be expected to be associated with a significant hemorrhagic potential. In addition, it is easy to see how these alterations in hemostasis could be superficially confused with DIC and secondary fibrinolysis.

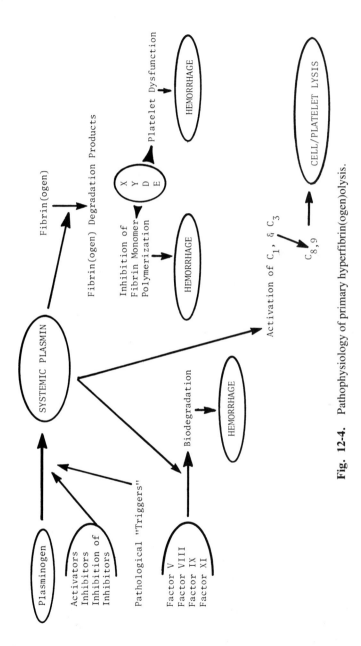

**Fig. 12-4.** Pathophysiology of primary hyperfibrin(ogen)olysis.

395

## Other Defects

Heparin rebound (the delayed recirculation of heparin) has received significant attention as a potential cause of CPB hemorrhage.[85,92-95] This was observed more often in earlier studies. With today's generally accepted doses of both heparin and protamine, both heparin rebound and inadequate heparinization are rarely, if ever, seen.[44,45,48] In fact, heparin rebound, as well as inadequate heparin neutralization,[39,41] have been poorly documented as actual causes of CPB hemorrhage. Similarly, protamine excess has occasionally been incriminated as a source of CPB hemorrhage; however, several carefully studied series have failed to note this phenomenon in a single patient undergoing CPB.[44,45,46,93,96] In addition, although protamine sulfate is a well-known in vitro anticoagulant,[97] it is unlikely that this agent is a cause of in vivo hemorrhage.

Several authors have reported that both coagulation defects and significant CPB hemorrhage may be associated with hypothermic perfusion;[29,35,37,85] our experience in comparing normothermic to hypothermic perfusions has led to the same conclusion.[76] Gomes and McGoon[70] and Porter and Silver,[34] however, have found no increased incidence of CPB hemorrhage as a consequence of hypothermic perfusion. Many patients undergoing coronary artery bypass grafting for coronary occlusive disease have been on warfarin-type drugs. Verska and associates[29] have noted that even though the prothrombin time had returned to normal prior to CPB, patients previously receiving warfarin-type therapy demonstrated more hemorrhage than those not on these agents. One study[29] noted that increased hemorrhage was associated with a repeat CPB procedure; others,[41,70] however, have noted that no increased hemorrhage was associated with a second procedure. In addition, patients undergoing CPB for correction of cyanotic heart disease appear to have more severe derangements in hemostasis during perfusion, and thus a propensity to hemorrhage, than those operated on for noncyanotic heart disease.[33,70]

## Summary of CPB Hemostasis Pathophysiology

Many conclusions regarding altered hemostasis and resultant hemorrhage during CPB are of questionable significance; for example, it appears that overheparinization, heparin rebound, inadequate protamine neutralization, and protamine excess, although receiving at least theoretical attention as potential sources of CPB hemorrhage, have not been clearly shown to be responsible for bleeding associated with bypass surgery. Similarly, thrombocytopenia, almost certainly a potential source of hemorrhage, is an inconsistent finding during CPB and most likely arises as a consequence of differences in pumping technique among cardiovascular teams and prolonged perfusion times. The finding of isolated coagulation defects during CPB has added little to our understanding of altered hemostasis during bypass surgery; most likely, these simply represent isolated measurements of the results of hyperfibrino(geno)lysis and systemic circulation plasmin.

Although DIC has been thought by some to occur during CPB, most carefully done studies have failed to document it. The significant doses of heparin used during CPB, the absence of consistent thrombocytopenia, and the general correction of hypofibrinogenemia, hypoplasminogenemia, and elevated FDP after heparin neutralization all suggest that the presence of DIC during CPB is a very rare event. This author has noted DIC in association with CPB only when another triggering event was provided, such as sepsis, shock, massive transfusions, or a frank hemolytic transfusion reaction.

**Table 12-8**
Hemorrhagic Syndromes
Associated with
Cardiopulmonary Bypass
(in Descending Order of
Probability)

---

Platelet functional defects
  CPB-induced
  Drug-induced
Primary hyperfibrin(ogen)olysis
Thrombocytopenia
Hyperheparinemia/heparin rebound?
DIC?

---

Predisposing factors which do seem to be associated with enhanced CPB hemorrhage are (1) long perfusion times, (2) prior ingestion of warfarin-type drugs, (3) cyanotic heart disease, and (4) the preoperative ingestion of drugs known to interfere with platelet function. More importantly, evidence suggests that the majority of patients undergoing CPB develop a primary hyperfibrin(ogen)olytic syndrome, although the exact triggering mechanisms involved remain unclear. However, the resultant secondary derangements in hemostasis will certainly create a potential for CPB hemorrhage. In addition, virtually all patients undergoing CPB develop a severe platelet functional defect. It is not clear if this defect is due to coating of platelet surfaces by FDP, membrane damage from the oxygenation mechanism, platelet damage from fast flow rates, or other unrecognized mechanisms. Whatever the triggering mechanism(s), it is quite clear that the most significant alterations in hemostasis associated with CPB are defective platelet function and primary hyperfibrin(ogen)olysis. These 2 defects, alone or in combination, certainly account for the majority of nonsurgical and nontechnical hemorrhage in patients undergoing CPB; platelet functional defects account for far more hemorrhagic episodes than the primary hyperfibrin(ogen)olytic syndrome.

## Diagnosis of CPB Hemorrhage

When bleeding occurs during or after bypass, it is obviously extremely important to define the defect as quickly as possible; only in this manner can specific and effective therapy be delivered.[98] As previously mentioned, many instances of CPB hemorrhage are clearly due to inadequate surgical technique, but alterations of hemostasis may also be responsible for accentuating CPB hemorrhage. This discussion will be limited to nontechnical causes of CPB hemorrhage. The types of hemorrhage which occur during CPB are somewhat limited, and are depicted in Table 12-8 in descending order of probability.

The primary distinction to be made is between strictly surgical bleeding, defects in hemostasis, or a combination of the two. This distinction becomes more difficult and more important after the patient has left the operating room; during this period, a decision must be made regarding reexploration and the adequacy of hemostasis for reexploration. In distinguishing between surgical and nonsurgical bleeding, many physical findings are helpful: Is the bleeding localized or systemic? If the patient is already in the recovery room, the recognition of hematuria in association with petechiae and ecchymoses, and oozing from intravenous sites in conjunction with increased chest tube blood loss usually means a defect in hemostasis, whereas increased chest tube blood loss alone often signifies a technical bleeding problem. While the patient is in the operating room, these same findings hold true; in addition, the surgeon will often note bleeding or oozing throughout the surgical field in nontechnical bleeding. It is imperative, therefore, that communication between the surgeon and the hematologist or internist occur.

As soon as CPB hemorrhage is seen or suspected, the following laboratory tests are ordered: prothrombin time, activated partial thromboplastin time, CBC and platelet count, examination of a peripheral smear, FDP, heparin assay by synthetic substrate, thrombin time, and plasminogen/plasmin levels by synthetic substrate. Evaluation of the heparin assay will provide rapid information regarding the status of heparin and its potential effects on other tests of hemostasis. The resultant clot from the thrombin time is always observed for 5 minutes for evidence of lysis, thus providing rapid additional information on the presence or absence of a clinically significant primary hyperfibrin(ogen)olytic syndrome. Additional evidence for or against primary lysis is obtained by noting the FDP level.[99] A peripheral blood smear and platelet count are invaluable to evaluate rapidly the potential for thrombocytopenic bleeding. Plasminogen and plasmin levels obtained by the synthetic substrate technique are not time-consuming, but are not used for an immediate diagnosis; however, they are invaluable in making decisions regarding antifibrinolytic therapy at a later time. If significant primary hyperfibrin(ogen)olysis is present, FDP will be significantly elevated, and hypoplasminogenemia and circulating plasmin will be detected. If, on the other hand, excess heparin is a potential problem, this will be noted by the heparin assay and the thrombin time will be markedly prolonged. If no significant clot lysis is observed in the clot formed during measurement of the thrombin time, and significant FDP elevation is not present, primary fibrinolysis should not be dwelled upon. All patients undergoing CPB display a functional platelet defect; when bleeding occurs, this author assumes that the problem is present, and even though it might not be the primary reason for hemorrhage, platelet dysfunction can be assumed to be additive to any other defect, whether surgical or due to altered hemostasis. No tests of platelet function are done, therefore, but platelets are immediately ordered for any patient who demonstrates postbypass hemorrhage. The time period during which hemorrhage occurs, that is, intraoperative, after heparin neutralization, or in the recovery room, appears to bear little relationship to the etiology of the primary hemostatic defect responsible for hemorrhage. Exceptions to this are thrombocytopenic bleeding, which usually occurs after the patient is in the recovery room, and a significant drug-induced platelet functional defect, which is usually manifested as significant oozing as soon as the operative procedure is done. Tests ordered for the differential diagnosis of the causes of hemorrhage are listed in Table 12-9.

## Management of CPB Hemorrhage

When one first sees a patient with CPB hemorrhage, whether intraoperative or postoperative, it is of prime importance (1) to note the type of bleeding (systemic versus local), (2) to order a stat laboratory screen as outlined previously, and (3) to administer 6–8 U of platelet concentrates as quickly as possible. Even though the use of platelet concentrates is somewhat empirical at this point, it is done for several sound reasons: (1) virtually all patients have a significant platelet functional defect, which may be the primary reason for hemorrhage (and usually is if it is a nontechnical bleed), or (2) this defect is

**Table 12-9**
Laboratory Evaluation of
CPB Hemorrhage

Platelet count and CBC
Blood smear evaluation
Prothrombin time
Activated partial thromboplastin time
FDP
Heparin assay (synthetic substrate)
Thrombin time: observe for lysis
Plasminogen/plasmin assay (synthetic substrate)

most likely accentuating bleeding from other causes, whether it be a surgical or defective hemostasis in origin. In this author's experience, the quick administration of platelet concentrates, while awaiting the aforementioned laboratory evaluation, will often stop or significantly reduce most instances of nontechnical CPB hemorrhage.

When bleeding begins immediately upon initiation of surgery, a platelet functional defect, usually drug-induced, can be assumed to be present until further laboratory investigation can be done. In this instance, the patient should be given 6–8 U of platelet concentrates as quickly as possible, and the surgical wound should be closed if this is feasible. If a platelet functional defect is found to be responsible for the hemorrhage (no laboratory evidence of significant fibrin(ogen)olysis or hyperheparinemia), 6–8 U of platelet concentrates should be repeated the evening after surgery and for 2 postoperative mornings. Thrombocytopenic CPB hemorrhage should be controlled in the same manner, although greater numbers of platelet concentrates may be needed as dictated by the initial platelet count, the site and severity of bleeding, and the response to platelet transfusions. Hyperheparinemia and heparin rebound, if thought to be a real clinical problem as documented by synthetic substrate assays, are managed by delivering 25 percent of the initial calculated protamine dose; this is repeated every 30–60 minutes until bleeding ceases. It should again be emphasized that hyperheparinemia and heparin rebound are not at all likely to be responsible for bleeding, and should not be dwelled upon unless concrete laboratory evidence of hyperheparinemia is present and evidence of primary fibrin(ogen)olysis is clearly absent. This author has seen many instances of excessive heparinization due to mistakes in calculations and solution preparation; not one of them was associated with significant hemorrhage. Similarly, protamine excess is rarely, if ever, a clinical problem. This situation should never require therapy and should not be dwelled upon at the risk of ignoring other potential defects in hemostasis.

Primary hyperfibrin(ogen)olysis is commonly present and may or may not be responsible for hemorrhage. This syndrome should not be treated empirically; antifibrinolytic therapy should be considered if the patient has failed to respond to platelet concentrates and there is documented laboratory evidence for this syndrome, as noted by the presence of hypoplasminogenemia, circulating plasmin, and elevated FDP. Primary hyperfibrin-(ogen)olytic bleeding is generally treated with epsilon aminocaproic acid as an initial 5–10-g slow intravenous push followed by 1–2 g/hr until bleeding ceases or slows to a non-life-threatening level. It should be recalled that EACA may be associated with ventricular arrhythmias, hypotension, hypokalemia, localized or diffuse thrombosis, and DIC. Thus, this agent should be injected slowly, and patients should be monitored carefully with respect to renal output, blood pressure, and electrolytes.

## THROMBOHEMORRHAGIC COMPLICATIONS OF PROSTHETIC DEVICES

Exposure of the blood to foreign surfaces is often linked with thrombosis, which provides a major clinical obstacle to the use of prosthetic devices. The use of prosthetic devices has become commonplace in the management of patients with cardiovascular disease, renal disease, or chemotherapy, for long-term parenteral hyperalimentation, and for common angiographic studies.[100] The hemostatic complications that follow the insertion of prosthetic devices include consumption of coagulation factors, other plasma protein, or platelets; the generation of microthrombi of little clinical consequence; and thrombosis or thromboembolism that gives rise to serious, life-threatening, or terminal vasoocclusion. Under normal circumstances, the blood remains fluid because of numerous obvious factors, including a nonthrombogenic endothelial surface, endogenous fibrinolytic activity, natural proteinase inhibitors such as ATIII, and the dilution and dispersion of procoagulant components of the blood;[101] all of these protective mechanisms are lost, to some degree, with the use of prosthetic devices. In general, slow flow rates are associated with local thrombotic events; however, fast flow rates are more commonly associated with a high shear force and embolization.[102] In addition, smooth prosthetic surfaces tend to favor little adhesiveness of a formed thrombus, and thus embolization is more likely to occur than with a rough surface, which tends to favor firm fibrin clot formation and eventual neoendothelialization.[103] When blood is exposed to prosthetic devices or any foreign surface, plasma proteins are immediately adsorbed, primarily fibrinogen, albumin, α- and β-globulins, γ globulin, factor VIII, factor XII (Hageman factor), factor XI, and thrombin.[104,104a] Factors XII and XI may be simply adsorbed or may be activated. Fibrinogen appears to be the major plasma protein adsorbed and promotes subsequent platelet adhesion, with platelets adhering as a monolayer and then aggregating. Platelet adhesion will be enhanced/induced not only by fibrinogen but also by γ globulin, thrombin, and subsequent factor XII-factor XI activation.[105] In addition, the activation of factors XII and/or XI may induce intrinsic coagulation, with further fibrin formation generating a platelet-fibrin thrombus. As thrombotic surfaces form and embolize in the aforementioned manner, they may eventually overwhelm the ability of the reticuloendothelial system to clear them; subsequent thromboembolization with vascular occlusion and subsequent end-organ infarction may occur.[106] The most common defects which may generally occur with prosthetic devices are as follows: (1) there may be frank coagulation factor and platelet consumption, with subsequent thrombocytopenia and resultant hemorrhage; (2) devices may cause partial platelet degranulation, with subsequent defective platelet function and resultant hemorrhage; (3) in cases of oxygenation/dialysis membranes, fibrin-platelet deposition will render the exchange ineffective and provide a focus for thromboembolus; and (4) micro- or macrothromboemboli of platelets and/or fibrin may give rise to serious clinical vasoocclusive events. The use of anticoagulants, including warfarin-type drugs, heparin, and platelet-suppressive agents, tends to minimize thrombotic and thromboembolic problems with prosthetic devices. However, the problem still remains clinically significant, especially during CPB surgery, hemodialysis, angiographic studies, prosthetic heart valve placement, long-term intravenous catheterization, and the use of LeVeen shunts.

Intra-arterial or intravenous catheters are coated with fibrin and/or platelet aggregates when used for angiographic studies, long-term chemotherapy, infusion of fluids, and long-term parenteral hyperalimentation.[107] Thromboembolism occurs in approximately 2 percent of individuals catheterized for angiographic studies.[108] An additional complication is that an existing atherosclerotic plaque may be disrupted and embolize. The thromboembolic complications of short-term or long-term catheterization are usually minimized by the use of low-dose intravenous heparin.

Intra-aortic balloon assistance is a widely utilized clinical procedure to control postmyocardial infarction cardiogenic shock and to stabilize selected patients following CPB surgery.[109,110] The balloons in common use are made of polyurethane. Minimal to moderate fibrin formation and minimal platelet aggregation are noted with these assist balloons.[111] However, clinically significant problems remain, including thrombosis, thromboembolism, vasoocclusive ischemic changes in the lower extremities (the balloon is usually introduced via the left common femoral artery), and potential injury to the aortic wall. An additional hematological complication with intra-aortic balloon assistance is hemolysis, which occurs in up to 10 percent of patients. However, the use of heparin or heparin in conjunction with platelet-suppressive therapy appears to have minimized the thrombotic and thromboembolic risks associated with intra-aortic balloon assistance.

Renal hemodialysis is the mainstay of therapy for acute and chronic renal failure, as well as for the alleviation of acute poisoning. However, the formation of fibrin-platelet thrombi on the dialysis membrane greatly reduces its efficiency and provides a focus for embolization, with subsequent potential complications. In addition, renal hemodialysis is commonly associated with neutrophil adherence and complement activation on the dialysis membrane.[112] Since thrombosis and thromboembolism remain major clinical problems associated with renal hemodialysis, systemic or regional heparinization is used. Regional heparinization consists of adding heparin to the arterial line as blood leaves the patient and neutralizing heparin with protamine in the venous lines as blood returns to the patient. Some have considered heparin rebound to be a clinical problem with regional heparinization.[113] Platelet-suppressive therapy has decreased platelet adhesion to dialysis membranes; however, antiplatelet agents must be used cautiously in uremic patients with already compromised platelet function.[114,115] Access shunts in the form of surgically created arteriovenous (AV) shunts or prosthetic AV shunts are necessary for hemodialysis patients, frequently transfused patients, patients undergoing long-term parenteral hyperalimentation, and selected patients undergoing long-term chemotherapy.[64,116] Surgically created AV shunts tend to have fewer thrombotic complications than prosthetic shunts.[117] Although thrombosis of the shunt remains the major significant problem with these devices, infection is also of concern. Prosthetic shunts as well as surgically created shunts are usually "declotted" by the use of surgery or streptokinase, with reasonably good success. Anticoagulant therapy has not become commonplace for patients with AV shunts; however, it has been shown that dipyridamole will correct decreased platelet survival and decreased platelet turnover in patients with these devices.[118] Aspirin alone will not decrease the incidence of shunt thrombosis.

Prosthetic vascular grafts are primarily constructed of Dacron with sufficient porosity to allow for neovascularization, thrombus organization, and nutrient flow. Thrombotic occlusion of prosthetic grafts is not well controlled with heparin or warfarin-type drugs and is now most commonly treated with platelet-suppressive therapy.

Peritoneovenous shunting using a LeVeen valve has become a palliative procedure for the treatment of intractable ascites associated with severe liver disease.[119,120] A generalized hemorrhagic diathesis is frequently seen with the use of Le Veen valves and appears to represent a straightforward DIC-type syndrome[121,122] associated with accelerated fibrinogen and platelet destruction.[123] The removal of ascitic fluid at the time of valve implantation, as well as the use of anticoagulants, have been advocated to abort DIC in patients receiving Le Veen valves.[124] Le Veen shunts are discussed further in Chapter 14.

This chapter has attempted to provide a review of the available literature regarding alterations of hemostasis associated with surgery, particularly CPB surgery. The key to prevention of surgical hemorrhage is to obtain an adequate preoperative workup. Of extreme importance is an adequate history with respect to bleeding tendencies in both the patient and the family; of equal importance is a careful history regarding the use of drugs affecting hemostasis, especially platelets. A careful physical examination, searching for clues of a real or potential bleeding diathesis, may also prevent catastrophic cases of surgical hemorrhage. An adequate presurgical laboratory screen must be performed. In addition to the usual prothrombin time, partial thromboplastin time, and platelet count, a standardized template bleeding time (and thrombin time in patients subjected to CPB) should be added. The use of these simple testing modalities will guard against significant defects in vascular and platelet function. Most instances of nontechnical surgical and heart surgery hemorrhage are due to several well-defined defects in hemostasis which should be readily controllable if approached in a logical manner and as a team effort involving surgeons, cardiac surgeons, pathologists, and hematologists. In addition, this chapter has attempted to highlight thrombohemorrhagic phenomena associated with numerous frequently used prosthetic devices.

## REFERENCES

1. Bick RL, Shanbrom E: A systematic approach to the diagnosis of bleeding disorders. Med Counterpoint 6:27–33, 1972
2. Bick RL: A systematic approach to the diagnosis of bleeding disorders, in Murano G, Bick RL (eds): Basic Concepts of Hemostasis and Thrombosis. Boca Raton, Fla, CRC Press, 1980, pp 81–88
3. Mielke CH, Kaneshiro MM, Maher LA, et al: The standardized normal Ivy bleeding time and its prolongation by aspirin. Blood 34:204–215, 1969
4. Bick RL: Difficult Diagnostic Problems in Hemostasis and Thrombosis. Chicago, American Society of Clinical Pathology No. 5549, 1980
5. Bick RL, Murano G: Primary hyperfibrino(geno)lytic syndromes, in Murano G, Bick RL (eds): Basic Concepts of Hemostasis and Thrombosis. Boca Raton, Fla, CRC Press, 1980, pp 181–204
6. Brecker G, Cronkite EP: Morphology and enumeration of human blood platelets. J Appl Physiol 3:365–377, 1950
7. Hougie C: Fundamentals of Blood Coagulation in Clinical Medicine. New York, McGraw-Hill, 1963, pp 241–243
8. Proctor RR, Rapaport SI: The partial thromboplastin time with kaolin. A simple screening test for first stage plasma clotting factor deficiencies. Am J Clin Pathol 36:212–219, 1961
9. Quick AJ, Stanley-Brown M, Bancroft FW: A study of the coagulation defect in hemophilia and in jaundice. Am J Med Sci 190:501–511, 1935
10. Bick RL: Vascular disorders associated with thrombohemorrhagic phenomena. Semin Thromb Hemostas 5:167–183, 1979
11. Bick RL: Current Concepts of Hemostasis and Thrombosis. Chicago, American Society of Clinical Pathology Manual No. 5548, 1980
12. Bick RL: Vascular disorders, in Murano G, Bick RL (eds): Basic Concepts of Hemostasis and Thrombosis. Boca Raton, Fla, CRC Press, 1980, pp 89–94

13. Bick RL: Alterations of hemostasis associated with malignancy: Etiology, pathophysiology, diagnosis, and management. Semin Thromb Hemostas 5:1–26, 1978

14. Cohen LS: Clinical pharmacology of acetylsalicylic acid. Semin Thromb Hemostas 2:146–175, 1976

15. Mustard JF, Packham MA: Factors influencing platelet function: Adhesion, release, and aggregation. Pharmacol Rev 23:97–187, 1970

16. Triplett DA: Qualitative or functional disorders of platelets, in Triplett DA (ed): Platelet Function. Chicago, American Society of Clinical Pathology, 1978, pp 123–160

17. Triplett DA: Platelet disorders, in Murano G, Bick RL (eds): Basic Concepts of Hemostasis and Thrombosis. Boca Raton, Fla, CRC Press, 1980, pp 95–148

18. Bick RL: Alterations of hemostasis during cardiopulmonary bypass: A comparison between membrane and bubble oxygenators. Am J Clin Pathol 73:300–301, 1980

19. Bick RL: Alterations of hemostasis associated with cardiopulmonary bypass: Pathophysiology, prevention, diagnosis, and management. Semin Thromb Hemostas 3:59–82, 1976

20. Bick RL, Schmalhorst WR, Shanbrom E: Prothrombin complex concentrates: Use in controlling the hemorrhagic diathesis of chronic liver disease. Am J Dig Dis 20:741–749, 1975

21. Bick RL: Disseminated intravascular coagulation (DIC) and related syndromes, in Murano G, Bick RL (eds): Basic Concepts of Hemostasis and Thrombosis. Boca Raton, Fla, CRC Press, 1980, pp 163–180

22. Bick RL: Disseminated intravascular coagulation and related syndromes: Etiology, pathophysiology, diagnosis and management. Am J Hematol 5:265–282, 1978

23. Bick RL: Disseminated intravascular coagulation and related syndromes, in Fareed J, Messmore H, Fenton J, et al (eds): Perspectives in Hemostasis. New York, Pergamon Press, 1981, pp 122–138

24. Bick RL: Treatment of bleeding and thrombosis in the patient with cancer, in Nealon T (ed): Management of the Patient with Cancer. Philadelphia, WB Saunders Co, 1976, pp 48–60

25. Mertins BF, Green LF, Bowie EJW, et al: Fibrinolytic split products and ethanol gelation test in preoperative evaluation of patients with prostatic disease. Mayo Clin Proc 49:642–646, 1974

26. Beall AC, Yow EM, Bloodwell RD, et al: Open heart surgery without blood transfusion. Arch Surg 94:567–570, 1967

27. Cordell AR: Hematological complications of extracorporeal circulation, in Cordell AR, Ellison RG (eds): Complications of Intrathoracic Surgery. Boston, Little, Brown, 1979, pp 27–34

28. Mammen EF: Natural proteinase inhibitors in extracorporeal circulation. Ann NY Acad Sci 146:754–761, 1968

29. Verska JJ, Lonser ER, Brewer LA: Predisposing factors and management of hemorrhage following open-heart surgery. J Cardiovasc Surg (Torino) 13:361–368, 1972

30. Graeff H, Beller FK: Fibrinolytic activity in whole blood, dilute blood, and euglobulin lysis time tests, in Bang N, Beller FK, Deutsch E, et al (eds): Thrombosis and Bleeding Disorders, Theory and Methods. New York, Academic Press, 1970, pp 328–331

31. Menon IS: A study of the possible correlation of euglobulin lysis time and dilute blood clot lysis time in the determination of fibrinolytic activity. Lab Pract 17:334–335, 1968

32. Kevy SV, Glickman RM, Bernhard WF, et al: The pathogenesis and control of the hemorrhagic defect in open-heart surgery. Surg Gynecol Obstet 123:313–318, 1966

33. Signori EE, Penner JA, Kahn DR: Coagulation defects and bleeding in open heart surgery. Ann Thorac Surg 8:521–529, 1969

34. Porter JM, Silver D: Alterations in fibrinolysis and coagulation associated with cardiopulmonary bypass. J Thorac Cardiovasc Surg 56:869–878, 1968

35. Tice DA, Worth MH: Recognition and treatment of postoperative bleeding associated with open heart surgery. Ann NY Acad Sci 146:745–753, 1968

36. Wright TA, Darte J, Mustard WT: Postoperative bleeding after extracorporeal circulation. Can J Surg 2:142–146, 1959

37. von Kaulla KN, Swan H: Clotting deviations in man during cardiac bypass: Fibrinolysis and circulating anticoagulant. J Thorac Surg 36:519–530, 1958

38. Blombäck M, Norén I, Senning A: Coagulation disturbances during extracorporeal circulation and the postoperative period. Acta Chir Scand 127:433–445, 1964

39. Deiter RA, Neville WE, Piffare R, et al: Preoperative coagulation profiles and posthemodilution cardiopulmonary bypass hemorrhage. Am J Surg 121:689–693, 1971

40. Penick GD, Averette HE, Peters RM, et al: The hemorrhagic syndrome complicating extracorporeal shunting of blood: An experimental study of its pathogenesis. Thromb Diath Haemorrh 2:218–225, 1958

41. Trimble AS, Herst R, Grady M, et al: Blood loss in open heart surgery. Arch Surg 93:323–326, 1966

42. Bick RL, Arbegast NR, Holtermann N, et al: Platelet function abnormalities in cardiopulmonary bypass. Circulation 50(suppl III):301, 1974 (abstract)

43. Bick RL, Schmalhorst WR, Crawford L, et al: The hemorrhagic diathesis created by cardiopulmonary bypass. Am J Clin Pathol 63:588, 1975 (abstract)

44. Bick RL, Arbegast NR, Crawford L, et al: Hemostatic defects induced by cardiopulmonary bypass. Vasc Surg 9:228–243, 1975

45. Bick RL, Schmalhorst WR, Arbegast NR: Alterations of hemostasis associated with cardiopulmonary bypass. Am J Clin Pathol 63:588, 1975 (abstract)

46. Casteneda AR: Must heparin be neutralized following open heart operations? J Thorac Cardiovasc Surg 52:716–724, 1966

47. de Vries SI, von Creveld S, Groen P, et al: Studies on the coagulation of the blood in patients treated with extracorporeal circulation. Thromb Diath Haemorrh 5:426–446, 1961

48. Müller N, Popov-Cenić S, Büttner W, et al: Studies of fibrinolytic and coagulation factors during open-heart surgery. II. Postoperative bleeding tendencies and changes in the coagulation system. Thromb Res 7:589–598, 1975

49. Holswade GR, Nachman RL, Killip T: Thrombocytopathies in patients with open-heart surgery. Preoperative treatment with corticosteroids. Arch Surg 94:365–369, 1967

50. Salzman EW: Blood platelets and extracorporeal circulation. Transfusion 3:274–277, 1963

51. Bick RL, Adams T, Schmalhorst WR: Bleeding times, platelet adhesion, and aspirin. Am J Clin Pathol 65:69–72, 1976

52. Bowie EJW, Owen CA, Thompson JH: Platelet adhesiveness in von Willebrand's disease. Am J Clin Pathol 52:69–77, 1969

53. Bowie EJW, Owen CA: The value of measuring platelet adhesiveness in the diagnosis of bleeding diseases. Am J Clin Pathol 60:302–308, 1973

54. Adams T, Schutz L, Goldberg L: Platelet function abnormalities in the myeloproliferative disorders. Scand J Haematol 13:215–224, 1975

55. Hellem AJ: The adhesiveness of human blood platelets in vitro. Scand J Clin Lab Invest Suppl 51:1–147, 1960

56. Bick RL, Fekete LF: Cardiopulmonary bypass hemorrhage: Aggravation by pre-op ingestion of antiplatelet agents. Vasc Surg 13:277–280, 1979

57. Kowalski E, Kopeć M, Wegrzynowicz Z: Influence of fibrinogen degradation products (FDP) on platelet aggregation, adhesiveness, and viscous metamorphosis. Thromb Diath Haemorrh 10:406–423, 1963

58. Kowalski E: Fibrinogen derivatives and their biologic activities. Semin Hematol 5:45–59, 1968

59. Harker LA, Malpass TW, Branson NE, et al: Mechanisms of abnormal bleeding in patients undergoing cardiopulmonary bypass: Acquired transient platelet dysfunction associated with selective $\alpha$-granule release. Blood 56:824–834, 1980

60. Stass S, Bishop C, Fosberg R, et al: Platelets as affected by cardiopulmonary bypass. Trans Am Soc Clin Pathol 35, 1976

61. Behrendt DM, Epstein SE, Morrow AG: Postperfusion nonthrombocytopenic purpura: An uncommon sequel of open heart surgery. Am J Cardiol 22:631–635, 1968

62. Bick RL, Comer TP, Arbegast NR: Fatal purpura fulminans following total cardiopulmonary bypass. J Cardiovasc Surg (Torino) 14:569–571, 1973

63. Derman UM, Rand PW, Barker N: Fibrinolysis after cardiopulmonary bypass and its relationship to fibrinogen. J Thorac Cardiovasc Surg 51:223–228, 1966

64. Bachmann F, McKenna R, Cole ER, et al: The hemostatic mechanism after open-heart surgery. I. Studies on plasma coagulation factors and fibrinolysis in 512 patients after extracorporeal circulation. J Thorac Cardiovasc Surg 70:76–85, 1975

65. Tsuji HK, Redington JV, Kay JH, et al: The study of fibrinolytic and coagulation factors during open heart surgery. Ann NY Acad Sci 146:763–776, 1968

66. Woods JE, Kirklin JW, Owen CA, et al: The effect of bypass surgery on coagulation sensitive clotting factors. Mayo Clin Proc 42:724–735, 1967

67. Gans H, Subramanian V, John S, et al: Theoretical and practical (clinical) considerations concerning proteolytic enzymes and their inhibitors with particular reference to changes in the plasminogen-plasmin system during assisted circulation in man. Ann NY Acad Sci 146:721–736, 1968

68. Palester-Chlebowzyk M, Strzyzewska E, Sitowski W, et al: Detection of the intravascular coagulation of blood clotting. II. Results of the paracoagulation test in patients undergoing open-heart surgery, with extracorporeal circulation. Pol Med J 11:59–66, 1972

69. Kladetsky RG, Popov-Cenić S, Büttner W, et al: Studies of fibrinolytic and coagulation factors during open-heart surgery. I. Fibrinolytic problems during open heart surgery with ECC. Thromb Res 7:579–588, 1975

70. Gomes MM, McGoon D: Bleeding patterns after open-heart surgery. J Thorac Cardiovasc Surg 60:87–97, 1970

71. Bick RL, Kovacs I, Fekete LF: A new two stage functional assay for antithrombin III (heparin cofactor): Clinical and laboratory evaluation. Thromb Res 8:745–756, 1976

72. Lackner H, Javid JP: The clinical significance of the plasminogen level. Am J Clin Pathol 60:175–181, 1973

73. Tsitouris G, Bellet S, Eilberg R, et al: Effects of major surgery on plasmin-plasminogen systems. Arch Intern Med 108:98–104, 1961

74. Wuelfing D, Brandau KP: Fibrinolytic activity after surgery. Minn Med 51:1503–1507, 1968

75. Ygge J: Changes in blood coagulation and fibrinolysis during the postoperative period. Am J Surg 119:225–232, 1970

76. Bick RL, Bishop RC, Warren M, et al: Changes in fibrinolysis and fibrinolytic enzymes during extracorporeal circulation. Trans Am Soc Hematol 109, 1971 (abstract)

77. Bick RL, Bishop RC, Shanbrom ES: Fibrinolytic activity in acute myocardial infarction. Am J Clin Pathol 57:359–363, 1972

78. Bishop RC, Ekert H, Gilchrist G, et al: The preparation and evaluation of a standardized fibrin plate for the assessment of fibrinolytic activity. Thromb Diath Haemorrh 23:202–210, 1970

79. Fareed J: New methods in hemostatic testing, in Fareed J, Messmore H, Fenton J, et al (eds): Perspectives in Hemostasis. New York, Pergamon Press, 1981, pp 310–347

80. Fareed J, Messmore HL, Bermes EW: New perspectives in coagulation testing. Clin Chem 26:1380–1391, 1980

81. Huseby RM, Smith RE: Synthetic oligopeptide substrates: Their diagnostic application in blood coagulation, fibrinolysis, and other pathologic states. Semin Thromb Hemostas 6:173–314, 1980

82. Naeye RL: Thrombotic state after a hemorrhagic diathesis: A possible complication of therapy with epsilon aminocaproic acid. Blood 19:694–701, 1962

83. Verska J: Letter to the editor. Ann Thorac Surg 13:87, 1972

84. Brooks DH, Bahnson HT: An outbreak of hemorrhage following cardiopulmonary bypass. J Thorac Cardiovasc Surg 63:449–452, 1972

85. O'Neill JA, Ende N, Collins IS, et al: A quantitative determination of perfusion fibrinolysis. Surgery 60:809–812, 1966

86. Pechet L: Fibrinolysis. N Engl J Med 273:966–973, 1965
87. Sharp AA: The significance of fibrinolysis. Proc R Soc Lond (Biol) 173:311–315, 1969
88. Sherry S, Fletcher AP, Alkjaersig N: Fibrinolysis and fibrinolytic activity in man. Physiol Rev 39:343–382, 1959
89. Larrieu MJ, Dray L, Ardaillou N: Biological effects of fibrinogen-fibrin degradation products. Thromb Diath Haemorrh 34:686–692, 1975
90. Alkjaersig N, Fletcher AP, Sherry S: Pathogenesis of the coagulation defect developing during pathological plasma proteolytic (''fibrinolytic'') states. II. The significance, mechanism, and consequences of defective fibrin polymerization. J Clin Invest 41:917–934, 1962
91. Latallo ZS, Fletcher AP, Alkjersig N, et al: Inhibition of fibrin polymerization by fibrinogen proteolysis products. Am J Physiol 202:681–686, 1962
92. Akkerman JW, Runne WC, Sixma JJ, et al: Improved survival rates in dogs after extracorporeal circulation by improved control of heparin levels. J Thorac Cardiovasc Surg 68:59–65, 1974
93. Ellison N, Beatty CP, Blake DR, et al: Heparin rebound: Studies in patients and volunteers. J Thorac Cardiovasc Surg 67:723–729, 1974
94. Gollub S: Heparin rebound in open-heart surgery. Surg Gynecol Obstet 124:337–346, 1967
95. Jaberi M, Bell WR, Benson DW: Control of heparin therapy in open-heart surgery. J Thorac Cardiovasc Surg 67:133–141, 1974
96. Ellison N, Ominsky AJ, Wollman H: Is protamine a clinically important anticoagulant? A negative answer. Anesthesiology 35:621–629, 1971
97. Ollendorff P: The nature of the anticoagulant effect of heparin, protamine, Polybrene, and toluidine blue. Scand J Clin Lab Invest 14:267–276, 1962
98. Soloway HB, Cornett BM, Donahoo JV, et al: Differentiation of bleeding diathesis which occurs following protamine correction of heparin anticoagulation. Am J Clin Pathol 60:188–191, 1973
99. Lewis HJ, Wilson HJ, Brandon JM: Counterelectrophoresis test for molecules immunologically similar to fibrinogen. Am J Clin Pathol 58:400–404, 1972
100. Forbes CD: Thrombosis and artificial surfaces, in Prentice CRM (ed): Thrombosis. Clin Haematol 10:653–668, 1981
101. Seegers WH: Basic principles of blood coagulation. Semin Thromb Hemostas 7:180–198, 1981
102. Salzman EW: The events that led to thrombosis. Bull NY Acad Med 48:225–234, 1972
103. Braunwald NS, Bonchek L: Prevention of thrombus formation on rigid prosthetic heart valves by the ingrowth of autogenous tissue. J Thorac Cardiovasc Surg 54:630–638, 1967
104. Bagnall RD: Absorption of plasma proteins on hydrophobic surfaces. II. Fibrinogen and fibrinogen-containing protein mixtures. Biomed Biomater Res 12:203–207, 1978
104a. Hubbard D, Lucas GL: Ionic charges of glass surfaces and other materials and their possible role in the coagulation of blood. J Appl Physiol 15:265–270, 1960
105. Mason RG: The interaction of blood hemostatic elements with artificial surfaces, in Spaet TH (ed): Progress in Hemostasis and Thrombosis. New York, Grune & Stratton, 1972, pp 141–164
106. Knieriem HJ, Chandler AB: The effect of warfarin sodium on the duration of platelet aggregation. Thromb Diath Haemorrh 18:766–772, 1967
107. Lessin LS, Jensen WH, Kelser GA, et al: Scanning electron microscopy of thrombogenesis on vascular catheter surfaces. N Engl J Med 286:139–140, 1972
108. Moore CH, Wolma FJ, Brown RW, et al: Complications of cardiovascular radiology. A review of 1204 cases. Am J Surg 120:591–593, 1970
109. Bolooki N: Clinical Application of Intra-aortic Balloon Pump. New York, Futura Publishing, 1977
110. Okada M, Shiozawa T, Iizuka M, et al: Experimental and clinical studies on the effect of

intra-aortic balloon pumping for cardiogenic shock following acute myocardial infarction. Artif Organs 3:271–276, 1979

111. Schoen FJ, DeLaria GA, Bernstein EF: Evaluation of intra-aortic balloon surfaces by scanning electron microscopy. Surg Forum 23:167–168, 1972

112. Kapplow LS, Goffinet JA: Profound neutropenia durng early phase of haemodialysis. JAMA 203:133–135, 1968

113. Hampers CL, Blanfox MD, Merrill JP: Anticoagulation rebound after hemodialysis. N Engl J Med 275:776–778, 1966

114. Lindsay RM, Prentice CRM, Davidson JF, et al: Hemostatic changes during dialysis, associated with thrombus formation on dialysis membranes. Br Med J 4:454–458, 1972

115. Woods HF, Ash G, Weston MJ: Sulfinpyrazone reduced deposition of fibrinon dialyser membranes. Thromb Haemostas 42:401, 1979 (abstract)

116. Williams BT, Blainey JD, Dawson-Edwards P, et al: Use of the Quinton-Scribner arteriovenous shunt in the management of aplastic anemia. Br Med J 2:484–485, 1967

117. Kuruvila KC, Beven EG: Arteriovenous shunts and fistulas for hemodialysis. Surg Clin North Am 51:1219–1242, 1971

118. Harker LA, Slichter SJ: Platelet and fibrinogen survival in man. N Engl J Med 287:999–1005, 1972

119. LeVeen HH, Christoudias G, Ip M, et al: Peritoneovenous shunting for ascites. Ann Surg 180:580–591, 1974

120. Reinhardt GF, Stanley MM: Peritoneovenous shunting for ascites. Surg Gynecol Obstet 145:419–424, 1977

121. Lerner RG, Nelson JC, Corines P, et al: Disseminated intravascular coagulation: Complication of LeVeen peritoneovenous shunts. JAMA 240:2064–2066, 1978

122. Harmon DC, Demirjian Z, Ellman L, et al: Disseminated intravascular coagulation with the peritoneovenous shunt. Ann Intern Med 90:774–776, 1979

123. Stein SF, Fulenwider JT, Ansley JD, et al: Accelerated fibrinogen and platelet destruction after peritoneovenous shunting. Arch Intern Med 141:1149–1151, 1981

124. Kitchens, C: Personal communication

Virginia H. Donaldson

# 13

# Hemorrhagic Disorders of Neonates

The coagulation mechanism of the newly born infant may be inadequate for the challenges of extrauterine life because of the balance that necessarily exists between the biosynthesis and utilization, or catabolism, of procoagulants in plasma. The immaturity of hepatic synthetic mechanisms may leave the infant with suboptimal amounts of certain procoagulants, and this situation may be worse in the prematurely born. The prematurely born is at an added disadvantage, because the permeability and fragility of its capillaries are increased as compared to the full-term infant.[1] The platelet count in the premature infant may also be normal or slightly low, with subnormal adenosine diphosphate (ADP)-induced aggregation, and prolonged bleeding time.[1-4] The bleeding time is, in fact, inversely related to the gestational age.[1] In a full-term normal infant, on the other hand, vascular fragility and permeability, as well as bleeding time, are normal.[1,5-7]

## PHYSIOLOGY OF THE COAGULATION MECHANISM IN THE NEWLY BORN

Coagulation factors do not appear to cross the placental barrier,[8,9] with the possible exception of factors IX (Christmas factor) and XIII (fibrin-stablizing factor).[1,9,10]

### Fibrinogen

The concentration of fibrinogen in the plasma of normal newborn infants is within the normal adult range, but the thrombin-induced clotting time of plasma obtained from the umbilical artery or vein is prolonged, and fibrin clots formed of cord plasma are resistant to compression.[11] The rate of polymerization of fibrin monomers derived from fibrinogen isolated from cord plasma is delayed as compared to polymerization of fibrin monomers from normal adult plasma fibrinogen,[12] and this difference is exaggerated with high salt concentrations.[13] This is probably due to a qualitative alteration in the fibrinogen synthesized by the fetus, for there may be a unique species of fetal fibrinogen. The nature of the alteration in the structure of this fibrinogen is not entirely clear. In some studies, peptide maps of tryptic digests of fetal fibrinogen differed from those of adult fibrinogen,[14] the phosphorus content of fetal fibrinogen was greater than that of adult fibrinogen,[15] and fetal fibrinogen was isoelectric at a higher pH than adult fibrinogen.[16] Some of the unusual properties of fibrinogen derived from cord plasma may be due to fragments of fibrinogen released by proteolytic activity such as fibrinolysis, for when blood was drawn from umbilical cord vessels into inhibitors of fibrinolysis, the coagulation abnormalities were not found.[17,18] A recent reevaluation of this problem, however, showed that polymerization of fibrin monomers from fibrinogen from umbilical cord blood differed from that of normal adult fibrinogen. This difference depended upon the ionic strength of the solvent used,[13] but no evidence was found that fibrinogen fragments released by proteolytic activity delayed the polymerization of fibrin monomers. In addition, no clear evidence of structural differences in fibrinogen chains between adult and fetal (cord) fibrinogens was found.[13] Nonetheless, the investigators favored the view that a genetically determined fetal fibrinogen does exist.[13]

Despite these impressive alterations in laboratory measurements of the last stage of clotting, there is no hemorrhagic state associated with the presence of fetal fibrinogen, and hemorrhage in the newborn should not be ascribed to it.

## Factors VIII (Antihemophilic factor, AHF) and V (Proaccelerin)

The factor VIII molecule is large and complex, and consists of functionally different subunits:[19]

Factor VIII coagulant activity; Factor VIII-related antigen (which does not have coagulant activity); and Factor VIII-ristocetin-cofactor activity (required for the aggregation of platelets by the antibiotic ristocetin).

All of these properties of the factor VIII molecule exist in higher concentrations in plasma from normal full-term infants than in normal adult plasma samples,[20] and the levels are elevated in maternal plasma during pregnancy as well. The electrophoretic mobility of the factor VIII-related antigen in plasma from normal full-term infants is normal.[20] There is no notable difference between the levels of factor VIII coagulant activity in infants delivered vaginally and those delivered by cesarean section.[20] In one survey, plasma from sick infants contained twice as much factor VIII-related antigen as plasma from healthy newborns, but the electrophoretic mobility of these antigens was normal.[20] Only in severely ill infants was the electrophoretic mobility of the factor VIII-related antigen more anodal than normal; these infants may have had intravascular clot-promoting activity, with diffuse intravascular coagulation and possibly secondary fibrinolytic activity.[20] In another study, qualitative abnormalities of factor VIII-related antigens, probably due to plasma proteolytic activity, were found in one-half of the cord blood samples from a group of newborn infants, but it is not clear that they were all normal.[21] Increased levels of factor VIII in plasma from newly born infants probably reflect increased release from the endothelium,[20] where it is synthesized.[22]

Factor V procoagulant activity in plasma from normal umbilical cord vessels is within the normal adult range of concentration.[23]

## Hageman Factor (Factor XII), Plasma Prekallikrein (Fletcher Factor), High Molecular Weight Kininogen (HMWK), and Plasma Thromboplastin Antecedent (Factor XI, PTA)

When coagulation is initiated in vitro by exposing plasma to a glass surface or certain negatively charged substances, Hageman factor, plasma prekallikrein, HMWK, and PTA interact to form clot-promoting activity and also to release vasoactive polypeptides, such as bradykinin.[24,25] Bradykinin is derived from HMWK, which also has clot-promoting activity.[26] The concentrations of each of these clotting factors are lower in plasma from the normal newborn infant than in adult plasma.[27,28] Maternal plasma levels of PTA are within the normal adult range during pregnancy,[26] but prekallikrein and Hageman factor levels are higher than those in normal adult plasmas.[29-31] The concentrations of the specific antigens of the Hageman factor and prekallikrein molecules were somewhat higher in plasma from normal newborns than were the procoagulant activities,[28] as if precursor molecules which do not yet have full procoagulant activity may exist in the newborn. It is also possible that the molecules may have been damaged in vivo, altering their procoagulant functions. Of this group of procoagulants, it is likely that the deficiency of Hageman factor, but not of the other 3 factors, contributes to the prolonged plasma clotting time characteristic of this age group.[28] However, since a hemorrhagic tendency is not associated with severe inherited deficiencies of Hageman factor, HMWK, or prekallikrein, these deficiencies should not play a direct part in any bleeding which occurs in the newborn infant. Neonatal PTA deficiency, on the other hand, may play a role.[27] The concentration of PTA gradually increases after birth, reaching normal adult levels in about 60 days.[27]

## Fibrinolysis

The concentration of plasminogen, the precursor of the fibrinolytic enzyme plasmin, is lower in plasma from newly born infants than in normal adult plasma[32] and may remain low for 6 weeks or more.[33] This deficiency may be exaggerated in the prematurely born. On the other hand, the inhibitory activity in plasma directed against plasmin may also be lower than that in adult plasma.[34] Therefore, an equilibrium may exist at these lowered concentrations of fibrinolytic components which permits activation under stressful conditions such as anoxia or exercise; both are known to provoke enhanced fibrinolytic activity in plasma. The blood plasma of the newborn may actually have increased fibrinolytic activity as compared to adult plasma,[35,36] but this activity decreases rapidly after birth.[37] The fact that fragments released from fibrinogen by the action of plasmin (fibrin split products, or FSP) are not elevated in umbilical vein or umbilical artery blood suggests that free fibrinolytic activity is not present to a measurable degree during delivery.[36,38,39]

## Inhibitors

Critical to the normal balance of the clotting and fibrinolytic mechanisms are the inhibitors which regulate the action of the enzymes which can evolve.

### Antithrombin III (AT III)

ATIII, an $\alpha$-globulin heparin cofactor[49] found in normal plasma, can inhibit factor Xa (Stuart-Prower factor),[40-42] thrombin,[43-47] factors IXa,[48] XIa,[47] and XIIa,[50] and plasmin.[51] Although the concentrations of ATIII in plasma of normal neonates are reduced to levels found in some individuals reported to have hereditary deficiencies of ATIII (about 50 percent of normal adult levels),[52] this does not apparently predispose the *normal* infant to thrombosis; however, it may do so in the sick neonate when clot-promoting activity is generated in the blood. When ATIII was isolated from cord blood from term and premature infants, it functioned just like the ATIII from normal adult plasma in inhibiting factor Xa and thrombin. Nor could it be distinguished from adult ATIII upon sodium dodecyl sulfate polyacrylamide gel electrophoresis, either in its heparin cofactor activity or in its molecular weight.[53] Therefore, there was no qualitative abnormality of ATIII in the cord plasmas of premature or term infants.

### α-2-Macroglobulin (α₂M)

$\alpha_2$M can inhibit a broad spectrum of proteases and is widely distributed in the body.[54] It is able to interact with several hemostatic enzymes in plasma and probably with most proteases, but in this process it is cleaved by the enzyme and forms a complex with it in which the enzyme may retain some activity.[54] $\alpha_2$M can thus interact with plasmin, but the complex still has esterase activity and some fibrinogenolytic activity.[55] $\alpha_2$M is found in high concentrations in plasma from infants; it may be 2.5 times as high in the plasma of infants as in that of adults,[56,57] and it increases during pregnancy[58] and in women on oral contraceptives.[59]

$\alpha_2$M can inhibit kallikrein,[60] the coagulant activity of thrombin,[61] and also some of the proteolytic properties of plasmin, including much of its fibrinogenolytic activity.[55,62]

### α₂-Antiplasmin (α₂PI)

$\alpha_2$PI is a more effective inhibitor of plasmin than $\alpha_2$M, and is an important regulator of fibrinolytic activity in plasma, for individuals with an inherited deficiency of $\alpha_2$PI have a bleeding tendency.[63,64] It can also inhibit plasma coagulants including activated Hageman factor, fragments of Hageman factor which activate prekallikrein, plasma kallikrein, activated PTA, and thrombin.[65] Its concentration in the plasma of the neonate has not been defined.

### C1̄ Inhibitor

C1̄ inhibitor, an $\alpha$-globulin found in normal human serum, is the only known inhibitor in plasma of the activated first component of complement, C1̄.[66,67] In addition, it inhibits plasma kallikrein (Fletcher factor), plasmin, activated Hageman factor, enzymatically active fragments of Hageman factor, and activated PTA (factor XIa),[68–70] but these substances are also regulated by other inhibitory substances in plasma.[67] Levels of C1̄ inhibitor activity often drop significantly during the second and third trimesters of pregnancy, but its concentration in the umbilical cord plasma or serum of normal infants is normal and remains so during the first 4 days of life.[71] A deficiency of this inhibitor is not associated with any tendency to thromboembolism; no such inclination has been reported in persons with hereditary angioneurotic edema, who have almost no C1̄ inhibitor activity in their serum,[72] and C1̄ inhibitor is not known to play a role in thromboembolism in infancy. In several infants who were later determined to have hereditary angioneurotic edema, trace amounts of C1̄ inhibitor activity were found in their serum in early infancy.[73] There is no evidence that this protein can cross the placental barrier.

*α₁-Antitrypsin*

$\alpha_1$-Antitrypsin is an $\alpha$-globulin in serum which inhibits trypsin[74] and elastase.[75] This may explain the tendency of persons with deficient function of this inhibitor to have pulmonary emphysema. Leukocytic elastases can also promote fibrinolysis.[76] In addition, they hydrolyze and inactivate factors VIII, XII, XIII, and fibrinogen, and partially inactivate factor V.[77] $\alpha_1$-Antitrypsin may therefore be important in regulating clot-promoting activity which may develop in the blood of the sick neonate, but there is presently no direct support for this possibility.

## DEVELOPMENT OF PROCOAGULANTS IN THE FETUS

Fetal tissues synthesize fibrinogen after as little as 5.5 weeks of gestation,[78] but plasminogen is not synthesized until 10 weeks of gestation.[78] At the end of the first trimester (11–12 weeks) fetal blood is coagulable,[79] and fibrinolytic activity can be found in fetal blood after 12 weeks of gestation.[36] In the second trimester the clotting time of fetal blood is actually shorter than that of normal adults.[80] Other coagulation factors have been identified in conceptuses after varying periods of gestation (Table 13-1). These and other related data have been summarized by others.[1,80–86] Table 13-1 describes the level of coagulants as a percentage of the normal adult level, arbitrarily defined as 100 percent, with the exception of fibrinogen levels, which are given in milligrams per deciliter. One must interpret the low levels of coagulation factors in the neonatal period with caution, for many of the assays were done without consideration of the relative polycythemia of the newborn and the consequent decrease in plasma volume when anticoagulants were added to blood samples. It should also be borne in mind that when umbilical cord blood samples are tested, the coagulant activity of the umbilical vein blood is higher than that of the umbilical artery, suggesting that the placental circulation contributes clot-promoting activity to the venous side of the umbilical circulation.[87]

Patterns of development of procoagulant activities in utero have been monitored in studies of fetal lambs.[88] There was a decrease in fibrinogen, prothrombin, and factor VII in fetal plasma during the last trimester of pregnancy, but the levels of factors V, VIII, IX, X, XI, and XIII increased during this period.[88] Further, the activities of factors VIII and IX increased during delivery.

## VITAMIN K-DEPENDENT COAGULATION FACTORS AND HEMORRHAGIC DISEASE OF THE NEWBORN

Vitamin K is essential for the synthesis of several clotting factors, for it enables the biosynthetic mechanism of the liver to carboxylate certain glutamic acid residues on the prothrombin molecule after it has been synthesized by the liver.[89,90] The $\gamma$-carboxyglutamic residues are essential to the function of the prothrombin molecule because of their ability to bind calcium and lipids; this calcium-binding region is absent from the prothrombin molecule in the plasma of persons taking coumarin anticoagulants.[91,92] Similar structural deficiencies in factors VII, IX, and X molecules synthesized in the presence of vitamin K antagonists have also been described[93–96] using immunologic techniques.

**Table 13-1**

Plasma Procoagulants During Gestation of the Human Fetus

| Factor | Gestation Time, Weeks | | | | | | Adult |
|---|---|---|---|---|---|---|---|
| | 20 | 24–31 | 27–31 | 32–35 | 36–39 | Term | |
| Fibrinogen (± 1 SD) | — | 282 ± 60 mg/dl | 256 ± 70 mg/dl | 260 ± 80 mg/dl | 230 ± 50 mg/dl | 215 ± 35 mg/dl | 315 ± 60 mg/dl |
| Factor V | 28 ± 10% | 73% | 91 ± 30% | 90 ± 12% | 85 ± 15% | 56—200% (cord blood) | 100% |
| Factor VIII-related antigen | 104 ± 28% | — | — | — | — | — | 100% |
| Coagulant antigen | 19 ± 7% | — | — | — | — | — | 100% |
| Coagulant activity | 12 ± 3% | 87% | 90% | 120% | 120% | 50 – 180% (cord blood) | 100% |
| Factor XII | — | — | — | — | — | 44 ± 13% (venous blood) | 100% |
| Factor XI | — | 20% | — | — | — | 31% (cord blood) | 100% |
| Prekallikrein (Fletcher factor) | | | | | | 36 ± 14% (venous blood) | 100% |
| High Molecular Weight Kininogen, HMWK | | | | | | 64 ± 10% (venous blood) | 100% |
| Vitamin K dependent | | | | | | | |
| Prothrombin antigen | 19 ± 3% | — | — | — | — | — | 100% |
| Prothrombin activity | — | 31% | 30 ± 8% | 33 ± 11% | 52 ± 20% | 54 ± 15% | 100% |
| Factor X | 19 ± 2% | — | — | — | — | — | 100% |
| Factor VII | 21 ± 6% | — | — | — | — | — | 100% |
| Factor X–VII complex | 29% | 29% | 38 ± 14% | 42 ± 20% | 43 ± 20% | 56 ± 16% | 100% |
| Factor IX | 5 ± 2% | 22% | 27% | 34 ± 14% | 43 ± 13% | 15 ± 42% (cord blood) | 100% |

Another vitamin K-dependent protein synthesized by the liver was recently described. Protein C[97] is a proteolytic zymogen which can be activated by thrombin[98] in the presence of an endothelial cell cofactor.[98] Once active, it can destroy the coagulant properties of factors VIII and V[99] and can enhance the fibrinolytic activity in human plasma.[100] There is presently no information available regarding protein C levels in plasma from neonates. A protein which is active in osteogenesis, called osteocalcin, also contains a peptide with essential glutamic acid residues dependent upon vitamin K for its production.[101,102] Although this protein is not active in hemostasis, interference with its synthesis in the fetus may play a role in the embryopathy induced by maternal ingestion of coumarin anticoagulants.

The deficiency of vitamin K-dependent plasma-clotting factors is the main reason for the occasional delayed clotting and prolongation of the prothrombin time in plasma from normal newborn infants. These factors include factors VII, IX (Christmas factor), X (Stuart-Prower factor), and prothrombin. Some investigators have suggested that vitamin K may not actually be deficient because the prothrombin time of the newborn is frequently within the normal adult range, and there is a suggestion of inadequate synthesis of the portions of the molecule not requiring vitamin K, which are then modified by vitamin K.[103,104] Nonetheless, when levels of vitamin K-dependent clotting factors are quantified in the newborn plasma, they are low. During the first few days of life, the already decreased levels of factors VII, IX, X, and prothrombin become progressively lower; this decrease can be prevented by administering vitamin K parenterally to the newborn infant.[6] Normal adult levels of vitamin K-dependent clotting factors may not be reached for several weeks in the normal neonate,[105] but in vitro measures of blood coagulation, including the plasma prothrombin time, may become normal before that period because the optimal hemostatic function determined by such a test occurs when these clotting factors are at about 50 percent of the normal level.[106]

To prevent a decrease in the concentration of vitamin K-dependent clotting factors during the first week of life, vitamin $K_1$, considered the drug of choice, should be administered to the newborn in a single parenteral dose of 0.5 or 1.0 mg, or in an oral dose of 1.0 or 2.0 mg. It may occasionally be necessary to repeat this dosage for therapeutic effect.[104,107] In one study, as little as 100 μg of vitamin K was as effective as 5 mg in preventing hemorrhage due to deficiencies of vitamin K-dependent clotting factors.[108] Since the effectiveness of vitamin K administered to the mother prior to delivery is variable, and since the appropriate dose, time of administration, and duration of treatment of the mother are uncertain, this prophylactic approach is not recommended, and the newborn infant should be given vitamin K directly.[107,109–111]

Table 13-2 describes some natural vitamin K compounds, and Table 13-3 designates some synthetic analogues used in prophylaxis and therapy for vitamin K deficiency of neonates. Care should be exercised in the use of menadione sodium diphosphate (Synkavite); because of the hemolysis and hyperbilirubinemia which it may induce, its use is discouraged.

## HEMORRHAGIC DISEASE OF THE NEWBORN

A self-limited hemorrhagic disease of the newly born infant was recognized in 1894,[110] and was noted to be distinct from the hereditary hemostatic disorders associated with lifelong disability. Characteristically, bleeding begins on the second or third day of life, but it may occur on the first day. The most common site of bleeding is the gastrointestinal tract, but occasionally bleeding from the nose or into the skin, internal organs, or umbilicus has

**Table 13-2**

Vitamin K Sources
Natural Compounds

| | Vitamin K$_1$ | Vitamin K$_2$ |
|---|---|---|
| | (2-methyl-3-phytyl-1,4 naphthoquinone) | (2-methyl-3-difarnesyl-1,4 naphthoquinone) |
| USP designation | Phytonadione | — |
| Solubility | Fat | Fat |
| Source | Green plants | Gastrointestinal bacterial flora |
| Preparations: | Phytonadione and Mephyton (oily preparations) for oral or intravenous administration | None |
| | Aquamephyton and Konakion (aqueous suspensions) for oral, subcutaneous, intramuscular, or intravenous administration | |

Data from the Report of the Committee on Nutrition, American Academy of Pediatrics. Pediatrics 28:501–505, 1961. With permission.

been observed. Hemorrhagic disease of the newborn is associated with a deficiency of vitamin K, and therefore of prothrombin, factor VII, factor X, and factor IX. It can be prevented by parenteral injection of vitamin K into the infant at the time of delivery.

The time of onset of bleeding and the nature of infant feeding influence the degree of the coagulation defect and the incidence of the hemorrhagic disorder. If milk feedings are begun 8 hours following delivery, rather than later, the levels of prothrombin in the infant's blood are higher at 3 days of life than they are if feedings are begun later.[111] Moreover, the use of cow's milk enhances the biosynthesis of vitamin K-dependent clotting factors, in part because cow's milk contains about 4 times as much vitamin K (6 μg/dl) as human breast milk (1.5 μg/dl).[112] The difference in the gastrointestinal flora in infants fed cow's milk rather than breast milk may be an important factor as an endogenous source of vita-

**Table 13-3**
Vitamin K Analogues

| Compound | USP Designation | Solubility | Route | Preparations Marketed (U.S.) |
|---|---|---|---|---|
| 2-Methyl 1,4-naphthoquinone | Menadione | Water | Intravenous Intramuscular | Menadione |
| 2-Methyl-2-sodium bisulfite-3-dehydro-1,4 naphthoquinone | Menadione sodium bisulfite | Water | Oral Intravenous Intramuscular | Hykinone, menadione sodium bisulfite |
| 2-Methyl-1,4-naphthalendiol tetrasodium diphosphate hexahydrate | Menadiol sodium diphospate | Water | Oral Intravenous Intramuscular | Synkavite, menadiol sodium diphosphate |

Data from the Report of the Committee on Nutrition, American Academy of Pediatrics. Pediatrics 28:501–505, 1961.

min K in infants on cow's milk formulas. In some studies, hemorrhagic disease of the newborn and associated hypoprothrombinemia appeared to be limited to breast-fed infants not given vitamin K.[108] Moreover, if cow's milk feedings were given without parenteral vitamin K, the prothrombinlike activity in the plasma of infants 24 hours after this feeding did not differ from that in infants given vitamin K at birth.[113] Cow's milk formulas thus have a preventive effect in hemorrhagic disease of the newborn.

The incidence of hemorrhagic disease in the newborn is tremendously variable. One group reported that 1.7 percent of infants not receiving vitamin K had moderate or severe bleeding;[108] on the other hand, 0.4 percent of those who had been given vitamin K had similar bleeding. Another estimate of the incidence of the disease places it between 1 in 200 and 1 in 400 births.[114] It should be suspected when hemorrhage occurs in an apparently healthy newborn infant who has no history of having received vitamin K at birth. Serious bleeding can involve the central nervous system and adrenal glands or the gastrointestinal tract, and anemia may occur rapidly because of hemorrhage.

Another factor that may increase the severity of this disease include the ingestion of anticonvulsant medication by the mother during pregnancy. Infants born of epileptic mothers who have received barbiturates, phenytoin, or primidone are extremely susceptible to hemorrhagic disease of the newborn,[103,115] and the mother with epilepsy requiring treatment should be given vitamin K orally for at least the last 2 months of pregnancy.[116] The infant of an epileptic mother receiving treatment who develops hemorrhagic disease of the newborn will require larger amounts of vitamin K than the normal infant to alleviate the hemostatic defect, and may require replacement tranfusion for active bleeding.[117]

## MATERNAL FACTORS PRESENTING A HEMOSTATIC RISK TO THE FETUS AND NEONATE

Hemorrhagic death has occurred in the offspring or fetuses of mothers taking coumarin anticoagulants.[118-120] When the drug is administered during pregnancy, it should be stopped at least 4 weeks before delivery.[121] Heparin should probably be used in preference to coumarin drugs whenever possible, and should certainly be substituted for coumarin drugs in the last months of pregnancy if anticoagulation is required.[117] Heparin therapy is preferable because this anticoagulant does not cross the placental barrier.[122-124] It should be used, however, with the knowledge that the incidence of maternal hemorrhage, stillbirth, fetal death, and fetal abnormalities is increased by this treatment.[125] Even so, the risk of pulmonary embolism in pregnant women with leg vein thrombosis is so high that treatment with heparin is indicated.[122] When heparin is used for the treatment of maternal thromboembolic disease, an initial intravenous injection of 10,000–15,000 U may be given, followed by intravenous injections of 10,000 U every 4–6 hours. Even more preferable is heparin given continuously as an intravenous infusion in an acute situation. The whole blood clotting time or the activated partial thromboplastin time should be measured before the administration of intravenous heparin, with the aim of extending the clotting time to 1.5–2.0 times the normal value.[120] The continuous infusion of heparin, particularly in acute thrombosis, has the obvious advantage of maintaining a steady level of anticoagulation; an increased incidence of bleeding during heparin therapy by bolus injections, rather than continuous intravenous injections, has been reported. Prolonged therapy with subcutaneous heparin given in doses of 20,000 U every 12 hours for 2 weeks, and then of 10,000 U every 12 hours for several weeks more in late pregnancy and into the postpartum period, has been successful but may harm the fetus.[118,125-127]

An additional theoretical risk to maternal ingestion of coumarin anticoagulants lies in the possibility that these drugs may appear in breast milk, and thereby place a breast-fed infant at risk.[128] This risk may not be significant, because the prothrombin time of plasmas from infants breast fed by mothers receiving therapeutic doses of anticoagulants are not prolonged[129] and the coumarinlike substances in breast milk may be inactive metabolites.[131] It is not clear if protein C or osteocalcin synthesis may be affected by coumarinlike substances which may be found in such breast milk.

The congenital malformations resulting from coumarin therapy during pregnancy can be devastating,[131] and fetal mortality resulting from hemorrhage into the fetus is about 50 percent.[124] A "warfarin embryopathy" may result from intrauterine hemorrhage in the fetus secondary to the coagulation defects induced by the drug, but it is likely that a deficiency of the vitamin K-dependent bone protein osteocalcin (page 415) also plays a role in these disorders.[101,102] Ingestion of coumarin anticoagulants during the first trimester of pregnancy may cause chondrodysplasia punctata, which is characterized by short stature, stippled epiphyses, saddle nose, nasal hypoplasia, and frontal bossing. Maternal coumarin ingestion is also associated with fetal cataracts, mental retardation, and flexure contractures, which are probably intrauterine sequelae to fetal hemorrhage during gestation.[132–134]

Intravascular clotting in the pregnant female affects the fetus, presumably because clot-promoting substances cross the placental barrier. In an experimental situation, when intravascular coagulation was induced in pregnant sheep, clot-promoting activity with laboratory evidence of intravascular coagulation could be observed in the fetus.[135] Indeed, human infants born of mothers with high-risk pregnancies, including preeclampsia, third trimester bleeding related to abruptio placenta, premature labor, and toxemia with hypertension, may have evidence of varying degrees of intravascular coagulation, including thrombocytopenia, in blood obtained from the umbilical cord vessels at birth. Cord blood samples should be examined in these situations; severe anemia secondary to impaired hemostasis may predispose the infant to the consequences of anoxia in the neonatal period, and this may require early treatment.[136] Otherwise, infants delivered of women having high-risk factors late in pregnancy merit careful observation in the newborn nursery. Once delivery is completed, further risk of transmitting maternal pathology to the infant is terminated.

When therapeutic abortion is induced by intra-amniotic injection of hypertonic saline, true disseminated intravascular coagulation appears to evolve in the maternal bloodstream.[136] This condition, however, is not usually associated with an obvious hemorrhagic tendency in the mother.[137]

Maternal causes of reductions in the platelet count of infants are discussed in a later section.

## BLEEDING IN THE SICK NEONATE

The causes of hemorrhage in the sick neonate differ from those in a healthy newborn infant, as summarized in Table 13-4.

### Disseminated Intravascular Coagulation

The hemostatic disasters associated with intravascular clotting have received much attention in recent years, and several reviews of this subject have been published with particular reference to newborns and children.[138–141] The process of intravascular coagulation may be widely disseminated in vivo, and the term *disseminated intravascular*

**Table 13-4**
Causes of Bleeding in Healthy and
Sick Neonates

Causes of bleeding in a healthy neonate
   Hemorrhagic disease of the newborn
   Hereditary deficiency of plasma clotting factors
   Vascular anomalies
   Trauma
   Thrombocytopenia
Causes of bleeding in a sick neonate
   Intravascular coagulation with:
      Fetal distress
      Anoxia
      Sepsis
      Erythroblastosis fetalis (severe)
      Respiratory distress syndrome
   Severe trauma (intraventricular, perirenal
      hemorrhage, etc.)

*coagulation* is frequently applied to the hemostatic disorder associated with circulating clot-promoting activity which leads to consumption of coagulation factors and a secondary major hemostatic defect. When this occurs, platelets, plasma-clotting factors including prothrombin, factors V, VIII, and XIII, fibrinogen, and plasminogen may be depleted in a consumptive process in which fibrin may be deposited in the capillaries, and plasminogen becomes activated secondarily. The infant or premature neonate, in particular, may be unable to adjust its biosynthetic mechanisms to correct these defects, and a bleeding syndrome results. Because of the deposits of fibrin and platelets in the small blood vessels, relative ischemia to various organs may then cause tissue necrosis and release of thromboplastic substances into the blood, thus worsening the situation. In addition, microangiopathic damage to the erythrocytes occurs because of intravascular fibrin that impairs their transport through the small vessels, leading to a morphologic change characterized by polymorphic fragmentation.

Intravascular coagulation on a widely disseminated basis is probably a complicating factor in most overwhelming illnesses. It may be initiated by damage to the endothelium, by endotoxin, by thromboplastic materials which gain access to the circulating blood, by proteolytic enzymes (certain venoms, for example), by injection of particulate matter, and by platelet aggregation from any of a number of causes. In the newborn infant, disseminated intravascular coagulation may occur to some degree in association with abruptio placentae or placenta praevia,[142] and if third trimester maternal bleeding has occurred, the newly born infant may have hemorrhagic shock and anemia. Asphyxia at birth, shock, and anemia can contribute to tissue damage and anoxia with acidosis, all of which can produce intravascular coagulation in the infant.[143] Infants with respiratory distress syndrome are also poorly oxygenated and may have intravascular coagulation.[144] Sepsis with bacterial infection or by viral agents may induce disseminated intravascular clotting,[145-148] and intravenous indwelling catheters used for parenteral alimentation may promote infection and coagulation.[149] The major factors which contribute to disseminated intravascular coagulation in the newborn thus include maternal complications, neonatal infections, and various other conditions including erythroblastosis fetalis,[150] giant hemangioma (Kasabach-Merritt syndrome),[151] hyperviscosity with hemoconcentration,[152] or relative polycythemia,[153] and purpura fulminans.[154] In fact, intravascular coagulaton in the Kasabach-Merritt syn-

**Table 13-5**
Causes of Intravascular Clotting
in the Neonate

Maternal disorders and
  obstetrical problems
    Pre-eclampsia, eclampsia
    Abruptio placentae
    Amniotic fluid embolism
    Dead twin fetus
    Fetal distress at delivery
Infections
  Gram-negative or gram-positive sepsis
  Toxoplasmosis
  Syphilis
  Disseminated herpes simplex
  Rubella
  Cytomegalovirus
Other diseases of the neonate
  Intravascular hemolysis-erythroblastosis fetalis
    (severe)
  Respiratory distress syndrome
  Acidosis, anoxia
  Giant hemangioma
  Renal vein thrombosis
  Indwelling catheters

Reproduced from Donaldson VH, Kisker CT: Blood co-
agulation in hemostasis, in Nathan DG, Oski FA (eds):
Hematology of Infancy and Childhood. Philadelphia,
WB Saunders Co, 1974, pp 561–625. With permission.

drome occurs in the hemangioma and is not really diffuse. When one of monochorionic twins dies in utero, the surviving fetus may have a consumptive coagulopathy because thromboplastic materials from the macerated twin may reach the circulation of the surviving twin through placental anastomoses in the circulation.[155] The causes of neonatal disseminated intravascular coagulation are summarized in Table 13-5. Recently, neonatal purpura fulminans has been related to homozygous deficiency to protein C (see page 41).[155a,155b]

Clinical evidence of the consumptive coagulopathy associated with intravascular coagulation is typically manifested by oozing at venipuncture sites in a sick infant. The infant may have petechiae; pulmonary, umbilical, intraventricular, or cerebral hemorrhages; diffuse ecchymoses; and bleeding from body orifices. The laboratory abnormalities associated with this disorder include thrombocytopenia of varying degrees; prolongation of the thrombin, partial thromboplastin, and prothrombin times; and evidence of hemolytic anemia with fragmented red cells in the peripheral blood. When specific coagulation factors are quantified, factor V is decreased and factor VIII and fibrinogen are also usually significantly reduced. Associated with the decrease in fibrinogen is the presence of fibrinogen-related antigens in the serum of such an infant, reflecting the fibrinolytic activity which develops secondarily in the face of intravascular coagulation in vivo. This fibrinolytic activity can cleave fibrin and fibrinogen molecules, releasing fragments that inhibit coagulation and persist in serum because they are not able to form polymers with normal thrombin-generated fibrin monomers and therefore are incoagulable.[156,157] In addition to these

**Table 13-6**
Differences Between DIC and Hemorrhagic Disease of the Newborn (HDN)

| Indication | HDN | DIC |
|---|---|---|
| Clinical | Healthy infant bleeding with trivial trauma | Sick infant: shock, sepsis, etc. |
| History | No vitamin K given; mother taking anticonvulsants | Vitamin K given |
| Laboratory | | |
|   Blood smear | Normal | Fragmented erythrocytes, often thrombocytopenia |
|   Partial thromboplastin time | Prolonged | Prolonged |
|   Prothrombin time | Prolonged | Prolonged |
|   Thrombin time | Normal for age group | Prolonged, usually |
|   Fibrinogen | Normal | Often low |
|   Factor V | Normal | Low |
|   Factor VIII | Normal | Often low |
|   Fibrinogen-related antigens in serum (FRA, FDP, or FSP) | Absent | Present |
| Effect of vitamin K: | Alleviates symptoms and laboratory abnormalities | Decreased response |

hemostatic abnormalities, the infant may, of course, demonstrate those associated with vitamin K deficiency. The two conditions should not be confused, however, for isolated vitamin K deficiency generally occurs in a healthy infant, whereas disseminated intravascular coagulation invariably accompanies illness. The coagulation defects in the sick neonate are more variable than in infants with vitamin K deficiency. There is often a prolonged bleeding time and evidence of increased capillary fragility, and the infant may have already received vitamin K. The distinguishing features of these two syndromes are summarized in Table 13-6.

Since fibrinolytic activity may sometimes be generated in the fetus during and shortly after birth, the finding of fibrinogen-related antigens in serum from umbilical cord or newborn blood vessels is insufficient evidence of pathologic intravascular clot-promoting activity in the newborn. Assays providing more direct evidence of the generation of thrombin have been devised. In one, the fibrin monomer that is formed following the release of fibrinopeptide A from fibrinogen by thrombin is quantified.[158] Although this method appears to quantify specifically the action of thrombin on fibrinogen, it is not readily available. In another approach, the fibrinopeptides released from fibrinogen by thrombin may be assayed,[159] and radioimmunoassay procedures are available for measurement of both fibrinopeptides A and B.[160,161]

The therapy for disseminated intravascular coagulation must be directed at correction of the underlying disease. Management of the hematologic abnormalities should receive secondary attention where necessary, but there are no control studies proving the effectiveness of attempts to repair hemostatic abnormalities in this situation. Correct diagnosis of the underlying cause is critical to appropriate therapy. Shock, acidosis, and sepsis thus must be treated appropriately with replacement of fluid and blood volume, adjustment of pH and electrolyte abnormalities, and antibiotics. In addition, adequate oxygenation and blood pressure should be maintained. The clot-promoting activity in vivo may be arrested by alleviating its underlying causes; the need to treat the coagulation abnormalities must depend upon clinical findings, not the laboratory abnormalities. If thrombosis can be identified in the infant, heparin may be given in doses of 100 U/kg of body weight in a loading dose, and then in doses of 50 U/kg every 4 hours. Heparin therapy should be aimed at keeping the 3-tube whole blood clotting time in the range of 30 minutes or the activated partial thromboplastin time between 60 and 70 seconds.[162] Heparin therapy should be continued until the process of disseminated intravascular coagulation has apparently been halted; this depends on the success in managing the underlying disease. When heparin has been discontinued, the platelet count, prothrombin time, activated partial thromboplastin time, and thrombin time should be determined after about four hours. If these determinations are within the normal range, and remain so after 6–8 hours, one can probably presume that the episode of intravascular coagulation has ceased, and heparin therapy may be stopped.

Physicians often feel the need for replacement therapy in this seemingly urgent situation and give platelets, concentrates of coagulation factors, and blood to such an infant. Because of the pathophysiologic state, none of these substances should be administered until the patient has been adequately heparinized, for premature administration of blood or fractions thereof may enhance the process of disseminated intravascular coagulation and induce thrombosis. If one unit of platelet concentrate (the amount of platelet derived from one unit of blood) is given per 5 kg of body weight, along with 10 ml/kg of fresh frozen plasma, most of the hemostatic abnormalities in this syndrome should be corrected.[107]

It is difficult to be precise in defining the correct treatment of disseminated intravascular coagulation. Infants usually recover without anticoagulation if the primary disease is successfully and readily treated. Nonetheless, the mortality in infants with this disorder has been as high as 60 percent[163,164] even with heparin therapy. Careful observation of an infant being treated for this disorder, with particular attention to changing levels of platelets, hemoglobin concentration, and peripheral blood smears for evidence of red cell fragmentation, is therefore important in making decisions regarding changes in therapy. Exchange transfusion with fresh heparinized blood has been used for the treatment of disseminated intravascular coagulation. This therapy is successful in anticoagulating the patient, as well as replacing the coagulation factors which have become depleted,[165] and removing the fibrin degradation products which impair the last stage of clotting. It is probably unwise to develop arbitrary guidelines in determining when, or if, an exchange transfusion or blood fraction infusions will be necessary for treatment of an infant with this disorder.

## BLEEDING IN APPARENTLY HEALTHY NEONATES

Neonatal bleeding may be due to an inherited deficiency of a coagulation factor other than vitamin K-dependent factors. Even though the majority of infants with significant inherited deficiencies of plasma procoagulants are usually asymptomatic early in life, some do have significant hemorrhage during the neonatal period.[166] In determining the etiology of such bleeding, the family or genetic history of the infant is of primary importance. The patterns of inheritance, form of bleeding, laboratory abnormalities, and antenatal history must be evaluated to establish a correct diagnosis.

### AHF (Factor VIII) and Christmas Factor
### (Factor IX) Deficiencies

Deficiencies of factors VIII and IX are both transmitted as X-linked traits, and are the cause of about 90 percent of hereditary coagulation defects. Of the two conditions, factor VIII deficiency is much more common. Bleeding from the umbilical cord stump does not occur in infants deficient in factors VIII or IX, but does occur in those deficient in factors V, VII, X, prothrombin, fibrinogen, or fibrin-stabilizing factor. It is surprising that relatively few males with either deficiency, even if severe, bleed in the neonatal period. Further, in several series of observations, only 30–40 percent of those with severe factor VIII or IX deficiency have any hemorrhage in this phase of life.[166–169] Even after circumcision, the incidence of bleeding in severe hemophilia is only about 43 percent,[169] and in mild hemophiliacs it is about 10 percent.[169] In another study,[170] 50 percent of severe hemophiliacs who had circumcision in the first 10 days of life bled, and 13 percent of those with a mild defect (greater than 1 percent factor VIII:C) bled.[170] When circumcision was delayed beyond 10 days of life, it was accompanied by more severe bleeding.[170] It is conceivable that the relatively low incidence of bleeding following immediate circumcision reflects the release of tissue thromboplastin into the area of trauma and the hemostatic effect of the circumcision clamp. It cannot be attributed to maternal factor VIII crossing the placenta, for there is no evidence that this occurs.

When bleeding does occur, it may be intracranial,[171,172] with disastrous consequences. Splenic hemorrhage, perirenal bleeding, cephalohematomata, umbilical or gastrointestinal bleeding, and bleeding about venipuncture sites may announce hemophilia in the neonate. It is more usual for the symptoms to appear when a child becomes ambulatory and therefore sustains frequent trauma.

When a diagnosis of classic hemophilia has been established, treatment with cryoprecipitated factor VIII should be initiated in the face of neonatal hemorrhage. The amounts of factor VIII preparations and the frequency of administration are given in Table 13-7. Since factor VIII levels are within the normal adult range in the neonate when measured in a specific assay for coagulant activity, the diagnosis in this age group is not difficult to establish.

The diagnosis of severe hereditary factor IX deficiency in the neonate can be made with a specific coagulation assay for factor IX activity. Despite the fact that decreased levels of factor IX are physiological in the neonate, levels much lower than 40 percent of those in normal adult plasma will be found in the plasma of a patient with a hereditary deficiency. Factor IX deficiency can be treated with plasma from stored blood, since factor IX is relatively stable during storage, but better therapeutic effects and higher plasma levels are produced by fresh frozen plasma.[107]

## Factor XIII (Fibrin-Stabilizing Factor, Fibrinase) Deficiency

A deficiency of the fibrin-stabilizing factor is characteristically manifested in the neonate with prolonged bleeding, delayed in onset, from the umbilical stump.[173–175] This form of bleeding is a characteristic expression of factor XIII deficiency; 80 percent of factor XIII-deficient neonates bleed from the umbilical cord stump days or weeks after birth.[165] Other forms of bleeding in this age group are uncommon.

This deficiency appears to be inherited as an autosomal recessive trait, and consanguinity among parents has been reported.[104,106] One report suggested X-linked inheritance in kindreds having only affected males.[176] Infants heterozygous for this defect do not bleed, but homozygous individuals may have severe bleeding and defective wound healing with keloid formation.

Patients with severe factor XIII deficiency have normal numbers of platelets; tests of plasma coagulation are normal, despite the significant bleeding they may sustain following injury. One must suspect this disorder, therefore, when umbilical stump bleeding occurs,

**Table 13-7**

Treatment of Coagulation Defects: Replacement Therapy

| Disorder | Intravascular Half-Life, hours | Increase in Plasma Concentration After 1 U/kg IV | Level Needed For: | | |
|---|---|---|---|---|---|
| | | | Hemostasis | Minor Trauma | Surgery and Major Trauma |
| Factor VIII deficiency | 8–12 | 2% | 10% | 20–30% | 50% |
| Factor IX deficiency | 24 | 1–1.5% | 5–10% | 15% | 25% |
| Factor VII deficiency | 5 | 1% | 5% | 10–15% | 20% |
| Factor X deficiency | 24–60 | 1% | 5% | 10% | 25% |
| Factor V deficiency | 36 | 1.5% | 5% | 10% | 25% |
| Von Willebrand's disease | 24–48 | 3% | 10% | 20–30% | 50% |
| Factor XI deficiency | 40–80 | 2% | 10% | 10–15% | 20% |
| Factor XIII deficiency | 72 | 1% | 2–3% | 2–3% | 2–3% |
| Afibrinogenemia | 56–82 | 1–1.5 mg/dl | 100 mg/dl | 150 mg/dl | 200 mg/dl |

Donaldson VH, Kisker CT: Blood coagulation in hemostasis, in Nathan DG, Oski FA (eds): Hematology of Infancy and Childhood. Philadelphia, WB Saunders CO, 1974, p 578. With permission.

**Table 13-8**
Replacement Therapy in Hemorrhagic States: Contents of Therapeutic Preparations

| Disease | Plasma | | Cryoprecipitated Proteins* | Concentrates |
| | Fresh Frozen | Aged | | |
|---|---|---|---|---|
| Factor VIII deficiency | + | + | + | In factor VIII concentrates |
| Factor IX deficiency | + | + | + | In Konȳne and similar concentrates |
| Factor VII deficiency | + | + | — | In Konȳne and similar concentrates |
| Factor X deficiency | + | + | — | In Konȳne and similar concentrates |
| Factor V deficiency | + | — | — | |
| Prothrombin deficiency | + | + | — | In Konȳne and similar concentrates |
| Von Willebrand's disease | + | + | + | Cryoprecipitates† |
| Factor XI deficiency | + | — | — | — |
| Factor XIII deficiency | + | — | — | — |
| Afibrinogenemia | + | + | + | Cryoprecipitates |

*+ = functional protein present in adequate amounts; — = functional protein absent or not present in adequate amounts.
†Highly purified concentrates do not shorten the bleeding time.

but tests of coagulant functions are normal. Its diagnosis can be presumptively established by determing the solubility of plasma, clotted with calcium chloride, in 5 $M$ urea or 1 percent monochloroacetic acid.[177,178] In normal plasma, factor XIII is activated by thrombin, and in the presence of calcium, fibrin stabilization occurs through the transpeptidase activity of factor XIII. Normal plasma clots are insoluble in 1 percent monochloroacetic acid or 5 $M$ urea, but in the absence of factor XIII, stabilization fails to occur, and the clots dissolve at room temperature within 24 hours in 6–7 volumes of either solution. The exact amount of factor XIII in plasma may be quantified by radiochemical methods in which the incorporation of radiolabeled glycine ethyl ester,[179] or dansyl cadaverine[180] into casein, for example, by the active factor XIII is measured.

Since fibrin-stabilizing factor is found in normal plasma, infusions of fresh frozen or unfrozen plasma will correct the deficiency (see Table 13-8). Since the half-life of factor XIII is about 12 days, and since low concentrations of it will correct defective fibrin formation, infrequent treatment with plasma may provide effective wound healing.[181]

## Factor V Deficiency

There is seldom overt bleeding even with a severe deficiency of factor V in the neonatal period. In one study, only 5 percent of deficient patients had neonatal bleeding as a manifestation of factor V deficiency.[182] The diagnosis of factor V deficiency may be considered when there is a family history of a bleeding disorder apparently inherited as an autosomal recessive trait,[183] but apparent autosomal dominant inheritance has occurred in several kindreds.[184] Although factor V is synthesized in the liver, it is not dependent upon vitamin K for its synthesis. Therefore, there is laboratory support for the diagnosis when the prolonged prothrombin time remains so following the administration of vitamin K, and when the prolonged prothrombin time of the plasma is corrected by fresh plasma from which vitamin K-dependent clotting factors have been removed, but not by plasma which has been incubated at 37°C for several hours, which causes factor V inactivation. At birth, the level of factor V is normally about equal to that in adult plasma. Bleeding from the umbilical cord may occur in the factor V-deficient neonate.

## Factor XI Deficiency (PTA)

The incidence of bleeding in the factor XI-deficient neonate was less than 5 percent in one study.[182] This disorder is transmitted as an autosomal recessive trait.[185,186] Since a disproportionately large number of affected kindred are Ashkenazi Jews,[187] it is wise to investigate this possibility in a Jewish kindred with a mild bleeding tendency or an asymptomatic abnormality of blood coagulation. Although bleeding is infrequent and mild in most cases of PTA deficiency, menorrhagia and postpartum bleeding have been observed,[188] and a spontaneous cerebral hemorrhage has been reported in an older individual.[189] Since the level of PTA is low in the normal neonate, unless the deficiency is severe a firm diagnosis may be difficult to make in this age group.

## Afibrinogenemia and Hypofibrinogenemia

In these conditions, there may be oozing from the umbilical stump, as there is with factor XIII deficiency, or unusual bleeding from ammoniacal dermatitis of the diaper area[191] in infants with afibrinogenemia. More usually, however, there is no significant bleeding in the neonatal period. It is remarkable that throughout life, individuals with a severe deficiency of plasma fibrinogen suffer hemorrhagic symptoms only upon sustaining trauma. In some cases, traces of fibrinogen may be found in plasma, and platelet fibrinogen probably aids in hemostasis in the face of markedly deficient plasma fibrinogen.[191,192] In this disorder, the inheritance pattern is that of an autosomal recessive trait; in some kindred the incidence of affected males exceeds that of females.[188] Since the plasma levels of fibrinogen vary widely in different physiologic states, it is likely that the heterozygous state may be obscured because the effect of a single gene may result in synthesis of a relatively normal amount of fibrinogen.[188] The blood is virtually incoagulable in congenital afibrinogenemia.

A number of abnormal fibrinogens have been identified in persons with hereditary dysfibrinogenemias,[193] and subaponeurotic bleeding and cephalohematomata due to birth trauma have been described in one case in the neonatal period.[194] The effect of abnormal fibrinogens upon hemostasis is variable, and little information on the neonatal consequences of these biosynthetic abnormalities is available.

## Von Willebrand's Disease

Von Willebrand's disease is classically characterized by a deficiency of factor VIII procoagulant activity, factor VIII-related antigen, a prolonged bleeding time, and a deficiency of a plasma cofactor required for the agglutination of platelets by the antibiotic ristocetin.[195–197] The etiology of the prolonged bleeding time is unclear, for restoration of the plasma factor VIII activity and antigen concentration need not correct the bleeding time.[198] The variability in the expression of von Willebrand's disease is wide, and understanding of the molecular mechanisms of this disease is incomplete at present. In contrast to classic hemophilia, this disease is inherited as an autosomal dominant trait, but there appear to be frequent sporadic cases. The bleeding symptoms may be mild throughout life, characteristically expressed as easy bruising, gastrointestinal bleeding, epistaxis, and gingival bleeding. Bleeding from dental extractions may be remarkable later in life, but significant bleeding in the neonate with this disorder is infrequent. Even so, epistaxis and tongue bleeding have been reported early in life in infants with von Willebrand's disease, and can be severe.[199,200]

## Hageman Factor, HMWK, and Fletcher Factor (Plasma Prekallikrein) Deficiencies

There is no evidence that individuals with severe deficiencies of any of these factors have a hemorrhagic tendency, and therefore it is not necessary to consider these possibilities in the diagnosis of an infant with a bleeding syndrome. Each of these factors is required for a normal activated partial thromboplastin time, but the deficiency of Fletcher factor (prekallikrein) is corrected in vitro when the plasma is incubated with an activating surface (kaolin, for example) for 8 minutes before recalcification of the plasma.[201]

Characteristic abnormalities of laboratory tests in hereditary deficiencies of plasma-clotting factors are summarized in Table 13-9, and the appropriate therapy for these disorders when hemorrhage is apparent is summarized in Tables 13-7 and 13-8. It is important to recognize that when there is a life-threatening hemorrhage in a neonate, such as may occur with intraventricular or pulmonary hemorrhage, it is extremely important to determine if there is a deficiency of factors VIII or IX so that appropriate treatment can be carried out for the period required for recovery and prevention of permanent damage to the infant.

Abnormalities of the quantity and quality of platelets will be considered in the next section.

## DIAGNOSIS AND MANAGEMENT OF THE BLEEDING INFANT

Widespread petechiae or obvious ecchymoses in the newborn infant demand diagnostic investigation. It is probably unnecessary to pursue extensive studies in the infant who demonstrates petechiae only over the areas of presentation during delivery, for this is a common cause of a petechial eruption. If obvious hemorrhage occurs from the gastrointestinal tract, one must decide whether this is maternal or infant blood. This determination can be made by hemolyzing the erythrocytes in water and exposing the hemoglobin solution to sodium hydroxide to determine if it contains adult or fetal hemoglobin. The adult hemoglobin readily denatures to a compound with a yellowish-brown color, whereas the fetal hemoglobin remains red under these circumstances.

If thrombocytopenia is not present, one must determine if the infant has received vitamin K; if it has not been administered, it should be. In addition, a history of prolonged anoxia during birth, prematurity, and traumatic delivery should be taken seriously, as an acquired bleeding syndrome may occur in any of these situations.

**Table 13-9**
Alterations in Hemostatic Tests in Some Hereditary Disorders of Coagulation

| Disorder | Activated Partial Thromboplastin time | Prothrombin Time | Thrombin Time | Serum Prothrombin | Bleeding Time | Other |
|---|---|---|---|---|---|---|
| Factor VIII deficiency | Long | Normal | Normal | High | Normal | |
| Factor IX deficiency | Long | Normal | Normal | High | Normal | |
| PTA (XI) deficiency | Long | Normal | Normal | High | Normal | |
| Fletcher trait | Long | Normal | Normal | Normal | Normal | Partial thromboplastin time shortened with prolonged exposure to Kaolin; no bleeding |
| HMWK deficiency | Long | Normal | Normal | High | Normal | No bleeding |
| Hageman factor (XII) deficiency | Long | Normal | Normal | High | Normal | No bleeding |
| Factor X deficiency | Long | Long | Normal | High | Normal | |
| Factor V deficiency | Long | Long | Normal | High | Normal | |
| Factor VII deficiency | Usually normal | Long | Normal | Normal | Normal | |
| Von Willebrand's disease | Variably long | Normal | Normal | Normal or high | Long | |
| Prothrombin deficiency | Usually long | Long | Normal | Low | Normal | |
| Afibrinogenemia | Infinite | Infinite | Infinite | Normal | Normal | Bleeding episodes |
| Factor XIII deficiency | Normal | Normal | Normal | Normal | Normal | Umbilical stump bleeding; Clot soluble in 5 M urea or 1 percent monochloroacetic acid |

Source: Donaldson VH, Kisker CT: Blood coagulation in hemostasis, in Nathan DG, Oski FA (eds): Hematology of Infancy and Childhood. Philadelphia, WB Saunders Co, 1974, p 573. With permission.

If the family history includes a tendency to an inherited disorder of hemostasis, one must determine whether this is apparently transmitted with relationship to sex (X-linked), or as an autosomal trait. Of the hereditary hemorrhagic syndromes, the deficiency of anti-hemophilic factor (factor VIII) is the most common X-linked inherited disorder, but factor IX deficiency, also X-linked, may also produce bleeding in the newly born. If the history suggests that a bleeding syndrome is inherited as an autosomal dominant trait, one must consider the possibility of von Willebrand's disease or PTA deficiency, for this disorder may also assume this pattern of inheritance in some kindreds.[187] Among the autosomal recessive traits, deficiencies of prothrombin, factors V, VII, X, XIII, and fibrinogen should be considered. A deficiency of Hageman factor, HMWK, or Fletcher factor is not associated with bleeding, and PTA (factor XI) deficiency is likely to be clinically inapparent in the neonate.

A maternal history of ingestion of drugs, including anticonvulsants or aspirin, and the preexistence of maternal diseases, including eclampsia or preeclampsia, should alert one to the possibility of complications of the disease as well as to the effect of treatment of the disorder upon the neonate.

## Physical Examination

Infants with hemophilia may have subcutaneous hematomas, joint or muscle hemorrhages, and, less commonly, cephalohematomas rather than petechiae or minute ecchymoses. If sufficiently deficient, these infants will also bleed from venipuncture sites. Infants with significant bloody oozing from the umbilical stump or following circumcision may have vitamin K deficiency or deficiencies of factor V or fibrinogen. When jaundice, hepatosplenomegaly, and diffuse bleeding are apparent, sepsis must be suspected. Diagnostic efforts should be made to exclude bacterial infection, cytomegalic inclusion disease, toxoplasmosis, herpes simplex, and syphilis. Syndactylism has been reported in association with factor V deficiency.[202]

## Laboratory Studies

A precise diagnosis requires laboratory evaluation. As noted elsewhere, a presumptive diagnosis of thrombocytopenia can be made on examination of a well-prepared cover slip smear of the peripheral blood or by direct platelet count. If the platelet count is decreased in association with a prolongation of the partial thromboplastin and prothrombin times, this is strongly suggestive of disseminated intravascular coagulation. In this case, the thrombin time will probably be prolonged compared to that of normal plasma; there will be a decreased concentration of factors V, VII, and fibrinogen; and there may be high levels of fibrinogen-related antigens in the serum from the blood of the patient. Red cell fragmentation on a peripheral blood smear, if present, is a prominent clue to this disorder. If the platelet count is normal and the prothrombin and partial thromboplastin times are prolonged, vitamin K deficiency is a likely possibility. Reassessment of laboratory studies within 4–8 hours after the administration of 1–2 mg of vitamin K will confirm this diagnostic impression if the coagulation defect is corrected. On the other hand, congenital deficiencies of other clotting factors synthesized by the liver, including factors V, X, and fibrinogen, will not respond to this medication and must be considered as diagnostic possibilities when vitamin K is ineffective in correcting the delayed prothrombin and activated partial thromboplastin times. If the prothrombin time alone is prolonged, a deficiency of, or defect in, prothrombin or factor VII must be entertained. If a long partial thromboplastin time is the only clearly demonstrable laboratory abnormality, deficiencies of factors VIII, IX, XI, XII, HMWK, or Fletcher factor should be considered, as well as von Willebrand's disease. One must recall that inadvertent administration of heparin may mimic all of these disorders.

One must bear in mind that extensive laboratory studies of the male infant to be circumcised are probably a futile exercise, for just as much information can be obtained by taking a careful history from the mother in the search for evidence of hereditary coagulation defects. On the other hand, if the infant is already beset with a hemorrhagic syndrome, correct diagnosis and treatment are necessary before this procedure is carried out.

## THROMBOCYTOPENIA

In the healthy newborn, a platelet count of 120,000–300,000/µl is usual.[203] In the otherwise healthy prematurely born infant, counts of less than 100,000/µl[3] have been reported, but it is unlikely that platelet numbers in healthy prematures vary significantly from those of full-term neonates. From the tenth to 20th day after birth, the platelet counts of premature infants, especially those of lowest birth weights, may drop to 50,000, and then reach a normal level by about 1 month of age, but the lowest platelet counts may have been associated with undetected infection or other complications or prematurity.[3,204] Therefore, any newborn infant with a platelet count of less than 100,000/µl probably merits investigation.[205,206]

The causes of thrombocytopenia in the neonate are basically those of thrombocytopenia in any age group: (1) decreased platelet production, (2) increased platelet destruction, or (3) both decreased production and increased utilization.

### Decreased Production of Platelets

The proof of decreased production of platelets in thrombocytopenic states rests on finding decreased numbers of megakaryocytes when the bone marrow is examined, or decreased cytoplasmic budding of the megakaryocytes, which may appear to be in nearly normal numbers, as if there were impaired release of platelets from them. Although megakaryocytes may be reduced in some cases of thrombocytopenia secondary to platelet antibodies or to sepsis, there are cases in which megakaryocytic failure is the primary cause.

#### Hereditary thrombocytopenias, (primary and secondary)

Rarely, an infant may have congenital thrombocytopenia with *megakaryocytic hypoplasia* as an isolated finding. In some of these instances, aplasia of the bone marrow has evolved.[207,208] In one report, a nonfamilial congenital thrombocytopenia involved male infants only[208] and progressed to pancytopenia. There is also a familial form of aplastic anemia.[209] Testosterone and corticosteroid therapy may improve these patients.[210]

Thrombocytopenia in association with *trisomy* has been reported in one child with D₁ trisomy and in 3 infants with E trisomy.[211] In the latter instance, 2 infants with E trisomy, and hypoplasia or absence of the radii and thumbs were observed[211] (see below).

#### Thrombocytopenia associated with other anomalies

A complex syndrome in which severe thrombocytopenia is associated with absent radii, called the TAR (thrombocytopenia and absent radii) syndrome,[212,213] may present with a variety of hemorrhagic symptoms ranging from a few petechiae to fatal intracranial hemorrhage. TAR may be associated with other limb abnormalities, producing a clinical syndrome of phocomelia;[214] congenital heart disease occurs in about 30 percent of these cases.[206] About two-thirds of patients with TAR die within the first year of life, but gradual improvement may occur near the end of the first year; a few patients have survived to adulthood. Bleeding may begin within the first few days of life, and platelet counts are often between 10,000 and 30,000/$\mu$l. An associated leukemoid blood picture with a total blood count as high as 140,000/$\mu$l and a shift to the left with occasional blastic cells in the peripheral blood is frequently present. Bone marrow examination reveals hyperplasia of the myeloid elements but an almost total absence of megakaryocytes.

The diagnosis of TAR should be considered with purpura in association with shortening of the forearms, elbow flexion, and obvious radial deviation of the wrist, or more extensive anomalies, including absence of the ulna and humerus, resembling bilateral phocomelia, which may be confirmed with radiologic studies.[214] Although this constellation of anomalies may resemble that seen in the infants of women who have taken thalidomide, thrombocytopenia was not found in those cases, nor were other hematologic abnormalities.

### Fanconi's syndrome

Thrombocytopenia is a concomitant of the pancytopenia found in Fanconi's anemia, which is also associated with other congenital anomalies such as a deformed radius or thumb or absence of both, and renal abnormalities.[215] These skeletal abnormalities resemble those of TAR, but cytogenetic abnormalities found in the Fanconi hypoplastic anemia, including chromatid breaks and endoreduplication, have not been observed in TAR.[216]

### Down's syndrome

Infants with Down's syndrome occasionally have a leukemialike disorder in the newborn period,[217] with profound thrombocytopenia, anemia, and a peripheral blood smear resembling acute granulocytic leukemia. These infants may have nodular skin infiltrations similar to those of true leukemia in the neonate; it is conceivable that this syndrome is truly a leukemia rather than a leukemoid state.[206] In this disorder, the hemorrhagic symptoms should be treated when necessary with platelet concentrates, but it is recommended that antileukemic therapy be withheld.[206]

### Osteopetrosis (Albers-Schoenberg disease)

Thrombocytopenia in association with osteopetrosis, in which there is extramedullary hematopoiesis and myelofibrosis, reflects failure of platelet production.[218] Occasionally, splenectomy leads to some improvement.[218]

In cases of microcephaly,[219,220] congenital hypoplastic thrombocytopenia rarely occurs concurrently. This has been reported in 2 members of a sibship. The thrombocytopenia in this instance persists beyond the first year of life and appears not to reflect a viral infection.

### Wiskott-Aldrich syndrome

Significant thrombocytopenia is characteristically found in patients who have Wiskott-Aldrich syndrome,[221,222] a disorder inherited as an X-linked trait and associated with eczema and a tendency to severe infection. In this disorder, the megakaryocytes are normal, but thrombocytopenia appears to result from impaired production and poor survival of defective platelets.[223] Recently, light has been shed on the etiology of this disease with the description of an apparent deficiency or absence of a normal membrane protein of the platelets and lymphocytes in the Wiskott-Aldrich syndrome.[224] An X-linked form of hereditary thrombocytopenia probably represents a form of the Wiskott-Aldrich syndrome.[225] Transfer factor or bone marrow transplantation may provide effective therapy for this disorder.[226,227]

### May-Hegglin anomaly

Patients with the May-Hegglin anomaly may have bleeding, but this is not a recognized problem in the neonatal period. In this disorder, the marrow megakaryocytes are normal, but autologous platelet survival is shortened.[228]

### Rubella syndrome

Some infants of mothers who had rubella in the first trimester of pregnancy[229–231] may have thrombocytopenia with congenital cardiac lesions, cataracts, and deafness, as well as pneumonia, giant cell hepatitis, hepatosplenomegaly, and bone lesions which may characterize the congenital rubella syndrome.

## Management of Thrombocytopenia Due to Decreased Platelet Production

Transfusion of platelets harvested in plastic equipment is necessary to control the hemorrhagic symptoms in most of these disorders. When this procedure is carried out, the platelets may continue to circulate in the blood for about 10 days, decreasing at a rate of about 10 percent per day.[206] When the platelets given disappear from the circulating blood at this rate, there is no increased rate of utilization, and when a drop in platelet count occurs more rapidly in such a patient, there is shortened survival. Splenectomy may allow some improvement in patients with osteopetrosis, but the prognosis for survival in this disease is poor.

## Thrombocytopenia Due to Shortened Platelet Life Span

Thrombocytopenia due to increased utilization of platelets may be found in sick newborns, but an immune thrombocytopenia may also result from a number of factors in an apparently healthy newborn. The thrombocytopenia in the sick newborn associated with intravascular coagulation has been discussed previously. Thrombocytopenia may also be seen with severe erythroblastosis fetalis, or following its therapy with exchange transfusion with platelet-deficient blood, but it need not be due to a shortened platelet life span. In addition, a number of infectious processes, including cytomegalic inclusion disease, disseminated herpes simplex infection, congenital toxoplasmosis, and congenital syphilis, are accompanied by thrombocytopenia, which is likely to be associated with intravascular clot-promoting activity.

## Immune Thrombocytopenias

About one-half of the newly born infants of mothers who have idiopathic thrombocytopenic purpura (ITP) have thrombocytopenia. Even though the mother may have had a remission following splenectomy, her newly born infant has an even chance of having thrombocytopenia.[232] Following *spontaneous* remission of ITP, however, the offspring of such a woman is unlikely to have thrombocytopenia. Similarly, newly born infants of women with systemic lupus erythematosus and associated thrombocytopenia are likely to be thrombocytopenic,[233] and antibody against platelets and a positive lupus erythematosus test have been demonstrated in serum from such infants during the first few days of life. In each instance, maternal antibody directed against platelets is probably transferred across the placenta to the infant.

The placental transfer of antibody is apparently an active process, and there are binding sites for the Fc portion of immunoglobulin G (IgG) molecules on placental cell membranes.[234,235] Once the antibody has gained access to the fetal circulation, its relatively slow catabolic rate allows it to persist for several weeks. Since the half-life of IgG is approximately 22 days in adults,[236,237] one may anticipate that detectable amounts of the etiologic agent will persist for at least one month in these neonates.

In infants of thrombocytopenic mothers, petechiae may be noted at birth but less often there is more severe bleeding characterized by ecchymoses, mucosal bleeding, and, rarely, bleeding into the central nervous system. The infants of mothers who are purpuric at the time of delivery are more likely to have severe bleeding symptoms themselves.[238] The platelet count may remain low for the first few days of life and the risk of hemorrhage is significant, but the hemorrhagic symptoms usually abate after 2 or 3 days in the neonate.

A transient thrombocytopenia in the newly born occasionally occurs even though the mother does not have a history or indication of thrombocytopenia. One opinion[239] holds that the thrombocytopenia in this situation may be due to immunization of the mother by the infant's platelets. The maternal antibodies then generated may cross the placenta and react with the infant's platelets, causing thrombocytopenia, but they do not react with maternal platelets.[240] A similar cause of thrombocytopenia in a newborn infant may be an unusual complication of erythroblastosis fetalis. It is possible that the platelets of an infant might become involved as innocent bystanders in an interaction between immune complexes involving maternal antibody and another antigen, for the Fc portions of IgG molecules in these complexes could bind to the platelet membrane.

### Diagnosis

Any infant of a woman with thrombocytopenia should be carefully evaluated for this condition and its complications whether or not hemorrhagic symptoms are apparent. The platelet count of such infants may be exceedingly low, and a presumptive diagnosis may be made on a carefully prepared cover slip smear of capillary blood. Bone marrow samples usually contain increased numbers of megakaryocytes which appear immature, precisely the condition found in ITP in older individuals. Occasionally, decreased numbers of megakaryocytes have been observed and this may be due to the effect of immune antibody on megakaryocytes.[239–241]

There have been many attempts to devise satisfactory laboratory tests for platelet antibodies. Unfortunately, these tests suffer from difficulties in interpretation, reliability, and execution. Some complement-fixing assays may provide evidence for an isoimmune form of thrombocytopenia in the neonate in a significant number of cases, but are also likely to be unhelpful in an equal number of instances, in part because some antibodies do not fix complement.[240] It is probably important to recognize that the significant antibody in these disorders is often that which resides on the platelet surface. Antibody in the circulating blood may not have a high affinity for platelet antigens, and therefore may not be the most offensive agent. A more precise double immune fixation diagnostic assay utilizes the fixation of complement by a preparation of antibody directed against platelet-bound antibody.[242] In another assay, radiolabeled antibody directed against IgG and the third component of complement, C3, has proved successful in quantifying antibody and C3 bound to platelets.[243]

## Management

Special treatment is not required in most cases of neonatal thrombocytopenia, but life-threatening hemorrhage demands treatment with corticosteroids and platelet infusions. It is unwise to perform a splenectomy on such an infant, in part because the splenectomized infant may be susceptible to overwhelming sepsis.

The risk of intracranial hemorrhage and the association of this disorder with a mortality of 12–14 percent[107] demand careful observation of such an infant and thoughtful use of therapeutic measures. The risk of spontaneous bleeding is probably increased only when the platelet count, measured directly, is lower than $10,000/\mu l$.[244] It may be wise, if possible, to obtain platelet counts from the fetal scalp during labor to decide if a cesarean section should be done when a female with a history of ITP is in labor.[244] Cesarean section has been recommended if the fetal platelet count is below $50,000/\mu l$[244] to avoid the risk of intracranial hemorrhage, which may be found in one-half of the stillborn infants of women with immune thrombocytopenia,[245] but there is not general agreement on this approach. Occasionally, exchange transfusion has been used to remove the platelet antibody from the infant, but this therapeutic maneuver does not always alleviate the thrombocytopenia. When a high serum bilirubin level evolves subsequent to hemorrhage in an infant with neonatal thrombocytopenia, exchange transfusion may be necessary to avoid the complications of neonatal jaundice.

The management of the mother with autoimmune thrombocytopenia may have a significant influence on her fetus. In a recent study, a majority of infants of mothers with autoimmune thrombocytopenia who were treated with steroids had adequate numbers of platelets in their peripheral blood within one hour of delivery.[245] In this series, the lowest platelet count was $65,000/\mu l$, and the overall data indicated that the mean platelet count at birth in these infants was 3.6 times that of infants born of thrombocytopenic mothers who had not received this treatment. Unfortunately, these assays do not determine the specificity of the immunoglobulin associated with the platelets and a significant amount of immunoglobulin is found on normal platelets using these techniques. Therefore, the meaning of data obtained with these assays is controversial. When a radiolabelled monoclonal antibody to the Fc portion of human IgG has been used to quantify immunoglobulins on platelets,[245a] lower concentrations were found on normal platelets than with other techniques, but an occasional patient with ITP exhibited a normal amount of platelet-associated antibody. This diagnostic approach may be helpful. In another study, there was a poor correlation between fetal and maternal platelet counts in women with thrombocytopenia.[244] The beneficial effects of steroids administered to a pregnant woman with immune thrombocytopenia suggest that the complications of a cesarean section and birth trauma may be alleviated by adequate treatment of mothers in this way.

In another recent study quantifying platelet antibodies in ITP during pregnancy, maternal platelet-associated IgG was not related to the risk of thrombocytopenia in the neonate,[243] but the level of maternal circulating antiplatelet antibody correlated with the presence and the extent of thrombocytopenia in her infant.[243] Significant in these observations was the finding that maternal plasma antibody levels did not correlate with maternal platelet counts in mothers treated with steroids or splenectomy.[243] The lack of correlation of platelet-associated antibody in maternal blood with the risk of thrombocytopenia in the neonate may indicate the specificity of the antibody for antigens on the maternal platelets which may be absent from the infant's platelets. On the other hand, the level of circulating antiplatelet IgG did correlate somewhat with the risk of neonatal thrombocytopenia, and this may indicate that the antibody in the circulating blood is directed against a more common antigen, also found on the infant's platelets.[243] The mothers with the highest levels of circulating antiplatelet antibodies produced neonates with the lowest platelet counts; their antibodies were broadly reactive with normal platelets and did not show human leukocyte antigen (HLA) or platelet antigen A1 (P1-A1) specificity.[243] This study confirms the previous observation that mothers who have ITP in clinical remission may not be in immunologic remission, and their infants may have serious thrombocytopenia with bleeding.

Despite the evidence that corticosteroid therapy for the mother with ITP may be helpful to her neonate,[245] this therapy may alter the biochemical topography of the platelet membrane so that the affinity of the maternal antiplatelet antibody for her platelets is decreased, freeing the antibody to cross the placenta. Indeed, the level of platelet-associated immunoglobulin in a woman so treated may decrease, and an increased level of plasma antibody apparently dissociated from the platelet can then occur. If the steroids do not protect the infant directly, this therapy might increase the antibody being delivered to the infant via the placenta. A conclusion which can be derived from this study[244] is that the level of free circulating antibody does have some cocrrelation with the development of neonatal thrombocytopenia when mothers have ITP either clinically evident or in remission. Therefore, if a method for measuring antibody in plasma against platelets of the infant is available, one may be able to identify the fetus at greatest risk, and therefore possibly in greatest need of delivery by cesarean section.[244]

## Thrombocytopenia in Neonates Associated with Antepartum Medications

Neonatal thrombocytopenia has been reported in the offspring of women who have received *thiazides* for prolonged periods as therapy for preeclampsia.[246] It may present soon after birth with purpura, gastrointestinal, and intraperitoneal bleeding. One such infant succumbed at 40 hours of age, with pulmonary and subdural hemorrhages. The platelet counts varied widely but were below $50,000/\mu l$. The duration of the therapy with the offensive drug was unrelated to the degree of purpura or thrombocytopenia, and the role of thiazides in such cases is difficult to prove. It is possible that a predisposing genetic mechanism plays a role, for in one study there was no relationship between thiazide intake and platelet counts;[247] neonatal thrombocytopenia recurred in a subsequent pregnancy in one instance of thiazide-induced thrombocytopenia.[247] In this case, the thrombocytopenia was due to decreased production of platelets, for the number of megakaryocytes was decreased when marrow aspirates were examined.

Transient thrombocytopenia in an infant of a diabetic woman taking *tolbutamide* may have been due to an effect of the tolbutamide on the production of platelets by the infant. The platelet count became normal within two weeks of delivery, and the serum levels of tolbutamide in the affected infant were initially elevated.[248] Renal venous thrombosis occurs more frequently in infants of diabetic mothers than in normal mothers and is often associated with thrombocytopenia.[249]

In some infants of mothers who have thrombocytopenia induced by taking *quinine,* neonatal thrombocytopenia may occur,[250] because the antibody induced in the maternal circulation can cross over into the fetal circulation. Exchange transfusion has been recommended in this instance if hemorrhage is suspected or obvious, and platelet concentrates may be given.

The management of these disorders hinges on identifying the etiologic agent and withdrawing it from the infant's environment. Supportive and replacement therapy may be necessary if symptomatology merits it.

## Other Conditions Associated with
## Neonatal Thrombocytopenia

One infant has been described who developed thrombotic thrombocytopenic purpura (TTP) on the third day of life which was associated with jaundice, hematuria, and melena with a platelet count of 4000/μl.[251] Although the infant improved following exchange transfusion, the thrombocytopenia persisted and the infant died at the age of 9 months with typical lesions of TTP.

Thrombocytopenia has been reported in infants with methylmalonic acidemia and ketotic glycinemia,[252] and with isovaleric acidemia[253] in association with other cytopenias. In the last instance, the hematologic alterations were corrected with a low leucine diet.

In one kindred, successive thrombocytopenic infants have been born of a hyperthyroid mother,[254] but the mechanism of platelet deficiency in this situation was unclear.

## Evaluation of the Thrombocytopenic Newborn

Once a deficiency of platelets has been detected in a neonate, it is essential to elicit a maternal and family history of previous bleeding or any symptoms of maternal thrombocytopenia at any time in the past. Specific questions regarding ingestion of drugs and exposure to rubella in the first trimester of pregnancy must be asked; lack of clinical rubella does not necessarily exclude the disease, for many patients have few symptoms. Previous delivery of thrombocytopenic infants with purpura may suggest an inherited thrombocytopenia. A peripheral blood smear and platelet count on the mother should be obtained.

In examining the thrombocytopenic newborn, if hepatosplenomegaly is accompanied by jaundice, an infectious process is most likely the cause of the platelet deficiency. Congenital leukemia, which is extremely rare, should be considered. Obvious deformities of the extremities, of course, suggest the possibility of the TAR syndrome, and hemagiomas, either multiple or large and single, suggest the Kassabach-Merritt syndrome. The presence of cataracts, microcephaly, and congenital heart lesions may indicate that the infant has a congenital rubella syndrome. The infants of women with autoimmune thrombocytopenia are likely to have purpura but appear otherwise healthy.

The laboratory evaluation should exclude deficiencies or abnormalities of other blood cells, and the marrow should be examined for the content and nature of its megakaryocytes. If these are decreased, a hypoplastic condition is suggested, but an immune disorder may also cause this picture. If reliable serologic tests for platelet antibodies are available, these studies should be performed on both the mother and the infant (see pages 433–434).

## Disorders of Platelet Function

Although a number of clinical syndromes result from disturbed platelet function, most of them do not provide a clinical problem for the neonate. Glanzmann's thrombasthenia, a rare disorder which can appear in the neonatal period, is associated with a prolonged bleeding time, defective clot retraction, and defective aggregation of platelets exposed to ADP.[255]

Increased levels of serum bilirubin (above 15–20 mg/dl) can, in some way, induce morphologic abnormalities of platelets and impair their clot-promoting and clot-retraction functions.[256] The impaired platelet function is apparently due to the free, or unconjugated, fraction of bilirubin.[257]

Platelet dysfunction in the neonates of mothers who have taken aspirin during preg-

**Table 13-10**
Etiologic Factor in Intraventricular
Hemorrhage in the Neonate

| |
| --- |
| Birth trauma |
| Hereditary bleeding disorder |
| Angiomatous vascular malformations |
| Hemorrhagic cerebral necrosis with infection |
| Acquired coagulation disorders |
|     Iatrogenic (heparin) |
|     Maternal (antenatal medications) |

nancy can be significant. Cephalohematoma, melena, and periorbital bleeding have occurred in infants of mothers who received aspirin antepartum, and an aspirinlike defect in platelet function was demonstrable in the newborns' platelets.[258,259]

## Hemorrhage Peculiar to the Neonate

Occasionally, a neonate may succumb to a massive pulmonary hemorrhage, usually during the first week of life.[259a] This hemorrhage is usually a complication of another illness, hypoxia, stress, perhaps the end stage of hyaline membrane disease,[260] oxygen toxicity,[261,262] airway obstruction, or hemorrhagic edema with left heart failure following chronic asphyxia. It is likely that many of these infants have disseminated intravascular coagulation, perhaps originating in the pulmonary circulation.[143,263-266]

Although disseminated intravascular coagulation may not actually be the cause of this disorder, it may complicate the syndrome and add to the tendency to hemorrhage. One study has indicated that correction of the deficiencies of platelets and fibrinogen increased the survival rate of such infants.[261] Other forms of supportive therapy, including pulmonary toilet and the prevention of hypoxia and acidosis, are important in the management of such a patient.

Intracranial (intraventricular) hemorrhage in the neonate, especially the prematurely born, may result from a number of causes (Table 13-10). This syndrome is a difficult clinical problem in perinatal medicine and occurs frequently enough to be a major problem. Among the most common events that predispose an infant to intraventricular hemorrhage are birth asphyxia or chronic hypoxia. Sequential studies with ultrasonography or computed tomography are very helpful in following such a patient.

Immaturity of the blood vessels in an infant probably increases the tendency toward intraventricular hemorrhage, for their rupture may follow an episode of hypoxia.[267,268] Immaturity of the blood vessels of the subependymal or germinal layer probably contributes to the susceptibility of these vessels to rupture. If heart failure follows hypoxia, the intracranial venous pressure may be increased, thus enhancing the likelihood of bleeding. Electrolyte disorders associated with iatrogenic factors such as the administration of excess alkali[269,270] may be implicated in the cause of intraventricular hemorrhage, and the impaired hemostatic effectiveness due to physiologically depressed coagulation factor functions in the newborn adds to the disaster. Evidence of disseminated intravascular coagulation has been more frequently found in infants with intraventricular hemorrhage than in those without this disorder.[263,271] The hemostatic abnormalities, manifested by prolonged prothrombin and partial thromboplastin times, do not appear to be causative, but the coagulation abnormalities exaggerate the bleeding tendency.[263,271]

The preventive management of this disorder with infusions of fresh frozen plasma (2 infusions of 10 ml/kg within the first 24 hours of age) appeared to reduce the incidence of intraventricular hemorrhage in a treated group as compared to an untreated group.[272] In other controlled studies, however, this favorable outcome has not been found.[273] Various plasma fractions, including stable factor concentrates, have been used, but in one such study there was actually an increase in the incidence of intraventricular hemorrhage in the treated group.[274] Prophylactic exchange transfusion has provided extremely variable results; therefore, this form of prophylaxis cannot be recommended.[117]

This serious problem persists. Hydrocephalus sometimes occurs following these intracranial hemorrhages, but a satisfactory neurologic outcome may be achieved in as many as 40 percent of infants who have sustained intraventricular hemorrhage as neonates.[275] It is likely that given the modern tools of ultrasonography and computed tomography, along with careful observation, the diagnosis and follow-up care of infants who are candidates for intraventricular hemorrhage will allow more satisfactory management in the future.

## REFERENCES

1. Bleyer WA, Hakami N, Shephard T: The development of hemostasis in the human fetus and newborn infant. Fetal Neonate Med 79:838–855, 1971
2. Hathaway WE: The bleeding newborn. Semin Hematol 12:175–188, 1975
3. Medoff HS: Platelet counts in premature infants. J Pediats 64:287–289, 1964
4. Aballi AJ, Prendes Z, Prez Alcover M, et al: Neuvos hallazgos para el prognostico del prematuro de poco peso. Rev Cubana Pediatr 27:679–690, 1955
5. Mull MM, Hathaway WE: Altered platelet function in newborns. Pediatr Res 4:229–237, 1970
6. Aballi AJ, DeLamerens S: Coagulation changes in the neonatal period and in early infancy. Pediatr Clin North Am 9:785–817, 1962
7. Lopez Banus V, deLamerens S: Estudio de la coagulacion sanguinea en el Ricinen Nacido termine en nuestro media hospitaliario. Rev Cubana Pediatr 28:381–414, 1956
8. Hrodek O: Blood platelets in the newborn: Their function in hemostasis and hemocoagulation. Univ Carolinae Monogr 22:1–119, 1966
9. Gitlin D, Kumate J, Urrusti J, et al: The selectivity of the human placenta in the transfer of plasma proteins from mother to fetus. J Clin Invest 43:1938–1951, 1964
10. Cade JF, Hirsh J, Martin M: Placental barrier to coagulation function: Its relevance to the coagulation defect at birth and to hemorrhage in the newborn. Br Med J 2:281–283, 1969
11. Burstein M, Lewi S, Walter P: Sur l'existence du fibrinogene foetal. Sang 25:102–107, 1954
12. Guillin M-C, Ménaché D: Fetal fibrinogen and fibrinogen Paris I. Comparative fibrin mono-mer aggregation studies. Thromb Res 3:117–135, 1973
13. Galankis DK, Mosesson MW: Evaluation of the role of in vivo proteolysis (fibrinogeno-lysis) in prolonging the thrombin time of human umbilical cord fibrinogen. Blood 48:190–198, 1976
14. Witt I, Muller H, Kunzer W: Evidence for the existence of foetal fibrinogen. Thromb Diath Haemorrh 22:101–109, 1969
15. Witt I, Muller H: Phosphorus and hexose content of human fetal fibrinogen. Biochim Biophys Acta 221:401–404, 1970
16. Aguerçif M, Giacometti N, Nigg OM, et al: Existe-t-il un fibrinogen foetal? Pediatrie 28:381–399, 1973
17. Larrieu MJ, Soulier JP, Minkowski A: Le sang du corden ombilical: Étude compléte da sa coagulabilité, comparaison avec le sang maternel. Etudes Neonat 1:39–60, 1952

18.  von Felten A, Straub PW: Coagulation studies of cord blood with special reference to "fetal fibrinogen." Thromb Diath Haemorrh 22:273–280, 1969

19.  Gralnick HR, Coller BS, Shulman NR, et al: Factor VIII. Ann Intern Med 86:598–616, 1975

20.  Johnson SS, Montgomery RR, Hathaway WE: Newborn factor VIII complex: Elevated activities in term infants and alterations in electrophoretic mobility related to illness and activated coagulation. Br J Haematol 47:597–606, 1981

21.  Fukui H, Takase T, Ikari H, et al: Factor VIII procoagulant activity, factor VIII related antigen and von Willebrand factor in newborn cord blood. Br J Haematol 42:637–646, 1979

22.  Jaffe EA, Nachman RL: Subunit structure of factor VIII antigen synthesized by cultured human endothelial cells. J Clin Invest 56:698–702, 1975

23.  Jurgens H, Gobel U, Bokelmann J, et al: Coagulation studies on umbilical arterial and venous blood from normal newborn babies. Eur J Pediatr 131:199–204, 1979

24.  Ratnoff OD, Rosenblum J: Role of Hageman factor in the initiation of clotting by glass. Am J Med 25: 160–168, 1958

25.  Margolis J: Activation of plasma by contact with glass: Evidence for a common reaction which releases plasma kinin and initiates coagulation. J Physiol 144:1–22, 1958

26.  Donaldson VH, Glueck HI, Miller MA, et al: Kininogen deficiency in Fitzgerald trait: Role of high molecular weight kininogen in clotting and fibrinolysis. J Lab Clin Med 87: 327–333, 1976

27.  Hilgartner MW, Smith CH: Plasma thromboplastin antecedent (factor XI) in the neonate. J Pediatr 66:747–752, 1965

28.  Gordon EM, Ratnoff OD, Saito H, et al: Studies on some coagulation factors (Hageman factor, plasma prekallikrein and high molecular weight kininogen) in the normal newborn. Am J Pediatr Hematol/Oncol 2:213–216, 1980

29.  Marcel GA, Caspar C, Sabatis C, et al: High prekallikrein levels during pregnancy. Pathol Biol 23(suppl):66–68, 1975

30.  Donaldson VH, Merriweather A, Wagner CJ: Unpublished observations

31.  Ratnoff OD: Personal communication

32.  Boisvert PL: The streptococcal antifibrinolysis test in clinical use. J Clin Invest 19:65–74, 1940

33.  Quie PG, Wannamaker WL: The plasminogen-plasmin system of newborn infants. Am J Dis Child 100:836–843, 1960

34.  Phillips LL, Skordelis J: A comparison of the fibrinolytic enzyme system in maternal and umbilical cord blood. Pediatrics 22:715–726, 1958

35.  Markarian M, Githins JH, Jackson JJ, et al: Fibrinolytic activity in premature infants: Relationship of the enzyme system to the respiratory distress syndrome. Am J Dis Child 113:312, 1967

36.  Ekelund H, Hedner U, Nilsson IM: Fibrinolysis in newborns. Acta Pediatr Scand 59:33–43, 1970

37.  Engström L, Kager L: Changes in plasma fibrinolytic activity of newborn infants during the first hour after birth. Acta Paediatr 53:326–328, 1964

38.  Chessels JM, Pitney WR: Fibrin split products in serum of newborn. Pediatrics 45:155, 1970 (letter)

39.  Karpatkin M: Fibrin split products in serum of newborn. Pediatrics 45:157–158, 1970 (letter)

40.  Seegers WH, Marciniak E: Inhibition of autoprothrombin C activity with plasma. Nature 193:1188–1190, 1962

41.  Biggs R, Denson KWE, Akman N, et al: Antithrombin III, antifactor Xa and heparin. Br J Haematol 19:283–305, 1970

42.  Yin ET, Wessler S, Stoll PJ: Identity of plasma activated factor X inhibitor with antithrombin III and heparin cofactor. J Biol Chem 246:3712–3719, 1971

43.  Seegers WH, Warner ED, Brinkhous KM, et al: Heparin and antithrombin activity of plasma. Science 96:300–301, 1942

44.  Abildgaard U: Purification of two progressive antithrombins of human plasma. Scand J Clin Lab Invest 19:190–195, 1967

45. Abildgaard U: Highly purified antithrombin III with heparin cofactor activity prepared by disc electrophoresis. Scand J Clin Lab Invest 21:89–91, 1968

46. Dombrose FA, Seegers WH, Sedensky JA: Antithrombin. Inhibition of thrombin and auto-prothrombin C(F-Xa) on a mutual depletion system. Thromb Diath Haemorrh 16:103–123, 1971

47. Rosenberg RD, Damus PS: The purification and mechanism of action of human antithrombin-heparin cofactor. J Biol Chem 248:6490–6505, 1973

48. Rosenberg JS, McKenna P, Rosenberg RD: Inhibition of human factor IXa by human antithrombin-heparin cofactor. J Biol Chem 250:8883–8888, 1975

49. Damus PS, Hicks M, Rosenberg RD: Anticoagulant action of heparin. Nature (Lond) 246:355–357, 1973

50. Stead N, Kaplan AP, Rosenberg RD: Inhibition of activated factor XII by antithrombin-heparin cofactor. J Biol Chem 251:6481–6488, 1976

51. Highsmith RF, Rosenberg RD: The inhibition of human plasmin by antithrombin-heparin cofactor. J Biol Chem 249:4335–4338, 1974

52. Hathaway WE, Neumann LL, Borden CA, et al: Immunologic studies of AT III heparin co-factor in the newborn. Thromb Haemost 39:624–630, 1978

53. McDonald MM, Hathaway WE, Reeve EB, et al: Biochemical and functional study of antithrombin III in newborn infants. Thromb Haemost 47:56–58, 1982

54. Harpel PC, Rosenberg RD: $\alpha_2$-Macroglobulin and antithrombin-heparin cofactor: Modulators of hemostatic and inflammatory reactions, in Spaet TH(ed): Progress in Hemostasis and Thrombosis, vol. 3. New York, Grune & Stratton, 1976, pp.145–189

55. Harpel PC, Mosesson MW: Degradation of human fibrinogen by plasma $\alpha_2$-macroglobulin–enzyme complexes. J Clin Invest 52:2175–2184, 1973

56. Ganrot PO, Schersten B: Serum $\alpha_2$-macroglobulin concentration and its variation with age and sex. Clin Chim Acta 15:113–120, 1967

57. James K, Johnson G, Fudenberg HH: The quantitative estimation of $\alpha_2$-macroglobulin in normal, pathological and cord sera. Clin Chim Acta 14:207–214, 1966

58. Ganrot PO, Bjerre B: $\alpha_1$-Antitrypsin and $\alpha_2$-macroglobulin concentration in serum during pregnancy. Acta Obstet Gynecol Scand 46:126–137, 1967

59. Horne CHW, Weir RJ, Howie PW, et al: Effect of combined oestrogen-progestogen con-traceptives on serum levels of $\alpha_2$-macroglobulin, transferrin, albumin, and IgG. Lancet 1:49–50, 1970

60. Harpel PC: Human plasma $\alpha_2$-macroglobulin, an inhibitor of plasma kallikrein. J Exp Med 132:329–352, 1970

61. Lanchantin GF, Plesset MC, Friedmann JA, et al: Dissociation of esterolytic and clotting activities of thrombin by trypsin-binding macroglobulin. Proc Soc Exp Biol Med 121:444–449, 1966

62. Ganrot PO: Inhibition of plasmin activity by $\alpha_2$-macroglobulin. Clin Chim Acta 16:328–329, 1967

63. Aoki N, Saito H, Kamiya T, et al: Congenital deficiency of $\alpha_2$-plasmin inhibitor associated with severe hemorrhagic tendency. J Clin Invest 63:877–884, 1979

64. Collen D: Identification of some properties of a new fast-reacting plasmin inhibitor in human plasma. Eur J Biochem 69:209–216, 1976

65. Saito H, Goldsmith GH, Moroi M, et al: Inhibitory spectrum of $\alpha_2$-plasmin inhibitor. Proc Natl Acad Sci USA 76:2013–2017, 1979

66. Pensky J, Levy L, Lepow IH: Partial purification of a serum inhibitor of C′1-esterase. J Biol Chem 236:1674–1679, 1961

67. Donaldson VH, Serum C1-inhibitor (C̄1-INH) in Bing DH (ed) The Chemistry and Physiol-ogy of Human Plasma Proteins. New York, Pergamon Press, 1979, pp 369-383

68. Ratnoff OD, Pensky J, Ogston D, et al: The inhibition of plasmin, plasma kallikrein, plasma permeability factor, and the C′1r subcomponent of the first component of complement by serum C′1-esterase inhibitor. J Exp Med 129:315–331, 1969

69. Forbes CD, Pensky J, Ratnoff OD: Inhibition of activated Hageman factor and activated plasma thromboplastin antecedent by purified serum C1-inactivator. J Lab Clin Med 76:809–815, 1970

70. Schreiber AD, Kaplan AP, Austen KF: Inhibition by C1̄-INH of Hageman factor fragment activation of coagulation, fibrinolysis and kinin generation. J Clin Invest 52:1402–1409, 1973

71. Donaldson VH: Serum inhibitor of C′1-esterase in health and disease. J Lab Clin Med 68:369–382, 1966

72. Donaldson VH, Evans RR: A biochemical abnormality in hereditary angioneurotic edema: Absence of serum C′1 esterase inhibitor. Am J Med 35:37–44, 1963

73. Donaldson VH: Unpublished observations

74. Laurell CB, Eriksson S: The electrophoretic $\alpha_1$-globulin pattern of serum in $\alpha_1$-antitrypsin deficiency. Scand J Clin Lab Invest 15:132–140, 1963

75. Meyer JF, Beith J, Metais P: On the inhibition of elastase by serum: Some distinguishing properties of $\alpha_1$-antitrypsin and $\alpha_2$-macroglobulin. Clin Chim Acta 62:42–53, 1975

76. Plow EF: Leukocyte elastase release during blood coagulation. A potential mechanism for activation of the alternative fibrinolytic pathway. J Clin Invest 69:564–572, 1982

77. Schmidt W, Egbring R, Haveman K: Effect of elastase-like and chymotrypsin-like neutral proteases from human granulocytes on isolated clotting factors. Thromb Res 6:315–319, 1975

78. Gitlin D, Biasucci A: Development of $\gamma$G, $\gamma$A, $\gamma$M, $\beta$1C/$\beta$1A, C′1 esterase inhibitor, ceruloplasmin, transferrin, hemopexin, haptoglobin, fibrinogen, plasminogen, $\alpha_1$-antitrypsin, orosomucoid, $\beta$-lipoprotein, $\alpha_2$-macroglobulin, and prealbumin in the human conceptus. J Clin Invest 48:1433–1446, 1969

79. Zilliacus H, Otterlin A-M, Maisson T: Blood clotting and fibrinolysis in human foetuses. Biol Neonate 10:108–112, 1966

80. Heikinheimo R: Coagulation studies with fetal blood. Biol Neonate 7:319–327, 1964

81. Terwiel JP, Veltkamp JJ, Bertina RM, et al: Coagulation factors in the human fetus of about 20 weeks of gestational age. Br J Haematol 45:641–650, 1980

82. Holmberg L, Henriksson P, Ekelund H, et al: Coagulation in the human fetus. Comparison with term newborn infants. J Pediatr 85:860–864, 1974

83. Vahlquist B, Westberg V, De las Heras M: Prothrombin and fibrinogen values in the young human fetus. Acta Soc Medic Upsallieusis 58:281–284, 1952

84. Firshein SI, Hoyer LW, Lazarchick J, et al: Prenatal diagnosis of classic hemophilia. N Engl J Med 300:937–941, 1979

85. Peake IR, Bloom AL, Giddings JC, et al: An immunoradiometric assay for procoagulant factor VIII-antigen. Results in haemophilia, von Willebrand's disease and fetal plasma and serum. Br J Haematol 42:269–281, 1979

86. Mibashan RS, Rodeck CH, Thumpston JK, et al: Prenatal plasma assay of fetal factor VIII and IX. Br J Haematol 41:611, 1979 (abstract)

87. Foley ME, Clayton JK, McNicol GP: Haemostatic mechanisms in maternal, umbilical vein and umbilical artery blood at the time of delivery. Br J Obstet Gynecol 84:81–87, 1977

88. Kisker CT, Robillard JE, Clarke WR: Development of blood coagulation—A fetal lamb model. Pediatr Res 15:1045–1050, 1981

89. Nelsestuen GL, Suttie JW: The mode of action of vitamin K. Isolation of a peptide containing the vitamin K-dependent portion of prothrombin. Proc Natl Acad Sci USA 70:3366–3370, 1973

90. Nelsestuen GL, Zytokovicz TH, Howard JB: The mode of action of vitamin K. Identification of $\gamma$-carboxyglutamic acid as a component of prothrombin. J Biol Chem 249:6347, 1974

91. Stenflo J: Vitamin K and the biosynthesis of prothrombin. III. Structural comparison of an $NH_2$-terminal fragment from normal and from Dicumarol-induced bovine prothrombin. J Biol Chem 248:6325–6350, 1973

92. Stenflo J, Fernlund P, Egan W, et al: Vitamin K dependent modifications of glutamic acid residues in prothrombin. Proc Natl. Acad Sci USA 71:2730–2733, 1974

93. Reekers PPM, Lindhout MJ, Kop-Klaassen BHM, et al: Demonstration of three anomalous

plasma proteins induced by a vitamin K antagonist. Biochim Biophys Acta 317:559–562, 1973

94. Hemker HC, Reekers PPM: Isolation purification of protein induced by vitamin K absence. Thromb Diath Haemorrh Suppl 57:83, 1974

95. Lindhout MJ, Kop-Klaassen BHM, Kop JMM, et al: Purification and properties of the phenprocoumon-induced decarboxyfactor X from bovine plasma. A comparison to normal factor X. Biochim Biophys Acta 533:302–317, 1978

96. Lindhout MJ, Kop-Klaassen BHM: Isolation and properties of the abnormal factor X induced by vitamin K antagonist. Thromb Diath Haemorrh 34:592, 1975

97. Stenflo J: A new vitamin K-dependent protein. Purification from bovine plasma and preliminary characterization. J Biol Chem 251:355–363, 1976

98. Esmon CT, Owen WG: Identification of an endothelial cell cofactor for thrombin-catalyzed activation of protein C. Proc Natl Acad Sci USA 28:2249–2252, 1981

99. Kisiel W, Canfield W, Ericsson L, et al: Anticoagulant properties of bovine plasma protein C following activation by thrombin. Biochemistry 16:5824–5831, 1977

100. Seegers WH, McCoy LE, Groben HD, et al: Purification and some properties of autoprothrombin II-A: An anticoagulant perhaps also related to fibrinolysis. Thromb Res 1:443–460, 1972

101. Price PA, Otuska AS, Poser JW, et al: Characterization of γ-carboxyglutamate-containing protein from bone. Proc Natl Acad Sci USA 73:1447–1451, 1976

102. Haushka P, Gallop PM: Purification and calcium-binding properties of osteocalcin, the γ-carboxyglutamate-containing protein of bone, in Wasserman RH, Corradino RA, Carafoli Z, et al (eds): Calcium Binding Proteins and Calcium Function. New York, Elsevier North-Holland, 1977, pp 338–347

103. Dam H, Dyggve H, Larsen H, et al: Vitamin K and hemorrhagic disease of the newborn. Adv Pediatr 5:129–153, 1952

104. Fresh JW, Ferguson JH, Stamey C, et al: Blood prothrombin, proconvertin and proaccelerin in normal infancy: Questionable relationships to vitamin K. Pediatrics 19:241–251, 1957

105. Dyggve H: Prothrombin and proconvertin in the newborn and during the first year of life. Acta Paediatr 47:251–259, 1958

106. VanCreveld S, Paulssen MMP, Eus JC, et al: Proconvertin content in blood of newborn full-term and premature infants. Etud Neonatal 3:53–61, 1954

107. Oski FA, Naiman JL: Blood coagulation and its disorders in the newborn, in Hematologic Problems in the Newborn (ed 2). Philadelphia, WB Saunders, 1972, pp 236–272

108. Sutherland JM, Glueck HI, Gleser G: Hemorrhagic disease of the newborn. Breast feeding as a necessary factor in the pathogenesis. Am J Dis Child 113:524–533, 1967

109. Aballi AJ, Lopez-Banus V, DeLamerens S, et al: Coagulation studies in the newborn period. I. Alterations of thromboplastin generation and effects of vitamin K on full term and premature infants. Am J Dis Child 94:594–600, 1957

110. Townsend CW: The hemorrhagic disease of the newborn. Arch Pediatr 11:559–565, 1894

111. Aballi A: The action of vitamin K in the neonatal period. South Med J 58:48–55, 1965

112. Dam H, Glavind J, Larsen H, et al: Investigations into the cause of physiological hypoprothrombinemia in newborn children. IV. The vitamin K content of women's milk and cows' milk. Acta Med Scand 112:210–216, 1942

113. Keenan WJ, Jewett T, Glueck HI: Role of feeding and vitamin K in hypoprothrombinemia of the newborn. Am J Dis Child 121:271–277, 1971

114. Smith CH: Aplastic anemia and bone marrow transplantation. in Miller D, Pearson HA (eds.): Blood Diseases of Infancy and Childhood. St. Louis, CV Mosby, 1960, pp 465–496

115. Mountain KR, Hirsh J, Gallus AS: Neonatal coagulation defect due to anticonvulsant drug treatment in pregnancy. Lancet 1:265–268, 1970

116. Seip M: Effects of antiepileptic drugs in pregnancy on the fetus and newborn infant. Ann Clin Res 5:205–207, 1973

117. Hathaway WE, Bonnar J: Perinatal Coagulation, New York, Grune & Stratton, 1978, pp 115–169, 171–200

118. Sacks JJ, Labate JS: Dicumarol in the treatment of antenatal thromboembolic disease. Report of a case with hemorrhagic manifestations in the fetus. Am J Obstet Gynecol 57:965–971, 1949

119. Fillimore SJ, McDevitt E: Effects of coumarin compounds on the fetus. Ann Intern Med 73:731–735, 1970

120. Gordon RR, Dean I: Fetal deaths from antenatal anticoagulant therapy. Br Med J 2:719–721, 1955

121. Bonnar J: Warfarin anticoagulation and pregnancy. Lancet 1:862–863, 1971

122. Flessa HC, Glueck HI, Dritschilo A: Thromboembolic disorders in pregnancy: Pathophysiology, diagnosis and treatment with emphasis on heparin. Clin Obstet Gynecol 17:195–235, 1974

123. Hirsh J, Cade JF, O'Sullivan EF: Clinical experience with anticoagulant therapy during pregnancy. Br Med J 1:270–273, 1970

124. Bonnar J: Long term self-administered heparin therapy for prevention of and treatment of thromboembolic complications in pregnancy, Kakkar VV, in Thomas DP (eds.): Heparin—Chemistry and Clinical Usage. London, Academic Press, 1976, pp 247–260

125. Hall JG, Pauli RM, Wilson KM: Maternal and fetal sequelae of anticoagulation during pregnancy. Am J Med 68:122–140, 1980

126. Bonnar J, Denson KWE, Biggs R: Subcutaneous heparin and prevention of thrombosis. Lancet 2:539–540, 1972

127. Salzman EW, Deykin D, Shapiro RM, et al: Management of heparin therapy: Controlled prospective trial. N Engl J Med 292:1046–1050, 1975

128. Douglas AS, McNicol GP: Anticoagulant therapy, in Biggs R (ed): Human Blood Coagulation, Haemostasis and Thrombosis (ed 2). Oxford, Blackwell Scientific Publications, 1976, pp 557–607

129. Hirsh J, Gentoh E, Hull R (eds.): Heparin, in Venous Thromboembolism. New York, Grune & Stratton, 1981, pp 155–183

130. Kwaan H, Bowie EW: Thrombosis. Philadelphia, WB Saunders Co, 1981, p 172

131. Bloomfield DK: Fetal deaths and malformations associated with the use of coumarin derivatives in pregnancy. A critical review. Am J Obstet Gynecol 107:883–888, 1970

132. Pettifor JM, Benson R: Congenital malformations associated with administration of oral anticoagulants during pregnancy. J Pediatr 86:459–462, 1975

133. Shaul WL, Emery H, Hall JG: Chondrodysplasia punctata and maternal warfarin use during pregnancy. Am J Dis Child 129:360–362, 1975

134. Warkany J, Bofinger M: Le role de la coumadine dans les malformations congenitales. Med Hyg 33:1454–1457, 1975

135. Bishop AJ, Israels LG, Chernick V, et al: Placental transfer of intravascular coagulation between mother and fetus. Pediatr Res 5:113–125, 1971

136. Stander RW, Flessa HC, Glueck HI, et al: Changes in maternal coagulation factors after intra-amniotic injection of hypertonic saline. Obstet Gynecol 37:660–666, 1971

137. Glueck HI, Flessa HC, Kisker CT, et al: Hypotonic saline-induced abortion. Correlation of fetal death with disseminated intravascular coagulation. JAMA 225:28–31, 1973

138. Abildgaard CF: Recognition and treatment of intravascular coagulation. J Pediatr 74:163–176, 1969

139. Lascari AD, Wallace PD: Disseminated intravascular coagulation in the newborn. Clin Pediatr 10:11–17, 1971

140. Karpatkin M: Diagnosis and management of disseminated intravascular coagulation. Pediatr Clin North Am 18:23–38, 1971

141. Whaun JM, Oski FA, Urmson J: Experience with disseminated intravascular coagulation in a children's hospital. Can Med Assoc J 107:963–967, 1972

142. Edson JR, Blaese RM, White JG, et al: Defibrination syndrome in an infant born after abruptio placentae. J Pediatr 72:342–346, 1968

143. Chessells JM, Wigglesworth JS: Coagulation studies in severe birth asphyxia. Arch Dis Child 46:252–256, 1971
144. Karpatkin M, Sacker I, Ackerman N: Respiratory distress syndrome and disseminated intravascular coagulation in two siblings. Lancet 1:102–103, 1972
145. Adner MM, Kauff RE, Sherman JD: Purpura fulminans in a child with pneumococcal septicemia two years after splenectomy. JAMA 213:1681–1683, 1970
146. Goldenfarb PB, Zucker S, Corrigan JJ Jr, et al: The coagulation mechanism in active bacterial infection. Br J Haematol 18:643–652, 1970
147. Corrigan JJ, Ray WL, May BS: Changes in the blood coagulation system associated with septicemia. N Engl J Med 279:851–856, 1968
148. McCracken GH, Dickerman JD: Septicemia and disseminated intravascular coagulation. Am J Dis Child 118:431–434, 1969
149. Prochazka JV, Lucas RN, Beauchamp CJ, et al: Systemic candidiasis with disseminated intravascular coagulation. A complication of total parenteral alimentation. Am J Dis Child 122:255–256, 1971
150. Mannucci PM, Lobina GF, Gaocci L, et al: Effect on blood coagulation of massive intravascular hemolysis. Blood 33:207–213, 1969
151. Kasabach HH, Merritt KK: Capillary hemangioma with extensive purpura. Am J Dis Child 59:1063–1070, 1940
152. Rivers RP: Coagulation changes associated with a high hematocrit in the newborn infant. Acta Pediatr Scand 64:449–456, 1975
153. Dennis LH, Stewart JL, Conrad ME: A consumption coagulation defect in congenital cyanotic heart disease and its treatment with heparin. J Pediatr 71:407–410, 1967
154. Allen DM: Heparin therapy of purpura fulminans. Pediatrics. 38:211–214, 1966
155. Benirshke K: Twin placenta in perinatal mortality. NY State Med J 61:1499–1508, 1961
155a. Branson HE, Katz J, Marble R, et al: Inherited protein C deficiency and coumarin-responsible chronic relapsing purpura fulminans in a newborn infant. Lancet 2:1165–1168, 1983
155b. Marciniak E, Wilson HD, Marlar RA: Neonatal purpural fulminans as expression of homozygosity for protein C deficiency. Blood 62:303a, 1983 (abstract)
156. Niewiarowski S, Latallo Z, Stachurska J: Apparition d'un inhibiteur de la thromboplastino-formation au cours de la protéolyse du fibrinogène. Rev Hematol 14:118–128, 1959
157. Fletcher AP, Alkjaersig N, Sherry S: The maintenance of a sustained thrombolytic state in man. I. Induction and effects. J Clin Invest 38:1096–1110, 1959
158. Kisker CT, Rush RR: Detection of intravascular coagulation. J Clin Invest 50:2235–2241, 1971
159. Nossel HL, Younger LR, Wilner GD, et al: Radioimmunoassay of human fibrinopeptide A. Proc Natl Acad Sci USA 68:2350–2353, 1971
160. Nossel HL, Yudelman I, Canfield RE, et al: Measurement of fibrinopeptide A in human blood J Clin Invest 54:43–53, 1974
161. Bilezikian SB, Nossel HL, Butler VP, et al: Radioimmunoassay of human fibrinopeptide B and kinetics of fibrinopeptide cleavage by different enzymes. J Clin Invest 56:438–445, 1975
162. Stuart RK, Michel A: Monitoring heparin therapy with activated partial thromboplastin time. Can Med Assoc J 104:385–388, 1971
163. Whaun JM, Urmson J, Oski FA: One year's experience with disseminated intravascular coagulation in a children's hospital. Prog Am Pediatr Soc 6, 1971
164. Whaun JM, Oski FA, Urmson J: Experience with disseminated intravascular coagulation in a children's hospital. Can Med Assoc J 107:963–967, 1972
165. Gross S, Melhorn DK: Exchange transfusion with citrated whole blood for disseminated intravascular clotting. J Pediatr 78:415–419, 1971
166. Schulman I: Pediatric aspects of the mild hemophilias. Med Clin North Am 46:93–105, 1962
167. Didisheim P, Lewis JH: Congenital disorders of the mechanisms for coagulation of blood. Pediatrics 22:478–493, 1958
168. Hartmann JR, Diamond LK: Hemophilia and related haemorrhagic disorders. Practitioner 178:179–190, 1957
169. Baehner RL, Strauss HS: Hemophilia in the first year of life. N Engl J Med 275:524–528, 1966

170. Strauss HS: Clinical pathological conference. J Pediatr 66:443–452, 1965
171. Struwe FE: Intracranial hemorrhage and occlusive hydrocephalus in hereditary bleeding disorders. Dev Med Child Neurol 112:(suppl 22):165–169, 1970
172. McCarthy JW, Coble LL: Intracranial hemorrhage and subsequent communicating hydro-cephalus in a neonate with classical hemophilia. Pediatrics 51:122–124, 1973
173. Losowsky MS, Miloszewski KJA: Annotation: Factor XIII. Br J Haematol 37:1–5, 1977
174. Duckert F, Jung E, Schmerling DH: A hitherto undescribed congenital hemorrhagic diathesis probably due to congenital fibrin stabilizing factor deficiency. Thromb Diath Haemorrh 5:179–186, 1960
175. Britten AF: Congenital deficiency of factor XIII (fibrin-stabilizing factor). Report of a case and review of the literature. Am J Med 43:751–761, 1967
176. Ratnoff OD, Steinberg AG: Inheritance of fibrin stabilizing factor deficiency. Lancet 1:25–26, 1968
177. Lorand L: Fibrin clots. Nature (Lon) 166:694–695, 1950
178. Lorand L: A study of the solubility of fibrin clots in urea. Hung Acta Physiol 1:192–196, 1948
179. Loewy AG: Enzymatic control of insoluble fibrin formation, Laki K (ed): in Fibrinogen. New York, Marcel Dekker, 1968, pp 185–223
180. Lorand L, Ong HH: Labelling of amine-acceptor cross-linking sites of fibrin by transpeptidation. Biochemistry 5:1747–1753, 1966
181. Miloszewski K, Losowsky MS: The half-life of factor XIII in vivo. Br J Haematol 19:685–690, 1970
182. Kunzer W: Die Blutgerinnung bie Neugeborenen und ihre Störungen. Wien Klin Wochenschr 80:150–156, 1968
183. Kingsley CS: Familial factor V deficiency: The pattern of heredity. Q J Med ns 23:323–329, 1954
184. Breederveld K, van Royen EA, tenCate JW: Severe factor V deficiency with prolonged bleed-ing time. Thromb Diath Haemorrh 32:538–548, 1974
185. Rosenthal RL, Dreskin OH, Rosenthal N: New hemophilia-like disease caused by deficiency of third plasma thromboplastin factor. Proc Soc Exp Biol Med 82:171–174, 1953
186. Cavins JA, Wall RL: Clinical and laboratory studies of plasma thromboplastin antecedent deficiency (PTA). Am J Med 29:444–448, 1960
187. Seligsohn U: High gene frequency of factor XI (PTA) deficiency in Ashkenazi Jews. Blood 51:1223–1228, 1978
188. Ratnoff OD (ed): Deficiency of plasma thromboplastin antecedent, in Bleeding Syndromes. Springfield, Ill, Charles C Thomas, 1960, pp 56–59
189. Henry EI, Rosenthal RL, Hoffman I: Spontaneous hemorrhages caused by plasma thrombo-plastin antecedent deficiency. Report of a case. JAMA 162:727–729, 1956
190. Kingsley CS: Familial factor V deficiency: The pattern of heredity. Q J Med ns 23:323–329, 1954
191. Gitlin D, Borges W: Studies on the metabolism of fibrinogen in two patients with congenital afibrinogenemia. Blood 8:679–686, 1953
192. Gugler E, Luscher EF: Platelet function in congenital afibrinogenemia. Thromb Diath Haemorrh 14:361–373, 1965
193. Ménaché D: Abnormal fibrinogens. A review. Thromb Diath Haemorrh 29:525–535, 1973
194. Aznar J, Fernandes-Pavon A, Reganon E, et al: Fibrinogen Valencia. A new case of congeni-tal dysfibrinogenemia. Thromb Diath Haemorrh 32:564–577, 1974
195. von Willebrand EA: Hereditary pseudohemophili. Finsk Lakarsallskapets Handlingar 68:87–112, 1926
196. Minot GR: A familial hemorrhagic condition associated with prolongation of the bleeding time. Am J Med Sci 175:301–306, 1928
197. Abildgaard CF, Suzuki A, Harrison J, et al: Serial studies in von Willebrand's disease: Vari-ability vs. variants. Blood 56:712–716, 1980
198. Ratnoff OD, Bennett B: Clues to the pathogenesis of bleeding in von Willebrand's disease. N Engl J Med 289:1182–1183, 1973
199. Larrieu M-J, Caen JP, Meyer DO, et al: Congenital bleeding disorders with long bleeding

time and normal platelet count. II. Von Willebrand's disease (report of thirty-seven patients). Am J Med 45:354–372, 1968

200. Cornu P, Larrieu M-J, Caen JP, et al: Maladie de Willebrand. Étude clinique, genetique et biologique. Nouv Rev Fr Haematol 1:231–262, 1961

201. Hathaway WE, Belhazen LP, Hathaway HS: Evidence for a new plasma thromboplastin factor. I. Case report, coagulation studies and physico-chemical properties. Blood 26:521–532, 1965

202. DeVries A, Matoth P, Shamir ZS: Familial congenital labile factor deficiency with syndactylism: Investigation on the mode of action of the labile factor. Acta Haematol 5:129–142, 1951

203. Albin AR, Kushuer JH, Murphy A, et al: Platelet enumeration in the neonatal period. Pediatrics. 28:822–824, 1961

204. Kaplan S, Klein SW: Thrombocytopenia and intestinal bleeding in premature infants. J Pediatr 61:17–23, 1962

205. Fogel BJ, Arias D, Kung F: Platelet counts in healthy premature infants. J Pediatr 73:108–110, 1959

206. Pearson HA, McIntosh S: Neonatal thrombocytopenia. Clin Haematol 7:111–122, 1978

207. Berry AM, Agarawal KN, Bajaj G: Congenital amegakaryocytic thrombocytopenia. J Indian Med Assoc 50:209–211, 1968

208. O'Gorman-Hughes DW: Neonatal thrombocytopenia: Assessment of etiology and prognosis. Aust Paediatr J 3:226–233, 1968

209. Estren S, Dameshek W: Familial hypoplastic anemia of childhood. Am J Dis Child 73:671–687, 1947

210. Mauer AM: The coagulation system: The Platelets, in Pediatric Hematology. New York, McGraw Hill, 1969, pp 411–442

211. Oski FA, Naiman JL: Thrombocytopenia in the newborn, in Schaffer AJ (ed): Hematologic problems in the newborn. Philadelphia, WB Saunders, 1972, pp 273–311

212. Emery JL, Gordon RR, Rendle-Short J, et al: Congenital amegakaryocytic thrombocytopenia with congenital deformities and a leukemoid blood picture in the newborn. Blood 12:567–576, 1957

213. Hall JG, Levin J, Kuhn JP, et al: Thrombocytopenia with absent radius. Medicine 48:411–439, 1969

214. Dignan P St J, Mauer AM, Frantz C: Phocomelia with congenital hypoplastic thrombocytopenia and myeloid leukemoid reactions. J Pediatr 70:561–573, 1967

215. Fanconi G: Familiare Infantile perniziosartig Anamie (pernizioses Blutbild und Konstitution). Jahrbuck Kinderheilk 117:257–280, 1927

216. Bloom GE, Warner S, Gerald PW, et al: Chromosomal abnormalities in constitutional aplastic anemia. N Engl J Med 274:8–14, 1966

217. Engel RR, Hammond D, Eitzman DV, et al: Transient congenital leukemia in seven infants with mongolism. J Pediatr 65:303–305, 1964

218. Besselman DM: Splenectomy in the management of the anemia and thrombocytopenia of osteopetrosis (marble bone disease) J Pediatr 69:455–457, 1966

219. Eisenstein EM: Congenital amegakaryocytic thrombocytopenic purpura. Clin Pediatr 5:143–147, 1966

220. Hoyeraal HM, Lamvik J, Moe PJ: Congenital hypoplastic thrombocytopenia and cerebral malformations in two brothers. Acta Paediatr Scand 59:185–191, 1970

221. Wiskott A: Familiarer angeborener Morbus Werlhofii? Mschr Kinderheilk 68:212–216, 1937

222. Aldrich RA, Steinberg AG, Campbell DC: Pedigree demonstrating a sex-linked recessive condition characterized by draining ears, eczematoid dermatitis, and bloody diarrhea. Pediatrics 13:133–139, 1954

223. Baldini M, Kim B, Steiner M, et al: Metabolic platelet defect in the Wiskott-Aldrich syndrome. Pediatr Res 3:377–378, 1969

224. Parkman R, Remold-O'Donnell E, Kenney DM, et al: Surface protein abnormalities in lymphocytes and platelets from patients with Wiskott-Aldrich syndrome. Lancet 2:1387–1389, 1981

225. Canales GL, Mauer AM: Sex-linked hereditary thrombocytopenia as a variant of the Wiskott-Aldrich syndrome. N Engl J Med 277:899–901, 1967

226. Spitler LE, Levin AS, Stites DP, et al: The Wiskott-Aldrich syndrome: Results of transfer factor therapy. J Clin Invest 51:3216–3224, 1972

227. August CS, Hathaway WE, Githins JH, et al: Improved platelet function following bone marrow transplantation in an infant with Wiskott-Aldrich syndrome. J Pediatr 82:58–64, 1973

228. Oski FA, Naiman JL, Allen DM, et al: Leukocyte inclusions—Dohle bodies—associated with platelet abnormality (the May-Hegglin anomaly). Report of a family and review of the literature. Blood 20:657–667, 1962

229. Hugh-Jones K, Mansfield PA, Brewer HF: Congenital thrombocytopenic purpura. Arch Dis Child 35:146–151, 1960

230. Korn D: Congenital hypoplastic thrombocytopenia. Am J Clin Pathol 37:405–413, 1962

231. Berge T, Brunnhage F, Nilsson LR: Congenital hypoplastic thrombocytopenia in rubella embryopathy. Acta Paediatr 52:349–352, 1963

232. Epstein RD, Lozner EL, Cobbey TS Jr, et al: Congenital thrombocytopenic purpura. Am J Med 9:44–56, 1950

233. Nathan DJ, Snapper I: Simultaneous placental transfer of factors responsible for L-E cell formation and thrombocytopenia. Am J Med 25:647–653, 1958

234. Kohler PF, Farr RS: Elevation of cord over maternal IgG immunoglobulin: Evidence for an active placental IgG transport. Nature 210:1070–1071, 1966

235. Schlamowitz M: Membrane receptors in the specific transfer of immunoglobulins from mother to young. Immunol Commun 5:481–500, 1976

236. Blaese RM, Strober W, Waldmann TA: Hypercatabolism of several serum proteins in the Wiskott-Aldrich syndrome. J Clin Invest 48:8a, 1969 (abstract)

237. Waldmann TA, Strober W, Blaese RM: Variations in the metabolism of immunoglobulins measured by turnover rates, in Merler E (ed): Immunoglobulins. Washington DC, National Academy of Sciences, 1970, pp 33–48

238. Robson HN, Walker CHM: Congenital and neonatal thrombocytopenic purpura. Arch Dis Child 26:175–183, 1951

239. Harrington WJ, Sprague CC, Minnich V, et al: Immunologic mechanisms in idiopathic and neonatal thrombocytopenic purpura. Ann Intern Med 38:433–469, 1953

240. Schulman I, Smith CH, Ando RE: Congenital thrombocytopenic purpura; observations on 3 infants of a non-affected mother; demonstrations of platelet agglutinins and evidence for platelet isoimmunization. Am J Dis Child 88:784–786, 1954

241. Desai RG, McCutcheon E, Little B, et al: Feto-maternal passage of leukocytes and platelets in erythroblastosis fetalis. Blood 27:858–862, 1966

242. Dixon R, Rosse W, Ebbert L: Quantitative determination of antibody in idiopathic thrombocytopenic purpura. Correlation of serum and platelet bound antibody with clinical response. N Eng J Med 292:230–236, 1975

243. Cines DB, Schreiber AD: Immune thrombocytopenia. Use of a Coombs antiglobulin test to detect IgG and C3 on platelets. N Engl J Med 300:106–111, 1979

244. Scott JR, Cruickshank DP, Kochenour NK, et al: Fetal platelet counts in obstetric management of immunologic thrombocytopenic purpura. Am J Obstet Gynecol 136:495–499, 1980

245. Karpatkin M, Porges RF, Karpatkin S: Platelet counts in infants of women with autoimmune thrombocytopenia. Effect of steroid administrations to the mother. N Engl J Med 305:936–939, 1981

245a. LoBuglio AF, Court WS, Vinocur L, et al: Immune thrombocytopenic purpura. Use of a [125]I-labelled antihuman IgC monoclonal antibody to quantify platelet-bound IgG. N Engl J Med 309:459–463, 1983

246. Rodriguez S, Leikin S, Hiller M: Neonatal thrombocytopenia associated with antepartum administration of drugs. N Engl J Med 270:881–884, 1964

247. Merenstein GB, O'Loughlin EP, Plunkett DC: Effects of maternal thiazides on platelet counts of newborn infants. J Pediatr 76:766–767, 1970

248. Schiff D, Aranda JV, Stern L: Neonatal thrombocytopenia and congenital malformation associated with administration of tolbutamide to the mother. J Pediatr 77:457–458, 1970

249. Hathaway WE, Bonnar J: Perinatal Coagulation. New York, Grune & Stratton, 1978, pp 191–194

250. Mauer AM, deVaux LO, Lahey ME: Neonatal and maternal thrombocytopenic purpura due to quinine. Pediatrics 19:84–87, 1957

251. Monnens LAH, Retera RJM: Thrombotic thrombocytopenic purpura in a neonatal infant. J Pediatr 71:118–123, 1967

252. Morrow G III, Barness LA, Auerbach VH, et al: Observations on the coexistence of methylmalonic acidemia and glycinemia. J Pediatr 74:680–690, 1969

253. Allen DM, Necheles TF, Rieker R, et al: Reversible neonatal pancytopenia due to isovaleric acidemia. Soc Prog Pediatr Res 156, 1959 (abstract)

254. Bowie EJW, Thompson JH Jr, Owen CA Jr: The blood platelet (including a discussion of qualitative platelet diseases). Proc Mayo Clin 40:625–651, 1965

255. Zaizov R, Cohen I, Matoth Y: Thromboasthenia. A study of two siblings. Acta Paediatr Scand 57:522–526, 1968

256. Suransri U, Cheung WH, Sawitsky A: The effect of bilirubin on the human platelet. J Pediatr 74:240–246, 1969

257. Maurer HM, Caul J: Bilirubin-induced platelet staining, aggregation, and adenine nucleotide release. Soc Pediatr Res 4:465, 1970 (abstract)

258. Bleyer WA, Au WY, Lange WA Sr, et al: Studies on the detection of adverse drug reactions in the newborn. I. Fetal exposure to maternal medication. JAMA 213:2046–2048, 1970

259. Bleyer WA, Breckenridge RT: Studies in the detection of adverse drug reactions in the newborn. II. The effects of prenatal aspirin on newborn hemostasis. JAMA 213:2049–2053, 1970

259a. McAdams AJ: Pulmonary hemorrhage in the newborn. Am J Dis Child 113:255–262, 1967

260. Rowe S, Avery ME: Massive pulmonary hemorrhage in the newborn. II. Clinical considerations. J Pediatr 69:12–20, 1966

261. DeSa DJ, MacLean BS: An analysis of massive pulmonary haemorrhage in the newborn infant in Oxford, 1848–1969. J Obstet Gynecol Br Commonw 77:158–163, 1970

262. Fedrirk J, Butler NR: Certain causes of neonatal death. IV. Massive pulmonary haemorrhage. Biol Neonate 18:243–262, 1971

263. Cole VA, Norman ICS, Reynolds EOR, et al: Pathogenesis of hemorrhagic pulmonary edema and massive pulmonary hemorrhage in the newborn. Pediatrics 51:175–187, 1973

264. Hathaway WE: Coagulation problems in the newborn infant. Pediatr Clin North Am 17:929–942, 1970

265. Roberts JT, Davies AJ, Bloom AL: Coagulation studies in massive pulmonary hemorrhage of the newborn. J Clin Pathol 19:334–338, 1966

266. Thomas DB: Survival after massive pulmonary hemorrhage in the neonatal period. Acta Paediatr Scand 64:825–829, 1975

267. Gruenwald P: Subependymal cerebral hemorrhage in premature infants and its relation to various injurious influences at birth. Am J Obstet Gynecol 61:1285–1292, 1951

268. Ross JJ, Dimmette RM: Subependymal cerebral hemorrhage in infancy. Am J Dis Child 110:531–542, 1965

269. Thomas DB: Hyperosmolality and intraventricular haemorrhage in premature babies. Acta Paediatr Scand 65:429–432, 1976

270. Wigglesworth JS, Keith IH, Girling DJ, et al: Hyaline membrane disease, alkali and intraventricular haemorrhage. Arch Dis Child 51:755–762, 1976

271. Gupta JM, Starr H, Fincher P, et al: Intraventricular haemorrhage in the newborn. Med J Aust 2:338–340, 1976

272. Gray OP, Ackerman A, Fraser AJ: Intracranial haemorrhage and clotting defects in low birth weight infants. Lancet 1:545–548, 1968

273. Hambleton G, Appleyard WJ: Controlled trial of fresh frozen plasma in asphyxiated low birth weight infants. Arch Dis Child 48:31–35, 1973

274. Waltl H, Födisch H, Kurz R, et al: Terminalisblutungen bei Frühgeborenen: Wirkungslosigkeit einer gerinnugsfördernden Prophylaxe (Eine kontrollierte Studie). Monatsschr Kinderheilk 122:192–197, 1974

275. Lorber J, Bhat US: Posthemorrhagic hydrocephalus. Diagnosis, differential diagnosis, treatment and long term results. Arch Dis Child 49:751–762, 1974

276. Report of the Committee on Nutrition, American Academy of Pediatrics. Pediatrics 28:501–507, 1961.

277. Donaldson VH, Kisker CT: Blood coagulation in hemostasis, in Nathan DG, Oski FA (eds): Hematology of Infancy and Childhood. Philadelphia, WB Saunders Co, 1974, pp 561–625

Oscar D. Ratnoff

# 14

# Hemostatic Defects in Liver and Biliary Tract Disease and Disorders of Vitamin K Metabolism

A generalized bleeding tendency has long been recognized as a concomitant of protracted biliary tract obstruction, chronic hepatic disease, and the severer forms of acute hepatitis, and may contribute significantly to morbidity and mortality.[1-3] Apparently spontaneous cutaneous purpura, epistaxis, and gastrointestinal, genitourinary, or gingival bleeding are disturbingly frequent. Impaired hemostasis may enhance bleeding from varices or peptic ulceration, and surgical procedures may be followed by devastating hemorrhage.

The principal cause of bleeding in obstructive jaundice is impaired absorption of vitamin K from the gastrointestinal tract. Other disorders of vitamin K metabolism are less common, but are clinically important. In hepatic disease, depressed synthesis of clotting factors, decreased clearance of activated clotting factors from the circulation, disseminated intravascular coagulation, fibrinolysis, or platelet disturbances may be responsible singly or in combination.

## THE VITAMIN K-DEPENDENT CLOTTING FACTORS

Prothrombin, factor VII, Stuart factor (factor X), and Christmas factor (factor IX), all of which participate in the clotting process, are synthesized only when vitamin K is available to the liver. Functional deficiencies of the first three of these factors are recognized in the laboratory by the presence of an abnormally long prothrombin time, and deficiency of Christmas factor by prolongation of the partial thromboplastin time.

*Vitamin K* is the generic name for a group of naphthoquinone derivatives with similar biological properties. It serves as a cofactor for a hepatic microsomal enzyme that is needed for posttranslational completion of the synthesis of the vitamin K-dependent clotting factors. This enzyme directs the insertion of carbon dioxide into the $\gamma$-carbon of certain glutamic acid residues in the protein precursors of these factors after their synthesis by hepatocytes.[4] The hepatic origin of these factors, suggested by their deficiency in hepatic disease and in experimental animals with damaged or extirpated livers, has been established by their synthesis by rat liver slices[5] and by the isolated, perfused rat liver.[6,7]

Deficiencies of single vitamin K-dependent clotting factors are almost invariably hereditary in nature and do not respond to therapy with vitamin K (Chapter 5); one exception is the deficiency of Stuart factor (factor X) that may complicate amyloidosis (Chapter 10). Disturbances of vitamin K metabolism, on the other hand, lead to deficiencies of all of the clotting factors that require this vitamin for synthesis. Multiple deficiencies, then, can come about from a lack of available vitamin K, from its malabsorption or from interference with its utilization by coumarin-like anticoagulants or by hepatic disease.

Compounds with vitamin K-like activity cannot be synthesized by mammals but are furnished by plant foods, particularly leafy green vegetables and legumes, and by intestinal flora. Natural vitamin K compounds are lipid soluble. As a consequence, their absorption from the gut is dependent upon the presence of bile salts.[8,9] Absorption in man takes place principally in the small intestine.[10]

When vitamin K is not absorbed from the gut or its utilization is inhibited by administration of coumarinlike anticoagulants (Chapter 16), functional clotting tests demonstrate deficiencies of the vitamin K-dependent factors. In fact, however, the protein precursors of these factors, lacking the full component of tricarboxylic glutamic acid residues, are synthesized by the liver and discharged into the bloodstream. There they can be recognized immunologically[11-14] or by abnormalities of their coagulant properties.[15,16]

In newborn infants, the concentration of the vitamin K-dependent clotting factors is less than in older infants or adults, and may decline during the first few days of life. Human milk is a poor source of vitamin K, but the vitamin is soon furnished by intestinal flora; cow's milk is considerably richer in vitamin K. Rarely, the deficiency of vitamin K may bring about so sharp a decline in the clotting factors dependent on this agent that a severe bleeding tendency results, hemorrhagic disease of the newborn, discussed more fully in Chapter 13. In contrast, in otherwise normal adults, deprivation of vitamin K for several weeks does not bring about a deficiency of the vitamin K-dependent factors unless oral antibiotics are simultaneously administered.[17] In patients with cirrhosis, however, interference with bacterial growth by administration of neomycin may impair vitamin K synthesis, as demonstrated by prolongation of the prothrombin time.[18]

Rarely, a patient in whom dietary intake of vitamin K is poor may develop deficiencies of the vitamin K-dependent factors, particularly if he is also under treatment with oral antibiotics. The patient is particularly vulnerable in the postoperative period. Antibiotic therapy, however, is not a requisite for the appearance of this syndrome, which is more likely to occur when bowel surgery has interfered with normal absorption of lipids. A deficiency of the vitamin K-dependent factors is an uncommon troublesome complication of disorders that impair absorption of this vitamin. For example, in non-tropical sprue the patient may come to medical attention because of the gradual appearance of ecchymoses and, in women, menorrhagia. The diagnosis depends on an accurate history, the presence of an otherwise unexplained long prothrombin time, and laboratory studies appropriate for the basic disorder.

Similarly, the absorption of vitamin K is impeded by therapy with cholestyramine,[19] which is used to suppress the itching caused by partial biliary tract obstruction and to reduce serum cholesterol in hypercholesterolemia. Cholestyramine binds bile salts, and as a consequence the absorption of vitamin K is reduced. In all these situations, intramuscular injection of 5 to 25 mg of vitamin $K_1$ will correct the defect within hours, but treatment must be continued until the basic disorder is corrected. If bleeding is alarming, temporary benefit until the effect of vitamin K is manifest may be provided by transfusion of plasma; a typical dosage is one liter to an adult.

These observations provide an understanding of the deficiency of the vitamin K-dependent clotting factors observed in patients with obstructive jaundice or parenchymal hepatic disease. During the first few days after biliary duct obstruction by stone, the titers of the vitamin K-dependent factors are normal or even elevated.[20] In more prolonged obstruction, the exclusion of bile salts from the gut impedes the absorption of vitamin K, so that the carboxylation of the vitamin K-dependent factors is incomplete. In this way, patients with either intra- or extrahepatic obstructive jaundice may develop evidence of a bleeding tendency, and the prothrombin time is prolonged.[21]

Oral administration of a combination of vitamin K and bile salts corrects the bleeding tendency when absorption of the vitamin is impaired.[22] Current practice, however, is to furnish the vitamin by parenteral injection.[23] As little as 5 mg/day of vitamin $K_1$ will shorten the prothrombin time to normal within a day or two in adults with obstructive jaundice uncomplicated by hepatic disease. Therapy with vitamin K has essentially eliminated the high risk of hemorrhage in patients undergoing surgery for extrahepatic biliary tract obstruction.[24] It is less effective in patients with intrahepatic obstructive jaundice, who usually have concomitant hepatic dysfunction. In an acute emergency, the transfusion of one liter of plasma to an adult may provide temporary hemostasis until the effect of vitamin K is manifested. Because the biological half-life of factor VII is only a few hours, the initial transfusion may need to be followed by additional plasma, for example, 200 ml every four hours. The use of commercial concentrates of the vitamin K-dependent factors is unnecessary and dangerous because the high risk of hepatitis and disseminated intravascular coagulation.

In parenchymal hepatic disease, the titers of all the vitamin K-dependent clotting factors may be depressed, as measured in clotting assays. In contrast to obstructive jaundice, these low titers are due almost entirely to decreased synthesis of the protein precursors of these factors.[11,25] Additionally, utilization of vitamin K for posttranslational carboxylation may be defective, so that the small fraction of the vitamin K-dependent factors that does reach the plasma may be incompletely carboxylated.[14] Low titers of the vitamin K-dependent factors account, in part, for the long prothrombin time that is commonplace in both acute and chronic hepatic disease.[26-29] A concomitant deficiency of proaccelerin (factor V) often contributes to the long prothrombin time.

On the average, the prothrombin time is longer in patients with hemorrhagic symptoms or in those whose prognosis is poor.[29,30-32] Unexpectedly, in chronic biliary cirrhosis, the concentration of the vitamin K-dependent factors may be above normal, as though protein synthesis were enhanced.[20,33]

Treatment of the bleeding tendency of patients with parenchymal hepatic disease with vitamin K is usually disappointing.[23,29,34-37] A trial of intravenous or intramuscular vitamin $K_1$, for example 10 mg daily for 3 days, should be attempted, but further therapy is not justified if the prothrombin time does not shorten. Occasional patients with parenchymal disease, usually those with severe jaundice, will respond to vitamin K therapy. In such cases, the deficiency of the vitamin K-dependent factors has been ascribed, at least in part, to intrahepatic biliary obstruction. This interpretation may be incomplete, as the amount of vitamin K needed to elicit a response is usually greater than that required in extrahepatic obstruction.[38] The suggestion has been made that a favorable response can be predicted by the detection in plasma of incompletely carboxylated forms of the vitamin K-dependent clotting factors, as measured in clotting assays.[39] Contrary evidence has been presented indicating that failure of therapy is associated with an inability to utilize the vitamin for carboxylation.[14]

When the bleeding tendency of patients with hepatic disease appears to be life-threatening, or when surgery is necessary, the transfusion of fresh-frozen plasma in the manner suggested for obstructive jaundice (page 453) may provide partial and transitory correction of deficiencies of the vitamin K-dependent factors and proaccelerin (factor V). Complete correction of the hemostatic abnormalities is usually not achieved.[40–42] The infusion of concentrates of the vitamin K-dependent factors has been recommended to maintain patients during hemorrhagic episodes or in preparation for liver biopsy or surgery. These preparations may be only partially effective,[42] and their use may be complicated by hepatitis[41,43] and by untoward thrombotic reactions.[44–46] The simultaneous administration of plasma and concentrates especially rich in factor VII has been proposed as preparation for liver biopsy,[42] but the generally benign nature of liver biopsy makes assessment of any prophylactic regimen difficult.[47]

Few patients with parenchymal hepatic disease require anticoagulant therapy for thromboembolic disease. Oral anticoagulants should be used with special care, as the response to these drugs may be exaggerated in such patients. Heparin therapy must also be used with circumspection, as many patients with hepatic disease have thrombocytopenia, which may enhance the action of heparin; also heparin itself occasionally induces thrombocytopenia.

Individuals with hereditary disorders of bilirubin metabolism, including Dubin-Johnson syndrome, Gilbert's syndrome, and Rotor syndrome, have, on the average, somewhat lower titers of factor VII than normal individuals.[48,49] In a few cases, in which the titer of factor VII was less than 20 percent of normal, mild bleeding manifestations have occurred. This striking abnormality is unexplained.

## PROACCELERIN (FACTOR V)

Proaccelerin is synthesized largely or exclusively in the liver, as demonstrated in the perfused rat liver.[7] Support for the liver as a source of proaccelerin comes from studies of patients and experimental animals with hepatic damage or subjected to partial or total hepatectomy, in whom the titer of this factor may be reduced. Although proaccelerin has been detected in hepatocytes,[50] some evidence suggests that its site of origin is the reticuloendothelial cell.[51]

An abnormally low titer of proaccelerin is found in many patients with acute or chronic hepatic disease,[20,27,52] in whom it contributes to the abnormally long prothrombin time. Recognition of proaccelerin deficiency rests on specific assays, a procedure seldom warranted in the diagnosis or treatment of hepatic disease. Some observers believe that a deficiency of proaccelerin is a more sensitive indicator of hepatic damage that the titer of the vitamin K-dependent factors. In contrast, the titer of proaccelerin is usually normal or elevated in patients with obstructive jaundice,[27,52] primary biliary cirrhosis,[20,52] or metastatic disease in the liver.

In most patients with hepatic disease, the likely pathogenesis of a decreased titer of proaccelerin is impaired synthesis. In some, however, a low titer may be due to the utilization of proaccelerin in disseminated intravascular coagulation. Proteolytic degradation of proaccelerin by plasmin has also been invoked to explain decreased titers of this factor, but evidence for this possibility is based largely on in vitro studies. Treatment of cirrhotic patients with epsilon aminocaproic acid, which impedes activation of plasmin, is ineffective.[53]

The degree to which proaccelerin deficiency contributes to the bleeding diathesis in hepatic disease is unclear. Hereditary deficiencies of proaccelerin, which are usually much more severe than those observed in hepatic disease, result in a mild bleeding tendency, ordinarily manifested only after injury. Perhaps, however, proaccelerin deficiency may exaggerate the hemostatic defect brought about by concurrent deficiencies of the vitamin K-dependent factors. Transfusion of fresh-frozen plasma in the manner described for obstructive jaundice or hepatic disease (page 453) may raise the titer of proaccelerin transiently. Vitamin K therapy is not indicated.

## CLOTTING FACTORS INVOLVED IN THE SURFACE-MEDIATED INITIATION OF CLOTTING

The early steps of the intrinsic pathway of thrombin formation involve the participation of Hageman factor (factor XII), plasma prekallikrein (Fletcher factor), high molecular weight kininogen (Fitzgerald, Flaujeac, or Williams factor), and plasma thromboplastin antecedent (PTA, factor XI). Synthesis of Hageman factor has been demonstrated in the perfused rat liver,[54] whereas the hepatic origin of the other three factors has been inferred from their low titers in patients with acute or chronic hepatic disorders.[55-57] The possibility has been raised that deficiency of prekallikrein in liver disease may be the result, in part, of its activation by Hageman factor and subsequent inactivation.[58]

The clinical significance of these defects in patients with hepatic disease is not clear. Individuals with isolated hereditary deficiencies of Hageman factor, plasma prekallikrein, or high molecular weight kininogen do not have a significant hemorrhagic tendency, and those with PTA deficiency have relatively minor bleeding symptoms. Perhaps, however, the milder abnormalities associated with liver disorders may augment the hemorrhagic problems brought about by deficiencies of other factors. Present evidence does not support this possibility.

In patients with primary biliary cirrhosis or early obstruction of the common bile duct by stone, the titer of Hageman factor may be modestly increased.[20]

## ANTIHEMOPHILIC FACTOR (FACTOR VIII)

Antihemophilic factor is a complex molecule composed of a subcomponent of relatively low molecular weight that participates in the intrinsic pathway of clotting (factor VIII:C) and a high molecular weight subcomponent that is concerned with the interaction of platelets and injured vascular walls (factor VIII:VWF). The low molecular weight subcomponent may be synthesized by the reticuloendothelial cells, as suggested by perfusion studies of the isolated rat liver,[51] whereas the high molecular weight subcomponent is probably synthesized in vascular endothelial cells.[59]

Surprisingly, the titer of antihemophilic factor is elevated as much as sevenfold in patients with acute and chronic hepatic disease[60,61] and in patients with metastases to the liver.[62] The titers of both the low and high molecular weight subcomponents are increased, the latter often disproportionately.[63] The mechanisms responsible for the elevated titer of antihemophilic factor are not known, but similar, although usually much less impressive, increases are seen with a variety of stresses in normal individuals and in such diverse disorders as diabetes mellitus, malignancy, and renal failure.[64] These observations suggest that the increased titer of antihemophilic factor in hepatic disease may be an acute-phase reaction. Alternatively, the liver may be one site of catabolism of this complex molecule, as has been suggested by experiments of Sodetz et al.[65] The clinical meaning of elevations in the titer of antihemophilic factor is uncertain.

Rarely, the titer of antihemophilic factor may be decreased in massive hepatic necrosis.[66] Whether this is the result of impaired synthesis or increased consumption during disseminated intravascular coagulation is not obvious.

## FIBRINOGEN, FIBRINOLYSIS, AND DISSEMINATED INTRAVASCULAR COAGULATION

Fibrinogen (factor I) appears to be synthesized exclusively in the liver, as was first suggested many years ago by Corin and Ansiaux[67] and later established in studies of the isolated, perfused liver by Miller et al.[68,69] Synthesis takes place in the hepatocyte, as demonstrated in liver slices,[70] and in cultures of human embryonal liver cells[71] and hepatoma cells.[72] Fibrinogen can be detected in the hepatocyte by immunologic techniques.[73]

In normal human plasma, the concentration of fibrinogen averages about 280 mg/dl, ranging in 1 series from about 165 to 485 mg/dl. Hypofibrinogenemia or afibrinogenemia may result from impaired synthesis, from consumption of fibrinogen during disseminated or localized intravascular coagulation, from intravascular fibrin(ogen)olysis, and, rarely, from uncompensated loss during massive hemorrhage.

The rate of synthesis of fibrinogen in hepatic disease is usually normal[74] or even increased.[75] Patients with cirrhosis, however, do not exhibit the usual rise in the concentration of fibrinogen that follows stresses such as infection.[76] In most cases of acute or chronic hepatic disease, the concentration of fibrinogen in plasma is normal or elevated; occasionally, it is moderately decreased.[28,75,76] In contrast to primary hepatic disorders, the concentration of fibrinogen is almost always elevated in metastatic disease in the liver[77] and may also be increased in obstructive jaundice.[78]

Severe hypofibrinogenemia or even afibrinogenemia is unusual in hepatic disease, and is most likely to be associated with fulminant hepatitis.[79,80] Whether in the reported cases this complication was the result of impaired synthesis or consumption of fibrinogen during disseminated intravascular coagulation is conjectural.

When hypofibrinogenemia that is thought to be due to impaired synthesis of fibrinogen appears to contribute to a bleeding tendency, temporary relief may be obtained by transfusion of cryoprecipitates of plasma such as those used for the treatment of classic hemophilia (factor VIII deficiency). Each bag of cryoprecipitate, prepared from 1 unit of blood, contains about 300 mg of fibrinogen; transfusion of about 1 bag of cryoprecipitate for each 3 kg of body weight will raise the plasma level of fibrinogen by about 200 mg/dl. Since about one-half of the transfused fibrinogen is metabolized in three or four days, a daily transfusion thereafter of 1 bag of cryoprecipitate per 15 kg of body weight should suffice to maintain the concentration of fibrinogen at normal levels.

### Disseminated Intravascular Coagulation

The belief that disseminated intravascular coagulation may be responsible for hypo- or afibrinogenemia stems from studies, originally performed by Wooldridge,[81] in which clot-promoting agents such as tissue thromboplastin are slowly infused intravenously into experimental animals. The consequences of such maneuvers include a gradual decline in the concentration of fibrinogen and other clotting factors, and the appearance of anticoagulant properties in plasma, thrombocytopenia, and, inconstantly, evidence of fibrinolytic phenomena. These changes are thought to be the result of intravascular clotting, with consumption of clotting factors and platelets and conversion of plasminogen to plasmin.

In recent years, considerable emphasis has been placed upon the possible role of disseminated intravascular coagulation in the pathogenesis of bleeding in hepatic disease.[75,82–87] Because patients with hepatic disease may, for other reasons, have decreased titers of many clotting factors and thrombocytopenia, the contribution of disseminated intravascular coagulation to a hemorrhagic tendency may be difficult to assess in any individual case.[88] Accelerated catabolism of fibrinogen,[89,90] prothrombin, and plasminogen[91] has been noted in some patients with cirrhosis and has been reversed by administration of heparin[88] even with low-dose schedules.[92] Accelerated catabolism of fibrinogen has also been described in acute hepatic necrosis, biliary tract obstruction, cholangitis, and contusion of the liver.[93,94] Accelerated catabolism, however, may be difficult to distinguish from other processes, such as the digestion of fibrinogen by plasmin or other proteases, rapid clearance of abnormal fibrinogen molecules, or the loss of clotting factors into extravascular spaces or through hemorrhage.

In patients believed to have experienced disseminated intravascular coagulation, the serum, which normally should be depleted of fibrinogen, may contain agents that are immunologically or chemically related to this protein.[94,95] These fibrin(ogen)-related antigens may represent incompletely aggregated fibrin monomers, degradation products of the action of plasmin or other proteases upon fibrinogen or fibrin (FDP), or complexes of fibrin monomer with fibrinogen or FDP. Most current tests for fibrin split products or FDP do not clearly distinguish among these possibilities. In any case, firm laboratory support for the presence of disseminated intravascular coagulation is not found in the great majority of patients with acute or chronic hepatic disease.[33,63,96]

Disseminated intravascular coagulation has also been invoked to explain some cases of hepatic disease in which the level of antithrombin III has been decreased, although this change may in fact reflect a decrease in the rate of synthesis of this protein. In a small series of cirrhotics, Hiller et al.[97] observed that decreased titers of antithrombin III and increased concentrations of fibrin(ogen)-related antigens were exaggerated in nearly all patients after the onset of severe esophageal hemorrhage, auguring a poor prognosis. Correction of antithrombin III deficiency by transfusion of this inhibitor increases the biological half-life of plasma fibrinogen, as if the deficiency contributed to the rapid turnover of fibrinogen in cirrhosis.[97a]

Few if any stigmata of intravascular coagulation are found at liver biopsy or autopsy. A few thrombi may be seen in the small blood vessels of the kidney, lung, or spleen, but their absence is not a bar to diagnosis of this syndrome.[86,98] Presumably, fibrinolysis by plasmin or other proteases may erase the anatomic evidence of disseminated intravascular clotting.

Several hypotheses, not mutually exclusive, have been offered to explain the occurrence of disseminated intravascular coagulation in hepatic disease. Perhaps, as Verstraete et al.[87] have proposed, necrotic hepatocytes may activate the clotting process within the circulating plasma. Defective hepatic or reticuloendothelial clearance of activated factors, combined with decreased titers of inhibitors of coagulation, may then foster the development of disseminated intravascular coagulation. Alternatively, perhaps clot-promoting endotoxins, liberated into the portal system, may induce intravascular coagulation.[94] In support of this possibility, experimental extirpation of the bowel is said to prevent hypofibrinogenemia after hepatectomy.[99] Evidence of disseminated intravascular coagulation is much more frequent or severe in cirrhosis complicated by septicemia than in the absence of infection. No firm conclusion about the role of endotoxins can be drawn, however, as controversy exists concerning the frequency with which these agents can be demonstrated in cirrhotic blood.[58,100–103] The pathogenesis of disseminated intravascular coagulation in cirrhosis thus remains a puzzle.

The treatment of disseminated intravascular coagulation in hepatic disease, as in other conditions, is difficult. If hypofibrinogenemia is severe, the administration of cryoprecipitates (page 456) may support the patient during a crisis, but at the same time provides more fibrinogen to be clotted. Similarly, the transfusion of concentrates of the vitamin K-dependent factors may enhance the intravascular clotting process.[97] Heparin therapy to halt intravascular coagulation has been suggested.[83,84,104] Its benefits have not been impressive,[105] but heparin therapy may perhaps be more effective if combined with transfusion of plasma.[84,93,104] Plasma may provide antithrombin III, the agent through which heparin's anticoagulant properties are mediated.[97] Heparin therapy is dangerous in the presence of thrombocytopenia, and should be avoided if active bleeding is present.

The origin of the disseminated intravascular coagulation that appears in patients who have undergone transfusion of ascitic fluid or peritoneovenous (LeVeen) shunting is more apparent.[106–108] The cells that are suspended in ascitic fluid appear to be clot-promoting.[108,109] Its intravenous infusion thus might reasonably be supposed to induce intravascular clotting. Cell-depleted ascitic fluid does not promote coagulation in vitro,[110] but ascitic fluid is a rich source of endotoxin that might contribute in vivo to disseminated thrombosis.[101,102]

After the placement of a shunt, transient or protracted alterations in plasma suggestive of disseminated intravascular clotting almost always take place, and occasionally life-threatening or lethal bleeding may ensue.[109,111] The concentration of fibrinogen and the platelet count are significantly increased, apparently reflecting a shortened survival of these agents.[111a] When disseminated intravascular coagulation seems minor, this complication is usually transient, but the presence of clinical symptoms demands that the shunts be interrupted. Therapy with heparin has not been helpful.

A recent report attributes the bleeding tendency of a small group of patients with biliary tract obstruction to disseminated intravascular coagulation.[112] In five of six patients, *Escherichia coli* or *Klebsiella* were cultured from the bile. In the absence of systemic infection, however, disseminated intravascular coagulation must be excessively rare in obstructive jaundice uncomplicated by hepatic disease.

## Abnormal Plasma Fibrinolytic Activity

In 1914, Goodpasture[113] reported that the clotted blood of patients with cirrhosis of the liver reliquefied upon incubation at body temperature. Accelerated fibrinolysis in vitro has been described many times by subsequent investigators in studies of clots formed from whole blood[76] or cell-depleted plasma of cirrhotics[114–116] or from the euglobulin (i.e., water-insoluble) fraction of plasma.[117,118] Rapid fibrinolysis is not usually seen in acute hepatic disease, carcinoma of the liver, primary biliary cirrhosis, or obstructive jaundice,[114,117,119] although apparent exceptions have been described.[80]

As Goodpasture recognized, fibrinolysis is the result of the digestion of fibrin by the plasma protease, plasmin. Plasmin can be generated from its precursor, plasminogen, in many ways, among them mechanisms intrinsic to the blood. Accelerated fibrinolysis, as measured in vitro, is observed in clots formed from the blood of individuals who are under stress or who have been injected with such vasoactive agents as nicotinic acid. Presumably, under these conditions, an activator of plasminogen is discharged into the circulation. Experimentally, one or more activators can be released from venous endothelium[120] or stimulated monocytes,[121] but whether these are responsible for rapid fibrinolysis in stressed individuals is uncertain. Plasminogen can also be activated in vitro by agents participating in the initial steps of the intrinsic pathway, including plasma kallikrein, activated PTA (factor $XI_a$) and, to a lesser degree, activated Hageman factor (factor $XII_a$). Conceivably, these clotting factors may contribute to the enhanced fibrinolysis that may accompany disseminated intravascular coagulation.

Plasma also contains inhibitors directed against the activation of plasminogen and the action of plasmin, of which the most important is $\alpha_2$-plasmin inhibitor,[122,123] backed up by $\alpha_2$-macroglobulin[122] (Chapter 9).

Some of the factors influencing the rate of fibrinolysis in vitro are the concentrations of plasminogen, its activators and inhibitors, and the fibrin content of the clot to be digested. Activation of plasminogen is more effective on the surface of a fibrin clot, to which it is adsorbed. As plasmin forms on the fibrin surface, it is inhibited stoichiometrically by $\alpha_2$-plasmin inhibitor. In vitro, fibrinolysis coincides with the depletion of this inhibitor in the surrounding serum.[124]

Plasmin can digest not only fibrin but also myriad other substrates, including fibrinogen and other clotting factors. Products of the digestion of fibrinogen and fibrin inhibit the formation and action of thrombin and the polymerization of fibrin monomers, and in this way may enhance a bleeding tendency. These so-called fibrin(ogen) split or degradation products may lengthen the thrombin time, that is, the clotting time of a mixture of thrombin and plasma, and can be recognized immunologically in the serum of individuals thought to have experienced fibrinolysis in vivo.

The mechanisms responsible for the enhanced fibrinolysis observed in vitro in cirrhosis are not completely defined. The titer of plasminogen is often depressed in both acute and chronic hepatic disease,[61,86,125] suggesting that the availability of this proenzyme is not an important factor in this phenomenon. The low titer of plasminogen may be due to either decreased synthesis or increased consumption during disseminated intravascular coagulation.[91,111a] In primary biliary cirrhosis or early common bile duct obstruction, the titer of plasminogen is normal or even elevated.[20] Fibrinolysis induced by exercise or by the intravenous injection of nicotinic acid is more rapid in cirrhotics than in normal subjects, as though the liver cannot remove the putative activators of plasminogen.[126–128] The concentration of $\alpha_2$-plasmin inhibitor is decreased in both acute and chronic hepatic disorders, as well as in obstructive jaundice, which again does not explain the differing behavior of clots in these situations. On the other hand, the depletion of plasmin inhibitors that occurs during incubation of clotted plasma, noted above, is more rapid in cirrhosis.[129] Recently, Lijnen et al.[130] reported that another plasma agent, histidine-rich glycoprotein, which inhibits fibrinolysis by reducing binding of plasminogen to fibrin, is reduced in the plasma of cirrhotics; the importance of this observation in the pathogenesis of enhanced fibrinolysis is not yet known. The concentrations of other inhibitors of plasmin are not reduced in hepatic disease. These random clues do not explain the absence of rapid fibrinolysis in acute hepatic disease.

The author has emphasized that rapid fibrinolysis in cirrhosis is a test tube phenomenon. Whether it is of importance in increasing the bleeding tendency of patients with this disease is not at all certain. Conceivably, in some patients, recurrent hemorrhage after variceal bleeding might result from dissolution of clots that may have formed, or hemostasis might be impeded by FDP that may be present in the patient's plasma or serum.[131–134] Were excessive fibrinolysis clinically important, a logical treatment would be administration of epsilon aminocaproic acid or tranexamic acid, which block the transformation of plasminogen to plasmin. These agents, however, have not been helpful[53,135] and are contraindicated when, as is often the case, disseminated intravascular coagulation is suspected.[82,90]

## The Thrombin Time in Hepatic Disease

The clotting time of a mixture of plasma and thrombin is often abnormally long in cirrhosis, and may be increased in other hepatic disorders and in obstructive jaundice.[136–139] In a few instances, the delay in clotting has been related to either marked decreases or increases in the concentration of fibrinogen in plasma.[137] In most cases, however, other mechanisms appear to be responsible for an abnormally long thrombin time.

A growing number of reports have recorded the presence of functionally abnormal variants of fibrinogen in patients with hepatic disease. The variants are recognized because fibrinogen extracted from the plasma coagulates abnormally slowly upon the addition of thrombin. This acquired dysfibrinogenemia was first recognized in cirrhosis of the liver,[136] and has since been described in association with hepatic carcinoma,[140] severe acute hepatitis,[141] and chronic aggressive hepatitis;[142] dysfibrinogenemia is distinctly rare in metastatic hepatic disease.[138] In most patients in whom the presence of an abnormal fibrinogen has been unequivocally demonstrated, the thrombin time has been 2–4 times that of control plasma.

The abnormal fibrinogens of acquired dysfibrinogenemia have been characterized in some cases by alterations in the carbohydrate content of the molecule, particularly an increase in sialic acid.[143,144] The pathogenesis of dysfibrinogenemia is not known; perhaps there is a posttranslational defect in the attachment of carbohydrate to fibrinogen. The functional result is a delay in the aggregation of fibrin monomers;[14] the long thrombin time has been shortened by removal of sialic acid from the abnormal fibrinogen.[96,143]

A more modest prolongation of the thrombin time, usually less than twice that of control plasma, is observed in many patients with hepatic disease or obstructive jaundice.[136,138,145] A variety of mechanisms may be responsible for the prolonged thrombin time in these patients. In some but not all such patients, aggregation of fibrin monomers has been impaired.[118,138,139,146] Perhaps, as was suggested some years ago, the plasma is deficient in some as yet undefined accelerator of fibrin aggregation.[136,137] In support of this, transfusion of fresh frozen plasma is said to shorten the thrombin time of cirrhotics.[40] Another possibility is that the fibrinogen in the plasma of some patients with hepatic disease is qualitatively abnormal, in a manner comparable to that described in the preceding paragraphs.[138,147] There is contradictory evidence on whether fibrinogen purified from such plasma clots in a normal time upon addition of thrombin.[147,148]

In other patients, circulating anticoagulants, whose nature is not yet understood, may be responsible for a long thrombin time.[149] Conceivably, some such anticoagulants are FDP[138] but this is by no means established.[132,139,150] In one interesting case of cytomegalovirus hepatitis, $\beta_2$-microglobulin seemed to delay the thrombin time.[151] The long thrombin time observed in hepatic disease cannot be ascribed to an excess of antithrombin III, which, in fact, is often decreased in titer in these disorders.[152,153]

The clinical significance of a long thrombin time is uncertain. Only a fraction of patients with *hereditary* dysfibrinogenemia have a bleeding tendency. Green et al.[138] noted that among patients who were bleeding from esophageal varices, those with evidence of abnormal fibrin polymerization had a much worse prognosis than those without this defect. This correlation, however, may merely have reflected the severity of the underlying hepatic disease.

## Fibrin-Stabilizing Factor (Factor XIII)

Fibrin-stabilizing factor (factor XIII) is the precursor of an enzyme that induces covalent cross-linkage between fibrin monomers, providing tensile strength to the clot. It also induces linkages between fibrin and $\alpha_2$-plasmin inhibitor, rendering it less susceptible to fibrinolysis.[154] One site of synthesis is probably the liver. The titer of fibrin-stabilizing factor is reportedly decreased[155-158] or normal[159] in acute and chronic hepatic disorders, particularly cirrhosis or metastatic disease in the liver; the differences in result appear to be due, in part, to differences in technique. The titer is normal in obstructive jaundice.[156] The pathogenesis and clinical significance of a partial deficiency in fibrin-stabilizing factor are not evident. The concentration of this protein is usually sufficient to provide adequate hemostasis, as judged by the response to transfusion of patients with hereditary deficiencies of this protein. Impaired cross-linking of fibrin, however, may increase the susceptibility of clots to fibrinolysis.[160]

## INHIBITORS OF COAGULATION AND FIBRINOLYSIS

The sites of synthesis of the recognized inhibitors of coagulation and fibrinolysis have been only partially elucidated. Antithrombin III, which inhibits all the serine proteases involved in these processes, is probably synthesized at least partly by the liver. The titer of antithrombin III is diminished in chronic liver disease, severe acute hepatic necrosis, and acute fatty liver of pregnancy, as assayed functionally or immunologically.[28,152,161-165] Uncertainty exists over whether the low titers are the result of diminished synthesis or increased utilization, as in disseminated intravascular coagulation.[166] In most cases of acute hepatitis, in contrast, the titer of antithrombin III is normal,[167] and in obstructive jaundice and primary biliary cirrhosis, it may be elevated.[20,152] The action of antithrombin III is greatly increased by heparin. In one interesting study, the apparent deficiency of antithrombin III in alcoholic chronic liver disease appeared to be corrected by addition of heparin to plasma.[168]

$\alpha_2$-Macroglobulin, which inhibits thrombin and plasmin, is known to be synthesized by macrophages[169] and by cultured human hepatoma cells;[170] the latter observation is not proof that normal liver cells have this function. Alterations in its concentration, usually minor elevations, have been described in cirrhosis and hepatitis,[152,171,172] severe acute hepatic failure,[163] active chronic hepatitis,[172,173] and hemochromatosis.[172]

$\alpha_2$-Plasmin inhibitor is synthesized by cultured human hepatoma cells.[174] This agent, the major inhibitor of plasmin in plasma,[122,123] is decreased in concentration in cirrhosis, primary and metastatic hepatic malignancies, intra- and extrahepatic obstructive jaundice, fulminant hepatitis, and some cases of chronic aggressive hepatitis.[175] The concentration of $\alpha_2$-plasmin inhibitor is normal in acute hepatitis and chronic persistent hepatitis.[175]

One site of synthesis of $\alpha_1$-antitrypsin is the liver, as demonstrated in cultures of embryonal cells[71] and hepatoma cells,[170] but this protein is also synthesized by monocytes.[176] Its titer is unaltered or increased in cirrhosis and hepatitis,[161,171,175] and is elevated in obstruction of the common duct by stone and primary biliary cirrhosis.[20]

## PLATELETS

Thrombocytopenia is a common complication of hepatic disorders, particularly cirrhosis, in which it may occur in as many as one-third or more of patients, in rough proportion to the severity of the disease.[28,90,177] Thrombocytopenia itself is seldom severe enough to induce hemorrhage, although it may perhaps abet other defects in hemostasis. The bleeding time is only occasionally elevated, not necessarily in correlation with the platelet count.[28,90,145]

The origin of thrombocytopenia in cirrhosis has been ascribed in most situations to the presence of portal hypertension, with its accompanying congestive splenomegaly.[178,179] The marrow contains normal or even increased numbers of megakaryocytes, as though platelet production were not impaired; although the platelet life span has been said to be normal, more recent studies suggest that it is significantly reduced.[89,111a,179] Normally, as many as one-third of platelets are in the spleen. In individuals with congestive splenomegaly, a greater proportion of platelets are sequestered, with the result that the platelet count in peripheral blood is diminished. Thrombocytopenia does not appear to be due to the presence of ''autoantibodies'' against platelets.

In an acute crisis, such as bleeding from the gastrointestinal tract, the transfusion of platelets may be helpful. Splenectomy is rarely indicated. If this procedure is performed, it should probably be combined with splenorenal anastomosis. Portocaval anastomosis, without splenectomy, corrects the thrombocytopenia in about one-third of the cases.[180]

Thrombocytopenia in cirrhosis may be a complication of transfusion therapy for severe gastrointestinal bleeding. Stored bank blood or packed red blood cells do not provide viable platelets or adequate amounts of antihemophilic factor (factor VIII) or proaccelerin (factor V). The large quantities of blood needed to maintain the circulation may thus deplete the patient's own supply of these agents and contribute to the breakdown in hemostasis. The modern practice of combined transfusion of packed red cells, platelets, and fresh-frozen plasma helps to avoid these problems.

Since patients with cirrhosis are often alcoholics, two additional causes of thrombocytopenia may be present. Some patients may be deficient in folic acid, either because of dietary inadequacy or increased metabolic need.[181] Folic acid, 1 mg daily by mouth or intramuscularly, may be helpful under these conditions. Further, heavy intake of alcohol by itself may result in thrombocytopenia.[182] In such individuals, the formation of platelets may be depressed, and those platelets that reach the circulation may be qualitatively abnormal and have a shortened life span.

Thrombocytopenia is occasionally observed in patients with acute viral or chemical hepatitis.[86] The decreased number of circulating platelets may result from several causes, such as, disseminated intravascular coagulation[93] or the presence of autoantibodies against platelets.[183] Thrombocytopenia in acute hepatitis is seldom severe enough to warrant therapy, which, in any case, is not obvious beyond transfusion of platelets. Profound thrombocytopenia, however, is found in those rare patients in whom aplastic anemia follows acute hepatitis, usually non-A, non-B. This complication, which is more common in males and may be manifested after the delay of a month or more, carries a more grave prognosis than the usual case of aplastic anemia.[184–186]

Besides these various causes of thrombocytopenia in liver disease, mention should be made of a case report of a lethal thrombotic thrombocytopenialike syndrome in a patient with alcoholic Laennec's cirrhosis.[187] The pathogenesis of this complication is unknown; therapy with inhibitors of platelet aggregation and plasmapheresis was without benefit.

Paradoxically, a few patients with portal hypertension may have strikingly increased platelet counts. The author has studied three patients with thrombocythemia, that is, a platelet count above 800,000/μl, a situation which may be complicated by a bleeding tendency. Two of these patients had been subjected to splenectomy, and the third had extrahepatic portal vein obstruction. Therapy for this complication is not clear; in thrombocythemia of other origins, marrow suppressants are often used.

Various qualitative platelet defects have been described.[188,189] In some patients with "hypersplenism," most often accompanying chronic active hepatitis or Laennec's cirrhosis, the volume of individual platelets is significantly reduced.[190] Among the functional defects reported in cirrhosis or fulminant hepatitis have been diminished clot retraction,[188] impaired aggregation of platelets by adenosine diphosphate (ADP), collagen, or thrombin,[145,191,192] and impaired agglutination by ristocetin.[193] The aggregation defect has been reproduced by addition of the patient's platelet-poor plasma to normal platelets. In a large series of cases of Wilson's disease, Owen et al.[194] noted that the great majority had impaired platelet aggregation. Impaired aggregation of platelets by ADP has been related to the presence of an abnormally long bleeding time.[145,192] Retention of platelets by glass bead columns through which blood has been filtered is said to be enhanced in fulminant hepatic failure and reduced in hepatic cirrhosis.[195] The significance of these qualitative platelet abnormalities in hepatic disease, all seemingly minor, is unclear. Further, in one recent study, both platelet aggregation by ADP and platelet retention by glass bead columns were said to be normal.[111a]

## REFERENCES

1. Ratnoff OD: Disordered hemostasis in hepatic disease, in Schiff L (ed): Diseases of the Liver (ed 5). Philadelphia, JB Lippincott, 1982, pp 237–258
2. Bick RL, Murano G: Primary hyperfibrino(geno)lytic syndromes, in Murano G, Bick RL (eds): Basic Concepts of Hemostasis and Thrombosis. Boca Raton, Fl, CRC Press, 1980, pp 181–204
3. Brozovíc M: Acquired disorders of blood coagulation, in Bloom AL, Thomas DP (eds): Haemostasis and Thrombosis. Edinburgh, Churchill Livingstone, 1981, pp 411–438
4. Stenflo J, Fernlund P, Egan W, et al: Vitamin K dependent modifications of glutamic acid residues in prothrombin. Proc Natl Acad Sci USA 71:2730–2733, 1974
5. Pool JG, Robinson J: In vitro synthesis of coagulation factors by rat liver slices. Am J Physiol 196:423–428, 1959
6. Mattii R, Ambrus JL, Sokal JE, et al: Production of members of the blood coagulation and fibrinolysin systems by the isolated perfused liver. Proc Soc Exp Biol Med 116:69–72, 1964
7. Olson JP, Miller LL, Troup SB: Synthesis of clotting factors by the isolated perfused rat liver. J Clin Invest 45:690–701, 1966
8. Hawkins WB, Brinkhous KM: Prothrombin deficiency the cause of bleeding in bile fistula dogs. J Exp Med 63:795–801, 1936
9. Smith HP, Warner ED, Brinkhous KM et al: Bleeding tendency and prothrombin deficiency in biliary fistula dogs. Effect of feeding bile and vitamin K. J Exp Med 67:911–920, 1938
10. Udall JA: Human sources of absorption of vitamin K in relation to anticoagulation stability. JAMA 194:127–129, 1956
11. Goodnight SH Jr, Feinstein DI, Østerud B, et al: Factor VII antibody-neutralization material in hereditary and acquired factor VII deficiency. Blood 38:1–8, 1971
12. Girolami A, Burul A, Cappellato G, et al: Electroimmunoassay of factor IX in patients with liver damage and vitamin K unresponsive coagulation disorder. Folia Haematol (Leipzig) 106:65–71, 1979

13. Girolami A, Patrassi G, Capellato G, et al: An immunological study of prothrombin in liver cirrhosis. Blut 41:61–66, 1980

14. Blanchard RA, Furie BC, Jorgensen M, et al: Acquired vitamin K-dependent carboxylation deficiency in liver disease. N Engl J Med 305:242–248, 1981

15. Hemker HC, Veltkamp JJ, Hensen A, et al: Kinetic aspects of the interaction of blood clotting enzymes. III. Demonstration of an inhibitor of prothrombin conversion in vitamin K deficiency. Thromb Diath Haemorrh 19:346–363, 1963

16. Corrigan JJ Jr, Earnest DL: Factor II antigen in liver disease and warfarin-induced vitamin K deficiency: Correlation with coagulant activity using Echis venom. Am J Hematol 8:249–255, 1980

17. Frick PG, Riedler G, Brögli H: Dose response and minimal daily requirement for vitamin K in man. J Appl Physiol 23:387–389, 1967

18. Sherlock S, Alpert L: Bleeding in surgery in relation to liver disease. Proc R Soc Med 58:257–259, 1965

19. Gross L, Brotman M: Hypoprothrombinemia and hemorrhage associated with cholestyramine therapy. Ann Intern Med 72:95–96, 1970

20. Cederblad G, Korstan-Bengsten K, Olsson R: Observation of increased levels of blood coagulation factors and other plasma proteins in cholestatic liver disease. Scand J Gastroenterol 11:391–396, 1976

21. Quick AJ, Stanley-Brown M, Bancroft FW: A study of the coagulation defect in hemophilia and in jaundice. Am J Med Sci 190:501–511, 1935

22. Brinkhous KM, Smith HP, Warner ED: Prothrombin deficiency and the bleeding tendency of obstructive jaundice and in biliary fistula. Effect of feeding bile and alfalfa (vitamin K). Am J Med Sci 196:50–57, 1938

23. Lord JW Jr, Andrus W deW: Differentiation of intrahepatic and extrahepatic jaundice. Response of the plasma prothrombin to intramuscular injection of menadione (2-methyl-1,4-naphthoquinone) as a diagnostic aid. Arch Intern Med 68:199–210, 1941

24. Andrus W DeW, Lord JW Jr: The physiology of plasma prothrombin and its relation to liver function. Surgery 12:801–827, 1942

25. Lechner K: Immune reactive factor IX in acquired factor IX deficiency. Thromb Diath Haemorrh 27:19–24, 1972

26. Mann JD: Plasma prothrombin in viral hepatitis and hepatic cirrhosis. Evaluation of the two stage method in 75 cases. Gastroenterology 21:263–270, 1952

27. Rapaport SI, Ames SB, Mikkelsen S, et al: Plasma clotting factors in chronic hepatocellular disease. N Engl J Med 263:278–282, 1960

28. Hallén A, Nilsson IM: Coagulation studies in liver disease. Thromb Diath Haemorrh 11:41–63, 1964

29. Spector I, Corn M: Laboratory tests of hemostasis. The relation to hemorrhage in liver disease. Arch Intern Med 119:577–582, 1967

30. Mindrum G, Glueck HI: Plasma prothrombin in liver disease: Its clinical and prognostic significance. Ann Intern Med 50:1370–1384, 1959

31. Colombi A, Thölen H, Engelhart G, et al: Blutgerinnungsfaktoren als Index für den Schweregrad einer akuten Hepatitis. Schweiz Med Wochenschr 97:1716–1721, 1967

32. Tygstrup N: The prognostic value of laboratory tests in liver disease. Scand J Gastroenterol 8(suppl 19):47–50, 1973

33. Ritland S, Skrede S, Blomhoff JP, et al: Coagulation factors as indicators of protein synthesis in chronic liver disease. Scand J Gastroenterol 8(suppl 19):113–117, 1973

34. Bollman JL, Butt HR, Snell AM: The influence of the liver on the utilization of vitamin K. JAMA 115:1087–1091, 1940

35. Allen JG, Julian OC: Response of plasma prothrombin to vitamin K substitute therapy in cases of hepatic disease. Arch Surg 41:1363–1365, 1940

36. Reid J: Prothrombin deficiency in disease of the liver and bile passages and its treatment with synthetic vitamin K. Br Med J 1:579–584, 1941

37. Aggeler PM, Lucia SP: The bleeding tendency in disease of the liver and biliary passages. Acta Med Scand 107:179–226, 1941

38. Steigmann F, Schrifter H, Yiotsas ZD, et al: Vitamin K therapy in liver disease: Need for a reevaluation. Am J Gastroenterol 31:369–375, 1959

39. Malia RG, Preston FE, Holdsworth CD: Clinical responses to vitamin K, in Suttie JW (ed): Vitamin K Metabolism and Aspects of Vitamin K in the Human. Baltimore, University Park Press, 1980, pp 342–347

40. Spector I, Corn M, Ticktin HE: Effect of plasma transfusions on the prothrombin time and clotting factors in liver disease. N Engl J Med 275:1032–1037, 1966

41. Gazzard BG, Henderson JM, Williams R: The use of fresh frozen plasma or a concentrate of factor IX as replacement therapy before liver biopsy. Gut 16:621–625, 1975

42. Mannucci PM, Franchi F, Dioguardi N: Correction of abnormal coagulation in chronic liver disease by combined use of fresh-frozen plasma and prothrombin complex concentrates. Lancet 2:542–545, 1976

43. Wyke RJ, Thornton A, Portmann B, et al: Transmission of non-A and non-b hepatitis to chimpanzees by factor IX concentrates after fatal complications in patients with chronic liver disease. Lancet 1:520–528, 1979

44. Gazzard BG, Lewis ML, Ash G, et al: Coagulation factor concentrate in the treatment of the haemorrhagic diathesis of fulminant hepatic failure. Gut 15:993–998, 1974

45. Blatt P, Roberts HR: Prothrombin-complex concentrates in liver disease. Lancet 2:189, 1975 (letter)

46. Marassi A, Manzullo V, di Carlo V, et al: Thromboembolism following prothrombin complex concentrates and major surgery in severe liver disease. Thromb Haemost 39:787–788, 1978 (letter)

47. Aronson DL: Factor IX complex. Semin Thromb Hemostas 6:28–43, 1979

48. Seligsohn U, Shani M, Ramot B, et al: Dubin-Johnson syndrome in Israel. II. Association with factor-VII deficiency. Q J Med ns39:569–584, 1970

49. Seligsohn U, Shani M, Ramot B: Gilbert syndrome and factor-VII deficiency. Lancet 1:1398, 1970 (letter)

50. Giddings JC: The immunological localization of factor V in human tissue. Br J Haematol 29:57–65, 1975

51. Shaw E, Giddings JC, Peake IR, et al: Synthesis of procoagulant factor VIII, factor VIII related antigen, and other coagulation factors by the isolated perfused rat liver. Br J Haematol 41:585–591, 1979

52. Owren PA: Diagnostic and prognostic significance of plasma prothrombin and factor V levels in parenchymatous hepatitis and obstructive jaundice. Scand J Clin Lab Invest 1:131–140, 1949

53. Lewis JH, Doyle AP: Effect of epsilon aminocaproic acid on coagulation and fibrinolytic mechanisms. JAMA 188:56–63, 1964

54. Saito H, Hamilton SM, Angel A, et al: Production and release of Hageman factor (HF, factor XII) by the isolated perfused rat liver. Clin Res 28:770A, 1980 (abstract).

55. Naeye RL: Hemophiloid factors. Acquired deficiencies in several hemorrhagic states. Proc Soc Exp Biol Med 94:623–627, 1957

56. Saito H, Poon M-C, Vicic W, et al: Human plasma prekallikrein (Fletcher factor) clotting activity and antigen in health and disease. J Lab Clin Med 92:84–95, 1978

57. Hathaway WE, Alsever J: The relation of 'Fletcher factor' to factor XI and XII. Br J Haematol 18:161–169, 1970

58. Vliet ACM van, Vliet HHDM van, Džoljić-Danilović G, et al: Plasma prekallikrein and endotoxemia in liver cirrhosis. Thromb Haemost 45:65–67, 1981

59. Jaffe EA, Hoyer LW, Nachman RL: Synthesis of antihemophilic factor antigen by cultured human endothelial cells. J Clin Invest 52:2757–2764, 1973

60. Meili EO, Straub PW: Elevation of factor VIII in acute fatal liver necrosis. Thromb Diath Haemorrh 24:161–174, 1970

61. Outryve M van, Baele G, DeWerdt GA, et al: Antihaemophilic factor A (F VIII) and serum fibrin-fibrinogen degradation products in hepatic cirrhosis. Scand J Haematol 11:148–152, 1973

62. Zetterqvist E, Francken I von: Koagulation faktorerna vid leversjukdom. Nord Med 69:81–84, 1963

63. Green AJ, Ratnoff OD: Elevated antihemophilic factor (AHF, factor VIII) procoagulant activity and AHF-like antigen in alcoholic cirrhosis of the liver. J Lab Clin Med 83:189–197, 1974

64. Ratnoff OD: Antihemophilic factor, in Gordon AS, Silber R (eds): The Year in Hematology—1977. New York, Plenum, 1977, pp 399–454

65. Sodetz JM, Pizzo SV, McKee PA: Relationship of sialic acid to function and in vivo survival of human factor VIII/von Willebrand factor protein. J Biol Chem 252:5538–5546, 1977

66. Roberts HR, Cederbaum AI: The liver and blood coagulation: Physiology and pathology. Gastroenterology 63:297–320, 1972

67. Ratnoff OD: Why do people bleed? in Wintrobe MM (ed): Blood, Pure and Eloquent. New York, McGraw Hill, 1980, pp 600–657

68. Miller LL, Bly CG, Watson ML, et al: The dominant role of the liver in plasma protein synthesis. A direct study of the isolated perfused rat liver with the aid of lysine-$\epsilon$-C$^{14}$. J Exp Med 94:431–453, 1951

69. Miller LL, Bale WF: Synthesis of all plasma protein fractions except gamma globulins by the liver. The use of zone electrophoresis and lysine-$\epsilon$-C$^{14}$ to define the plasma proteins synthesized by the isolated perfused liver. J Exp Med 99:125–132, 1954

70. Straub PW: A study of fibrinogen production by human liver slices in vitro by an immuno-precipitin method. J Clin Invest 42:130–136, 1963

71. Gitlin D, Biasucci A: Development of $\gamma$G, $\gamma$A, $\gamma$M, $\beta_1/\beta_{1a}$, C$'$1 esterase inhibitor, ceruloplasmin, transferrin, hemopexin, haptoglobin, fibrinogen, plasminogen, $\alpha_1$-antitrypsin, orosomucoid, $\beta$-lipoprotein, $\alpha_2$-macroglobulin, and prealbumin in the human conceptus. J Clin Invest 48:1433–1446, 1969

72. Knowles BB, Howe CC, Aden DP: Human hepatocellular carcinoma cell lines secrete the major plasma proteins and hepatitis B surface antigen. Science 209:497–499, 1980

73. Forman WB, Barnhart MI: Cellular site for fibrinogen synthesis. JAMA 187:128–132, 1964

74. Volwiler W, Goldsworthy PD, MacMartin MP, et al: Biosynthetic determination with radioactive sulfur of turn-over rates of various plasma proteins in normal and cirrhotic man. J Clin Invest 34:1126–1146, 1955

75. Grün M, Liehr H, Brunswig D, et al: Regulation of fibrinogen synthesis in portal hypertension. Thromb Diath Haemorrh 32:292–305, 1974

76. Ham TH, Curtis FC: Plasma fibrinogen response in man. Influence of the nutritional state, induced hyperpyrexia, infectious disease and liver damage. Medicine 17:413–445, 1938

77. Rubin RN, Kies MS, Posch JJ Jr: Coagulation profiles in patients with metastatic liver disease. Blood 52(suppl 1):193, 1978 (abstract).

78. Walls WD, Losowsky MJ: The hemostatic defect of liver disease. Gastroenterology 60:108–109, 1971

79. Stefanini M, Petrillo E: The relative importance of plasmatic and vascular factors of hemostasis in the pathogenesis of the hemorrhagic diathesis of liver dysfunction. Acta Med Scand 134:139–145, 1949

80. Jacobson RJ, Wagner S, Weinberg R, et al: Bleeding complications in fulminant hepatitis. Lancet 2:1426, 1971 (letter)

81. Wooldridge LC: Ueber intravasculäre Gerinnungen. Arch Anat Physiol (Physiol Ab) 397–399, 1886

82. Bergstrom K, Blombäck B, Kleen G: Studies on the plasma fibrinolytic activity in a case of liver cirrhosis. Acta Med Scand 168:291–305, 1960

83. Zetterqvist E, Francken I: von. Coagulation disturbances with manifest bleeding in extrahepatic portal hypertension and in liver cirrhosis. Preliminary results of heparin treatment. Acta Med Scand 173:753–760, 1963

84.  Johansson S-A: Studies on blood coagulation factors in a case of liver cirrhosis. Remission of the hemorrhagic tendency on treatment with heparin. Acta Med Scand 175:177–183, 1964
85.  Hörder MH: Consumption coagulopathy in liver cirrhosis. Thromb Diath Haemorrh Suppl 36: 313–318, 1969
86.  Hellenbrad P, Parboo SP, Jedrychowski A, et al: Significance of intravascular coagulation and fibrinolysis in acute hepatic failure. Gut 15:83–88, 1974
87.  Verstraete M, Vermeylen J, Collen D: Intravascular coagulation in liver disease. Ann Rev Med 25:447–455, 1974
88.  Straub PW: Diffuse intravascular coagulation in liver disease. Semin Thromb Hemostas 4:29–39, 1977
89.  Brodsky I, Siegel NH, Kahn SB, et al: Simultaneous fibrinogen and platelet survival with [$^{75}$Se] selenomethionine in man. Studies in diseases with normal coagulation and in hepatocellular disease with abnormal coagulation. Br J Haematol 18:341–355, 1970
90.  Tytgat G, Collen D, Verstraete M: Metabolism of fibrinogen in cirrhosis of the liver. J Clin Invest 50:1690–1701, 1971
91.  Collen D, Rouvier J, Chamone DAF, et al: Turnover of radiolabelled plasminogen and prothrombin in cirrhosis of the liver. Eur J Clin Invest 8:185–188, 1978
92.  Coleman M, Finlayson N, Bettigole RE, et al: Fibrinogen survival in cirrhosis. Improvement by ''low dose'' heparin. Ann Intern Med 83:79–81, 1975
93.  Rake MO, Flute PT, Panell G, et al: Intravascular coagulation in acute hepatic necrosis. Lancet 1:533–537, 1970
94.  Wardle EN: Fibrinogen in liver disease. Arch Surg 109:741–746, 1974
95.  Coccheri S, Palareti G, Dalmonte PR, et al: Investigations on intravascular coagulation in liver disease: Soluble fibrin monomer complexes in liver cirrhosis. Haemostasis 8:8–18, 1979
96.  Gralnick HR, Givelber H, Abrams E: Dysfibrinogenemia associated with hepatoma. N Engl J Med 299:221–226, 1978
97.  Hiller EJ, Hegemann F, Possinger K: Hypercoagulability in acute esophageal variceal bleeding. Thromb Res 22:243–251, 1981
97a. Schipper HG, Cate JWten: Antithrombin III transfusion in patients with hepatic cirrhosis. Br J Haematol 52:25–33, 1982
98.  Oka K, Tanaka K: Intravascular coagulation in autopsy cases with liver diseases. Thromb Haemostas 42:564–570, 1979
99.  Rutherford RB, Hardaway RM III: Significance of the rate of decrease in fibrinogen level after total hepatectomy in dogs. Ann Surg 163:51–59, 1966
100. Wilkinson SP, Moodie H, Stamatakis JD, et al: Endotoxaemia and renal failure in cirrhosis and obstructive jaundice. Br Med J 2:1415–1418, 1976
101. Clemente C, Bosch J, Rodés J, et al: Functional renal failure and haemorrhagic gastritis associated with endotoxaemia in cirrhosis. Gut 18:556–560, 1977
102. Tarao K, So K, Moroi T, et al: Detection of endotoxin in plasma and ascitic fluid of patients with cirrhosis: Its clinical significance. Gastroenterology 73:539–542, 1977
103. Editorial: Endotoxin and cirrhosis. Lancet 1:318–319, 1982
104. Rake MO, Shilkin KB, Winch J, et al: Early and intensive therapy of intravascular coagulation in acute liver failure. Lancet 2:1215–1218, 1971
105. Gazzard BG, Clark R, Borirakchanyavat V, et al: A controlled trial of heparin therapy in the coagulation defect of paracetamol-induced hepatic necrosis. Gut 15:89–93, 1974
106. Parbhoo SP, Ajdukiewicz A, Sherlock S: Treatment of ascites by continuous ultrafiltration and reinfusion of protein concentrate. Lancet 1:949–952, 1974
107. Harmon DC, Demirjian Z, Ellman L, et al: Disseminated intravascular coagulation with the peritoneovenous shunt. Ann Intern Med 90:774–776, 1979
108. Phillips LL, Rodger JB: Procoagulant activity of ascitic fluid in hepatic cirrhosis in vivo and in vitro. Surgery 86:714–721, 1979
109. Lerner RG, Nelson JC, Corines P, et al: Disseminated intravascular coagulation. Complication of peritoneovenous shunts. JAMA 240:2064–2066, 1978

110.  Salem HH, Koutts J, Handley C, et al: The aggregation of human platelets by ascitic fluid: A possible mechanism for disseminated intravascular coagulation complicating LeVeen shunts. Am J Hematol 11:153–157, 1981

111.  Matsche JW: Fatal disseminated intravascular coagulation after peritoneovenous shunt for intractable ascites. Mayo Clin Proc 53:526–528, 1978

111a. Stein SF, Harker LA: Kinetic and functional studies of platelets, fibrinogen, and plasminogen in patients with hepatic cirrhosis. J Lab Clin Med 99:217–230, 1982

112.  Takeda S, Takaki A, Ohsato K: Occurrence of disseminated intravascular coagulation (DIC) in obstructive jaundice and its relation to biliary tract infection. Jap J Surg 7:82–89, 1977

113.  Goodpasture EW: Fibrinolysis in chronic hepatic insufficiency. Bull Johns Hopkins Hosp 25:330–336, 1914

114.  Ratnoff OD: Studies on a proteolytic enzyme in human plasma. IV. The rate of lysis of plasma clots in normal and diseased individuals, with particular reference to hepatic disease. Bull Johns Hopkins Hosp 84:29–42, 1949

115.  Beaumont JL, Beaumont V, Domart A: Recherches sur l'activité fibrinolytique spontanée du plasma dans les cirrhose du foie. Rev Fr Etud Clin Biol 1:667–673, 1956

116.  Kwaan HC, McFadzean AJS, Cook J: Plasma fibrinolytic activity in cirrhosis of the liver. Lancet 1:132–136, 1956

117.  deNicola P, Soardi F: Fibrinolysis in liver diseases: Study of 109 cases by means of the fibrin plate method. Thromb Diath Haemorrh 2:290–299, 1958

118.  Dettori AG, Ponari O, Civardi E, et al: Impaired fibrin formation in advanced cirrhosis. Haemostasis 6:137–148, 1977

119.  Jedrychowski A, Hillenbrand P, Ajdukiewicz AB, et al: Fibrinolysis in cholestatic jaundice. Br Med J 1:640–642, 1973

120.  Todd AS: The histological localisation of fibinolysin activator. J Pathol Bacteriol 78:281–283, 1959

121.  Unkeless JC, Gordon S, Reich E: Secretion of plasminogen activator by stimulated macrophages. J Exp Med 139:834–850, 1974

122.  Collen D: Identification and some properties of a new fast reacting plasmin inhibitor in human plasma. Eur J Biochem 69:209–216, 1976

123.  Moroi M, Aoki N: Isolation and characterization of $\alpha_2$-plasmin inhibitor from human plasma. A novel proteinase inhibitor which inhibits activator-induced clot lysis. J Biol Chem 251:5956–5964, 1976

124.  Collen D: On the regulation and control of fibrinolysis. Thromb Haemostas 43:77–89 1980

125.  Mowat NAG, Brunt PW, Ogston D: The fibrinolytic enzyme system in acute and chronic liver injury. Acta Haematol 52:289–293, 1974

126.  Das PC, Cash JD: Fibrinolysis at rest and after exercise in hepatic cirrhosis. Br J Haematol 17:431–443, 1969

127.  Fletcher AP, Biederman O, Moore D, et al: Abnormal plasminogen-plasmin system activity (fibrinolysis) in patients with hepatic cirrhosis: Its causes and consequences. J Clin Invest 43:681–695, 1964

128.  Tytgat G, Collen D, deVreeker R, et al: Investigations on the fibrinolytic system in liver cirrhosis. Acta Haematol 40:265–274, 1968

129.  Ratnoff OD: Studies on a proteolytic enzyme in human plasma. III. Some factors controlling the rate of fibrinolysis. J Exp Med 88:401–416, 1948

130.  Lijnen HR, Jacobs G, Collen D: Histidine-rich glycoprotein in a normal and a clinical population. Thromb Res 22:519–523, 1981

131.  Niléhn JE, Nilsson IM: Demonstration of fibrinolytic split products in human serum by an immunologic method in spontaneous and induced fibrinolytic states. Scand J Haematol 1:313–330, 1964

132.  Merskey C, Kleiner GJ, Johnson AJ: Quantitative estimation of split products of fibrinogen in human serum, relation to diagnosis and treatment. Blood 28:1–18, 1966

133. Fisher S, Fletcher AP, Alkjaersig N, et al: Immunoelectrophoretic characterization of plasma fibrinogen derivates in patients with pathological plasma proteolysis. J Lab Clin Med 70:903–922, 1967

134. Thomas DP: A comparative study of four methods for detecting fibrinogen degradation products in patients with various diseases. N Engl J Med 283:663–668, 1970

135. Tytgat GN, Collen D, Verstraete M: Metabolism of fibrinogen in cirrhosis of the liver. J Clin Invest 50:1690–1701, 1971

136. Ratnoff OD: An accelerating property of plasma for the coagulation of fibrinogen by thrombin. J Clin Invest 33:1175–1182, 1954

137. Jim RTS: A study of the plasma thrombin time. J Lab Clin Med 50:45–60, 1957

138. Green G, Thomson JM, Dymock IW, et al: Abnormal fibrin polymerization in liver disease. Br J Haematol 34:427–439, 1976

139. Lane DA, Scully MF, Thomas DP, et al: Acquired dysfibrinogenaemia in acute and chronic liver disease. Br J Haematol 35:301–308, 1977

140. Felten A von, Straub PW, Frick PD: Dysfibrinogenemia in a patient with primary hepatoma. First observation of an acquired abnormality of fibrin monomer aggregation. N Engl J Med 280:405–409, 1969

141. Soria J, Soria C, Samama M, et al: Dysfibrinogénémiés acquises dan les atteintes, hépatiques sévères. Coagulation 3:37–44, 1970

142. Lipinski B, Lipinska I, Nowak A, et al: Abnormal fibrinogen heterogeneity and fibrinolytic activity in advanced liver disease. J Lab Clin Med 90:187–194, 1977

143. Mester L, Szabados L: Structure défectueuse et biosynthèse des fractions glucidiques dans les variants pathologiques du fibrinogène. Nouv Rev Fr Hematol 10:679–684, 1970

144. Higuchi A, Sakurada K, Miyazaki T: Acquired dysfibrinogenemia associated with liver disease. Proc 18th Congr Int Soc Hematol 247, 1980 (abstract).

145. Ballard HS, Marcus AJ: Platelet aggregation in portal cirrhosis. Arch Intern Med 136:316–319, 1976

146. Green G, Poller L, Thomson JM, et al: Association of abnormal fibrin polymerization with severe liver disease. Gut 18:909–912, 1977

147. Palascak JE, Martinez J: Dysfibrinogenemia associated with liver disease. J Clin Invest 60:89–95, 1977

148. Weinstein MJ, Deykin D: Quantitative abnormality of an Aα chain molecular weight form in the fibrinogen of cirrhotic patients. Br J Haematol 40:617–630, 1978

149. Conley CL, Hartmann RC, Morse WI II: Circulating anticoagulants: A technique for their detection and clinical studies. Bull Johns Hopkins Hosp 84:255–268, 1949

150. Braunstein KM, Kinard HB, Hepfer TW, et al: Regulation of the thrombin time in cirrhosis. Thromb Res 9:309–317, 1976

151. Hammerschmidt DE, Moldow CF: Impaired fibrin polymerization in viral hepatitis. Report of a case: Probable identity of the inhibitor with $\beta_2$-microglobulin. J Lab Clin Med 92:1002–1008, 1978

152. Hensen A, Loeliger EA: Antithrombin III: Its metabolism and its function in blood coagulation. Thromb Diath Haemorrh 9(suppl 1):1–84, 1963

153. Kaulla E von, Kaulla KN von: Antithrombin III and its disorders. Am J Clin Pathol 48:69–80, 1967

154. Sakata Y, Aoki N: Cross-linking of $\alpha_2$-plasmin inhibitor to fibrin by fibrin-stabilizing factor. J Clin Invest 65:290–297, 1980

155. Nussbaum N, Morse B: Plasma fibrin stabilizing factor activity in various diseases. Blood 23:669–677, 1964

156. Walls WD, Losowsky MS: The hemostatic defect of liver disease. Gastroenterology 60:108–119, 1971

157. Mandel EE, Minn SK: Factor XIII activity of platelets and plasma in health and disease. Thromb Res 3:437–450, 1973

158. Lechner K, Niessner H, Thaler E: Coagulation abnormalities in liver disease. Semin Thromb Hemost 4:40–56, 1977
159. Hedner U, Henriksson P, Nilsson IM: Factor XIII in a clinical material. Scand J Haematol 14:114–119, 1975
160. Bickford AF Jr, Sokolow M: Fibrinolysis as related to the urea solubility of fibrin. Thromb Diath Haemorrh 5:480–488, 1961
161. Abildgaard U, Fagerhol MK, Egeberg O: Comparison of progressive antithrombin activity and the concentrations of three thrombin inhibitors in human plasma. Scand J Clin Lab Invest 26:349–354, 1970
162. Hedner U, Nilsson IM: Antithrombin III in a clinical material. Thromb Res 3:631–641, 1973
163. Damus PS, Wallace GA: Immunologic measurement of antithrombin III-heparin cofactor and $\alpha_2$-macroglobulin in disseminated intravascular coagulation and hepatic failure coagulopathy. Thromb Res 6:27–38, 1975
164. Rubin RN, Kies MS, Posch JJ: Antithrombin III determinations in patients with hepatic and non-hepatic coagulopathies. Clin Res 27:305A, 1979 (abstract)
165. Laursen B, Mortensen JZ, Frost L, et al: Disseminated intravascular coagulation in hepatic failure treated with antithrombin III. Thromb Res 22:701–704, 1981
166. Bick RL, Dukes ML, Wilson WL, et al: Antithrombin III (AT-III) as a diagnostic aid in disseminated intravascular coagulation. Thromb Res 10:721–729, 1977
167. Mannucci PM: Estimation of prothrombin in liver disease. J Clin Pathol 23:291–295, 1970
168. Gavrilis P, Lerner RG, Goldstein R: Plasma factor Xa-inhibitory activity in alcoholic liver disease and the effect of heparin. Thromb Res 4:335–343, 1974
169. Hovi T, Mosher D, Vaheri A: Cultured human monocytes synthesize and secrete $\alpha_2$-macro-globulin. J Exp Med 145:1580–1589, 1977
170. Knowles BB, Howe CC, Aden P: Human hepatocellular carcinoma cell lines secrete the major plasma proteins and hepatitis B surface antigen. Science 209:497–499, 1980
171. Miesch F, Bieth J, Metais P: The $\alpha_2$-macroglobulin content and the protease-inhibiting capacity of normal and pathological sera. Clin Chim Acta 31:231–241, 1971
172. Murray-Lyon IM, Clarke HGM, McPherson K, et al: Quantitative immunoelectrophoresis of serum proteins in cryptogenic cirrhosis, alcoholic cirrhosis and active chronic hepatitis. Clin Chim Acta 39:215–220, 1972
173. Housley J: Alpha-2-macroglobulin level in disease in man. J Clin Pathol 21:27–31, 1968
174. Saito H, Goodnough LT, Aden DP, et al: Synthesis and secretion of $\alpha_2$-plasmin inhibitor ($\alpha_2$-PI) by human liver cell lines. Blood 58(suppl 1):225a, 1981 (abstract)
175. Aoki N, Yamanaka T: The $\alpha_2$-plasmin inhibitor levels in liver diseases. Clin Chim Acta 84:99–105, 1978
176. Wilson GB, Walker JH Jr, Watkins JH Jr, et al: Determination of subpopulations of leukocytes involved in the synthesis of $\alpha_1$-antitrypsin in vitro. Proc Soc Exp Biol Med 164:105–114, 1980
177. Hedenberg L, Korstan-Bengsten K: Clotting tests and other tests of the haemostatic mechanism in cirrhosis of the liver and their diagnostic significance. Acta Med Scand 173:229–235, 1962
178. Tocantins LM: The hemorrhagic tendency in congestive splenomegaly (Banti's syndrome); its mechanism and management. JAMA 136:616–625, 1948
179. Aster RH: Pooling of platelets in the spleen: Role in the pathogenesis of "hypersplenic" thrombocytopenia. J Clin Invest 45:645–657, 1966
180. Sullivan BH Jr, Tumen HJ: The effect of portacaval shunt on thrombocytopenia associated with portal hypertension. Ann Intern Med 55:598–603, 1961
181. Jandl JH, Lear AA: The metabolism of folic acid in cirrhosis. Ann Intern Med 45:1027–1044, 1956
182. Cowan DH: Effect of alcoholism on hemostasis. Semin Hematol 17:137–147, 1980
183. Karpatkin S, Strick N, Karpatkin MB, et al: Cumulative experience in the detection of antiplatelet

antibody in 234 patients with idiopathic thrombocytopenic purpura, systemic lupus erythematosus and other clinical disorders. Am J Med 52:776–785, 1972

184. Rubin E, Gottlieb C, Vogel P: Syndrome of hepatitis and aplastic anemia. Am J Med 45:88–97, 1965

185. Editorial: Infectious hepatitis and aplastic anaemia. Lancet 1:844–845, 1971

186. Ajlouni K, Doeblin TD: The syndrome of hepatitis and aplastic anemia. Br J Haematol 27:345–355, 1974

187. Nally JV, Metz EN: Acute thrombotic thrombocytopenic purpura. Another cause for hemolytic anemia and thrombocytopenia in cirrhosis. Arch Intern Med 139:711–712, 1979

188. Breddin K: Hämorrhagische Diathesen bei Leberkrankungen unter besonderer Berücksichtung der Thrombocytenfunktion. Acta Haematol 27:1–16, 1962

189. Ordinas A, Maragall S, Castillo R, et al: A glycoprotein I defect in the platelets of three patients with severe cirrhosis of the liver. Thromb Res 13:297–302, 1978

190. Karpatkin S, Freedman ML: Hypersplenic thrombocytopenia differentiated from increased peripheral destruction by platelet volume. Ann Intern Med 89:200–203, 1978

191. Thomas DP, Ream VJ, Stuart RK: Platelet aggregation in patients with Laennec's cirrhosis of the liver. N Engl J Med 276:1344–1348, 1967

192. Rubin MH, Weston MJ, Bullock G, et al: Abnormal platelet function and ultrastructure in fulminant hepatic failure. Q J Med ns 46:339–352, 1977

193. Castillo R, Maragall S, Rodés J, et al: Increased factor VIII complex and defective ristocetin-induced platelet aggregation in liver disease. Thromb Res 11:889–906, 1977

194. Owen CA, Goldstein NP, Bowie EJW: Platelet function and coagulation in patients with Wilson disease. Arch Intern Med 136:148–152, 1976

195. Langley PG, Hughes RD, Williams R: Platelet adhesiveness to glass beads in liver disease. Acta Haematol 67:124–127, 1982

Peter A. Castaldi

# 15

# Hemostasis and Kidney Disease

Acute and chronic renal failure are complicated by a bleeding tendency that may be mild or sometimes life-threatening. The severity of hemostasis is related to the degree of azotemia and reverses when the metabolic disorder is corrected. It results from the effect of accumulated plasma factors that are probably dialyzable, as this treatment favorably influences bleeding. The precise identity of these retained products has not been determined, nor has the nature of an associated vascular defect. It is believed that the retained products adversely affect platelet function and interfere with the platelet–vessel endothelial interaction. There are qualitative abnormalities of in vitro tests of platelet function, and the bleeding time is prolonged. There may be an acquired imbalance in platelet and vascular prostaglandin metabolism and some failure of platelet secretion in modulating vascular responses.[1] These unsolved problems make the cause of uremic bleeding a question of continuing interest.

The involvement of platelets and coagulation factors in various forms of renal disease represents another area in which hemostasis may be disturbed apart from the influence of retained uremic products. Immune complexes are frequently the cause of glomerulonephritis, and may also lead to platelet activation and sequestration. The most dramatic example of disturbed hemostasis due to thrombocytopenia complicating renal failure occurs in the hemolytic-uremic syndrome (HUS) and thrombotic thrombocytopenic purpura (TTP). These conditions are discussed more fully in Chapters 4 and 8, but will be considered here because of the importance of the disturbance in vessel–platelet interaction leading to uninhibited platelet aggregation that occurs. The serious combination of bleeding and arterial thrombosis that results may respond to plasma infusion or exchange, suggesting a deficiency of some plasma component required for vascular prostacyclin production. This possibility is the subject of much current research. Although the nephrotic syndrome is often associated with thrombosis and renal transplant patients have an increased incidence of myocardial infarction and other thrombotic disorders, the mechanism of the increased thrombosis is not known. Again, there may be some disturbance of vascular prostaglandin unrelated to any metabolic disturbance.

Supported by the National Health and Medical Research Council of Australia and the Life Insurance Medical Research Fund of Australia and New Zealand.

**Table 15-1**
Hemostatic Disorders in Renal
Disease Investigations

Bleeding time
Platelet function
    Aggregation with ADP, collagen, epinephrine
    Adhesion in vivo and in vitro
    Release reaction: PF 3, PF 4, βTG, growth factor
Prostaglandins
    Platelets
    Vascular prostacyclin
Factor VIII complex
Deficiencies of factors IX and XII
Fibrinogen-fibrin secretion

## THE HEMOSTATIC DISORDER IN UREMIA

Patients in severe acute or chronic renal failure develop bruising and bleeding of the skin, muscles, and mucosal surfaces. This is associated with prolongation of the bleeding time and abnormalities in tests of platelet function. (Table 15-1.)

## BLEEDING TIME

The bleeding time has been shown to provide a reliable indication of the severity of the hemostatic defect.[2,3] The Ivy or template bleeding time is the most reliable of the methods available, and there have been a number of studies documenting bleeding in relation to this and other tests of platelet function. It is of interest that conventional tests of platelet aggregation with collagen, adenosine diphosphate (ADP), and adrenalin may show little impairment when the bleeding time is quite prolonged. This suggests that there is an imbalance in platelet–endothelial interaction that is not reflected in conventional tests of platelet function. This disturbance may be the result of a deficiency of plasma factors that regulate platelet–vessel wall interaction. The possibility that vascular prostacyclin production may be disturbed, or the balance between platelet and vascular prostaglandins altered, is the subject of much current research.

The principal currently known factors involved in maintenance of the bleeding time include the platelet surface glycoprotein component known as GPI, recognized by its inherited deficiency in the Bernard-Soulier syndrome, and factor VIII-von Willebrand factor (factor VIII-vWF), a plasma component, produced in vascular endothelium and presumably secreted, which is required for platelet–vessel wall adhesion and is recognized by its deficiency in the von Willebrand syndrome. These two factors, GPI and vWF, react with exposed subendothelial collagen and/or microfibrils in adhesion, which may also involve secreted granule proteins such as the granule glycoprotein (GPG) and fibrinogen liberated after platelet stimulation with α-thrombin or collagen. The rate and extent of adhesion are shear-related. There is currently no evidence to suggest that any of these components is altered or deficient in patients with renal disease, but it is certainly possible that defects in their interaction may contribute, and further work to explore this possibility needs to be done. It is known that factor VIII coagulant activity (factor VIII:C) may be elevated, particularly in patients with glomerulonephritis. There is also some correlation between increased factor VIII (antihemophilic factor) and thrombosis in these patients, which also points to the importance of these interactions. This is a developing area, however, requiring some complex methods or protein separation and identification, yet to be applied to many clinical disorders of bleeding.

There is further possibility, about which little is known, concerning the contribution of platelets to endothelial and vessel integrity. The nature of this relationship may depend on secreted platelet products, such as β-thromboglobulin (βTG), platelet factor 4 (PF 4, antiheparin), and the mitogenic platelet growth factor (PGF) or by some process of platelet incorporation into endothelium, although evidence for this is lacking. However, there is now some evidence,[4] based on studies of prostaglandin production in cultured vascular endothelial cells, that platelet proteins may modulate prostacyclin (PGI$_2$) production. This raises the important possibility of a direct contribution of platelets to vessel wall response and suggests possible roles for secreted platelet proteins. These relationships may also be altered in the uremic state and contribute to prolongation of the bleeding time.

## PLATELET ADHESION AND AGGREGATION

Standard tests of platelet adhesion correlate with the prolonged bleeding time in many patients with renal failure. Glass bead retention and the in vivo techniques of Borchgrevink[5] both reflect this abnormality and tend to be corrected as the uremia is treated by peritoneal dialysis. Since factor VIII is normal or even elevated in these patients and there is no known abnormality of platelet surface proteins, the adhesion defect must reflect the influence of dialyzable products on platelet–vessel reactions. Turney et al.[6] have described elevated levels of factor VIII and increased fibrinogen concentration in dialyzed uremic patients whose platelets showed a depressed agglutination response to ristocetin. They also induced this abnormality in normal platelets suspended in dialyzed uremic plasma. They therefore suggested the existence of an inhibitor of the interaction between factor VIII and GPI that may cause prolongation of the bleeding time. It seems unlikely that this inhibitor could have any relation to the accelerated atherogenesis found in patients with uremia undergoing regular dialysis, but it is certainly relevant to the platelet adhesion defect.

Abnormalities in platelet aggregation with ADP, collagen, and adrenalin are inconstant. They tend to occur in most severely affected patients, although the defects may be mild even with a prolonged bleeding time. In the study of Steiner et al.[3] impaired collagen-induced aggregation was significantly correlated with both increased bleeding time and the degree of azotemia. Platelet aggregation abnormalities, however, did not discriminate between bleeding and nonbleeding groups of patients, whereas the bleeding time was consistently related to bleeding. Earlier studies in a well-defined group of patients[7] did show a favorable effect of dialysis treatment on platelet aggregation responses. These studies may be more helpful in following the progress of treatment than in determining the severity of the bleeding tendency. It is also important that the patients under study be carefully examinied to exclude the effects of immune complexes which may, under certain conditions, lead to activation of circulating platelets, a release reaction, and so induce a relative refractory state in in vitro responses to collagen and other inducers.

## PLATELET RELEASE REACTION

Products of platelet activation may be detected in patients with chronic renal failure. βTG levels have been shown to be elevated, and to correlate with the creatinine level and with abnormalities of platelet aggregation and prolongation of the bleeding time.[8] Even more marked release was found during hemodialysis, reflecting increased platelet activation. However, Guzzo et al.[9] have also shown accumulation of secreted platelet proteins in chronic renal failure and suggested that impaired handling by the diseased kidney was the most important mechanism. It is probable that, as circumstances vary in background pathology, in vivo release may be a more constant phenomenon in some, but not all, forms of chronic renal disease. It is clearly important in immune complex glomerulonephritis and renal graft rejection but less so in other forms of indolent or late-stage disease. This aspect will be considered further below.

PF 3, the lipid procoagulant released from activated platelets, has been much studied as an indicator of the uremic defect. Both the prothrombin consumption test and kaolin-activated PF 3 release have been used; the former test has been advocated as one of the most reliable markers of the qualitative platelet disorder. It was suggested[7] that the bleeding time and the prothrombin consumption test were the best combination to use in assessing the likelihood of bleeding when renal biopsy was indicated in a patient with renal failure. Others have used the Stypven time of kaolin-stimulated platelet-rich plasma (PRP) to measure this release defect, and Horowitz et al.[10] related defective PF 3 release to uremic bleeding.

## THE UREMIC MOLECULES CAUSING BLEEDING

Much effort has been expended on the search for metabolites that could be held responsible for the bleeding tendency in renal failure. Infusions of urea in volunteers caused headache but did not prolong the bleeding time,[11] although a slight inhibitory effect was seen in PRP at high concentrations of added urea.[12] Guanidinosuccinic acid (GSA) was shown by Horowitz et al.[13] to be present in increased concentration in uremic plasma and to inhibit the second wave of aggregation with ADP when added to normal PRP. Aggregation with collagen and ADP-induced PF 3 release were also inhibited, as was the centralization of granules characteristic of the normal response to low concentrations of ADP. There was no effect observed on the platelet-dense tubular system, and the morphological effects were likened to those observed with acetylsalicylic acid (ASA). The inhibitory effects of GSA were overcome by increasing the concentration of the aggregating agents, unlike those of ASA. It thus seems possible that GSA may be an important factor, but it has not been possible to determine whether other products, such as phenol and phenolic acid[14] or the so-called uremic middle molecules described by Gallice et al.[15] may not also contribute. The former study demonstrated that concentrations of phenolic acid encountered in uremic plasma impaired kaolin-activated PF 3 and primary aggregation with ADP when tested in PRP. Bleeding times were not done in this investigation, but dialysis, which lowers the phenol concentration, corrected the functional abnormalities. It can only be concluded that these unfavorable influences contribute to uremic bleeding, but more recent work describing changes in the balance between vascular and platelet prostaglandins indicates that the functional disturbances may have a much more complex basis.

## PROSTAGLANDINS IN CHRONIC RENAL DISEASE

The recognition of a central role for prostaglandins in platelet function, following the work of Moncada and Vane[16] and others, has given a new direction to the study of disorders of hemostasis. It has become apparent in recent years[17] that vascular and platelet prostaglandins have an important influence in the microcirculation and in the development of some forms of glomerulonephritis. The balance between proaggregatory thromboxanes and antiaggregatory endoperoxides such as $PGE_2$ and $PGI_2$ working through the platelet adenylcyclase system is important to normal hemostasis. There is accumulating evidence that alteration in this balance is a cause of bleeding in renal failure and an important factor in microvascular thrombosis in HUS and TTP. Furthermore, it seems possible that plasma factors, possibly produced in the kidney, influence this balance by acting on endothelial production of prostacyclin. The opportunity to test these hypotheses is now available through the technique of culture of vascular endothelium, allowing models to be established for the measurement of $PGI_2$ production under the influence of normal and uremic plasma fractions. De Gaetano and his group[18] have used inhibition of platelet aggregation as an assay for prostacyclinlike activity and produced results supporting the hypothesis that vascular prostacyclin may have an important role in uremic bleeding. They showed both that uremic plasma stimulated prostacyclin production and that venous tissues from patients with acute and chronic renal failure generated more $PGI_2$-like activity than material from normal subjects. After repeated washings, when this activity could no longer be detected in control samples, inhibitory activity was still present in samples of venous tissue from uremic patients. They correlated prolonged bleeding times and return to normal on restoration of renal function with vascular prostacyclin production. This work, and that of Janson et al.[19] on the treatment of uremic bleeding with plasma fractions, point to the need for greater clarification of the roles of the prostaglandin products and the circulating influences that control their synthesis.

## COAGULATION FACTORS

Deficiency of coagulation factors is an uncommon occurrence in renal failure. The ill patient with acute renal failure in a hospital setting with intravenous fluids and antibiotics is certainly at risk of vitamin K deficiency, but other specific deficiencies are rare events. The massive proteinuria of the nephrotic syndrome has led to deficiency of factor IX (Christmas factor) and factor XII (Hageman factor) and, at least in the latter case, coagulation factor activity was identified in the urine. The reason for this development is unclear, as it must result from altered turnover of the lost protein with failure of a compensatory increase in production. Factor VIII imbalance has been recognized to be a not uncommon event in some patients with chronic renal disease. Elevated levels of factor VIII:C have been found and must result from some disturbance in factors regulating production of this factor VIII component. In view of the potential for altered $PGI_2$ production, this change in factor VIII activity represents a vascular synthetic response that needs further exploration. The situation is complex, however, since some authors have described a disturbed factor VIII–platelet glycoprotein interaction in uremic plasma and have detected inhibitory activity for this reaction in dialyzed uremic plasma.[6]

Other coagulation factors such as prekallikrein and fibrinogen-fibrin may be found in the urine of patients with renal failure. There is no evidence that altered fibrinolytic activity or surface-related activation of the kinin system contributes to uremic bleeding, but it is possible that excretion of their products may reflect the occurrence of local coagulation and provide evidence of ongoing glomerular damage.

## THROMBOCYTOPENIA

Thrombocytopenia is a serious complication of renal disease and may make its investigation by renal biopsy hazardous. In the steady state in chronic renal failure, the platelet count is not reduced and platelet survival time as measured with [51]Cr is within normal limits. It is the qualitative abnormality, described above, that is the usual cause of bleeding. There are a number of acute or transient influences, however, that may enhance platelet turnover and lead to thrombocytopenia, especially when renal failure accompanies a systemic disorder. Immune thrombocytopenia is a rare association of renal disease, but immune complexes are readily adsorbed by the platelet Fc receptor and their clearance may lead to increased turnover and sometimes thrombocytopenia. This is a poorly documented area and needs much further investigation. This is especially true since knowledge is accumulating about heparin-related thrombocytopenia and the frequent need to use heparin in chronic hemodialysis. There is evidence[20] that heparin greatly potentiates the action of immune complexes in causing platelet aggregation. Heparin was shown to cause aggregation in stirred PRP of some patients with circulating immune complexes. Heparin was also shown to induce thromboxane $B_2$ synthesis, which was inhibited by indomethacin. These findings suggest that heparin may aggravate platelet sequestration in patients with glomerulonephritis when immune complexes may be involved. It therefore seems likely that heparin may in fact contribute to the thrombotic tendency associated with regular hemodialysis and justifies attempts to inhibit platelet activation with inhibitors such as sulfinpyrazone and prostacyclin.

Thrombocytopenia, usually profound, is an integral part of HUS, TTP, and the severe forms of preeclamptic toxemia (PET) (Chapter 8). In each of these conditions, there is evidence that an imbalance has developed in the production or release of vascular prostacyclin. These conditions are considered below.

Thrombocytopenic episodes have been recognized in patients wtih well-functioning renal allografts and are believed to have an immune basis since immunosuppressive treatment and rejection processes could be excluded as pathogenic factors.[20a] There is some evidence that these thrombocytopenic episodes, although never severe, were due to increased platelet consumption, as the proportion of large platelets was inversely related to the platelet count. This phenomenon needs further study with more precise tests for platelet antibody and platelet-associated immunoglobulin.

## ACUTE RENAL FAILURE

The bleeding disorder of uremia is seen in its most florid form in severe acute renal failure, especially when this is complicated by anemia, infection, or another systemic disorder. The principal features are mucosal and gastrointestinal bleeding with a qualitative platelet defect and a prolonged bleeding time. The condition is reversible with dialysis[7,11] and is attributed to retained metabolic products. There may also, however, be a

**Table 15-2**

Hemostatic Disorders in Clinical Syndromes
of Renal Disease

---

Acute Renal Failure—Renal tubular necrosis, Acute GN
  HUS, TTP, Preeclamptic toxemia (PET)
Glomerulonephritis
Nephrotic Syndrome
Renal transplants and allograft rejection
Treatment of Bleeding
  Dialysis, heparin, and hemodialysis
  Plasma and cryoprecipitate
  Platelet transfusion
  Prostacyclin

---

disturbance of the prostaglandin balance because of a deficiency of some renal factor which modifies or inhibits vascular production of prostacyclin and/or platelet endoperoxide and thromboxane synthesis. This would result in disturbed control of platelet cyclic adenosine monophosphate (cAMP) levels and a state refractory to aggregation stimulants. (Table 15-2)

HUS and TTP are related conditions with severe thrombocytopenia and renal failure associated with hemolysis and organ damage resulting from microvascular thrombosis with platelet aggregates. The latter are sometimes detectable in superficial biopsies or are even visible in the retinal circulation, but the clinical syndrome is so striking that negative biopsies do not preclude the diagnosis. A less severe variant of this disorder may be the cause of PET. The major hemostatic disorder in HUS and TTP is thrombocytopenia. A functional defect in aggregation with epinephrine (adrenalin) during the thrombocytopenic phase of the former condition has been described,[21] but this could have resulted from in vivo release. There has been much interest in recent years in the etiology of these conditions based on observations of recovery associated with the use of inhibitors of platelet aggregation, plasmapheresis, and plasma exchange or infusion. The possible role of some plasma factor, a deficiency of which has allowed platelet aggregation to occur, is strongly suggested, and the lack of prostacyclin ($PGI_2$), a potent antiaggregant, has been proposed. Coupled with the in vitro observation that TTP plasma induces aggregation of normal platelets, the evidence for some plasma deficiency is accumulating. Until reliable assays for plasma prostacyclin are applied to the study of HUS and TTP, the evidence rests on tests of aggregation to detect a prostacyclinlike effect. In addition, there are reports of a favorable effect of antithrombin III (ATIII) on the course of postpartum HUS developing after PET,[22] indicating either that a single deficiency may not be the cause or that the ATIII preparation contained the same factor that is supplied in normal plasma. These are important observations and indicate the need for vigorous treatment with plasma in these patients if a favorable outcome is to be achieved.

The hypothesis that the cause of HUS and TTP is the absence of a plasma factor needed for $PGI_2$ production or the acquisition of a circulatory inhibitor needs exploration. There are now numerous instances in which plasma infusion or plasmapheresis has been effective and the platelet count elevated coincident with a return of $PGI_2$-stimulating activity, as measured in vitro in various endothelial cultures of aortic ring incubation experiments. The renal functional abnormality may not be reversed, and many patients require long-term dialysis. In several cases, the plasma of patients and their relatives have been shown to lack $PGI_2$ stimulatory factor. This suggests that the deficiency may be inherited, predisposing to an exaggerated platelet aggregation response to some immune, infective, or other initiating stimulus.

## GLOMERULONEPHRITIS

Hemostatic defects are not a feature of glomerulonephritis unless renal failure is severe or untreated, but this group of conditions is accompanied by changes in some coagulation and platelet components that may contribute to the renal lesions. Since chronic glomerulonephritis may be associated with thrombosis, the cause and effects of these hemostatic changes become even more significant in our understanding of these conditions.

Circulating immune complexes are found more commonly than in control subjects in patients with acute glomerulonephritis, renal allografts, polyarteritis nodosa, and lupus nephritis. These immune complexes are responsible for platelet activation and release, products of which, such as serotonin and βTG, may be detectable in the plasma. This platelet activation may also lead to an increase in circulating platelet aggregates and possibly to an added stimulus to small vessel thrombosis, contributing to the renal glomerular capillary lesions. There have been attempts to influence the course of renal lesions in such patients by the use of antiplatelet drugs, and effects have been demonstrated on the number of circulating platelet aggregates. It cannot yet be determined, however, if the renal disease has been modified.[23] Fibrin deposition is a feature of many forms of glomerulonephritis, being detectable in crescents and possibly contributing to extracapillary cell proliferation, especially if platelet growth factors are locally released. Thus coagulation imbalance must be an important component. In fact, "hypercoagulation" in nephritis has been associated with an accelerated clotting time in some screening tests of coagulation, possibly indicating the presence of activated clotting intermediaries. In one large study of this phenomenon, Salem et al.[24] could detect patients with enhanced factor VIII coagulant activity which correlated with shortened partial thromboplastin times and occurred in a group of patients with a higher incidence of thrombotic complications. Other patients were found to have an imbalance in the components of factor VIII but no coagulation activator, and were free of thrombosis. It is therefore possible that patients at risk for thrombosis may be identifiable and could be protected with anticoagulants or antiplatelet agents.

## NEPHROTIC SYNDROME

Perhaps more than any other form of chronic renal disease, the nephrotic syndrome is recognized to be associated with thrombosis and with occasional marked changes in some coagulation factors. Both platelet aggregation and the release of βTG have been shown to be enhanced in the nephrotic syndrome in relapse and to improve with remission. Improvement in the nephrotic syndrome has also been observed when thrombocytopenia intervened, supporting a pathogenic role of platelet aggregates. Protein loss in the urine can produce changes in both thrombotic and hemostatic potential. ATIII loss has been demonstrated and clearly related to thrombotic episodes, and it is possible that this defect has not been recognized in all cases in which it may play a contributing role. Conversely, coagulation factors IX and XII have been lost through urine excretion in a number of patients. The deficiency of factor IX may be sufficient to induce a mild bleeding tendency. The mechanism of this coagulation factor loss is of interest and has not been determined. There must be some associated production defect that leads to failure to compensate for the increase in turnover.

## RENAL TRANSPLANTS AND ALLOGRAFT REJECTION

Mild thrombocytopenia is well recognized in patients with functioning renal allografts. Thrombocytopenia is not sufficiently severe to cause bleeding, and probably has an immune basis related to clearance of immune complexes.[16] Large platelets are seen, as might be expected, if these cells were released into the circulation in an attempt to compensate for increased turnover.

Graft rejection is associated with enhanced platelet aggregation and probably also involves enhancement of coagulation, as experiments in factor-deficient animals have shown some protection when the defect was in the intrinsic clotting system. Antiplatelet agents have also been shown to have a role in preventing graft rejection but must be combined with immunosuppressive treatment. Recent work has also been done on the use of prostacyclin in the treatment of hyperacute graft rejection in presensitized dogs.[25] This work indicates a central role for platelets, at least in this situation, and points to the possible use of this approach in grafted patients.

## TREATMENT OF BLEEDING IN RENAL FAILURE

Patients with acute or chronic renal failure require hemostatic control for a variety of indications. The management of bleeding in acute renal failure can be an urgent requirement and is not dependent solely on correction of the uremic state by dialysis. Peritoneal dialysis is probably more effective in reversing the laboratory defects of platelet function since the extracorporeal manipulations needed for hemodialysis, together with the use of heparin, will induce a certain amount of platelet activation in the circuit. In terms of control of bleeding, however, there is no real evidence to suggest that one form of dialysis is superior to the other. This allows for the use of regional heparinization in some situations and the current trend to exploit antiplatelet agents such as prostacyclin[26] and sulfinpyrazone,[27] especially in patients undergoing chronic hemodialysis.

Platelet transfusions may be of benefit when bleeding is severe, and it is possible that transfused plasma components may play a role. It is possible that plasma deficiency of some factor of renal origin, regulating vascular prostacyclin or influencing the balance between platelet and vascular prostaglandin on platelet cAMP levels, may contribute to the bleeding. Janson et al.[19] reported an improvement in the bleeding time 1–12 hours after cryoprecipitate was given to patients for control of bleeding. There was no influence on qualitative tests of platelet function, but bleeding times were corrected and invasive procedures could be done without bleeding. This observation has not yet been made by others, but it does indicate the need to explore this approach.

Patients undergoing chronic hemodialysis have an increased risk of thrombotic disease but also experience abnormal bleeding in relation to dialysis episodes. Generally, tests of platelet function in these patients do not show any abnormalities,[28] so that some other cause, such as the influence of medications, infection, or even anemia, must be sought. There have been some reports of serious bleeding, such as hemarthrosis occurring with systemic heparin administration. These problems can be overcome with regional heparinization or the addition of agents such as prostacyclin, which may allow reduction in the heparin dose.

## REFERENCES

1. Malpass TW, Harker LA: Acquired disorders of platelet function. Semin Hematol 17:242–258, 1980
2. Harker LA, Slichter SJ: The bleeding time as a screening test for evaluation of platelet function. N Engl J Med 287:155–159, 1972
3. Steiner RW, Coggins C, Carvalho ACA: Bleeding time in uremia: A useful test to assess clinical bleeding. Am J Hematol 7:107–117, 1979
4. Hope W, Martin TJ, Chesterman CN, et al: Human beta thromboglobulin inhibits PGI$_2$ production and binds to a specific site in bovine aortic endothelial cells. Nature 282:210–212, 1979
5. Borchgrevink CF: A method for measuring platelet adhesiveness in vivo. Acta Med Scand 168:157–164, 1960
6. Turney JHH, Woods HF, Fewell MR, et al: Factor VIII complex in uremia and effects of hemodialysis. Br Med J 282:1653–1656, 1981
7. Stewart JH, Castaldi PA: Uremic bleeding: A reversible platelet defect corrected by dialysis. Q J Med ns 36:409–423, 1967
8. Akizawa T, Nishiyama H, Koshikawa S: Plasma beta-thromboglobulin levels in chronic renal failure patients. Artif Organs 5:54–58, 1981
9. Guzzo N, Niewiarowski S, Musial J, et al: Secreted platelet proteins with antiheparin and mitogenic activities in chronic renal failure. J Lab Clin Med 96:102–113, 1980
10. Horowitz HI, Cohen BD, Martinez P, et al: Defective ADP-induced platelet factor 3 activation in uremia. Blood 30:331–340, 1967
11. Castaldi PA, Rozenberg M, Stewart JH: The bleeding defect in uremia: A qualitative platelet defect. Lancet 2:66–68, 1966
12. Somer JB, Steward JH, Castaldi PA: The effect of urea on the aggregation of normal human platelets. Thromb Diath Haemorrh 19:64–69, 1968
13. Horowitz HI, Stein IM, Cohen BD, et al: Further studies on the platelet-inhibitory effect of guanidinosuccinic acid and its role in uremic bleeding. Am J Med 49:336–345, 1970
14. Rabiner SF, Molinas F: The role of phenol and phenolic acids on the thrombocytopathy and defective platelet aggregation of patients with renal failure. Am J Med 49:346–351, 1970
15. Gallice P, Fournier N, Crevat A, et al: "In vitro" inhibition of platelet aggregation by uremic middle molecules. Biomedicine 33:185–188, 1980
16. Moncada S, Vane JR: Arachidonic acid metabolites and the interactions between platelets and blood vessel walls. N Engl J Med 300:1142–1147, 1979
17. Editorial: Platelets, endothelium and renal disease. Lancet 2:890–891, 1979
18. de Gaetano G, Remuzzi G, Mysliwiec M, et al: Vascular prostacyclin and plasminogen activator activity in experimental and clinical conditions of disturbed hemostasis or thrombosis. Haemostasis 8:300–311, 1979
19. Janson PA, Jubelirer, SJ, Weinstein MJ, et al: Treatment of the bleeding tendency in uremia with cryoprecipitate. N Engl J Med 303:1318–1322, 1980
20. Chong B, Bull H, Castaldi PA: Human platelet prostaglandin synthesis by immunological stimuli. Proc Aust Soc Med Res 15:25, 1981
20a. Landis TF, von Felten A, Berchtold H: Thrombocytopenic episodes in patients with well-functioning renal allografts. Inverse relationship between platelet count and platelet size pointing to intermittent platelet destruction. Acta Haematol (Basel) 61:2–9, 1979
21. Kaplan BS, Fong JS: Reduced platelet aggregation in hemolytic-uremic syndrome. Thromb Haemost 43:154–157, 1980

22. Brandt P, Jespersen J, Gregersen G: Post partum hemolytic-uremic syndrome treated with antithrombin-III. Nephron 27:15–18, 1981
23. Woo KT, Whitworth JA, Kincaid-Smith P: Effect of anti-platelet agents on circulating platelet aggregates in patients with glomerulonephritis. Thromb Res 20:663–668, 1980
24. Salem HH, Whitworth JA, Koutts J, et al: Hypercoagulation in glomerulonephritis. Br Med J (Clin Res) 282:2083–2085, 1981
25. Mundy AR, Bewick M, Moncada S, et al: Short term suppression of hyperacute renal allograft rejection in presensitized dogs with prostacyclin. Prostaglandins 19:595–603, 1980
26. Turney JH, Williams LC, Fewell MR, et al: Platelet protection and heparin sparing with prostacyclin during regular dialysis therapy. Lancet 2:224–226, 1980
27. Bern MM, Cavaliere BM, Lukas G: Plasma levels and effects of sulfinpyrazone in patients requiring chronic hemodialysis. J Clin Pharmacol 20:107–116, 1980
28. Jorgensen KA, Ingeberg S: Platelets and platelet function in patients with chronic uremia on maintenance hemodialysis. Nephron 23:233–236, 1979

Michael J. Mackie
A. Stuart Douglas

# 16

# Drug-Induced Disorders of Coagulation

Clinical disorders of blood coagulation result from oral anticoagulants (coumarin derivatives), heparin, and ancrod (derived from the Malayan pit viper venom). These are preparations in common clinical usage as antithrombotic agents.

In other chapters, the reader will find descriptions of drug actions on platelets and the fibrinolytic enzyme system.

The only addition to coumarins, heparin, and ancrod described in this chapter is L-asparaginase, which reduces the levels of plasma fibrinogen and factors IX (Christmas factor) and XI (plasma thromboplastin antecedent, PTA).

In the routine practice of clinical medicine, it is the patient on long-term coumarin therapy who is most likely to present with a significant hemorrhagic problem—and often with associated diagnostic difficulty. Many of the patients receiving heparin and ancrod are in the hospital; hemorrhage arises in a situation in which it is not unexpected, and medical staff is available to manage the situation. In the patient on long-term coumarin therapy, the practitioner may not recognize that the current problem is due to hemostatic failure. A small amount of bleeding into a critical site can be more serious than a large gastrointestinal blood loss—for example, a subdural hematoma or bleeding into the wall of the small intestine, with consequent intestinal obstruction.

## ORAL ANTICOAGULANTS

Warfarin the most commonly used oral anticoagulant and is the agent of choice. Other coumarin derivatives such as phenprocoumon or acencoumarol differ only in their pharmacokinetics, and therefore in duration of action. Phenindione, an indanedione derivative, is now rarely prescribed because of the incidence of allergic side effects, some of which can be serious, even fatal. The major part of this section therefore deals with warfarin. In order to appreciate the hemorrhagic hazards of warfarin, a brief account will be given of the mode of action, pharmacology, and control of warfarin therapy, followed by the incidence, sites of bleeding, and factors predisposing to hemorrhage.

## Mechanism of Action

Recent research on the mechanism of action of warfarin indicates that it interferes with the synthesis of the vitamin K-dependent clotting factors (factors II [prothrombin], VII, IX, and X [Stuart factor]), with the resultant production of proteins which are immunologically similar to the naturally occurring factors but functionally markedly abnormal. The evidence is that the vitamin K-dependent proteins possess carboxylglutamyl residues that are crucial for their clotting function and, in particular, for their ability to bind calcium and phospholipid.[1] Warfarin probably blocks that part of the cycle of vitamin K metabolism concerned with regeneration of the active hydroxyquinone form of vitamin K, which is intimately involved in the carboxylation of the glutamic acid residues.[2] Warfarin thus reduces the synthesis of normally functioning vitamin K-dependent clotting factors, but has no effect on their subsequent metabolism. Therefore, the level of the various vitamin K-dependent factors in the blood, following institution of oral anticoagulant therapy, is related to the half-life of the appropriate factor. This is variable, ranging from approximately 7 hours for factor VII to around 60 hours for factor II. It can thus be estimated that some 3–5 days of therapy are required before all the vitamin K-dependent factors reach their lowest levels.

These considerations have important practical implications for the safe and effective use of oral anticoagulants. The effect of warfarin on the coagulation system is conventionally measured by the prothrombin time, which is sensitive to reductions in factors VII and X and, to a lesser extent, factor II, but which is insensitive to alterations in factor IX. The early fall in factor VII following institution of warfarin therapy will therefore be reflected in a prolongation of the prothrombin time. Although the patient might appear well anticoagulated according to the laboratory test, the full antithrombotic effect of therapy is probably not achieved until all the vitamin K-dependent factors have fallen to their nadir. Indeed, work carried out over 20 years ago, involving the inhibition of experimentally produced venous thrombi, demonstrated that the attainment of an antithrombotic effect using oral anticoagulants was not achieved until several days after the prothrombin time was in a specified so-called therapeutic range.[3,4] It has thus become customary to overlap heparin and warfarin for three or more days before stopping the heparin to allow the full antithrombotic effect of the oral anticoagulant to become established.

The understanding of the mechanism of action of warfarin involves implications for the mode of initiating therapy. Until recently, this has usually been commenced with a large bolus loading dose. However, O'Reilly and Aggeler[5] demonstrated that this did not result in a more rapid reduction in factors II, VII, IX, and X than commencement of therapy with smaller repeated doses. Indeed, administration of a large loading dose may cause a precipitous fall in factor VII, exposing the patient to the possible risk of hemorrhage[6] because of the "overshoot." Most authorities thus now agree that it is safer and no less effective to inititate warfarin therapy with (for example) 10 mg daily on the first two days, after which the dose is adjusted according to the prothrombin time.

## Pharmacology

Warfarin is well absorbed orally and is highly bound to plasma albumin. Commercial warfarin is a racemic mixture of two isomers, $R^+$ and $S^-$. The latter is 3–5 times more potent than the former but is more rapidly eliminated.[7] Metabolism of warfarin is achieved by hepatic microsomal enzymes. $S^-$ warfarin is metabolized to 7-hydroxywarfarin, whereas

$R^+$ warfarin is eliminated via warfarin alcohols. The rate of metabolism of each isomer can thus be established, a procedure particularly useful when studying mechanisms of drug interaction (see below).

Warfarin can cross the fetoplacental barrier but is probably not excreted into breast milk in clinically important quantities.[8] The levels of vitamin K-dependent coagulation factors in the healthy newborn infant, however, are less than in the adult, and there is the possibility of a response to even small amounts of drug. There can be clinical situations in which this is an acceptable hazard.

## Control of Oral Anticoagulant Therapy

Optimal anticoagulant control is achieved theoretically when as complete an antithrombotic effect as possible is attained while exposing the patient to the least risk of hemorrhage. After 35 years of clinical use, the method of achieving this balance should become clear from scrutinizing the well-conducted clinical trials designed to demonstrate the relationship between the intensity of anticoagulation, the risk of recurrent thrombosis, and the incidence of hemorrhage. Evaluation of the available trial data, however, is fraught with difficulties. For example, few studies have randomized patients to different intensities of treatment; also, double-blinding has obvious practical difficulties, although it is not impossible to organize, using two observers.

Apart from problems relating to adequate trial design, a major difficulty concerns the exact methodology used in the laboratory to control the therapy. Although the prothrombin time is used most commonly, the results can be expressed in different ways. A number of trials use the Thrombotest, which attempts to assess all the vitamin K-dependent clotting factors. More recently, experience has been gained using chromogenic substrates to assay factors II and X. A reasonable correlation was found between these assays and conventional clotting tests performed on patients receiving long-term anticoagulant therapy.[9,10] However, the most important variable which makes inter-trial comparisons difficult has been the use of different types of thromboplastin in the 1-stage prothrombin time test. Rabbit thromboplastin, commonly used in North America, is less sensitive to the warfarin effect than is human thromboplastin, which is used in the United Kingdom (see Chapter 3). Kelton and Hirsh (1980)[11] determined the prothrombin times of 43 patients on warfarin using both Simplastin (a rabbit thromboplastin) and British Comparative Thromboplastin (a human thromboplastin). Over 80 percent of the test results which were within the therapeutic range (1.5–2.0 times the control value) using Simplastin were outside the therapeutic range (2–3 times the control value) with the British reagent.

In the United Kingdom, there has been a determined attempt to standardize methodology, in particular the thromboplastin time.[12,13] Initially, this was achieved by most laboratories evaluating their own thromboplastin against a standard (British Comparative Thromboplastin), supplied by the National (UK) Reference Laboratory for Anticoagulant Reagents and Control, Manchester, UK. This was done by testing a number of normal plasmas and plasma from patients treated with warfarin with both reference thromboplastin and the laboratory's local thromboplastin. Results could be expressed as a ratio of the patients' time to the control time for each thromboplastin. A graph could be constructed using the ratio obtained with the British Comparative Thromboplastin as one axis and the ratio obtained with the local thromboplastin as the other. Several methods for drawing the line through the various points obtained have been proposed. Many laboratories draw the calibration line by eye, but it can also be calculated by regression.

The approach favored by international organizations (1979)[14] was slightly different. They recommended the establishment of a mean value line, which is a line drawn through two points, one of which is the origin. The coordinates of the other line are the mean ratio of all coumarin plasmas established with the reference plasma as the abscissa, and the mean ratio obtained with the local thromboplastin as the ordinate. This approach allows subsequent results obtained with the laboratory's particular thromboplastin to be expressed in terms of the value that would have been expected if the reference thromboplastin had been used; this extrapolated value in the United Kingdom has been termed the British corrected ratio. More meaningful comparisons of results from different laboratories have thus been made possible. Even more recently, there has been an increasing tendency for laboratories in the United Kingdom to use the standardized thromboplastin prepared in Manchester as the routine reagent. This is obviously more convenient and allows results to be expressed as a ratio directly. To sustain this policy, however, a plentiful supply of standard thromboplastin must be available.

## Incidence of Hemorrhage

Initially, it might seem relatively easy to determine accurately the incidence of hemorrhage related to the use of oral anticoagulants. Much of the available data, however, are derived from poorly designed trials; few are prospective and controlled, and it is difficult to utilize a double-blind type of randomization. There is relatively little information relating the intensity of anticoagulation to the incidence of hemorrhage; furthermore, in view of differences in the methodology of anticoagulant control, inter-trial comparisons are difficult.

### Incidence in Inpatients (Short-Term) and Outpatients (Long-Term)

General reviews of the incidence of bleeding have reported varied findings. Pastor et al.[15] documented a 10 percent incidence of hemorrhage in hospitalized patients, with the figure approaching 40 percent for outpatients; however, serious hemorrhage was said to occur in only 2–10 percent of these groups. Mosley et al.[16] carried out a retrospective review of 978 patients on long-term oral anticoagulants; 22 percent had minor hemorrhage which required no hospital treatment, whereas 1.5 percent suffered major bleeding. Another retrospective study of 3862 patients on treatment found bleeding complications in 6.8 percent.[17]

### Other Identifiable Factors Affecting Incidence—Age and Intensity of Therapy

Bleeding has been found to be more common in older patients and in those whose therapy was initiated with a large loading dose.[17a] As might be expected, patients with relatively severe anticoagulation also had a higher incidence of bleeding. This is supported by the findings of Moschos et al.[18] who randomized patients prospectively to three groups of varying intensity of anticoagulation and found that the frequency of hemorrhage correlated directly with the degree of anticoagulation. Sevitt and Innes[19] also documented a similar relationship.

### Incidence of Hemorrhage in Hip Surgery and the Reluctance of Orthopedic Surgeons to use Prophylaxis with Coumarins

Sevitt and Gallagher[20] demonstrated the value of coumarin drugs in the prophylaxis of deep venous thrombosis in hip surgery. Sevitt and Innes,[19] as mentioned above, demonstrated the relationship of the degree of anticoagulation to hemorrhage. In the Sevitt and

Gallagher study,[20] there was an increased incidence of minor (20 versus 8 percent) and major (3.3 versus 1.3 percent) hemorrhage in the treated group compared to the controls. This incidence of hemorrhage no doubt accounts for the general reluctance of orthopedic surgeons to use anticoagulants in their patients with fractured neck of the femur.[21] A more recent prospective randomized controlled study has again demonstrated the prophylactic efficacy of an oral anticoagulant (warfarin) in reducing thrombotic episodes[22] in patients with fractured femurs. However, minor (10 versus 6 percent) and major (10 versus 3 percent) bleeding was more common in the treated patients compared to the control groups, although there was no evidence that the overall mortality differed as a consequence. Delaying the introduction of prophylactic anticoagulation in 1950 patients undergoing hip arthroplasty until five days postoperatively resulted in a 4.1 percent incidence of hemorrhage, the majority of episodes being wound hematomata.[23] Major bleeding, requiring surgical intervention, occurred in one percent, but there were no fatalities.

### Incidence of Hemorrhage in other Surgical Procedures

Less bleeding has been noted when oral anticoagulants have been used prophylactically in general surgical[24] and gynecological patients.[25] Presumably the hemostatic challenge involved in these particular types of surgery is less than in operations on the hip joint.

### Incidence of Hemorrhage in Long-term Use in Heart Disease

Anticoagulants have been used for many years in patients with rheumatic heart disease, thought to be at risk from atrial thrombus formation, especially those who have undergone valve replacement. Fleming and Bailey[26] followed 500 patients with mitral valve disease for 2000 patient years and found that minor hemorrhage occurred in 8.3 percent, with major bleeding in 7.4 percent. Forfar[27] studied 501 outpatients who received oral anticoagulant therapy, usually for valvular heart disease. During a study period equivalent to 1199 patient years of treatment, hemorrhage severe enough to cause the patient to seek medical aid occurred in 8.2 percent of patients.

### Incidence of Hemorrhage in Long-term Use in Ischemic Heart Disease and Transient Ischemic Attacks

Anticoagulants have been used extensively in patients with ischemic heart disease. Among 1091 patients followed for a mean of 22.4 months, there were hemorrhagic complications in one-fifth;[28] there were 6 hemorrhagic deaths, 4 of which were due to cerebral hemorrhage. Bjerklund[29] reported a frequency of bleeding of one event during eight years of treatment per patient, but the incidence of cerebral bleeding was no more frequent in the treated group than in the controls. As might be expected, however, those who had a cerebral bleed while on anticoagulants had a higher mortality rate. Several groups have reported the incidence of bleeding in postmyocardial infarction patients on long-term therapy. In a group preselected for suitability for anticoagulant therapy, Loeliger et al.[30] documented one bleed per ten patient treatment years, with no fatalities. One double-blind series reported no serious bleeding during a follow-up period of two years.[31]

The use of anticoagulants in patients with transient ischemic attacks might be expected to be complicated by an increased incidence of cerebral hemorrhage. Siekert et al.[32] found an incidence of 7.4 percent fatal cerebral hemorrhage in treated patients compared to 4.4 percent in controls. Among 60 patients selected as being suitable for anticoagulant therapy, another study reported that no deaths occurred secondary to therapy and that treatment had to be stopped in only 1 case because of bleeding.[33]

## Sites of Hemorrhage

Certain groups are at risk of hemorrhage from a particular site; for example, an increased incidence of wound hematomata might be expected in postoperative patients[23] and an increased risk of cerebral hemorrhage in those with cerebral vascular disease.[32] In most reports concerning general medical patients, hematuria, bruising, and gastrointestinal bleeding are the most common hemorrhagic complications of anticoagulant therapy.[15,28,34] The most common site of fatal hemorrhage is intracranial, the next most frequent site is the gastrointestinal tract, usually from a peptic ulcer. Askey,[35] reviewing 1626 patients on long-term oral anticoagulants, reported 30 instances of intracranial hemorrhage.

### Subdural Hematoma

It has become clear that a subdural hematoma is the most common manifestation of intracranial hemorrhage in those on long-term anticoagulants.[36,37] A survey of the literature revealed that subdural hematomata accounted for 102 of the 124 intracranial bleeds reviewed, and intracerebral bleeding for the remainder.[36] Indeed, the incidence of anticoagulant-induced subdural hematomata among all cases of subdurals varied from 12[38] to 38 percent.[39] The diagnosis of subdural hematoma in a patient on oral anticoagulants may be difficult, as a history of head trauma is obtained in only a minority and physical findings may be scanty. A high index of suspicion is required, as is complete investigation, utilizing especially computed tomography.

### Other Less Common Sites of Hemorrhage

Many other less common complications have occurred secondary to bleeding due to anticoagulant therapy. These are listed with references in Table 16-1 and have been reviewed by Loeliger.[40] Interstitial pulmonary hemorrhage may be confused radiologically with recurrence of pulmonary embolism, and the warfarin dose increased instead of decreased. Hemorrhagic cutaneous necrosis occurs when bleeding into skin leads to sloughing and a raw area requiring skin grafting. This occurs most commonly on the breast or thigh and may be symmetrical. Bleeding into the rectus sheath can present as an acute abdomen. An intramural bowel hematoma can present as acute intestinal obstruction.

Sometimes a patient on long-term warfarin has been known to be stable for years on follow-up at the anticoagulant clinic. When such a patient becomes hemorrhagic, a complication should be sought as an explanation. For example, a patient with mitral valve disease may have developed subacute bacterial endocarditis.

## Factors Predisposing to Hemorrhage

Much effort has been made to identify factors which predispose to hemorrhage. Patient reliability is of paramount importance in achieving and keeping good anticoagulant control. The patient's ability to cooperate should be assessed before he is placed on therapy. Unreliable patients (e.g., abusers of alcohol) should not normally be started on warfarin unless the drug is going to be administered solely by a nurse or other attendant. The presence of potential bleeding sites is always cause for concern. If possible, measures should be taken to diminish the risk, for example, by identifying and treating peptic ulcer or reducing high blood pressure. Certain conditions, such as recent cerebral hemorrhage, would contraindicate therapy. Patients with a preexisting hemorrhagic diathesis, either congenital or acquired, would also not usually receive an anticoagulant.

Abnormalities of vitamin metabolism would be expected to interfere with the action

**Table 16-1**
Less Common Sites of Hemorrhage in Patients on
Oral Anticoagulants

| Site | References |
|---|---|
| Respiratory | |
| Larynx | Kiviranta (1967)[139] |
| | Simon et al. (1969)[140] |
| | Hamaker et al. (1969)[141] |
| Interstitial pulmonary haemorrhage | |
| Cardiac | |
| Hemopericardium | Aarseth and Lange (1958)[142] |
| | Fell et al. (1965)[143] |
| Neurological | |
| Lower limb palsy | Lange (1966)[144] |
| Spinal epidural hemotoma | Spurny et al. (1964)[145] |
| | Harik et al. (1977)[146] |
| Endocrine | |
| Adrenal | Amador (1965)[147] |
| | McDonald et al. (1966)[148] |
| Corpus luteum | Dacus (1968)[149] |
| | Wong and Gillett (1977)[150] |
| Skin and soft tissue | |
| Skin necrosis | Robin et al. (1963)[151] |
| | Nalbandian et al. (1965)[152] |
| | Verhagen (1954)[152a] |
| Musculoskeletal | |
| Rectus abdominis | Borkovich and Stafford (1966)[153] |
| Joints | McLaughlin et al. (1966)[154] |
| Intraabdominal | |
| Intramural bowel hematoma | Herbert (1968)[155] |
| Retroperitoneal | Lowe et al. (1979)[156] |

of warfarin and therefore potentially predispose to hemorrhage. Patients on oral anticoagulants given a vitamin K-deficient diet experience an increased anticoagulant effect.[41] Malabsorption of vitamin K may not always lead to increased anticoagulant responsiveness, as there is often concomitant reduced absorption of the anticoagulant itself. The influence of antibiotics on gut bacterial flora which synthesize vitamin K will be discussed in the following section.

## Drug Interactions with Oral Anticoagulants

The ability of a large number of drugs to interfere with oral anticoagulants has long been appreciated. Patients tend to be on anticoagulants for some months at least, and thus there is ample time for exposure to other drugs. The literature on the subject tends to be confusing, abounding with anecdotal cases reports. The patients discussed have often been on multiple drug regimens, making identification of the offending drug causing the interaction difficult. The mechanism underlying a supposed drug interaction is also often ill-defined; even if a pharmacological interaction occurs, its in vivo significance in an individual patient has to be established.

There is little doubt about the potential magnitude of the problem. Koch-Weser[42]

**Table 16-2**

Drugs Likely to Cause Significant Interference with Anticoagulant
Control and/or Hemorrhage*

| Drug | Proposed Mechanism | Reference |
|------|--------------------|-----------| 
| Barbiturates | Induction of hepatic microsomal enzymes | MacDonald and Robinson (1968);[47] Johansson (1968);[46] Starr and Petrie (1972);[44] Udall (1975);[48] Hansten (1979)[45] |
| Rifampin | Induction of hepatic microsomal enzymes | O'Reilly (1974)[6] |
| Glutethimide | Induction of hepatic microsomal enzymes | Udall (1975)[48] |
| Phenylbutazone | Inhibition of S⁻ isomer | Aggeler et al. (1967);[77] Lewis et al. (1974)[75] |
| Cimetidine | Inhibition of S⁻ isomer | Serlin et al. (1979);[157] Wallin et al. (1979);[158] Silver and Bell (1979);[159] Barnett and Hancock (1975);[142] Hassall et al. (1975)[83] |
| Cortrimoxazole | Inhibition of S⁻ isomer | O'Reilly and Motley (1979);[85] O'Reilly (1979)[84] |
| Metronidazole | Inhibition of S⁻ isomer | O'Reilly (1976)[86] |
| Anabolic steroids | Unknown | Longridge et al. (1971);[161] De Oyar et al. (1971)[162] |
| Glucagon | ? Increased receptor site affinity | Koch-Weser (1970)[163] |
| Aspirin | See text | See text |

*Concurrent use of these drugs with oral anticoagulants should be generally avoided.

reported that drug interactions were implicated in 25 percent of the bleeding episodes recorded in 500 hospitalized patients studied prospectively. In another prospective series of 277 patients, 183 were taking drugs other than the anticoagulant. A theoretical interaction was documented in 94 of the drug courses given.[43] Starr and Petrie[44] noted a theoretical drug interaction of prescribed drugs with warfarin in 33 percent of 254 patients; a potential interaction was also observed in 30 percent involving self-administered drugs. The evidence showed that a genuine adverse reaction, involving loss of anticoagulant control, occurred only in 9 percent of patients.

Much work has been done to determine various potential mechanisms of drug interaction, some of which are thought to be clinically more relevant than others. Drugs are thought to have the potential for interference with the action of oral anticoagulants and/or to increase the risk of hemorrhage by altering the following:

1. Drug absorption
2. Protein binding
3. Receptor-site affinity
4. Metabolism and excretion
5. Additional parameters of the hemostatic mechanism

Tables 16-2 and 16-3 list the drugs reported in the literature to interact with oral anticoagulants and the mechanism by which this is thought to occur. No such list is ever complete; it needs continuous revision as new data become available. An attempt has been made to separate the drugs that are known to cause clinical problems with anticoagulant control

**Table 16-3**
Drugs Reported to Interact with Oral Anticoagulants*

| Allopurinol | Inhibition of metabolism | Rawlins and Smith (1973)[164] |
|---|---|---|
| Amiodarone | ? | Rees et al. (1981)[165] |
| Antipyrine | Induction of metabolism | Whitfield et al. (1973)[166] |
| Azapropazone | ? | Powell-Jackson (1977)[78] |
| Carbamazepine | Induction of metabolism | Hansen et al. (1971)[167] |
| Chloribrate | ? | Starr and Petrie (1972)[44] |
| Chloramphenicol | Inhibition of metabolism | Christensen and Skorsted (1976)[87] |
| Cholestyramine | Inhibition of absorption | Koch-Weser and Sellers (1971)[168] |
| Diflunisal | ? | Tempero et al. (1977)[80] |
| Disulfiram | Inhibition of metabolism | Rothstein (1968);[169] O'Reilly (1973)[170] |
| Ethacrynic acid | Displacement | Sellers and Koch-Weser (1970);[50] Petrick (1973)[171] |
| Ethchlorvynol | Induction of metabolism | Johanssen (1968)[46] |
| Griseofulvin | Induction of metabolism | Cullen and Catalano (1967)[89] |
| Mefenamic acid | Displacement | Sellers and Koch-Weser (1970)[50] |
| 6-Mercaptopurine | ? | Spiers and Mibasham (1974)[172] |
| Phenformin | ? | Hamblin (1971)[173] |
| Phenyramidol | Inhibition of metabolism | Carter (1965)[174] |
| Phenytoin | ? | Nappi (1979)[175] |
| Proproxyphene | ? | Orme et al. (1976)[79] |
| Quinidine | ? Decreased synthesis of Vitamin K-dependent factors | Koch-Weser (1968)[176] |
| Sulindac | ? | Carter (1979);[80] Ross and Beeley (1979)[34] |
| Sulfinpyrazone | ? | Davis and Johns (1978);[177] Gallus and Burkett (1980)[178] |
| Thyroxine | Increased catabolism of Vitamin K-dependent factors | Owens et al. (1962)[179] |

*The mechanism and clinical significance of interaction of these drugs are less clearly defined than those of the drugs listed in Table 16-2.

and bleeding from those drugs in which no clinical effect has yet been fully established. It is wise, however, to be particularly vigilant when any drug is introduced to or removed from the regimen of a patient stabilized on oral anticoagulant therapy. It is at these times of change that anticoagulant control is likely to be disturbed and the patient exposed to the risk of hemorrhage. Ideally, a patient on anticoagulants should take as few additional medications as possible. Indeed, difficulty in anticoagulant control, as manifested by the number of changes in dose per month, can be correlated directly with the number of additional drugs consumed.[43] The patient himself should be instructed to take only medications approved by his physician.

We do not intend to discuss every drug listed in Table 16-2; individual references are given, and Hansten[45] has recently reviewed the literature extensively. However, certain commonly prescribed groups of drugs which have long caused problems in anticoagulant usage are worthy of more detailed review.

*Hypnotics/Sedatives*

Barbiturates can increase the activity of the hepatic microsomal enzymes which metabolize warfarin. They will thus diminish its hypoprothrombinemic effect, necessitating an increased dosage to secure an adequate therapeutic action of concurrently administered warfarin. The main hazard, however, is that when the barbiturate is stopped, often at discharge of the patient from hospital, no simultaneous reduction in anticoagulant dosage is made; the patient is thus exposed to significant hypoprothrombinemia and risk of hemorrhage. This is a clinically significant problem and has been frequently reported; see Table 16-2.[44–48]

The clinical importance of this type of interaction is particularly well demonstrated in the study of McDonald and Robinson.[47] They documented 67 bleeding episodes occurring in patients on oral anticoagulants and found drugs causing enzyme induction to be involved in 14. The decreased anticoagulant response usually commences within 10 days of starting barbiturates and is maximal at 2–3 weeks. When the barbiturates are stopped, the effect is diminished for the next 7–10 days, and there is little residual enzyme induction by 2–3 weeks. Thus, although the long-term use of a relatively stable dose of barbiturates, as prescribed to epileptics, does not appear to interfere significantly with anticoagulant control,[43] barbiturates are generally best avoided in patients on oral anticoagulants. In any event, there is a consensus that barbiturates, because of their addictive effect, should not be prescribed as hypnotics at all. Benzodiazepine derivatives (nitrazepam, diazepam, flurazepam) are a more appropriate choice, as they can be used safely with anticoagulants.[45]

Chloral hydrate can also be used safely in patients on warfarin, although it still regularly appears in lists of drugs which potentiate oral anticoagulants.[49] This demonstrates the necessity of establishing the clinical importance of any drug interaction which may seem to have a firm pharmacological base. Although chloral hydrate can displace warfarin bound to plasma protein and may cause transient hypoprothrombinemia in some subjects,[50] long-term studies have failed to demonstrate a significant problem in regard to anticoagulant control.[51,52] This presumably reflects the complex nature of the kinetics of oral anticoagulants and, as Breckenridge[53] suggests, any increase in the concentration of free drug may result in an increased rate of its metabolism, thus tending to counteract the initial increase in plasma levels.

### Aspirin and other Analgesics

Most patients on oral anticoagulant therapy must periodically take an analgesic. The most commonly consumed analgesic is aspirin, which is marketed not only alone but also as a constituent of many proprietary preparations which are frequently bought without a medical prescription. The patient is often unaware that the product he buys for his pain contains aspirin. There are a number of ways in which aspirin ingestion can be potentially hazardous to a patient taking a drug such as warfarin. Aspirin in large doses (2–3 g/day) can exert a modest hypoprothrombinemic effect; it may displace warfarin from its binding sites; it certainly has an antiplatelet action (Chapter 4), thus contributing an additional hemostatic defect to that already created by the anticoagulant. Lastly, and possibly most important, is the local action of aspirin on the gastric mucosa.

Some of these points require discussion. It is thought that salicylate interference with the synthesis of coagulation factors by the liver is unlikely to be of clinical significance in the normal individual unless the salicylate level exceeds 30 mg/dl.[54] It is conceivable, however, that in patients whose vitamin K-dependent factors are already reduced, any further depression might be expected to cause increased risk of hemorrhage. Indeed, the four cases of 'aspirin-induced hypoprothrombinemia' described by Fausa[55] were likely to have an underlying degree of hypoprothrombinemia (secondary to congestive cardiac failure in one, partial gastrectomy and probably malabsorption in three cases) that was accentuated by heavy aspirin ingestion. Aspirin has also been reported by one group to elevate the whole blood fibrinolytic activity.[56] This work, however, awaits general confirmation, and its clinical relevance is questionable.

Aspirin has long been known to affect in vitro tests of platelet aggregation[57,58] and to prolong the bleeding time.[59,60] The basis of this antiplatelet action is the irreversible acetylation of the platelet enzyme cyclooxygenase,[61] which is required for the production of prostaglandin endoperoxides. The data regarding the bleeding time have become more controversial recently in that some authors have demonstrated a shortening of the bleeding time with higher doses of aspirin (generally 3–4 g),[62,63] although not all investigators agree with these data.[64] Fundamental to this debate is the hypothesis that higher doses of aspirin inhibit the formation of prostacyclin ($PGI_2$) in the vessel wall in addition to the production of thromboxane $A_2$ by the platelet, reflecting a possible differential sensitivity of the cyclooxygenase in platelets and vascular intima to aspirin.

It is of major relevance that patients with congenital cyclooxygenase deficiency have a bleeding problem.[65] Thus, even if aspirin were to inhibit cyclooxygenase totally in the vessel wall and the platelet, it seems likely that the hemostatic–thrombotic balance would still be in favor of hemorrhage rather than thrombosis. Furthermore, the vessel wall recovers from the aspirin effect, whereas the cyclooxygenase inhibitor in the platelet is permanent throughout the life of that platelet. In addition, aspirin ingestion causes a significantly more prolonged bleeding time in hemophiliacs than in control subjects.[66]

Most clinical hemorrhagic problems with aspirin are related to gastrointestinal blood loss. The site of blood loss is usually the stomach, and it is thought that aspirin changes the permeability of the gastric mucosa so that there is back diffusion of hydrogen ions, which are irritating to the mucosa.[67] Indeed, 50 percent of individuals ingesting aspirin at a low pH were observed at endoscopy to have hemorrhagic lesions.[68] Stubbé[69] found that 70 percent of controls and patients with rheumatic disorders had a positive fecal occult blood test related to consumption of 750 mg–3 g of aspirin daily. Patients with a known but quiescent focus of bleeding do not appear to bleed more frequently while on aspirin, but blood loss is augmented if a lesion is actively bleeding.[70] A large retrospective survey has demonstrated a correlation between regular aspirin usage (ingestion on 4 days or more per week), admission to a hospital for gastrointestinal bleeding, and either a benign gastric ulcer or the absence of a demonstrable lesion to account for the hemorrage.[71] Interestingly, there was no correlation between regular aspirin intake and gastrointestinal hemorrhage associated with an uncomplicated or bleeding duodenal ulcer.

The failure of intravenously administered aspirin to cause excess blood loss provides evidence of the primary local effect of aspirin in the pathogenesis of gastrointestinal bleeding,[72] although Grossman et al.[70] did notice increased blood loss following parenteral administration. The loss, however, was less than that documented following oral therapy, and a number of their patients had active peptic ulcers.

Despite the potential hemorrhagic hazards of using aspirin with warfarin, this combination of drugs has received attention because of its possible synergistic antithrombotic effect. Dale et al.[73] produced reasonable evidence that combined aspirin and oral anticoagulant therapy was more effective than the latter alone in preventing embolism from prosthetic cardiac valves. The incidence of bleeding, however, was significantly higher in the group with combined therapy (13.9 versus 4.7/100 patients/year). Analysis of the hemorrhagic episodes revealed that the bleeding excess was due almost entirely to gastrointestinal hemorrhage, again suggesting the importance of the local effect of aspirin. A similar earlier study had also shown an increased incidence of melena in a group treated with aspirin and oral anticoagulants.[74] It would thus seem wise to avoid the use of aspirin in patients on oral anticoagulants unless this practice is part of a well-conducted trial involving fully informed patient volunteers. It is of interest that another antiplatelet drug, dipyridamole, has also been used in combination with warfarin to prevent thromboembolic complications after cardiac valve replacement.[75] In this study, however, there was more gastrointestinal hemorrhage in the group treated only with warfarin, although there were 2 hemorrhagic deaths in the combined-treatment group.

There still remains the choice of an analgesic in patients on coumarin therapy. Unfortunately, a number of other preparations used particularly in the field of rheumatology should be avoided in patients on oral anticoagulants. Phenylbutazone has been shown to potentiate the anticoagulant action of racemic warfarin by inhibiting the metabolism of its potent $S^-$ isomer.[76] This is a clinically important interaction, and cases of resultant hemorrhage have been reported;[45,77] phenylbutazone and oxyphenylbutazone should thus be avoided. Azapropazone, which resembles phenylbutazone, has been documented on one occasion to augment the action of warfarin.[78] Similarly, mefenamic acid,[50] dextropropoxyphene,[79] diflunisal,[80] and sulindac[34,81] have all been reported to potentiate oral anticoagulants. However, the documentation of the clinical significance of the interaction involving the latter drugs is not so comprehensive and well-validated as it is in the case of phenylbutazone. At present, acetaminophen (paracetamol) can be recommended[45] to those on oral anticoagulants. With paracetamol there have been occasional reports of immune thrombocytopenia; the additive effect of these two abnormalities on hemostasis could be dangerous. Fortunately, this effect of paracetamol is extremely rare, and a widely acceptable, milder alternative analgesic is not available.

### Antimicrobial Agents

At some stage, it is common for a patient on long-term anticoagulant therapy to be given a short course of antibiotics. Broad-spectrum antibiotics have long been claimed to enhance anticoagulation by reducing the gut flora which synthesize vitamin $K_1$. However, closer inspection of the relevant data reveals that this is probably a misconception. Although patients on anticoagulant therapy given a vitamin K-deficient diet developed enhanced hypoprothrombinemia, the administration of neomycin to suppress gut flora had little effect on the prothrombin time.[41] This suggests that, providing dietary vitamin K is adequate, prevention of endogenous synthesis of vitamin K will have little effect.

A number of antibiotics, however, can interfere with the action of oral anticoagulants, usually by exerting an effect on the hepatic microsomal enzymes. Cotrimoxazole has been known for some time to potentiate warfarin.[82,83] In 1 of the 6 cases reported by Hassall et al.[83] bleeding occurred. It now seems clear that cotrimoxazole selectively inhibits the metabolism of the more potent $S^-$ isomer of racemic warfarin,[84,85] causing enhanced hypoprothrombinemia. A similar stereoselective effect involving the $S^-$ isomer of warfarin has also been described with metronidazole.[86] Chloramphenicol[87] and chlortetracycline[88] have been reported to inhibit drug metabolism, so that theoretically they could potentiate warfarin. Griseofulvin[89] and rifampin,[6] by contrast, are inducers of enzyme activity and thus would be expected to diminish the effect of oral anticoagulants. The hemorrhagic hazard is the same, in principle, as that encountered with barbiturates. Initially, the dose of anticoagulant would have been increased to compensate for the induction of the hepatic enzymes. If the inducing agent was stopped and the anticoagulant was continued at the same dosage, the patient would be subjected to a distinct hemorrhagic risk.

The above examples emphasize the most important principles to keep in mind when considering drug interactions with oral anticoagulants. It is obviously important to be aware of the possibility of such interactions and to be particularly vigilant in assessing anticoagulant control when there is any change in the patient's drug regimen. If a drug has been reported to interact with oral anticoagulants, then the wisest policy is to avoid that drug. In the small number of instances in which there is no suitable alternative to a drug known to interact, then, provided the mechanism of the interaction is known, it should be possible to use the drug in question with reasonable safety by making appropriate alterations in the dose of oral anticoagulant. Hopefully, it should be clear that the danger periods for loss of anticoagulant control occur when a drug is removed and when a new drug is added to the medications of a patient stabilized on oral anticoagulant therapy.

## Management of Excessive Anticoagulation and Bleeding in Patients on Oral Anticoagulant Therapy

A number of situations have to be considered, bearing in mind differing degrees of excessive anticoagulation and the overall features. One commonly encountered situation involves the patient who is found on follow-up to have a prothrombin time outside the therapeutic range, but who has no obvious bleeding problem. Such an individual should stop his anticoagulant for 24–48 hours, after which the prothrombin time should be rechecked. The patient should be questioned closely about any changes in medication which might have resulted in loss of control. A small oral dose of vitamin $K_1$ (2.5 mg) can also be given in this situation if the excess prolongation of the prothrombin time is substantial. This will ensure rapid correction of the abnormal prothrombin time but will not make the patient resistant to subsequent reintroduction of an anticoagulant effect.

If the patient is bleeding and has a prolonged prothrombin time, then the measures which should be taken depend on the clinical severity of the bleeding episode. In any event, the oral anticoagulant should be stopped. If the bleeding is not judged to be major, vitamin $K_1$ in a dose of 10 mg intravenously can be administered. This should correct a prolonged prothrombin time in 6–12 hours. Doses greater than this will render the patient difficult to anticoagulate with warfarin for 1–2 weeks thereafter.

Excessive anticoagulation in the presence of life-threatening hemorrhage requires more rapid correction of the coagulation defect. This can be achieved by the administration of fresh frozen plasma or a prothrombin–complex concentrate. Most hemorrhagic situations during coumarin therapy can be managed without resort to such preparations. This is fortunate, because they can be thrombogenic. A search should be made, if appropriate, for a local lesion to account for the occurrence of bleeding. Oral administration of vitamin $K_1$ is also effective but may be marginally slower in correcting the bleeding. Minor allergic reactions can occur with intravenous vitamin $K_1$.

## HEPARIN

Heparin affects hemostasis primarily by interfering with the coagulation mechanism, but it can also cause thrombocytopenia[90,91] (see Chapter 4).

## Mode of Action

Heparin exerts its anticoagulant action in the presence of an $\alpha_2$-globulin, antithrombin III (ATIII). Heparin binds to lysyl groups of ATIII, thereby inducing a conformational change in the latter which vastly enhances its inhibitory action on the serine centers of factors XIIa, XIa, IXa, Xa, and thrombin.[92]

## Routes and Objectives of Heparin Administration

Heparin is used clinically in two situations in which there is a thrombotic problem. It may be a given in a low dose prophylactically, in the absence of evidence of actual thrombosis, or it may be used in larger doses to prevent further thrombosis and embolism in patients who already have established thrombosis. When administered in small doses prophylactically, heparin is usually given subcutaneously. With an established thrombotic event it should be given intravenously, either by continuous infusion or intermittent injection. Intramuscular injection of heparin is to be avoided because of the real hazard of muscle hematoma formation.

## Laboratory Control

The question of laboratory control of heparin therapy remains controversial. The controversy concerns not only the selection of the best test available but also whether laboratory test results are helpful in predicting either recurrent thrombosis or bleeding complications. There are two groups of tests available for the evaluation of heparin therapy. The first group, represented by the activated partial thromboplastin time (APTT) and the whole blood clotting time (WBCT), are sensitive to all the coagulation factors that heparin inhibits. These global tests, however, will also be sensitive to factors (e.g., factor VIII) which are not altered by heparin. The second group represents tests which are more specific, in that they reflect the action of heparin on particular coagulation proteins (e.g., thrombin clotting time and various heparin assays). These latter tests are not, of course, sensitive to factors such as factor VIII which are not altered by heparin therapy. Elevation of factor VIII, which can occur in a variety of clinical situations, may result in a shorter APTT than might be expected.[93] The thrombin clotting time, however, has been criticized because its relationship to the level of heparin is linear over only a small range. Because of the expense of chromogenic substrates, heparin assays by that technique are not in routine use.

The most commonly used test is the APTT.[94] Its advantages are that it is routinely available, relatively inexpensive, and done in the laboratory. The last point highlights one of the major problems with the WBCT, which necessitates the presence at the bedside of a technician and his equipment, including a water bath. A very prolonged result can be expensive in technician time. There are potential problems, however, with the APTT. Choice of the anticoagulant used for APTT estimation is important; oxalate samples are less sensitive to the presence of heparin than citrate.[95] There is a theoretical objection that this test does not reflect the influence of platelets on the effect of heparin. The choice of the partial thromboplastin time reagant is most important. The use of a satisfactory reagent should result in a linear response to increasing concentrations of heparin. Not all commercially available reagents, unfortunately, demonstrate this type of response. Ts'ao et al.[96] evaluated six commercially available partial thromboplastin reagents and found that only three gave a linear response to an increasing concentration of heparin. Similar findings have been made by other workers.[97] Obviously, each laboratory using this technique should ensure that the partial thromboplastin it uses is properly evaluated with respect to linearity of the response to heparin.

## Hemorrhage During Heparin Therapy

The correlation of laboratory test results with the incidence of bleeding has led to conflicting data. Few trials, however, have randomized comparable groups to varying intensities of therapy or compared the bleeding in patients given a fixed dose of heparin without control with that in a group given a variable dose to keep the laboratory test within a predetermined potentially therapeutic range. In the clinical judgment of some investigators, patients with excessively prolonged clotting times tend to bleed.[98,99]

The Urokinase Pulmonary Embolism Trial[100] demonstrated a relationship between the intensity of treatment and the incidence of bleeding. In this test, 20 percent of patients who had a clotting time in excess of 60 minutes bled compared to 5 percent of those with a clotting time between 30 and 60 minutes. There was no bleeding in patients with a clotting time of less than 30 minutes. However, Basu et al.[101] found no correlation between control and the incidence of bleeding in 234 patients studied prospectively and given a continuous heparin infusion. Pitney et al.[102] also failed to demonstrate a close correlation between clotting times and bleeding complications. In a study of 50 patients treated with intermittent doses of heparin, 4 of the 6 patients who bled had APTT results outside the therapeutic ranges; however, a further 5 patients were cited whose APTT was also considerably prolonged, but who did not bleed. Salzman et al.[103] randomized patients prospectively to intermittent injections of heparin, one group of patients being given a fixed dose and the other a dose to keep the APTT within a therapeutic range. There was no difference in the incidence of major hemorrhage between the two groups, which were thought to be comparable in terms or risk factors (see below).

## Risk Factors Associated with Susceptibility to Bleeding in Patients Treated with Heparin

The incidence of hemorrhage in the published series of trials using full doses of heparin varies from 1 percent[103] to 33 percent.[104] It is natural to look for risk factors to explain these widely varying figures. Factors examined relate to the dose and method of administration of the heparin itself, and also to various patient characteristics which might predispose to bleeding. A number of host factors have been recognized. In the study of Jick et al.[105] 32 percent of women bled compared to 15 percent of men. Elderly females appear to be at particular risk.[105-108] Previous surgery also increased the risk of bleeding; the overall incidence of bleeding reported by Basu et al.[101] was 8 percent. Among those patients in their series who had undergone surgery (and were considered separately), the incidence was 13.4 percent; this increased bleeding was not necessarily at the operative site. This finding has been supported by the study of Norman and Provan[109] Intramuscular injections should be avoided, as extensive hemorrhage tends to occur at the injection site.[108] As might be expected, patients who have a defective hemostatic mechanism before commencement of heparin bleed more frequently. Only 7.6 percent of patients with a normal hemostatic mechanism prior to treatment bled, whereas 90 percent of those with a preexisting defect had a hemorrhagic complication.[102] Thus, patients who are known to have a preexisting impairment of hemostasis should be anticoagulated only rarely and with extreme caution.

### *Low-Dose Heparin*

In this account, an evaluation is needed of the risk of hemorrhage associated with heparin administered in a low dose as prophylaxis. The primary aim of the trials utilizing this heparin regimen has been to document any reduction in the incidence of venous thromboembolism. The objective recording of hemorrhagic complications has thus been very variable. Kelton and Hirsh[11] have reviewed the design of these trials, stressing particularly the importance of objective criteria to assess bleeding. Two double-blind randomized studies have prospectively assessed bleeding complications. Kiil et al.[110] studied

1296 general surgical patients randomized to heparin or a placebo. Preoperative and post-operative transfusion requirements were similar; increased bleeding at surgery was reported in 1.4 percent of the heparinized group and 2.6 percent of those receiving saline. There were two deaths in the heparin group and three in the placebo group attributable to bleeding. In the other prospective double-blind trial, involving orthopedic surgical patients, the incidence of perioperative bleeding was similar in the two groups.[111]

A number of other studies have assessed blood loss in prospective controlled trials using objective endpoints, but because they were non-blinded there was liability to observer bias. Four of these trials involving general surgical patients found no difference in transfusion requirement or significant blood loss,[24,111a,112,113] whereas two studies demonstrated increased transfusion requirements and a postoperative fall in hematocrit.[114,115] In similarly designed and conducted trials of low-dose heparin in patients undergoing orthopedic surgery, the majority have shown no difference in transfusion requirements or perioperative blood loss,[116–118] although one reported increased blood loss and transfusion requirements.[119] Although the majority of trials of low-dose heparin utilize a twice-daily dose of 5000 U, there is no evidence that this dose given 3 times a day results in significantly increased blood loss.[115,120] However, some trials employing a thrice-daily heparin regimen in surgical patients have documented an increased incidence of wound hematomata.[111a,115] Another variable which has been compared is the relative hemorrhagic risk between sodium and calcium salts. Berquist and Hallbook[121] reported the occurrence of large hematomas at the site of injection of calcium heparin, although overall there was no difference in clinically significant bleeding. This study was in agreement with earlier work.[122] Thorngren, however,[120] documented a higher transfusion requirement in those receiving sodium heparin. Thus, although the data are somewhat controversial, it seems likely that neither of the available salts of heparin causes more significant bleeding than the other.

### Aspirin Plus Heparin

A number of studies have reported on the incidence of bleeding when aspirin has been administered with heparin. One double-blind study compared the effect of heparin alone, aspirin alone, and aspirin plus heparin in three randomized groups of general surgical patients.[123] No difference in blood loss was noted. Other less well designed trials have produced conflicting results. Bleeding complications were similar when 75 patients undergoing hip surgery were randomized to aspirin, aspirin plus heparin, or a control group.[124] The majority of patients undergoing hip surgery and receiving heparin plus aspirin studied by Yett et al.,[125] however, had serious bleeding problems. Thus, although, as might be expected in theory, examples of bleeding apparently due to a combination of low-dose heparin and aspirin can be found in the literature, the results of better-designed trials do not suggest that excess hemorrhage is a major problem of the combined therapy. It seems reasonable, however, to be particularly vigilant when using aspirin and heparin in combination.

### Incidence of Hemorrhage Using Conventional
### Intravenous Administration

Conventional doses of heparin are commonly administered intravenously by two main methods: continuous infusion or intermittent injection. A number of prospective randomized trials have compared bleeding complications in patients receiving either intermittent or continuous therapy. Two studies have shown a significantly reduced incidence of hemorrhage in the group receiving heparin by continuous infusion. Salzman and colleagues[103] documented a 1 percent incidence of hemorrhage in a group given heparin by continuous infusion, whereas 8 percent bled in the intermittent group. Although the group on intermittent therapy received slightly more heparin, that difference was not significant. The groups were said to be comparable as far as risk factors for hemorrhage were concerned. These results were confirmed by Glazier and Cromwell,[104] who noted a 33 percent incidence of bleeding in the group receiving heparin by intermittent injection, whereas no major hemorrhage occurred in the continuous infusion group. Again, the groups were said to be comparable for risk factors, but more heparin was administered to the patients receiving the drug by intermittent injection. A more recent study reported no significant difference in the number of bleeding complications, although there were more instances of hemorrhage in the group given heparin by intermittent injection.[99] Mant et al.[107] also found no significant difference in the incidence of hemorrhage between patients randomized to intermittent and continuous therapy; in this trial, however, more heparin was generally given to the patients on continuous infusion.

Wilson et al.[126] randomized 118 patients with venous thrombosis to heparin therapy either by continuous infusion or by intermittent injection. No difference in the incidence of hemorrhage was noted if patients judged to be at high risk of bleeding were not included in the analysis. If such patients were included, however, more bleeding was found in those receiving heparin by intermittent injection. It was again noted that patients in the latter group tended to receive a higher dose of heparin. In regard to the risk of hemorrhage, the balance of evidence is marginally in favor of continuous infusion of heparin. No one knows whether one regimen is better or worse then the other in the prevention or treatment of deep venous thrombosis and pulmonary embolism.

## Management of Hemorrhage Due to Heparin Therapy

If bleeding is major, heparin therapy should be stopped and the coagulation times checked. Heparin, an acidic substance, can be neutralized if necessary by basic protamine sulfate. A 1 mg dose of protamine sulfate neutralizes 1 mg (100 U) of heparin. As the half-life of heparin is only about 60 minutes, however, the dose of protamine is reduced according to how long after the heparin injection it is given (e.g., only a 50 percent calculated dose after 1 hour). Protamine has to be given intravenously and should be injected slowly.

Factors should be identified which would predispose to hemorrhage in the patient on heparin. As mentioned previously, intramuscular injections and invasive procedures should be avoided.

The decision to restart heparin after an episode of bleeding depends on the severity of the bleed and the estimated risk of mortality and morbidity from recurrent thromboembolism. If the bleeding is life-threatening (e.g., gastrointestinal, cerebral), heparin should not be restarted. In this situation, some authorities recommend consideration of inferior caval interruption to prevent embolism in major thrombosis, or monitoring of calf vein thrombosis by leg screening or impedance plethysmography.[11]

## ANCROD

Ancrod is an enzyme purified from the venom of the Malayan pit viper. Its use as an antithrombotic agent was suggested by the observation that bites from the viper caused hypofibrinogenemia but little bleeding.[127,128] The proteolytic effect of ancrod on fibrinogen differs from that of thrombin in that ancrod cleaves only fibinopeptide A from the fibrinogen molecule.[129] The resultant fibrin is more susceptible to fibrinolysis, presumably because it is not cross-linked and contains degraded α-chains. In addition, ancrod does not appear to activate factor XIII,[130] nor does its administration result in the reduction of factors V, VIII, IX, or X.[131] Fibrin degradation products rise during the first 36 hours of treatment and then rapidly return to normal. Following the cessation of therapy, fibrinogen takes 2–3 weeks to reach normal levels.[132]

Ancrod must be given parenterally, the intravenous route being preferred, as resistance to therapy is often encountered when the drug is given intramuscularly. Although a number of protocols have been proposed for the administration of ancrod,[133–135] the low-dose regimen proposed by Barrie et al.[136] can be recommended. This consists of 1 U/kg body weight given intravenously over the first 12 hours, followed by 0.5 U/kg every 12 hours thereafter; this results in moderate hypofibrinogenemia ( ± 50 mg/dl). The effect of ancrod is monitored either by measuring the fibrinogen level itself or by using the fibrinogen titer as a guide. A fibrinogen level of 50 mg/dl or a titer of 1:2 or less is considered satisfactory.[134,137] Evaluation of the incidence of bleeding in trials using ancrod is made difficult by the use of differing dosage regimens, degrees of hypofibrinogenemia obtained, and length of treatment. Kakkar et al.[134] randomized 30 patients to heparin, streptokinase, and ancrod. Bleeding occurred in two of the ten patients on heparin and in three of those given streptokinase, but only in one of the ten who received ancrod.

In a randomized double-blind trial of 33 patients given either heparin or ancrod, hemorrhage was documented in 2 of the heparin group but in none of those on ancrod.[133] A similar low incidence of hemorrhagic problems was noted by Tibbutt et al.,[137] who randomized patients to ancrod or streptokinase. Of the 18 patients on the latter drug, 12 bled from venipuncture sites and there was 1 case of retroperitoneal hemorrhage. Only 2 subjects out of 16 in the ancrod group bled excessively from venipuncture sites. Sharp et al.[135] encountered more bleeding with ancrod in their patients (6/19), but the bleeding occurred in cases with recent surgical wounds, and the degree of defibrination was more severe than that used in the other trials discussed.

Thus, based on this evidence, the use of ancrod does not result in frequent hemorrhagic complications. If these complications do occur, they can be controlled by replacement of fibrinogen and an antivenom is available.

## L-ASPARAGINASE

L-Asparaginase is an antitumor drug used in the treatment of acute lymphoblastic leukemia. Sensitive tumor cells are unable to synthesize L-asparagine and are therefore more dependent than normal cells on an exogenous supply of this amino acid. This is reduced by the administration of L-asparaginase, which hydrolyzes L-asparagine. It is now appreciated that L-asparaginase has marked, predictable effects on coagulation factors. These effects were well documented by Ramsay et al.,[138] who performed serial coagulation studies on 26 children with acute lymphoblastic leukemia. Frequent prolongation of the screening tests was observed, especially the thrombin clotting time (21/26). The latter reflected the hypofibrinogenemia which was documented in all cases. Reduction in the levels of factors IX and XI was also recorded. The coagulation abnormalities disappeared when the L-asparaginase alone was discontinued, although the patients continued to receive other antileukemic agents. Despite the profound abnormalities of coagulation associated with L-asparaginase, no bleeding episodes were recorded, possibly because the patients' platelet counts were relatively high when the coagulation defect was at its maximum. The reduction in coagulation factors is thought to be related to diminished synthesis.

## REFERENCES

1. Suttie JW: Oral anticoagulant therapy: The biosynthetic basis. Semin Hematol 14:365–374, 1977
2. Gallop PM, Lian JB, Hauschka PV: Carboxylated calcium-binding proteins and vitamin K. N Engl J Med 302:1460–1466, 1980
3. Deykin D, Wessler S, Reimer SM: Evidence of an antithrombotic effect of Dicumarol. Am J Physiol 199:1161–1164, 1960
4. Jewell P, Pilkington T, Robinson B: Heparin and ethylbiscoumacetate in prevention of experimental venous thrombosis. Br Med J 1:1013–1016, 1954
5. O'Reilly RA, Aggeler PM: Studies on coumarin anticoagulant drugs. Initiation of warfarin therapy without a loading dose. Circulation 38:169–177, 1968
6. O'Reilly RA: Interaction of sodium warfarin and rifampin. Studies in man. Ann Intern Med 81:337–340, 1974
7. Breckenridge A: Oral anticoagulants—The totem and the taboo. Br Med J 1:419–423, 1976
8. Baty JD, Breckenridge A, Lewis PJ: May mothers taking warfarin breast feed their infants? Br J Clin Pharmacol 3:969, 1976 (abstract)
9. Axelsson G, Korsan-Bengtsen K, Waldenstrom J: Prothrombin determination by means of a chromogenic peptide substrate. Thromb Haemost 36:517–524, 1976
10. Latello ZS, Thomson JM, Poller L: Oral anticoagulant control and chromogenic substrates. Br J Haematol 45:174, 1980 (abstract)
11. Kelton JG, Hirsh J: Bleeding associated with antithrombotic therapy. Semin Hematol 17:259–291, 1980
12. Poller L: Progress in laboratory control of anticoagulant treatment, in Poller L (ed): Recent Advances in Blood Coagulation. London, Churchill, 1969, pp 137–154
13. Poller L: The British system for anticoagulant control. Thromb Haemost 33:157–162, 1975
14. ICTH/ICSH: Prothrombin time standardization: Report on the expert panel on oral anticoagulant control. Thromb Haemost 42:1073–1114, 1979
15. Pastor BH, Resnick ME, Rodman T: Serious hemorrhagic complications of anticoagulant therapy. JAMA 180:747–751, 1962
16. Mosley DH, Schatz IJ, Breneman GM, et al: Long term anticoagulant therapy. Complications and control in a review of 978 cases. JAMA 186:914–916, 1963
17. Coon WW, Willis PW: Hemorrhagic complications of anticoagulant therapy. Arch Intern Med 133:386–392, 1974
17a. Rods J, van Joost HE: The cause of bleeding during anticoagulant treatment. Acta Med Scand 178:129–131, 1965
18. Moschos CB, Wong PCY, Sise HS: Controlled study of the effective level of long term anticoagulation. JAMA 190:799–805, 1964
19. Sevitt S, Innes D: Prothrombin-time and Thrombotest in inured patients on prophylactic anticoagulant therapy. Lancet 1:124–129, 1964
20. Sevitt S, Gallagher NG: Prevention of venous thrombosis and pulmonary embolism in injured patients. A trial of anticoagulant prophylaxis with phenindione in middle aged and elderly patients with fractured necks of femur. Lancet 2:981–989, 1959
21. Morris GK, Mitchell JRA: Prevention and diagnosis of venous thrombosis in patients with hip fractures. A survey of current practice. Lancet 2:867–869, 1976
22. Morris GK, Mitchell JRA: Warfarin sodium in prevention of deep venous thrombosis and pulmonary embolism in patients with fractured neck of femur. Lancet 2:869–872, 1976
23. Coventry MB, Nolan DR, Beckenbaugh RD: "Delayed" prophylactic anticoagulation: A

study of results and complications in 2012 total hip arthroplasties. J Bone Joint Surg (Am) 55A:1487–1492, 1973

24. Van Vroonhoven TJMV, Van Zijl J, Muller H: Low dose subcutaneous heparin versus oral anticoagulants in the prevention of postoperative deep venous thrombosis. Lancet 1:375–378, 1974

25. Taberner DA, Poller L, Burslem RW: Oral anticoagulants controlled by the British comparative thromboplastin versus low dose heparin in prophylaxis of deep vein thrombosis. Br Med J 1:272–274, 1978

26. Fleming HA, Bailey SM: Mitral valve disease, systemic embolism and anticoagulants. Postgrad Med J 47:599–604, 1971

27. Forfar JC: A 7 year analysis of haemorrhage in patients in long term anticoagulant treatment. Br Heart J 42:128–132, 1979

28. Nichol ES, Keyes JN, Borg JF, et al: Long term anticoagulant therapy in coronary atherosclerosis. Am Heart J 55:142–152, 1958

29. Bjerkelund CJ: The effect of long term treatment with dicoumarol in myocardial infarction. Acta Med Scand Suppl 330:1–212, 1966

30. Loeliger EA, Hensen A, Kroes F: A double blind trial of long term anticoagulant treatment after myocardial infarction. Acta Med Scand 182:549–566, 1967

31. Meuwissen OJAT, Vervoorn AC, Cohen O, et al: Double blind trial of long term anticoagulant treatment after myocardial infarction. Act Med Scand 186:361–368, 1969

32. Siekert RG, Whisnant JP, Millikan CH: Surgical and anticoagulant therapy of occlusive cerebrovascular disease. Ann Intern Med 58:637–641, 1963

33. Baker RN, Schwartz WS, Rose AS: Transient ischemic strokes: A report of a study of anticoagulant therapy. Neurology 16:841–847, 1966

34. Ross JRY, Beeley L: Sulindac, prothrombin time and anticoagulants. Lancet 2:1075, 1979 (letter)

35. Askey JM: Hemorrhage during long term anticoagulant drug therapy. I. Intracranial hemorrhage. Calif Med 140:6–10, 1966

36. Iizuka J: Intracranial and intraspinal hematomas associated with anticoagulant therapy. Neurochirurgia (Stuttg) 15:15–25, 1972

37. Silverstein A: Neurological complications of anticoagulant therapy. A neurologist's review. Arch Intern Med 139:217–220, 1979

38. Weiner LN, Nathanson M: The relationship of subdural hematoma to anticoagulant therapy. Arch Neurol 6:282–286, 1962

39. Sreerama U, Ivan LP, Dennergy JM, et al: Neurological complications of anticoagulant therapy. Can Med Assoc J 108:305–307, 1974

40. Loeliger EA: Anticoagulant induced hemorrhage, in Girdwood RH (ed): Blood Disorders Due to Drugs and Other Agents. Amsterdam, Excerpta Medica, 1973, pp 221–240

41. Udall JA: Human sources and absorption of vitamin K in relation to anticoagulant stability. JAMA 194:127–129, 1965

42. Koch-Weser J: Hemorrhagic reactions and drug interactions in 500 warfarin-treated patients. Clin Pharmacol Ther 14:139, 1973 (abstract)

43. Williams JRB, Griffin JP, Parkins A: Effect of concomitantly administered drugs on control of long term anticoagulant therapy. Q J Med 45:63–73, 1976

44. Starr KJ, Petrie JC: Drug interactions in patients on long term oral anticoagulant and antihypertensive adrenergic neuron blocking drugs. Br Med J 4:133–135, 1972

45. Hansten PD: Oral anticoagulant drug interactions, in Clinical Drug Interactions (ed 4). London, Henry Kimpton, 1979, pp 33–68

46. Johansson S-A: Apparent resistance to oral anticoagulant therapy and influence of hypnotics of some coagulation factors. Acta Med Scand 184:297–300, 1968

47. MacDonald MG, Robinson DS: Clinical observations of possible barbiturate interference with anticoagulation. JAMA 204:97–100, 1968

48.  Udall JA: Clinical implications of warfarin. Interactions with five sedatives. Am J Cardiol 35:67–71, 1975

49.  British National Formulary: Drug Interactions. London, Pharmaceutical Press, 1981, p 323

50.  Sellers EM, Koch-Weser J: Displacement of warfarin from human albumin by diazoxide and ethacrynic, mefenamic, and nalidixic acids. Clin Pharmacol Ther 11:524–529, 1970

51.  Griner PF, Wiesner PJ: Chloral hydrate and warfarin interaction: Clinical significance? Ann Intern Med 74:540–543, 1971

52.  Udall JA: Warfarin-chloral hydrate, interaction, pharmacological activity and clinical significance. Ann Intern Med 81:341–344, 1974

53.  Breckenridge A: Oral anticoagulant drugs: Pharmacokinetic aspects. Semin Hematol 15:19–26, 1978

54.  Rothschild BM: Hematologic perturbations associated with salicylate. Clin Pharmacol Ther 26:145–152, 1979

55.  Fausa O: Salicylate-induced hypoprothrombinemia. A report of four cases. Acta Med Scand 188:403–408, 1970

56.  Moroz LA: Increased blood fibrinolytic activity after aspirin ingestion. N Engl J Med 296:525–529, 1977

57.  O'Brien JF: Effect of salicylates on human platelets. Lancet 1:779–783, 1968

58.  Stuart RK: Platelet function studies in human beings receiving 300 mg of aspirin per day. J Lab Clin Med 75:463–471, 1970

59.  Mielke CH Jr, Kaneshiro MM, Maher IA, et al: The standardized normal Ivy bleeding time and its prolongation by aspirin. Blood 34:204–215, 1969

60.  Quick AJ: Salicylates and bleeding: The aspirin tolerance test. Am J Med Sci 252:264–269, 1966

61.  Roth GJ, Stanford N, Majerus PW: Acetylation of prostaglandin synthetase by aspirin. Proc Natl Acad Sci USA 72:3073–3076, 1975

62.  O'Grady J, Moncada S: Aspirin: A paradoxical effect on bleeding-time. Lancet 2:780, 1978 (letter)

63.  Rajah SM, Penny A, Kester R: Aspirin and bleeding-time. Lancet 2:1104, 1978 (letter)

64.  Godal HC, Eika C, Dybdahl JH, et al: Aspirin and bleeding-time. Lancet 1:1236, 1979 (letter)

65.  Malmsten C, Hamberg M, Svensson J, et al: Physiological role of an endoperoxide in human platelets: Hemostatic defect due to platelet cyclooxygenase deficiency. Proc Natl Acad Sci USA 72:1446–1450, 1975

66.  Kasper CK, Rapaport SI: Bleeding times and platelet aggregation after analgesics in hemophilia. Ann Intern Med 77:189–193, 1972

67.  Page IH: Salicylate damage to the gastric mucosal barrier. N Engl J Med 276:1307–1312, 1967

68.  Thorsen WB, Western D, Tanaka Y, et al: Aspirin injury to the gastric mucosa. Gastrocamera observations of the effect of pH. Arch Intern Med 121:499–506, 1968

69.  Stubbé L Th FL: Occult blood in feces after administration of aspirin. Br Med J 2:1062–1066, 1958

70.  Grossman MI, Matsumoto KK, Lichter RJ: Fecal blood loss produced by oral and intravenous administration of various salicylates. Gastroenterology 40:383–388, 1961

71.  Levy M: Aspirin use in patients with major upper gastrointestinal bleeding and peptic ulcer disease. N Engl J Med 290:1158–1162, 1974

72.  Leonards JR, Levy G: The role of dosage form in aspirin-induced gastrointestinal bleeding. Clin Pharmacol Ther 8:400–408, 1969

73.  Dale J, Myhre E, Loew D: Bleeding during acetylsalicylic acid and anticoagulant therapy in patients with reduced platelet reactivity after aortic valve replacement. Am Heart J 99:746–752, 1980

74.  Altman R, Boullon F, Rouvrier J, et al: Aspirin and prophylaxis of thrombotic complications in patients with substitute heart valves. J Thorac Cardiovasc Surg 72:127–129, 1976

75.  Sullivan JM, Harker DE, Gorlin R: Pharmacologic control of thromboembolic complications of cardiac valve replacement. N Engl J Med 284:1391–1394, 1971

76.  Lewis RJ, Trager WF, Chan KK, et al: Warfarin. Stereochemical aspects of its metabolism and the interaction with phenylbutazone. J Clin Invest 53:1607–1617, 1974

77.  Aggeler PM, O'Reilly RA, Leong L, et al: Potentiation of anticoagulant effect of warfarin by phenylbutazone. N Engl J Med 276:496–501, 1967

78.  Powell-Jackson RR: Interaction between azapropazone and warfarin. Br Med J 1:1193–1194, 1977

79.  Orme M, Breckenridge A, Cook P: Warfarin and Distalgesic interaction. Br Med J 1:200, 1976

80.  Tempero KF, Cirillo VJ, Steelman SL: Diflunisal: A review of pharmacokinetic and pharmacodynamic properties, drug interactions, and special tolerability studies in humans. Br J Clin Pharmacol 4:315–365, 1977

81.  Carter SA: Potential effect of sulindac on response of prothrombin time to oral anticoagulants. Lancet 2:698–699, 1979

82.  Barnett DB, Hancock BW: Anticoagulant resistance: an unusual case. Br Med J 1:608–609, 1975

83.  Hassall C, Feetam CL, Leach RH, et al: Potentiation of warfarin by cotrimoxazole. Lancet 2:1155–1156, 1975

84.  O'Reilly RA: Stereoselective interaction of trimethoprim-sulfamethoxazole (TMP-SMZ) with the enantiomers of warfarin in man. Blood 54(suppl 1):295a, 1979 (abstract)

85.  O'Reilly RA, Motley CH: Racemic warfarin and trimethoprim-sulfamethoxazole interaction in humans. Ann Intern Med 91:34–36, 1979

86.  O'Reilly RA: The stereoselective interaction of warfarin and metronidazole in man. N Engl J Med 295:354–357, 1976

87.  Christensen LK, Skovsted L: Inhibition of drug metabolism by chloramphenicol. Lancet 2:1397–1399, 1976

88.  Peters MA, Fouts JR: The inhibitory effect of Aureomycin (chlortetracycline) pretreatment on some rats liver microsomal enzyme activities. Biochem Pharmacol 18:1511–1517, 1969

89.  Cullen SI, Catolano PM: Griseofulvin-warfarin antagonism. JAMA 199:582–583, 1967

90.  Bell WR, Tomasulo PA, Alving BM, et al: Thrombocytopenia occurring during the administration of heparin. Ann Intern Med 85:155–160, 1976

91.  Powers PJ, Cuthbert D, Hirsh J: Thrombocytopenia found uncommonly during heparin therapy. JAMA 241:2396–2397, 1979

92.  Rosenberg RD: Actions and interactions of antithrombin and heparin. N Engl J Med 292:146–151, 1975

93.  Edson RJ, Krivit W, White JG: Kaolin partial thromboplastin time: High levels of procoagulants producing short clotting times or masking deficiencies of other procoagulants or low concentrations of anticoagulants. J Lab Clin Med 70:463–470, 1967

94.  Poller L, Thomson JM, Yee KF: Heparin and partial thromboplastin time. An international survey. Br J Haematol 44:161–165, 1980

95.  Soloway HB, Cox SP, Donahoo JV: Sensitivity of activated partial thromboplastin time to heparin. Effect of anticoagulant used for sample collection. Am J Clin Pathol 59:760–762, 1973

96.  Ts'ao C-H, Galluzzo TS, Lo R, et al: Whole blood clotting time, activated partial thromboplastin time, and whole blood recalcification time as heparin monitoring tests. Am J Clin Pathol 71:17–21, 1979

97.  Triplett DA, Harms CS, Koepke JA: The effect of heparin on the activated partial thromboplastin time. Am J Clin Pathol 70:556–559, 1978

98.  O'Sullivan EF, Hirsh J, McCarthy RA, et al: Heparin in the treatment of venous thromboembolic disease. Med J Aust 2:153–159, 1968

99.  Wilson JR, Lampman J: Heparin therapy: A randomized prospective study. Am Heart J 97:155–158, 1979

100. Urokinase Pulmonary Embolism Trial: A national co-operative study. Circulation 47(suppl 11):1–108, 1973
101. Basu D, Gallus A, Hirsh J, et al: A prospective study of the value of monitoring heparin treatment with the activated partial thromboplastin time. N Engl J Med 287:324–327, 1972
102. Pitney WR, Pettit JE, Armstrong L: Control of heparin therapy. Br Med J 4:139–141, 1970
103. Salzman EW, Deykin D, Shapiro RM, et al: Management of heparin therapy. Controlled prospective trial. N Engl J Med 292:1046–1050, 1975
104. Glazier RL, Crowell EB: Randomized prospective trial of continuous versus intermittent heparin therapy. JAMA 236:1365–1367, 1976
105. Jick H, Slone D, Borda IT, et al: Efficacy and toxicity of heparin in relation to age and sex. N Engl J Med 279:284–289, 1968
106. Kernohan RJ, Todd C: Heparin therapy in thromboembolic disease. Lancet 1:621–623, 1966
107. Mant MJ, O'Brien BD, Thong KL, et al: Haemorrhagic complications of heparin therapy. Lancet 1:1133–1135, 1977
108. Vieweg WVR, Piscatelli RL, Houser JJ, et al: Complications of intravenous administration of heparin in elderly women. JAMA 213:1303–1306, 1970
109. Norman CS, Provan JL: Control and complications of intermittent heparin therapy. Surg Gynecol Obstet 145:338–342, 1977
110. Kiil J, Kiil J, Axelson F, Andersen D: Prophylaxis against post-operative pulmonary embolism and deep-vein thrombosis by low-dose heparin. Lancet 1:1115–1116, 1978
111. Williams JW, Eikman EA, Greenberg SH: Failure of low dose heparin to prevent pulmonary embolism after hip surgery or above the knee amputation. Ann Surg 188:468–478, 1978
111a. International Multicentre Trial: Prevention of postoperative pulmonary embolism by low doses of heparin. Lancet 2:45–51, 1975
112. Nicholaides AN, Dupont PA, Desai S: Small doses of subcutaneous sodium heparin in preventing deep venous thrombosis after major surgery. Lancet 2:890–893, 1972
113. Sagar S, Massey J, Sanderson JM: Low dose heparin prophylaxis against fatal pulmonary embolism. Br Med J 4:257–259, 1975
114. Gallus AS, Hirsh J, Tuttle RJ: Small subcutaneous doses of heparin in prevention of venous thrombosis. N Engl J Med 288:545–551, 1973
115. Gallus AS, Hirsh J: Prevention of venous thromboembolism. Semin Thromb Hemostas 2:232–290, 1976
116. Morris GK, Henry APJ, Preston BJ: Prevention of deep vein thrombosis by low dose heparin in patients undergoing total hip replacement. Lancet 2:797–799, 1974
117. Sagar S, Nairn D, Stamatakis JD, et al: Efficacy of low-dose heparin in prevention of extensive deep-vein thrombosis in patients undergoing total-hip replacement. Lancet 1:1151–1154, 1976
118. Venous Thrombosis Clinical Study Group: Small doses of subcutaneous sodium heparin in the prevention of deep vein thrombosis after elective hip operations. Br J Surg 62:348–350, 1975
119. Mannucci PM, Citerio LE, Panajotopoulos N: Low dose heparin and deep vein thrombosis after total hip replacement. Thromb Haemost 36:157–164, 1976
120. Thorngren S: Optimal regimen of low dose heparin prophylaxis in gastrointestinal surgery. Acta Chir Scand 145:87–93, 1979
121. Bergquist D, Hallbook T: A comparison between low dose sodium and calcium heparin. Acta Chir Scand 144:339–342, 1978
122. Abou-Addallah E, Rousis C, Loup P, et al: Étude comparative heparinate de sodium et de calcium dans la prophylaxie des maladies thromboemboliques en chirurgie. Helv Chir Acta 42:691–694, 1975
123. Loew D, Brocke P, Simma W: Acetylsalicylic acid, low dose heparin, and a combination of both substances in the prevention of postoperative thromboembolism. A double blind study. Thromb Res 11:81–86, 1974
124. Shondorf TH, Hey D: Combined administration of low dose heparin and aspirin as prophylaxis of deep vein thrombosis after hip joint surgery. Haemostasis 5:250–257, 1976

125. Yett S, Skillman JJ, Salzman EW: The hazards of aspirin plus heparin. N Engl J Med 298: 1092, 1978 (letter)

126. Wilson JE, Bynum LJ, Parkey RW: Heparin therapy in venous thromboembolism. Am J Med 70:808–816, 1981

127. Reid HA, Thean PC, Chan KE, et al: Clinical effects of bites by Malayan viper *(Ankistrodon rhodostoma)*. Lancet 1:617–621, 1963

128. Reid HA, Chan KE, Thean PC: Prolonged coagulation defect (defibrination syndrome) in Malayan Viper bite. Lancet 1:621–626, 1963

129. Ewart MR, Hatton MWC, Basford JM, et al: The proteolytic action of arvin on human fibrinogen. Biochem J 118:603–609, 1970

130. Pizzo SV, Schwartz ML, Hill RL, et al: Mechanism of ancrod anticoagulation. A direct proteolytic effect on fibrin. J Clin Invest 51:2841–2850, 1972

131. Bell WR, Bolton G, Pitney WR: The effect of arvin on blood coagulation factors. Br J Haematol 15:589–602, 1968

132. Bell WR, Pitney WR, Goodwin JF: Therapeutic defibrination in the treatment of thrombotic disease. Lancet 1:490–493, 1968

133. Davies JA, Merrick MV, Sharp AA, et al: Controlled trial of ancrod and heparin in treatment of deep vein thrombosis of lower limb. Lancet 1:113–115, 1972

134. Kakker VV, Flanc C, Howe CT, et al: Treatment of deep vein thrombosis. A trial of heparin, streptokinase, and arvin. Br Med J 1:806–810, 1969

135. Sharp AA, Warren BA, Paxton AM, et al: Anticoagulant therapy with purified fraction of Malayan pit-viper venom. Lancet 1:493–499, 1968

136. Barrie WW, Wood EH, Crumlish P, et al: Low-dosage ancrod for prevention of thrombotic complications after surgery for fractured neck of femur. Br Med J 4:130–133, 1974

137. Tibbutt DA, Williams EW, Walker MW, et al: Controlled trial of ancrod and streptokinase in the treatment of deep vein thrombosis of lower limb. Br J Haematol 27:407–414, 1974

138. Ramsay NKC, Coccia PF, Krivit W, et al: The effect of L-asparaginase on plasma coagulation factors in acute lymphoblastic leukemia. Cancer 40:1398–1401, 1977

139. Kiviranta UK: Laryngeal hematomas due to coagulopathies. J Laryngol Otol 81:503–513, 1967

140. Simon HB, Daggett WM, Desanctis RW: Hemothorax as a complication of anticoagulant therapy in the presence of pulmonary infarction. JAMA 208:1830–1834, 1969

141. Hamaker WR, Buchman RJ, Cox WA, et al: Hemothorax. A complication of anticoagulant therapy. Ann Thorac Surg 8:564–569, 1969

142. Aarseth S, Lange HF: The influence of anticoagulant therapy on the occurrence of cardiac rupture and hemopericardium following heart infarction. I. A study of 89 cases of hemopericardium (81 of them cardiac ruptures). Am Heart J 56:250–256, 1958

143. Fell SC, Rubin IL, Enselberg CD, et al: Anticoagulant induced hemopericardium with tamponade: Its occurrence in the absence of myocardial infarction or pericarditis. N Engl J Med 272:670–674, 1965

144. Lange LS: Lower limb palsies with hypoprothrombinaemia. Br Med J 2:93–94, 1966

145. Spurny OM, Rubin S, Wolf JW, et al: Spinal epidural hematoma during anticoagulant therapy. Report of two cases. Arch Intern Med 114:103–107, 1964

146. Harik SI, Raichle ME, Reis DJ: Spontaneously remitting spinal epidural hematomas in a patient on anticoagulants. N Engl J med 284:1355–1357, 1971

147. Amador E: Adrenal hemorrhage during anticoagulant therapy. A clinical and pathological study of ten cases. Ann Intern Med 63:559–571, 1965

148. McDonald FD, Myers AR, Pardo R: Adrenal hemorrhage during anticoagulant therapy. JAMA 198:1052–1056, 1966

149. Dacus RM: Massive intraperitoneal hemorrhage from a corpus luteum hematoma in women taking anticoagulants. Report of two cases. Obstet Gynecol 31:471–474, 1968

150. Wong KP, Gillett PG: Recurrent hemorrhage from corpus luteum during anticoagulant therapy. Can Med Assoc J 116:388–390, 1977

151. Robin GC, Levin SM, Freund M: Breast hemorrhage and gangrene during anticoagulant therapy. Br J Surg 50:773–774, 1963

152. Nalbandian RM, Mader IJ, Barrett JL, et al: Petechiae, ecchymoses and necrosis of skin induced by coumarin congeners. JAMA 192:603–608, 1965

152a. Verhagen H: Local haemorrhage and necrosis of the skin and underlying tissues during anticoagulant therapy with Dicumarol or Dicumacyl. Acta Med Scand 148:453–467, 1954

153. Borkovich KH, Stafford ES: Acute anemia and abdominal tumor due to hemorrhage in rectus abdominis sheath following anticoagulant therapy. Arch Intern Med 117:103–107, 1966

154. McLaughlin GE, McCarty DJ, Segal BL: Hemarthrosis complicating anticoagulant therapy. Report of three cases. JAMA 196:1020–1021, 1966

155. Herbert DC: Anticoagulant therapy and the acute abdomen. Br J Surg 55:353–357, 1968

156. Lowe GDO, McKillop JH, Prentice AG: Fatal retroperitoneal haemorrhage complicating anti-coagulant therapy. Postgrad Med J 55:18–21, 1979

157. Serlin MJ, Mossman S, Sibeon RG, et al: Cimetidine: Interaction with oral anticoagulants in man. Lancet 2:317–319, 1979

158. Wallin BA, Jacknowitz A, Raich PC: Cimetidine and effect of warfarin. Ann Intern Med 90:993, 1979 (letter)

159. Silver BA, Bell WR: Cimetidine potentiation of the hypoprothrombinemic effect of warfarin. Ann Intern Med 90:348–349, 1979

160. Sullivan JM, Harken DE, Gorlin R: Pharmacologic control of thromboembolic complications of cardiac valve replacement. N Engl J Med 284:1391–1394, 1971

161. Longridge RGM, Gillam PMS, Barton GMG: Decreased anticoagulant tolerance with oxymethalone. Lancet 2:90, 1971

162. De Oya JC, Del Rio A, Noya M, et al: Decreased anticoagulant tolerance with oxymethaline in paroxysmal nocturnal haemoglobinuria. Lancet 2:259, 1971 (letter)

163. Koch-Weser J: Potentiation by glucagon of the hypoprothrombinemic action of warfarin. Ann Intern Med 72:331–335, 1970

164. Rawlins MD, Smith SE: Influence of allopurinol on drug metabolism in man. Br J Pharmacol 48:693–698, 1973

165. Rees A, Dalal JJ, Reid PG, et al: Dangers of amiodarone and anticoagulant treatment. Br Med J 282:1756–1757, 1981

166. Whitfield JB, Moss DW, Neale G, et al: Changes in plasma α-glutamyl transpeptidase activity associated with alterations in drug metabolism in man. Br Med J 1:316–318, 1973

167. Hansen JM, Siersboek-Nielsen E, Skovsted L: Carbamazepine induced acceleration of diphenylhydantoin and warfarin metabolism in man. Clin Pharmacol Ther 12:539–543, 1971

168. Koch-Weser J, Sellers EM: Drug interactions with coumarin anticoagulants. N Engl J Med 285:487–498, 547–558, 1971

169. Rothstein E: Warfarin enhanced by disulfiram. JAMA 206:1574–1575, 1968

170. O'Reilly RA: Interaction of sodium warfarin and disulfiram (Antabuse) in man. Ann Intern Med 78:73–76, 1973

171. Petrick RJ: Interaction between warfarin and ethacrynic acid. JAMA 231:843–844, 1975

172. Spiers ASD, Mibashan RS: Increased warfarin requirement during mercaptopurine therapy: A new drug interaction. Lancet 2:221–222, 1974 (letter)

173. Hamblin TJ: Interaction between warfarin and phenformin. Lancet 2:1323, 1971 (letter)

174. Carter SA: Potentiation of the effect of orally administered anticoagulant by phenyramidol. N Engl J Med 273:423–426, 1965

175. Nappi JM: Warfarin and phenytoin interaction. Ann Intern Med 90:852, 1979 (letter)

176. Koch-Weser J: Quinidine-induced hypothrombinemic hemorrhage on patients in chronic warfarin therapy. Ann Intern Med 68:511–517, 1968

177. Davis JW, Johns LE Jr: Possible interaction of sulfinpyrazone with coumarins. N Engl J Med 299:955, 1978 (letter)

178. Gallus A, Birkett D: Sulfinpyrazone and warfarin: A probable drug interaction. Lancet 1:535–536, 1980

179. Owens JC, Neely WB, Owen WR: Effect of sodium dextrothyroxine in patients receiving anticoagulants. N Engl J Med 266:76–79, 1962

H. Alistair Reid

# 17

# Clinical Hemostatic Disorders Caused by Venoms

In 1635 Nierembergius wrote that victims bitten by the viper "haemorrhum" (probably *Bothrops atrox)* bled profusely through all the orifices and wounds of the body. Two hundred years ago in Italy, Fontana noted that blood remained fluid in animals killed by viper venoms. In 1860, Mitchell in the United States reported the same phenomenon following bites by rattlesnakes. In 1895, Martin found that injection of Australian snake venom given in minute amounts intravenously and in larger amounts subcutaneously caused intravascular coagulation with death from circulatory stasis. With lower venom concentrations no clotting occurred. The blood became incoagulable; a "negative phase" had been established, and further venom failed to cause clotting. In 1909, Mellanby in England showed that slow injection of viper venom caused defibrination; the negative phase resulted from the "precipitation" of fibrinogen, and fibrin was removed from the circulation. In the 1930s, Macfarlane reported a powerful thromboplasticlike action of *Vipera russelii* venom. Eagle, followed in the 1950s by Didisheim and Lewis, experimentally classified venoms into fibrinolytic, thrombic, thromboplastic, and fibrinogenolytic categories. Clinicians dealing with patients bitten or stung by venomous creatures have usually ignored these important observations. The first comprehensive study of blood coagulation in human victims of reliably identified viper bite with an adequate number of patients was carried out 25 years ago in Malaya. The general well-being of patients with nonclotting blood following bites by the Malayan viper *Agkistrodon rhodostoma* was remarkable and prompted development of the author's own concept of therapeutic defibrination.

Many venoms, particularly snake venoms, cause hemostatic disorders. Our main concern, however, will be with viper venoms.

## GENERAL CLASSIFICATION OF SNAKES

Most of the 2700 species of snakes are nonvenomous, having no fangs (Aglypha). In this group, the colubrid family includes the majority of species. A few colubrid snakes are technically venomous, having a venom gland connecting with a solid fang at the back of the mouth (Opisthoglypha). Their bites, although venomous to prey, are usually harmless

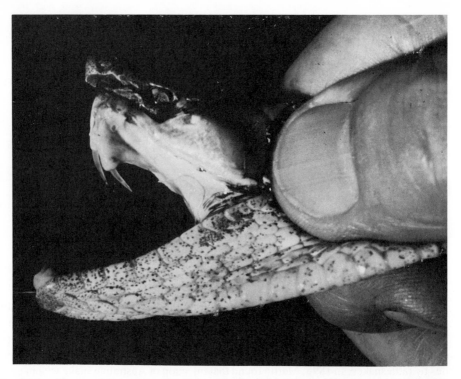

**Fig. 17-1.** The parotid or venom gland of a viper lies behind the eye (the skin over the gland has been removed) and is connected by a duct along the upper gum to an opening at the top of the canalized fang, which is long, mobile, and easily seen when erected. (Copyright Dr. H. Alistair Reid).

to man. Back-fanged colubrid snakes, however, should not be carelessly handled since, on rare occasions, bites by colubrids such as the African boomslang *Dispholidus typus* have caused serious, even fatal hemorrhagic poisoning. The venomous snakes have a venom gland behind the eye (Fig. 17-1) connecting with a venom duct which runs along the upper gum to hollow fangs at the front of the mouth (Proteroglypha). There are 3 families of venomous snakes: Elapidae, Hydrophiidae, and Viperidae. Elapids are land snakes with short, nonmobile fangs 3–5 mm long in adults; they include cobras, mambas, kraits, coral snakes, and the Australian venomous land snakes. Sea snakes (Hydrophiidae) have very short, fixed fangs and characteristic flat, rudderlike tails. Vipers have long, mobile fangs 10–30 mm long. They are easy to see when erected (Fig. 17-1), but when folded back against the upper gum, they can be very difficult to recognize. Vipers are subdivided into pit vipers (Crotalinae), which have heat-sensing pits between the eye and nose, and viperine vipers (Viperinae), which do not have these pits. Elapids and sea snakes bite their victims sometimes tenaciously, whereas vipers strike and immediately retract. Viper bites are much more common than elapid bites except in the Pacific-Australian area, where vipers do not naturally occur. Sea snake bites are common among fishing folk of Asian and Western Pacific coastal areas. In human victims, sea snake venoms are predominantly myotoxic; most elapid venoms have a selective neuromuscular blocking action on muscles for vision, swallowing, speaking, and breathing. In sea snake and elapid envenomings, there are no clinically significant hemostatic effects (except in some of the Pacific Australian elapid envenomings). In contrast, hemostatic upset is the predominant clinical effect of viper venoms. Viper bite poisoning will therefore be the main consideration of this chapter.

Although there are many different species of venomous snakes, only a few are known to be of medical importance. Some venomous snakes have a fearsome reputation, mainly because they are large and, when milked, can yield substantial amounts of highly toxic venom. For example, the bushmaster, *Lachesis muta,* is often described as deadly yet the author has been unable to discover a single medical report of its bite. Geographically, the foremost medically important vipers are *Crotalus atrox* (North America), *Bothrops atrox* (Central and South America), *Bitis arietans* (Africa), *Echis carinatus* (Africa, Asia), *Vipera russelii* (Asia), and *Agkistrodon* (or *Calloselasma) rhodostoma* (Southeast Asia). *E. carinatus* can justifiably be labeled the most dangerous snake in the world to man. Because of its vast distribution and abundance in farming areas, good camouflage in its natural habitat, irritability, lightning strike, and toxic venom, it causes more deaths and serious poisoning than any other snake.

## EPIDEMIOLOGY OF SNAKEBITE

Snakebite statistics are usually based on hospital cases and, for a number of reasons, are misleadingly fallacious. Most snakebite victims, particularly in the tropics where snakebite is common, rarely go to a hospital. They prefer treatment from a traditional healer. For example, in Nigeria a traditional healer treats several hundred snakebite patients each year, his dwelling/clinic being only about one mile from the university teaching hospital, which records about five cases a year. A high incidence of snakebite is often related to the prevalence of one particular snake species—for example, *A. rhodostoma* in Southeast Asia; *E. carinatus* in west Africa, Pakistan, and northwest India; and *V. russelii* in Burma and other areas of Asia. Adjacent to these areas of high snake prevalence may be similar terrain, yet the snake species is rare or absent and snakebite is correspondingly uncommon. A prospective three-year study in Malaya confirmed statistically that snakebite is mainly a rural and occupational hazard, most bites occurring in males during daylight when more people are exposed to risk. The severity of poisoning has shown no significant variation according to the time of the bite (in the light or dark), the part of the body bitten, the age of the victim, or the breeding habits of the snakes.

The recent development of an enzyme-linked immunosorbent assay (ELISA) enabling reliable identification and sensitive quantification of both venom and venom antibody is greatly advancing epidemiological and clinical studies of snakebite. Rural surveys complemented by ELISA have objectively confirmed the medically important species. In the savannah of Nigeria, the annual incidence of snakebite was estimated to be 497/100,000 population, resulting in about 10,000 deaths per year, mainly caused by *E. carinatus*. In the Waorani tribe of eastern Ecuador, 78 percent of the population had serum positive for venom antibody, chiefly against *Bothrops* species. Mouse protection tests indicated that these natural antibodies had neutralizing ability. This important finding was clinically confirmed in Nigeria by two patients who recovered unusually rapidly from a second bite with initially very severe poisoning. Specific venom antibody can be detected in the patient's serum one week after the bite. It rises to a maximum one year later, and may then fall to low levels three years after the bite. In some cases, however, specific venom antibody has been detected 40 years after the bite.

A very important finding of these epidemiological research studies is that over one-half of victims bitten by potentially lethal venomous snakes escaped with little or no poisoning. Similar findings have been recorded in the United States and other countries. This is a reassuring statistic for the physician, but one should remember that snakebite in its early stages can be very unpredictable. All victims should be observed closely for at least 12 hours, to assess the severity of poisoning and to ensure rational treatment.

## PATHOPHYSIOLOGY OF VIPER BITE POISONING

Viper venoms contain a complex mixture of enzymes such as phospholipase, proteases, and so on. It was previously thought that these enzymes accounted for the harmful effects of envenoming. More recently, peptides and low molecular weight proteins—so-called hemorrhagins, neurotoxins, cardiotoxins, myotoxins, and so on—have been isolated; they can have very specific chemical and biological actions. However, some experimental findings are not relevant to the clinical problem of envenoming in man and may indeed mislead the clinician. For example, a potent ''neurotoxin'' has been isolated from *Vipera xanthina* venom; yet when man is poisoned by this venom, no neurological effects have been observed. Envenoming in man undoubtedly involves multiple toxic reactions and release of autopharmacological substances by activation of coagulation, fibrinolytic, kinin, and complement systems. But the outstanding clinical effect of viper venom in man is on the hemostatic system, particularly capillary endothelium. Locally, this results in rapidly developing swelling of the part bitten (Fig. 17-2). Massive swelling of the whole limb may ensue over the next 48–72 hours. This swelling is often misinterpreted as due to venous thrombosis or inflammation (or both), but necropsy in such cases has revealed patent veins and no evidence of inflammation. The swelling is presumably caused by venom diffusing through the subcutaneous tissues and affecting vascular and lymphatic permeability from the outside, since the ''head'' of the swelling progresses up a limb in a uniform manner and is not necessarily prevented by an arterial tourniquet (which is *not* recommended). The increased permeability results in exudation, either of plasma or of whole blood, and in the latter case there is subsequent discoloration of the skin. Experimentally, hemorrhage may result either from rhexis through endothelial gaps or through intercellular junctions by diapedesis. Previously, the hemorrhage was ascribed to a proteolytic venom activity, but experimentally the ''hemorrhagin'' of *Trimeresurus flavoviridis* venom has been found to be devoid of proteolytic activity. A curious clinical anomaly of hemorrhagic venom toxins is that some have mainly local effects, whereas others are mainly systemic. For example, in bites by *Vipera berus,* spontaneous systemic hemorrhage is very rare, whereas discoloration of the bitten limb due to local hemorrhage is typical; the reverse is true with *E. carinatus* envenoming.

Local necrosis in viper bites appears to be mainly ischemic, usually developing slowly over weeks and presenting as ''dry gangrene'' (which almost inevitably becomes infected later). Presumably, a relatively high local concentration of venom results in the formation of intracapillary or pericapillary fibrin, which prevents the passage of oxygen to the tissue. Local necrosis in cobra bites is clinically different, more like ''wet gangrene,'' developing rapidly within a few days and with a characteristic putrid smell; presumably, it is caused mainly by direct cytolytic venom action. Because bacterial pathogens can often be recovered from the mouths and venom of snakes, the local features of snakebite poisoning have been attributed to bacterial infection introduced at the time of the bite (therefore, prophylactic antibiotics have been recommended in treatment). Local swelling, redness, increased warmth, and so on in viper bites develop within minutes of the bite, far too rapidly to be caused by bacteria. Antibiotics neither prevent the progression of these features nor expedite their resolution. When local necrosis has occurred, the dead tissue, as with burns,

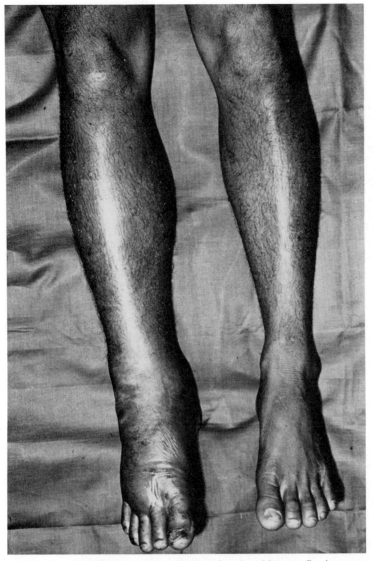

**Fig. 17-2.** Local swelling follows within minutes of a viper bite, confirming venom injection (vipers often bite without injecting venom). (Copyright Dr. H. Alistair Reid).

provides ideal culture for anaerobes; bacteria, of course, are found after necrosis has developed. In a series of 47 proven Malayan cobra bites, however, over one-half of the victims had distinct fang marks and yet developed no local reaction, thereby excluding the likelihood that bacteria from the snake's mouth are a primary factor in the necrosis which ensued in 20 of the 47 patients.

Systemic absorption of viper venoms is usually via the lymphatics and is generally slower than the absorption of elapid venoms, which have a lower molecular weight. Preliminary studies using ELISA in patients bitten by *E. carinatus* indicated that serum venom concentrations rose to a maximum 6–24 hours after the bite; at this time, the urine showed significant amounts of venom. Very *early* systemic symptoms, however, are common with bites of some vipers, such as *V. berus* and *V. xanthina*. Within a few minutes of the bite, vomiting, abdominal pain, explosive diarrhea, and collapse with unrecordable blood pressure can occur (but usually resolve spontaneously within 30–60 minutes). This early collapse suggests activation of the kinin system, followed by inhibition of released bradykinin. Shock, which starts later, is a main cause of death in viper bites. Hypovolemia from loss of blood and plasma into the swollen limb is one causal factor. But shock may develop before the limb becomes grossly swollen, and intravenous antivenom can be dramatically beneficial in these patients without causing any significant change in the size of the bitten limb. Further causal factors in shock (Fig. 17-3) must also be important, such as pulmonary intravascular clotting (which, of course, can be rapidly reversed by powerful natural fibrinolysis), pulmonary edema, and cardiac effects, as evidenced by an abnormal electrocardiogram and elevated serum enzyme levels.

Spontaneous hemorrhage into a vital organ, especially the brain, is the usual cause of death in viper bites. This lethal systemic capillary oozing may be delayed until several days after the bite. Clinical research in *E. carinatus* victims confirms that antivenom can temporarily stop abnormal bleeding and restore clotting to normal. ELISA no longer detects venom in the serum, and yet venom can still be found in blister aspirates at the bite site. Local swelling and blebs probably constitute a venom depot to which antivenom has poor access and from which further venom may be released to cause delayed poisoning effects and even fatal hemorrhage. In the Malayan viper *(A. rhodostoma)* envenoming, the earliest sign of spontaneous bleeding is hemoptysis, with the pulmonary endothelium being damaged by venom hemorrhagin before the systemic circuit. Blood-stained sputum was produced as early as 20 minutes after the bite and always preceded coagulation changes in blood aspirated from veins draining the bitten limb. It is important, especially on admission, to ask the patient to cough hard in order to produce sputum from the lungs; otherwise, this valuable sign may be overlooked. The tourniquet test becomes positive within 1 hour of the bite, and discoid ecchymoses (Fig. 17-4) start to appear about 3 hours after the bite. They are circular, 3–15 mm in diameter, and slightly raised. They may be explained by the effect of hemorrhagin emboli on vertical arterioles joining the superficial network in the corium with the subcutaneous plexus. In *E. carinatus* envenoming, oozing from the gums is usually the first sign of abnormal systemic bleeding.

Spontaneous oozing is not necessarily related to the coagulation defect also caused by certain viper venoms. The bleeding is mainly due to direct endothelial damage by a venom component (hemorrhagin) which does not affect coagulation. That the coagulation defect, defibrinogenation, is not the primary cause of bleeding is shown by the following:

1. Bleeding occurs with viper venoms which do not affect coagulation (e.g., in bites by the puff adder *Bitis arietans*).
2. Bleeding may occur before coagulation becomes abnormal.
3. Complete defibrinogenation can persist for many days, yet no spontaneous bleeding occurs.
4. The procoagulant factor isolated from ''clotting'' venoms does not cause spontaneous bleeding in man whether this factor acts, like Arvin from *A. rhodostoma* venom, directly on fibrinogen, or indirectly, like prothrombin activation by Ecarin from *E. carinatus* venom.

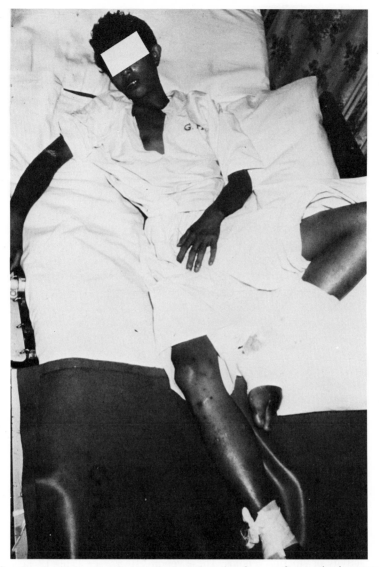

**Fig. 17-3.** Shock with hypotension may be an early or late feature of systemic viper envenoming. Shock responds well to specific antivenom therapy. (Copyright Dr. H. Alistair Reid).

Virtually all viper venoms have effects on coagulation and platelet function in in vitro and animal experiments, provided the venom concentration is high enough (in some experiments, unrealistically high in relation to the venom dose likely to be injected into man). It is interesting that coagulant crotaline venoms act directly on fibrinogen, whereas coagulant viperine venoms act indirectly by activating prothrombin or factor X (Stuart factor). When acting on fibrinogen, most coagulant crotaline venoms split off only fibrinopeptide A; this activity is not affected by heparin. In contrast, heparin inhibits the

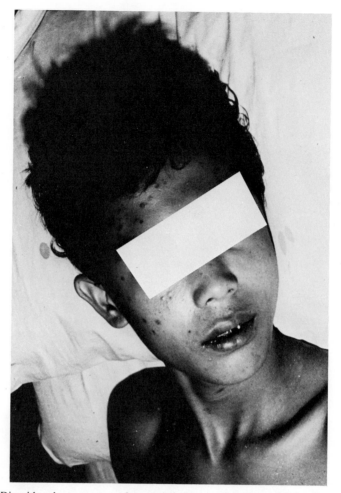

**Fig. 17-4.** Discoid ecchymoses are a characteristic feature of the hemorrhagic effects of some viper venoms. (Photograph by Dr. H. Alistair Reid).

coagulant activity of viperine venoms. These venom effects (see Table 17-1) constitute in vitro "procoagulant" activity. In vivo, if the venom dose is large, as for example, when the viper attacks prey for food, massive intravascular clotting stops the circulation and causes very rapid death. With smaller doses of venom, such as those injected subcutaneously into human victims, there is a continual action on fibrinogen to produce a fibrin more susceptible to lysis than natural fibrin. The venom thus eliminates fibrinogen more quickly than the liver provides it, and although these venoms are "coagulant" by in vitro and intravenous animal tests, the effect in human victims is nonclotting or poorly clotting blood, because of absent or very low fibrinogen (Table 17-1). The latter is not the primary cause of bleeding, although it will, of course, aggravate bleeding from endothelial damaged by venom or by harmful treatment measures.

Most of the venoms affecting coagulation in man are strongly procoagulant. Nonclotting blood is therefore a simple, very sensitive bedside test of systemic envenoming, warn-

**Table 17-1**
Defibrinogenating Activity of Snake Venoms

| Species | Clotting in Seriously Envenomed Patients | In Vitro Effects on Fibrinogen/Plasma |
|---|---|---|
| Crotaline vipers | | |
| Agkistrodon acutus (hundred-pace snake) | Nonclotting | Clots fibrinogen |
| A. bilineatus (cantil) | No record | Conflicting |
| A. contortrix (copperhead) | Normal clot | Conflicting |
| A. halys (Mumushi snake) | No record | No action |
| A. piscivorus (cottonmouth) | Nonclotting | Conflicting |
| A. rhodostoma (Malayan pit viper) | Nonclotting | Clots fibrinogen |
| Bothrops atrox (pit viper) | No record | Clots fibrinogen |
| B. asper alternatus (wutu) | No record | Clots fibrinogen |
| B. bilineatus (Amazon tree viper) | No record | Clots fibrinogen |
| B. jararaca (jararaca) | No record | Clots fibrinogen |
| B. jararacussu (jararacussu) | No record | Clots fibrinogen |
| H. nasutus (horned hog-nosed viper) | No record | No action |
| H. neuwiedi (jararaca pintada) | No record | Clots fibrinogen |
| H. schlegelii (Schlegel's palm viper) | No record | Clots fibrinogen |
| Crotalus adamanteus (Eastern diamondback rattlesnake) | Nonclotting | Clots fibrinogen |
| C. atrox less than 1 year old (Western diamondback rattlesnake) | Nonclotting | Clots fibrinogen |
| C. atrox more than 1 year old (Western (diamondback rattlesnake) | Normal clot | No action |
| C. basiliscus (Mexican west coast rattlesnake) | No record | Clots fibrinogen |
| C. durissus terrificus (South American rattler) | No record | Clots fibrinogen |
| C.h. horridus (timber rattler) | Nonclotting | Clots fibrinogen |
| C.m. molossus (Northern black-tail rattlesnake) | Normal clot | No action |
| C. scutellatus (Mohave diamondback rattlesnake) | Poor clotting | No action |
| C. viridis helleri (Southern Pacific rattlesnake) | No record | Conflicting |
| C.v. viridis (prairie rattlesnake) | No record | No action |
| Lachesis muta (Bushmaster) | No record | Clots fibrinogen |
| Timeresurus albolabriserythrurus (white-lipped tree viper) | Nonclotting | Clots fibrinogen |
| T. flavoviridis (Okinawa habu snake) | Normal clot | No action |
| T. mucrosquamatus (Chinese habu snake) | No record | No action |
| T. stejnegeri (Chinese green tree viper) | No record | Clots fibrinogen |
| T. purpureomaculatus (shore pit viper) | Nonclotting | Clots fibrinogen |
| T. wagleri (temple snake) | Normal clot | No action |
| Viperine vipers | | |
| Bitis arietans (puff adder) | Normal clot | No action |
| B. atropos (Berg adder) | Normal clot | No evidence |
| B. gabonica (Gaboon viper) | Normal clot | Conflicting |
| B. nasicornis (rhinoceros horned viper) | No record | No action |
| Causus maculatus (forest rhombic night adder) | Normal clot | No action |

*(continued)*

*Table 17-1 (continued)*

| Species | Clotting in Seriously Envenomed Patients | In Vitro Effects on Fibrinogen/Plasma |
|---|---|---|
| *Cerastes cerastes* (desert horned viper) | No record | Conflicting |
| *Echis carinatus* (saw-scaled viper) | Nonclotting | Clots plasma |
| *E. coloratus* (saw-scaled viper) | Nonclotting | Clots plasma |
| *Vipera ammodytes* (long-nose viper) | Normal clot | Conflicting |
| *V. aspis* (European asp) | No record | Clots plasma |
| *V. berus* (common European viper) | Normal clot | No action |
| *V. lebetina* (Levantine viper) | No record | No action |
| *V. russelii* (Russell's viper) | Conflicting | Conflicting |
| *V. xanthina* (Palestinian viper) | Normal clot | No action |
| Colubrid snakes | | |
| *Atractaspis dahomeyensis** (mole viper) | Normal clot | No evidence |
| *A. engaddensis* (oasis mole viper) | Normal clot | No evidence |
| *A. microlepidota* (Northern mole viper) | Normal clot | No evidence |
| *Dispholidus typus* (African boomslang) | Nonclotting | Clots plasma |
| *Rhabdophis subminiatus* (rear-fanged Asiatic keelback) | Nonclotting | Clots plasma |
| *R. tigrinus* (Oriental tiger snake) | Nonclotting | Clots plasma |
| *Thelotornis kirtlandii* (bird snake) | Nonclotting | Clots plasma |
| Australian Pacific elapid snakes | | |
| *Acanthophis antarcticus* (death adder) | Normal clot | Conflicting |
| *Austrelaps superba* (Australian copperhead) | No record | No action |
| *Notechis scutatus* (tiger snake) | Conflicting | Clots plasma |
| *Oxyuranus microlepidotus* (small-scaled snake) | Nonclotting | Clots plasma |
| *O. scutellatus* (taipan) | Nonclotting | Clots plasma |
| *Pseudechis australis* (white-nosed snake) | Normal clot | No action |
| *P. papuanus* (New Guinea mulga) | Conflicting | No action |
| *P. porphyriacus* (Australian black snake) | No record | Clots plasma |
| *Pseudonaja nuchalis affinis* (Western brown snake) | Conflicting | No evidence |
| *P. textilis* (Eastern brown snake) | Nonclotting | Clots plasma |

*The African burrowing snake *Atractaspis,* although front-fanged, is now classified in the colubrid family.

ing that abnormal bleeding may follow. A few venoms are only weakly procoagulant, such as the venom of juvenile *C. atrox;* in these cases, nonclotting blood suggests a high, potentially lethal dose. Nonclotting blood can also be used by the clinician to differentiate the cause of envenoming. For example, *E. carinatus* envenoming in Africa causes nonclotting blood, whereas *B. arietans* envenoming does not. This can facilitate the choice of an appropriate antivenom and can be used to monitor antivenom response.

In Table 17-1, in addition to vipers, a few colubrid species are included because fatal hemorrhage has been recorded, usually in freak accidents. Some Australian Pacific elapid venoms also affect hemostasis, although they are predominantly neurotoxic or myotoxic.

Increased fibrinolytic activity usually follows procoagulant envenoming. There is increased lysis of unheated fibrin plates by the patient's plasma euglobulin. This is probably due to release of plasminogen activator secondary to venom effect. Inhibitors such as epsilon aminocaproic acid have been observed not to benefit patients. Although venoms have anticoagulant effects in vitro, these are of no clinical importance in man. Viper bite hemorrhage may be accompanied by a depressed platelet count, although this is often normal. The low platelet count is probably due to consumption of platelets attempting to repair endothelial damage from hemorrhagin activity.

Hemolytic activity is rarely important clinically, except possibly as a factor in renal failure, which appears to be unusually common in *V. russelii* bites. Ischemic effects of fibrin deposition in the kidneys and direct damage by a venom nephrotoxin may be involved. Anemia due to viper bites is not common, and depends on the loss of erythrocytes externally from oozing blood vessels and internally into the local exudate of the bitten limb, behind the peritoneum, and so on.

## CLINICAL FEATURES OF VIPER BITE

### Fright

The most common symptom following viper bites is fear, often the fear of rapid and unpleasant death. Emotional symptoms start within minutes of the bite, whereas collapse due to systemic poisoning rarely develops until 30 or 60 minutes afterward. The frightened patient may appear semiconscious, with cold, clammy skin, feeble pulse, and rapid, shallow breathing. These symptoms resolve dramatically after a placebo injection. Early collapse with hypotension, however, is sometimes due to venom effects and not to fright (as recorded above).

### Early Features of Viper Envenoming

Local swelling (Fig. 17-2) starts within a few minutes of a viper bite if venom is injected. It is a very valuable sign, because if swelling is absent and one knows that the biting snake was a viper, then poisoning can be immediately excluded. Local pain also follows venom injection and may be severe for several days, but this sign is extremely variable and unreliable in diagnosis. Fang marks are also variable. Regional lymph nodes are sometimes tender.

Early signs of systemic viper envenoming include (1) vomiting, (2) hypotension (Fig. 17-3), which may also develop later, (3) abnormal bleeding, (4) nonclotting blood (Table 17-1), and (5) neutrophilic leukocytosis. Abnormal bleeding may start within 20 minutes of the bite. It is usually first observed as oozing from the bite site or wound, blood-stained sputum, or bleeding gums. Discoid ecchymoses (Fig. 17-4) and a positive tourniquet test are common early findings. Nonclotting blood is detected either in a venous sample (amount unimportant) left in a test tube at room temperature for 20 minutes or in finger-prick blood in a plain capillary tube kept horizontal for 20 minutes and then raised vertically. Nonclotting blood runs out of its own accord or can be easily blown out. This yes/no clot test is a bedside test for defibrinogenation which can be competently done by medical aides after brief teaching. Neutrophilic leukocytosis suggests serious poisoning (but the leukocyte count may be normal even in severe poisoning). Platelet counts may be normal or depressed, but the levels do not correlate with clinical severity.

## Later Features

The local swelling can increase both in extent (involving the whole limb and spreading to the trunk) and in amount 48–72 hours after the bite. The swelling is tense and can be massive. The bitten limb may now be cold and arterial pulses (not surprisingly) impalpable, suggesting that surgical intervention is necessary to prevent necrosis. If adequate specific antivenom is infused, however, recovery is usually uneventful. In such cases, ultrasound techniques have confirmed that the circulation is adequate despite appearances daunting to clinicians inexperienced in the natural history of such cases. Blebs around the site of the bite are not important, but if they extend beyond the bite, they suggest a higher venom dose which may cause necrosis. Necrosis is also shown by local darkening of the skin a few days after the bite. Later, an offensive putrid smell indicates secondary infection. Cerebral oozing can be delayed until at least a week after the bite if effective antivenom is not given. It presents as subarachnoid hemorrhage or deepening coma or, less frequently, as hemiplegia; it is often, though not inevitably, fatal. Shock is shown by prostration, sweating, cold extremities, tachycardia, hypotension, and sometimes electrocardiographic and serum enzyme abnormalities. Fever is unusual. Occasionally, victims exhibit reactions such as urticaria and fever in the absence of antivenom or other antiallergic medications. Presumably, these symptoms are caused by venom allergy.

## Diagnosis and Prognosis

The diagnostic importance of local swelling and nonclotting blood has already been stressed. Even when the swelling becomes massive, it will resolve completely, as a rule, within a few weeks, provided there is no underlying necrosis. Local necrosis often entails prolonged, even permanent, disability. The early signs of systemic poisoning have also been noted. Usually, the minority of victims who receive a venom dose large enough to cause systemic poisoning will already have signs of it by the time they see a physician. If the patient is seen soon after the bite, within the latent period between the bite and the possible onset of systemic symptoms (generally 1–2 hours), he should be observed every half-hour by the physician for these early systemic signs.

Viper bite poisoning is severe if, within 1–2 hours of the bite, swelling appears above the knee or elbow, shock is evident, or hemorrhagic signs other than hemoptysis develop (gum bleeding, ecchymoses, a positive tourniquet test, and so on, do not usually appear for 3 or more hours). A neutrophilia exceeding $20,000/\mu l$ and electrocardiographic changes (T-wave inversion and ST-segment deviation) also indicate severe poisoning. The average time of death in viper bites is 2–3 days after the bite. In patients who recover without receiving specific antivenom, shock and hemorrhagic features generally resolve within a week, but in bites by some vipers, coagulation changes may persist for up to four weeks. Complications of viper bites are rare. Acute renal failure usually responds to treatment. Neglected local necrosis can result in chronic osteomyelitis, with sinus discharges for years and extensive scarring.

## TREATMENT

### First-Aid and Prehospital Procedure

First-aid comprises the measures taken by the victim or his associates before medical treatment is received. Recommendations (only rarely will the physician apply them personally) should be short, simple, practical, and more helpful than harmful. Reassurance is important; aspirin* or alcohol in moderation are helpful for their calming effects. The site of the bite should be wiped to remove any venom on surrounding skin. Incision has, in experiments, been interpreted as both helpful and harmful, but clinical observations in man record only harmful effects. Bleeding is aggravated, especially in bites causing nonclotting of blood; nerves and tendons have been severed, infection introduced, and healing delayed.

If significant venom has been injected, it may be absorbed and cause generalized poisoning. Absorption can be delayed by the use of a compression bandage. This is not necessary if hospital treatment with antivenom facilities is available within 30 minutes. Otherwise, a broad and firm but not tight crepe bandage (as for a sprain) should be applied over the bite site and up the entire limb. The bandage should not be released during transit.

If the snake has been killed, it should be taken to the hospital. Otherwise, it should generally be left alone since attempts to find or kill it have resulted in further bites. On no account should the snake be handled even if it is judged to be dead. Decapitated head reactions can persist for up to one hour, and resulting bites have caused near-fatal poisoning.

All victims should be taken to the hospital, preferably directly to one with antivenom and intensive care facilities. Movement of the body generally and the bitten limb in particualar should be minimal, because movement can spread the venom even when a compressive bandage has been applied. If retching or vomiting occurs, the victim should be turned onto the side to prevent inhalation of vomit.

### Hospital Treatment

It is important neither to panic (there is abundant time to administer antivenom if indicated) nor to dismiss a case of snakebite as trivial without proper observation. Reassurance is fortified by tetanus toxoid or by a placebo injection—unless antivenom is already indicated. Except for cases in which there is no possibility of significant poisoning ensuing, the patient should be carefully observed, preferably in an intensive care unit, at least until the next day. The following should be monitored and charted:

1. Hourly: abnormal bleeding, blood pressure, pulse, and respiration rate
2. Yes/no clot test and, later, the clot quality test (Fig. 17-5)
3. Local swelling (circumference compared with that of the unbitten limb)
4. Electrocardiogram, leukocyte count, hemoglobin, creatine phosphokinase or serum glutamic oxaloacetic transaminase, twice daily or more often in severe poisoning
5. Urine output and specific gravity, blood urea, or creatinine
6. Local necrosis, if relevant (extent of blebs and skin darkening)

---

*In view of the impairment of platelet function by aspirin, acetaminophen may be more appropriate.

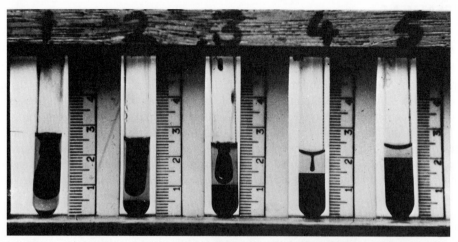

**Fig. 17-5.** Clot quality, judged after contraction by the size of the remaining clot and the volume of extruded cell deposit, is a simple bedside test used to assess defibrinogenation. It is particularly useful in monitoring the adequacy of the antivenom dosage. (Copyright Dr. H. Alistair Reid).

### General Measures

If a tourniquet or bandage has been applied, it should be released. After cleansing (if necessary), the site of the bite should be left uncovered. Local dressings increase secondary infection; oozing soon stops after effective antivenom therapy. Blebs should be left undisturbed to break spontaneously. They will then quickly heal without infection, provided there is no underlying necrosis. Cryotherapy aggravates necrosis. Antibiotics are not helpful unless and until local necrosis is clinically evident. Sloughs should then be excised. Necrosis, however, is usually confined to the subcutaneous tissues; tendons and muscles are rarely involved, although muscles may appear necrotic. They should not be excised, as they virtually always heal with little permanent ill effect. Normal saline is the best dressing after excision of sloughs. At this stage, systemic antibacterial drugs such as metronidazole may be helpful, and skin grafting should be carried out early rather than late.

Fasciotomy rarely benefits and may permanently harm snakebite patients. It should be obvious that this is contraindicated in patients with nonclotting blood. The local effects of envenoming, including massive swelling, usually resolve very satisfactorily after adequate antivenom treatment. In rare cases, muscle necrosis of the anterior tibial compartment syndrome type develops, suggesting that surgical intervention might be beneficial. In such cases, the decision to use fasciotomy should be based on objective measurements of impaired blood flow by ultrasound, rather than on purely clinical signs, which can be misleading in intensely swollen bitten limbs.

As recorded above, heparin does not affect the procoagulant activity of crotaline venoms (Table 17-1). Heparin has been advocated in viper envenoming for two reasons. First, experimentally, heparin prevents death from massive intravascular clotting. In man, however, this form of death is extremely rare. Further, if it occurred, it would happen far too quickly for heparin to be used. The second reason is the theoretical assumption that the effects of procoagulant venom factors, namely, low fibrinogen and platelet levels, are the main cause of spontaneous bleeding. As already discussed, this assumption is wrong, and clinical trials in *E. carinatus* envenoming confirm no benefit from heparin adjuvant therapy. Indeed, heparin has aggravated hemorrhage in patients bitten by snakes such as *V. berus,* whose venom does not affect coagulation (Table 17-1).

Fibrinogen infusions do not help defibrinogenated snakebite patients because the infused fibrinogen is rapidly consumed by unneutralized venom and the resultant increase in degradation products may aggravate hemorrhage. In contrast to these measures, coagulation returns permanently to normal within a few hours of adequate antivenom treatment. Platelet counts may take several days to reach normal levels, but this appears to be of no clinical importance.

Blood transfusion is helpful in viper bite shock, especially if the victim was anemic before the bite. Infusion of plasma, plasma substitutes, or even saline will often improve the shocked patient temporarily (and credit may be given to steroids if given at the same time), but shock is likely to recur if venom is not neutralized. Adequate antivenom therapy is usually dramatically successful in shock and hemorrhage in viper bite patients. A controlled trial of steroids showed that prednisone helped neither the local nor systemic symptoms of viper bite.

## Antivenom

In systemic snakebite poisoning, specific antivenom is the most effective therapeutic agent available. If used correctly, it can reverse systemic poisoning if it is given hours or even days after the bite. It is therefore not only safe but highly desirable to wait for clear clinical evidence of systemic poisoning before giving antivenom. It should not be given routinely in all cases of snakebite because it is expensive and can cause reactions. Immediate reactions occur in about 15 percent of patients when the antivenom is unrefined; rarely, reactions have been fatal. To prevent or minimize local effects of envenoming, especially local necrosis, antivenom should also be considered if the patient presents within four hours of the bite and has clear signs of poisoning, such as swelling spreading beyond the wrist or ankle.

To be effective, antivenom should generally be specific. In Africa, nonclotting blood is very useful in diagnosing *Echis* envenoming from that of other vipers such as the puff adder, and indicating the specific antivenom if available. In many countries, only polyvalent antivenom is stocked. A serum sensitivity test is not advisable when antivenom is indicated, because all such tests are unreliable and confusing. Instead, all patients given antivenom treatment should be regarded as likely to have a reaction. A known allergic history contraindicates the use of antivenom unless the risk of death from envenoming is high. In that rare event, two intravenous drips of isotonic saline should be set up, one containing antivenom and the other epinephrine. Small amounts of epinephrine are infused first, followed by the antivenom. According to the patient's progress, alternate amounts of antivenom are increased and epinephrine decreased.

Antivenom should always be given by intravenous infusion, which is the safest, most effective route. Epinephrine should be immediately available in a syringe for anaphylactoid reactions, when the drip should be temporarily stopped and 0.5 ml of epinephrine in a 1:1000 solution injected intramuscularly. If epinephrine is injected at the first sign of anaphylactoid reaction (often yawning or apprehension), it is almost always quickly effective and the drip can be cautiously restarted. In some cases, several injections of epinephrine are needed. Depending on the potency of the antivenom being used, 20–50 ml should be diluted in three volumes of isotonic saline. In severe poisoning, 100–150 ml of antivenom would be a suitable initial dose. The dose for children is the same as that for adults. The speed of infusion administration is progressively increased from the initial 15 drops/min, so that the infusion is completed within about an hour. If, by then, there has been little significant improvement, further antivenom should be given. Monitoring and charting as detailed above should continue until envenoming has resolved. In bites involving defibrinogenation, the clot quality test (Fig. 17-5) is very useful in monitoring the adequacy of the antivenom dosage.

## HEMORRHAGIC PHENOMENA ASSOCIATED WITH ENVENOMING OTHER THAN SNAKEBITE

Leeches have been used therapeutically for bloodletting from time immemorial. These annelid worms subsist by sucking blood from unwilling mammalian hosts to which they attach themselves. Their saliva contains agents that inhibit blood coagulation by one or another mechanism. The saliva of *Hirudo medicinalis* contains *hirudin,* a polypeptide that blocks the coagulant action of thrombin; that of *Haementeria ghilianii* digests fibrinogen; and that of Brazilian blood-sucking leech, *Haementeria lutzii,* converts plasminogen to the fibrinolytic enzyme plasmin. Other blood-sucking species, such as ticks and tsetse flies, also possess mechanisms for inhibiting the coagulation of ingested blood, whereas the saliva of vampire bats strongly inhibits platelet aggregation.

Bee sting anaphylaxis may be associated with epicardial hemorrhage, cutaneous, mucosal, and visceral petechiae, and intraventricular hemorrhage. These changes are presumably part of the picture of profound anaphylactic shock (see Chapter 8). Scorpion stings may also be followed by such evidence of a bleeding tendency as bloody tears and urine. Hemorrhage, however, does not appear too important in the lethal outcome that follows the sting of some species; some venoms contain anticoagulant agents.

Since few adequate clinical studies of envenoming other than by snakebite are available, these will not be further considered.

## BIBLIOGRAPHY

Lee C-Y: Snake Venoms, vol. 52. New York, Springer-Verlag, 1979
Reid HA: Animal poisons, in Manson-Bahr PEC, Apted FIC (eds). Manson's Tropical Diseases (ed18). London, Bailliere Tindall. 1982, pp 544–566
Theakston RDG: The application of immunoassay techniques to snake venom research. Toxicon 21:341–352, 1983

Gordon D. O. Lowe

# 18

## Vascular Disease and Vasculitis

Small blood vessels comprise arterioles, capillaries, and venules. Arterioles have muscular walls. Contraction of smooth muscle cells of the walls changes the arteriolar caliber. This regulates not only total peripheral circulatory resistance but also local distribution of flow. Arteriolar tone is influenced by adrenergic nerves and epinephrine, by local hormones, by hypoxia, and by accumulated products of cell metabolism. Arterioles contribute to hemostasis by contraction, which temporarily prevents extravasation of blood. Contraction also promotes platelet deposition, accumulation of coagulation factors, and fibrin formation. Platelet secretion of epinephrine, serotonin, and thromboxane $A_2$ may promote vasoconstriction in hemostasis. On the other hand, secretion of prostacyclin from the endothelial lining of the vessel wall may promote vasodilation and prevent platelet deposition under normal circumstances.

Capillaries and venules are tubes of endothelium which lack supporting muscular walls. The endothelium allows exchange of water, nutrients, metabolites, and proteins between blood and the interstitial fluid environment of tissue cells. Outside the endothelial basement membrane lie supporting cells (pericytes) and collagen fibers that run both around and along the vessels. The minimum diameter of capillaries is 3 μm, this being the smallest size of vessel which deformable red and white blood cells can traverse. Postcapillary venules have diameters of 12–15 μm.

Blood cells do not normally leave blood vessels, except in certain organs such as lymph nodes. Vessel integrity depends on several factors. Interaction with normal platelets and coagulation factors results in hemostasis in severed vessels. Platelets may also play a role in maintaining endothelial integrity in the absence of overt trauma.[1,2] The endothelium and basement membrane constitute the initial barrier to blood cell extravasation; both are increasingly recognized as highly complex structures.[3] Some basement membrane components are synthesized by endothelial cells, namely, collagen,[4] glycosaminoglycans, and fibronectin, a glycoprotein which may also be important in maintaining cell-to-cell contact.[5] Pericytes may contribute to vascular integrity, although their function is poorly understood.[6] Perivascular collagen[7] protects against vessel rupture, especially in the skin, where shearing forces are commonly encountered. Collagen fibers may also promote basement membrane formation by protecting glycosaminoglycans against degradation.[8]

**Table 18-1**
Classification of Vascular Abnormalities

| | |
|---|---|
| Congenital disorders | |
| Vascular malformations | Hereditary hemorrhagic telangiectasia |
| | Angiokeratoma corporis diffusum |
| | Cavernous hemangioma |
| Connective tissue disorders | Ehlers-Danlos syndrome |
| | Pseudoxanthoma elasticum |
| | Osteogenesis imperfecta |
| | Marfan's syndrome |
| Acquired purpuras | |
| Mechanical purpuras | Purpura from increased venous pressure |
| | Suction purpura |
| | Factitial purpura |
| | Abuse by others |
| Purpura due to decreased supporting tissue | |
| (atrophic purpuras) | Senile purpura |
| | Scurvy |
| | Excess corticosteroids |
| | Amyloid |
| Purpura due to drugs and chemicals | |
| Purpura due to infections | Purpura fulminans |
| Vasculitis | Henoch-Schönlein purpura |
| Bleeding due to vascular obstruction | |
| (anoxic purpuras) | DIC |
| | Fat embolism |
| | Leukostasis |
| | Paraproteinemia |
| | Proliferative retinopathy |
| Idiopathic purpuras | Simple easy bruising |
| | Progressive pigmented purpura |
| | Autoerythrocyte sensitization |
| | Autosensitivity to DNA |

## CLASSIFICATION, CLINICAL FEATURES, AND DIFFERENTIAL DIAGNOSIS

Vascular causes of bleeding are classified in Table 18-1. Congenital disorders may be grouped into vascular malformations (telangiectasias, hemangiomas) and hereditary disorders of connective tissue. The latter group bleed from tears in the weakened skin and other tissues. Acquired disorders usually present with purpura—extravasation of blood into the skin. In the acute phase, purpura is evident as a red or purple patch in the skin which does not blanch on external pressure. This response differentiates purpura from telangiectasia and erythema, red skin patches due to dilated vessels, which do blanch on pressure since the blood is still intravascular. Small purpuric spots (less than 3 mm in diameter) are termed petechiae, and larger lesions are called ecchymoses or bruises. Extravasated red cells may enter lymphatics, or may be consumed by tissue macrophages and converted into hemosiderin. If extravasation is chronic, hemosiderin accumulates, causing pigmentation.

Purpura from whatever cause tends to occur most often in the lower limbs, since this is the site of maximum venous back pressure on the capillaries. Purpura confined to the head and neck is produced by certain mechanical stresses, fat embolism, and amyloid.

Vascular purpura must be distinguished from purpura due to thrombocytopenia or platelet dysfunction (including von Willebrand's disease). Clinically, platelet disorders commonly cause bleeding from the mucous membranes of the nose, mouth, or gut—"wet" purpura—a medical emergency since fatal bleeding such as intracranial hemorrhage may result.[9] In vascular purpuras, bleeding is usually confined to the skin—"dry" purpura. The bleeding gums of scurvy are an exception. Platelet disorders are excluded by routine performance of a platelet count, blood film, and skin bleeding time. The bleeding time is usually prolonged in platelet disorders but normal in vascular purpuras, provided that platelet function is unimpaired and that the patient is not severely anemic. In doubtful cases, mild von Willebrand's disease should be excluded by measurement of factor VIII properties (VIIIC, VIIIR:Ag, and VIIIR:RCo).

Capillary fragility tests increase intracapillary pressure by obstructing venous flow with an arm sphygmomanometer[10,11] or increase extracapillary negative pressure by applying a suction cup to the skin.[12,13] The number of petechiae induced by these mechanical stresses within a certain area is counted. Increased petechiae may be observed in some patients with vascular purpuras, but the tests are insensitive. They are also nonspecific, since increased numbers of petechiae are also found in patients with platelet disorders and in subjects who do not have spontaneous purpura—especially normal females and diabetics.[14] Like others,[14,15] we rarely use such tests.

Differential diagnosis of vascular purpuras (Table 18-1) depends principally on a careful history and a physical examination. The site of the lesions and the presence of associated inflammation or skin necrosis (which suggest vasculitis) should be noted. The family history, history of trauma, and history of exposure to drugs or chemicals are important. Clinical features of child abuse, scurvy, Cushing's syndrome, systemic infection, and systemic vasculitis (Table 18-2) should be sought. The erythrocyte sedimentation rate (ESR) and plasma or serum viscosity are useful screening tests for infections, amyloid, vasculitis, and paraproteinemias. Further immunological investigations and skin biopsy may be indicated in selected patients (Table 18-3).

## HEREDITARY VASCULAR MALFORMATIONS

### Hereditary Hemorrhagic Telangiectasia (Osler-Weber-Rendu Disease)

This is the most common inherited vascular bleeding disorder. Transmission is autosomal dominant; hence, a family history of bleeding in both sexes is common. Bleeding occurs from telangiectases—malformations of dilated small vessels in the skin and mucosae. These abnormal vessels are the size of small veins, but like capillaries, they have thin walls without smooth muscle. When traumatized, they therefore bleed readily. They also contract ineffectually, resulting in prolonged bleeding.

The lesions are not prominent in childhood, but increase in size and number during adult life. Bleeding usually starts in the second or third decade, becoming more common as the lesions grow larger and more numerous. Epistaxis and alimentary bleeding are the most common symptoms. Chronic blood loss results in iron deficiency anemia, which may be the presenting feature if bleeding is occult.

**Table 18-2**

Clinical Features of Systemic Vasculitis

Fever
Arthritis—pain, erythema, swelling, effusion
Glomerulonephritis—proteinuria, hematuria, casturia, uremia
Intestinal upset—colic, vomiting, diarrhea, bleeding
Pleurisy, pleural effusion, lung infiltrates
Pericarditis
Iritis, retinal hemorrhage
Neurological disorders
Psychiatric disorders

Examination usually reveals characteristic lesions in the mouth (lips, tongue, and palate), face (particularly cheeks and ears), hands, and feet (Fig. 18-1). The lesions are 1–3 mm in diameter and red to purple in color. They may be raised or flat, round or spiderlike. They blanch easily on pressure.

The skin lesions must be distinguished from other common telangiectasias. Vascular spiders appear on the upper half of the body in healthy young subjects, and are more numerous with pregnancy, estrogen consumption, and acute or chronic liver disease. Cough venules are distended veins found along the costal margin in chronic bronchitis. Cherry hemangiomas (senile hemangiomas, Campbell de Morgan spots) are small, round, bright red lesions which do not blanch on pressure and occur on the trunk of many older healthy people. In the uncommon disease of scleroderma, telangiectases occur usually on the hands and face.

In some subjects with nasal or gastrointestinal bleeding, skin and oral lesions are not apparent. Rhinoscopy may then reveal nasal lesions, and endoscopy may reveal gastrointestinal lesions. In some patients with intestinal bleeding of unknown origin, vascular malformations may be diagnosed only by mesenteric angiography. Less commonly, bleeding occurs from lesions in the uterus, lungs, urinary tract, eye, brain, liver, or spleen.

Coagulation studies are usually normal. Some patients have evidence of chronic, low-grade disseminated intravascular coagulation (DIC), which may become acute.[16] Occasionally, the condition coexists with classic hemophilia or von Willebrand's disease.

Treatment is symptomatic and often disappointing. Regular oral iron therapy is usually required, and parenteral iron or blood transfusion may be indicated for resistant anemia. Acute epistaxis is treated by local measures (digital pressure, nasal packing or balloon

**Table 18-3**

Laboratory Findings in
Vasculitis

Increased ESR
Increased plasma and serum viscosity
Hypergammaglobulinemia—IgG, IgA, IgM
Rheumatoid factor, antinuclear factor
Cryoglobulinemia
Hypocomplementemia
Immune complexes
Skin biopsy—leukocytoclastic vasculitis

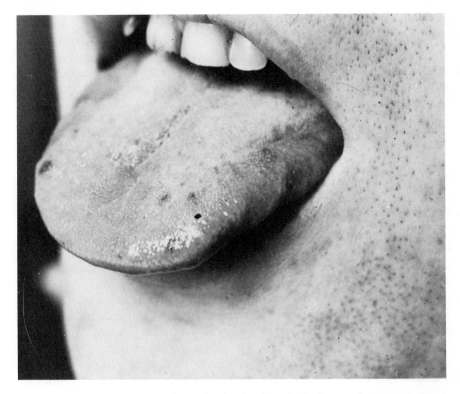

**Fig. 18-1.** Hereditary hemorrhagic telangiectasia. Lesions on the tongue.

compression, topical hemostatic agents). Nasal cautery may be of temporary benefit but can cause mucosal atrophy and septal damage, and lesions commonly recur. Systemic estrogens, which cause squamous metaplasia of the nasal mucosa, have been advocated.[17] Their efficacy has not been established by randomized trials. Side effects are both nasal and systemic,[18] including increased risk of thrombosis. Nasaseptal dermatoplasty has given good results[19] and should be considered in patients with frequent troublesome bleeds. Grafting of human amniotic membrane to replace excised nasal mucosa has also been attempted.[20] Recurrent gastrointestinal bleeding and recurrent hemoptysis have been treated by surgical resection, but even if the radiologically proven site of bleeding is excised, bleeding may recur from other lesions.

## Angiokeratoma Corporis Diffusum (Fabry's disease)[21,22]

This disorder is due to absence of the enzyme trihexosyl ceramide galactosyl hydrolase from skin fibroblasts. The inheritance is X chromosome-linked. Telangiectases, red or blue, are grouped in clusters on the abdomen, hips, thighs, scrotum, elbows, and mouth. They are covered by a thin scale. Other features of the disease are vasomotor disturbances of the limbs (pains, paresthesias, decreased sweating, scanty hair), corneal opacitiy, and occlusion of small vessels by lipid deposits (cerebral, cardiac, and renal). Diagnosis is by urine polaroscopy, which reveals "Maltese cross" material, or by assay of skin fibroblasts for the enzyme.

## Cavernous Hemangioma with Intravascular Coagulation (Kasabach-Meritt Syndrome)

Cavernous or "strawberry" hemangiomas are soft vascular malformations which usually develop during the first month after birth, enlarge during the first year to a size varying from 0.5 to 10 cm, and then slowly regress before adolescence. They occur in the skin or internal organs such as the liver or spleen. Occasionally, intravascular coagulation occurs. If the lesion is not cutaneous, then bleeding from consumption coagulopathy may be the presenting feature (see Chapter 8).

## HEREDITARY CONNECTIVE TISSUE DISORDERS[7,23]

### Ehlers-Danlos Syndrome[24]

This syndrome includes several rare types of collagen abnormality with different types of transmission. The clinical features are hyperextensible skin, hypermobile joints, fragile tissues, and bleeding. Bleeding is particularly common in type IV disease (ecchymotic or arterial type), in which type III collagen is defective,[25] and transmission is autosomal dominant. Possible causes of bleeding include mechanical tears in the fragile skin, other tissues, and major arteries; defective capillary structure (decreased perivascular collagen and increased elastin); and structural and functional abnormalities of platelets.[26,27]

Skin bruising and bleeding into skin tears to form subcutaneous hematomas are characteristic. Thin, pigmented scars are the chronic result of these lesions. Bleeding from the alimentary tract, hemoptysis, and prolonged bleeding after dental extraction also occur. Elective surgery should be avoided if possible, since bleeding and delayed wound healing are likely to occur.

### Pseudoxanthoma Elasticum[28]

In this rare disease, the elastic fibers of the skin and arterial tunica media are structurally and functionally abnormal.[29] Transmission is usually autosomal recessive. Clinically, the skin is lax, contains telangiectases, and bruises easily. Angioid streaks are seen in the optic fundus. Bleeding occurs in the skin, eyes, brain, kidneys, alimentary tract, and uterus. Calcification and occlusion of limb arteries are seen at radiology.

### Osteogenesis Imperfecta

In the lethal type of this disease, type I collagen is defective. Transmission is autosomal dominant. Fractures and deformity result from defective bone matrix. Bleeding manifestations include purpura, epistaxis, hemoptysis, and intracranial bleeding.

### Marfan's Syndrome[30]

This autosomal dominant disorder may be due to defective cross-linking of collagen, which renders it abnormally soluble.[31] The clinical features are long extremities, spidery fingers, dislocation of the lens, and weakness of the aortic root, leading to aortic incompetence and dissecting aneurysm. Spontaneous bruising and operative bleeding may occur, due to defective vessels or possibly to defective platelet function.

## MECHANICAL PURPURA

Mechanical factors probably play a role in initiating and localizing purpura due to generalized vascular or platelet defects. These factors include gravity, stretching of skin over extensor surfaces, trauma, and coughing or vomiting, which increase back pressure in the superior vena cava. Mechanical forces can also be sufficient to induce petechiae or bruising when vessels and platelets are apparently normal. Pressures of 380 mmHg are required to induce purpura in healthy young adults. There is a linear fall in capillary resistance with age, to 150 mmHg by 75 years.[12]

*Increased venous back pressure* causes purpura of the face, head, or neck following violent coughing, vomiting, seizures, strangling, crush injuries to the chest, or superior vena caval occlusion by intrathoracic tumor. At the lower end of the body, purpura from increased venous pressure may be due to tight garters or varicose veins (orthostatic purpura). Purpura and postpurpuric hemosiderin pigmentation are common components of varicose eczemas. This is probably due to trauma (scratching of the itchy lesions), as well as to vessel changes of acute inflammation or chronic thinning of the skin.

*Skin suction* causing petechiae or bruising, is perhaps most commonly encountered as a result of making love. The lesions are elliptical or round, and teeth marks may be present. Common sites are the neck, shoulder, breasts, abdomen, thighs, and buttocks. These souvenirs are termed "hickeys" or "love bites." Similar lesions may be self-induced. Factitial purpura[32] occur in accessible areas such as the shoulders, arms, or breasts. Factitial purpura can also be induced by sucking air from a glass placed over the face.[33] Entertaining children by sticking a sucker toy on the forehead may result in a characteristic round lesion—"purpura cyclops"[34] or the "sucker daddy" syndrome.[35,36]

The type of self-abuse known as *factitial purpura* is discussed in Chapter 19. Abuse of others also occurs. A sad fact of life is that many people batter their relations. Adult victims may seek medical attention for their bruises or for symptoms arising from general anxiety or misery, but initially they deny ill treatment. Young children are particularly vulnerable. The appearance of the child and his lesions may tell a story that he is too young or frightened to tell. The general and cutaneous features of battered or abused children, as well as the management of suspected cases, are described and illustrated in several recent publications.[37,40] All doctors who deal with children should be familiar with these works.

The lesions are often multiple and of different ages. Bite marks; marks from fingers grasping the cheeks, arms, or shoulder; marks of straps, belts, or cords; black eyes; and bruising of the cheeks, ears (from slaps), or toes (from stamping) should all arouse suspicion. Burns (e.g., from cigarettes), scalds, and injuries to the head, eyes, teeth, and bones commonly coexist. A telltale sign of battering is the presence of an abrasion over the ecchymotic area.

Battered children are commonly malnourished, dirty, and infested, and may have an extensive diaper rash. A haunting, reproachful regard has been called "the knowing and wise look of a much older person"[41] and "frozen watchfulness."[42] On admission to the hospital, the child may become more cheerful—the opposite of the normal reaction. The parents may delay bringing the child to hospital, give an inappropriate or evasive history, and be reluctant to permit an examination. Factors in the social background include young or immature parents, marital unhappiness or violence, alcohol or drug abuse, poverty, debt, isolation, and a single parent.

## PURPURA DUE TO DECREASED SUPPORTING TISSUE (ATROPHIC PURPURAS)

### Senile Purpura[43]

These characteristic lesions of old age are usually attributed to progressive loss of collagen in the dermis and vascular wall.[44] Defective cross-linking of collagen may be involved.[45] Capillary fragility increases with age,[12] but there is no increase in the bleeding time to suggest any change in platelet function.[46]

The purpura usually occurs on the backs of the hands, wrists, and forearms; lesions are large and well demarcated (Fig. 18-2). The increased collagen loss at these sites has been attributed to exposure to sunlight or, alternatively, to shearing forces. The skin is thin, and the extensor tendons are easily seen. The dorsal veins have fragile walls, and venipuncture frequently results in rapidly spreading purpura. The shear forces of minor trauma easily rupture small vessels, producing spontaneous bruises. The lesions resolve slowly. Some suggest that this results from decreased infiltration by phagocytic macrophages,[43] but others disagree.[47]

There is no specific treatment. Pressure should be applied for 5 minutes after venipuncture in elderly patients, and the possibility of scurvy should be considered (see below).

### Scurvy[48]

Ascorbic acid (vitamin C) activates the enzyme proline hydroxylase, which hydroxylates proline and lysine residues in collagen and thus stabilizes its helical structure. Deficiency of the vitamin results in a decreased quantity and quality of collagen.[7,49] Bleeding is usually attributed to defective collagen in small vessel walls. In addition, some workers have described decreased platelet adhesiveness in patients[50] and in experimental scurvy.[51] Other studies have reported normal platelet aggregation and platelet plug formation in experimental scurvy.[52,53]

Skin hemorrhages tend to be perifollicular and are most commonly seen on the legs (Fig. 18-3). Gingival congestion and bleeding is seen between the teeth. In children, subperiosteal bleeding causing tenderness and swelling at the distal ends of long bones may be the presenting feature. Internal bleeding occurs in severe cases, and gastrointestinal or intracranial hemorrhage may be fatal. Other features of scurvy include follicular hyperkeratosis of the limbs, and anemia which may be normocytic, microcytic due to iron deficiency, or macrocytic due to folate deficiency.[54]

The deficiency is usually nutritional, and groups at risk in developed countries include the young and old (especially those living alone), alcoholics, and food faddists. Leukocyte ascorbic acid estimations are time-consuming, and the diagnosis is best confirmed by the clinical response to replacement therapy (250 mg daily). The average daily requirement for prevention of scurvy is 50 mg. Treatment in the aged should not be delayed because of the risk of sudden death.

### Corticosteroid Excess[55]

Patients on long-term corticosteroid therapy in immunosuppressive doses, or who have excess endogenous secretion (Cushing's syndrome), commonly have thin skin and purpura. This is most prominent on the arms and legs. Bleeding also occurs into the char-

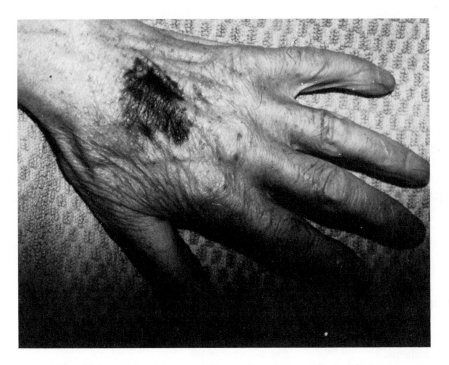

**Fig. 18-2.** Senile purpura. Lesions on the extensor surface of the hand.

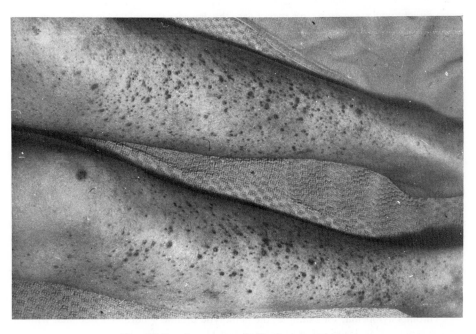

**Fig. 18-3.** Scurvy—perifollicular hemorrhages.

acteristic purple striae which are partial skin tears on the lower abdomen, loins, or thighs. These lesions are thought to result from increased catabolism of collagen, and possibly decreased collagen synthesis and deficient red cell phagocytosis.[55] Posttraumatic bleeding may be excessive.

### Amyloid[56]

Purpura is a common feature of amyloidosis, particularly primary amyloid and amyloid complicating myeloma. Amyloid fibrils are deposited in the walls of capillaries and arterioles, weakening the vessel wall and resulting in hemorrhage. In marked contrast to vasculitis and many other purpuras, amyloid purpura involves the face (especially the eyelids), neck, and upper trunk. The lesions are large and can be induced by applying pressure or by stroking the skin for 1 minute.

Amyloidosis, both primary and secondary, may also be complicated by a bleeding tendency associated with deficiencies of factor X (Stuart factor) and other clotting factors (Chapter 10).

## PURPURA DUE TO DRUGS AND CHEMICALS

Drugs and chemicals may cause purpura and internal bleeding by several mechanisms.

*Direct toxicity to blood vessels* is an uncommon but well-recognized effect of coumarin anticoagulants.[57] Large, spreading areas of hemorrhagic necrosis occur on the trunk, especially over fatty tissues such as breasts or lipomas. This is thought to be an idiosyncratic direct toxicity reaction. In a recent case the disorder was related to hereditary partial deficiency of protein C[57a] (see page 41). Heparin may be of therapeutic value.[58] Some components of snake venom are directly vasculotoxic[59] (see Chapter 17).

*Vasculitis* is discussed below.

*Thrombocytopenia* and platelet dysfunction are described in Chapter 4.

Disseminated intravascular coagulation is presented in Chapter 8.

Corticosteroid-induced collagen deficiency has previously been covered (page 534).

## PURPURA DUE TO INFECTIONS

Like drugs, infections may cause purpura and internal bleeding by several mechanisms (see also Chapter 11).

Direct vessel damage by organisms can occur. Purpura is characteristic of infections such as meningococcemia,[60] rickettsial diseases,[61] and Argentine hemorrhagic fever,[62] in which the offending agents have been demonstrated at the site of vascular damage.

Direct vessel damage by toxins is another possibility. Endotoxins are toxic to endothelium, particularly meningococcal endotoxin, which may partly explain the frequency of purpura in meningococcal septicemia.[63]

Vasculitis is discussed below (page 537).

Thrombocytopenia, for example, the hemolytic-uremic syndrome associated with shigella dysentery,[64] is described in Chapters 4 and 11.

Disseminated intravascular coagulation, for example, septicemia and purpura fulminans, is covered in Chapter 8.

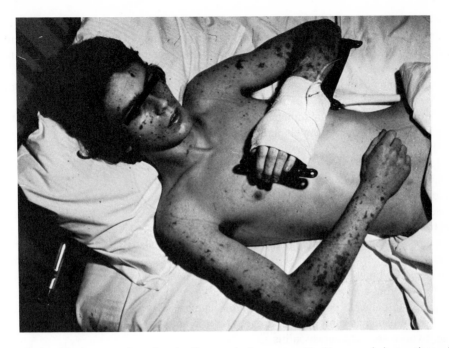

**Fig. 18-4.** Meningococcal septicemia. Symmetrical purpura with skin necrosis in a patient with circulatory shock.

Purpura fulminans[65] is an acute, severe form of purpura with necrotizing vasculitis, which arises as a complication of certain infections and which is usually associated with DIC. Underlying infections include meningococcal septicemia, septicemia due to gram-negative rods, streptococcal infections, and childhood fevers such as scarlet fever, measles, rubella, varicella, and diphtheria (see Chapter 8)

There is usually an acute onset of fever, circulatory and renal failure, and rapidly spreading purpura with skin necrosis. The purpura tends to affect the extremities and is usually symmetrical (Fig. 18-4). Examination of the blood usually shows evidence of consumption coagulopathy and microangiopathic hemolysis. the mortality is high despite intensive treatment with antibiotics, steroids, and sometimes heparin. At autopsy the skin lesions are composed of hemorrhage, necrosis, vasculitis, and thrombosis.[66] Similar findings may be present in internal organs, including renal cortical necrosis.

Purpura fulminans bears some similarity to the Shwartzman reaction induced in experimental animals.[67] In this model, intradermal injection of endotoxin produces local inflammation. After 24 hours, intravenous injection of endotoxin produces aggregation of white cells and platelets, particularly at the site of local injection. This reaction can be decreased by prior depletion of granulocytes[68] or by anticoagulation.[69] Recently, purpura fulminans in the newborn has been ascribed to homozygous protein C deficiency[69a,69b] (see page 41).

## VASCULITIS[70-72]

The term *vasculitis* literally means vascular inflammation. Since vascular inflammation occurs in most diseases, however, the term is now applied to vascular inflammation due to immune disturbance. Vascular lesions caused directly by physical agents, chemicals or toxins, or infections are excluded. Vasculitis commonly affects the skin and is a common cause of vascular purpura. These skin lesions commonly coexist with systemic vasculitis of internal organs and may be the presenting feature of several chronic systemic disorders of connective tissue, neoplasia, or infections such as subacute bacterial endocarditis. The most common type of vasculitic purpura is the self-limiting Henoch-Schönlein syndrome, which occurs particularly in children and young adults.

Four types of abnormal immune reaction are recognized. There is little evidence that type I (anaphylactic, immunoglobulin E-mediated) or type II (antibody-dependent cytotoxic) mechanisms are involved in the production of vasculitis. The type IV reactions (cellular delayed hypersensitivity) may produce vasculitis; histologically, the cellular infiltrate is lymphocytic. The most common type of immune reaction, however, is type III (antigen–antibody complex; Arthus reaction). Antigen–antibody complexes are formed locally on vessel walls or deposited from the circulation. These complexes can be demonstrated as electron-dense material between and under endothelial cells.[73] Complex deposition is followed by activation of the complement system and accumulation of granulocytes, which release lysosomal enzymes. These enzymes destroy the vessel wall, resulting in extravasation of blood. Light microscopy of skin biopsy specimens shows "cuffing" of small vessels by numerous granulocytes—leukocytoclastic vasculitis *(LCV)*. This infiltrate is palpable clinically—"palpable purpura." Endothelial damage may result in platelet adhesion, aggregation, and microthrombosis. Progressive vasculitis may result in necrosis of skin or other tissues—necrotizing vasculitis.

Clincally, vasculitis presents as purpura with associated inflammation, which may be macular, papular (palpable purpura), or urticarial. Urticarial lesions may last for 1–3 days, in contrast to classical urticaria, which lasts for a few hours. In the later stages, nodules, vesicles, or bullae (often hemorrhagic), and necrotic or ulcerative lesions occur (Fig. 18-5). Skin necrosis is apparent as gray or black patches, surrounded by purpura and inflammation. The dead skin eventually sloughs off, leaving ulcers. Vasculitic lesions are typically symmetrical, distal, and dependent. Common sites are the buttocks, lower legs and feet, elbows, and extensor surfaces of the arms. The face and trunk are uncommon sites. Systemic vasculitis may be apparent (Table 18-3), as may fever and skin edema.

The etiology of vasculitis is often unclear. Some cases may be ascribed to specific drugs, chemicals, infections, or neoplasms; insect bites, house-dust mites, and cold exposure have also been implicated. In some patients, skin vasculitis is part of a recognizable systemic disorder of connective tissue (Table 18-4). In rheumatoid arthritis, vasculitis usually occurs in patients with rheumatoid nodules and a high titer of rheumatoid factor. Vasculitis also causes leg ulcers and digital necrosis (e.g., nail fold infarcts, and nail bed infarcts which were formerly termed *splinter hemorrhages)*. Vasculitis is now thought to account for many features of subacute bacterial endocarditis, which were previously believed to be embolic—nail bed infarcts, glomerulonephritis, and Osler's nodes, which are due to vasculitis of the glomus body.[74] Purpuric vasculitis may occur.[75]

Immunological abnormalities in the blood are frequently found in vasculitis (Table 18-3). Three such abnormalities have been used to to define syndromes—hypergammaglobulinemia, cryoglobulinemia, and hypocomplementemia. Whether or not such laboratory findings should be used to define subgroups of vasculitis is debatable.[76]

Hypergammaglobulinemic purpura was first described by Waldenström.[77] The increased globulins cause elevation of the ESR and plasma or serum viscosity. Serum protein electrophoresis shows a diffuse increase in gamma globulins, indicating a polyclonal overproduction. The increase is usually in IgG; IgA levels may also be raised, and IgM is variable. In most patients, rheumatoid factor, anti-gamma globulin IgG, and immune com-

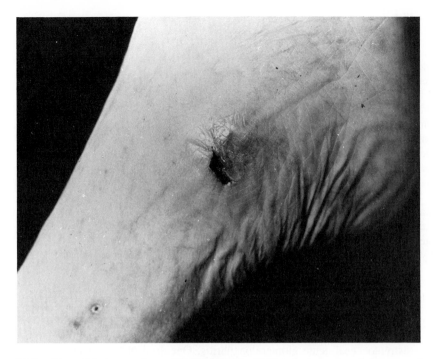

**Fig. 18-5.** Vasculitis in a patient with rheumatoid arthritis. A gray area of skin necrosis with petechial hemorrhages lies on a raised, erythematous base. The necrotic skin is sloughing off anteriorly to leave an ulcer with a hemorrhagic base.

plexes are detectable. Some patients develop Sjögren's syndrome, systemic lupus erythematosus, other collagen disorders, or hemoproliferative disorders.[78,79] This polyclonal gammopathy-purpura syndrome should be distinguished from Waldenström's macroglobulinemia,[80] in which there is a monoclonal increase in IgM paraprotein. Purpura and internal bleeding occur in macroglobulinemia, but are probably due to hyperviscosity and interference with platelets and coagulation (see the section on bleeding due to vascular obstruction, page 540).

Cryoglobulinemia is found occasionally in vasculitis by routine methods, but frequently by quantitative metods.[81] Cryoglobulins may be IgG, IgM, or mixed. Disease associations include connective tissue disorders, myeloma, and hepatitis B.[82,83] Raynaud's syndrome is common. The purpura may be induced by cold, and in some patients may be produced by holding an ice-cube on the skin.

Hypocomplementemia is commonly found in systemic lupus erythematosus, but may also occur in other types of vasculitis. Rheumatoid factor, antinuclear factor, and immune complexes are often associated.

## Henoch-Schönlein Purpura (Allergic or Anaphylactoid Purpura)

This syndrome is an acute vasculitis involving the skin, kidneys, gut (described by Henoch), and joints (described by Schönlein). Streptococcal infections have been suspected as a precursor, since there is commonly a history of upper respiratory tract infection 1–3 weeks prior to the onset of purpura; an association analogous to that of rheumatic fever

**Table 18-4**
Etiology of Cutaneous Vasculitis

---

Drugs and chemicals
   Blood products (serum sickness)
   Penicillins, erythromycin, tetracyclines, sulfonamides, streptomycin, isoniazid
   Aspirin, phenacetin, penicillamine, gold, colchicine, iodides
   Barbiturates, phenothiazines, chloral hydrate, amphetamines
   Thiazide diuretics
   Subcutaneous heparin[107]
   Herbicides, insecticides, azo dyes
Infections
   Streptococcal infections, hepatitis B, cat-scratch fever, malaria, leprosy, yellow fever, subacute
      bacterial endocarditis
Neoplasms
   Carcinoma, hemoproliferative disorders
Systemic connective tissue disorders
   Systemic lupus erythematosus, polyarteritis nodosa, rheumatoid arthritis, Wegener's
      granulomatosis
Miscellaneous
   Cold, insect bites, house-dust mite protein

---

For sources, see references 70–72 and 91.

and poststreptococcal acute glomerulonephritis. One-third of the patients have a raised antistreptolysin O titer, but this is not significantly different from the situation in control groups.[84,85] About one-half of the patients have elevated serum levels of IgA,[86] and IgA deposits have been identified in the skin and kidney.[70,87,88]

The syndrome may occur at any age but is most common in children aged 2–10 years. An increased incidence in the spring has been described. There is an acute onset of moderate fever and a macular or urticarial rash on the buttocks, legs, and arms. The rash rapidly becomes purpuric (Fig. 18-6), and crops of lesions are common. Edema of the legs, hands, scalp, and eyes is often seen. The gut, joints, and kidneys are each involved clinically in about one-half of cases.[89] Intestinal symptoms include colic, vomiting, diarrhea, bleeding, and intussusception in children. Joint symptoms are usually confined to polyarthralgia, but frank arthritis may occur. Kidney involvement is usually manifested as proteinuria, hematuria, and casturia; hypertension, renal failure, or nephrotic syndrome may occasionally develop. In such cases, renal biopsy may show various types of glomerulonephritis.[90] Pleurisy, pericarditis, iritis, and neurological disorders are sometimes seen.

Most patients recover witin a month, but relapses are frequent and progressive renal failure is an uncommon complication. Treatment is symptomatic. Penicillin is often given; corticosteroids may be used when systemic symptoms are marked; and cytotoxic drugs have been given to some patients with progressive glomerulonephritis. The value of such therapies is unknown.

## BLEEDING DUE TO VASCULAR OBSTRUCTION (ANOXIC PURPURAS)

Purpura may result from microcirculatory obstruction by microthrombi in DIC; by fat droplets in fat embolism; and by rigid myeloblasts in myeloblastic leukemia (leukostasis). Neurological features commonly coexist in these disorders, possibly due to similar micro-

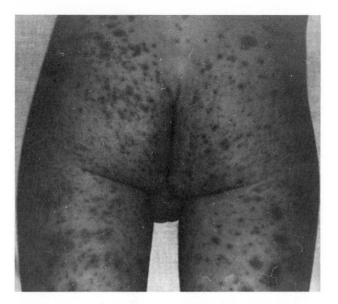

**Fig. 18-6.** Henoch-Schönlein purpura. Typical lesions on the buttocks.

circulatory obstruction in the central nervous system.[91] Bleeding and neurological features are also seen in paraproteinemias, in which the high plasma viscosity probably produces a functional, rheological obstruction to microcirculatory blood flow. Hyperviscosity has also been associated with the proliferative, hemorrhagic retinopathy of diabetes and retinal vein thrombosis.

## Disseminated Intravascular Coagulation (DIC)

Fibrin microthrombi are frequently present in the skin circulation in DIC[66] and may contribute to purpura. Thrombocytopenia and increased fibrinogen-fibrin degradation products also predispose to bleeding (see Chapter 8).

## Fat Embolism

Fat embolism usually results from recent fractures of long bones and presents as confusion, dyspnea, fever, and purpura. Petechiae usually involve the upper half of the body and are commonly seen in the conjunctivae. They may result from microcirculatory obstruction by fat droplets, but vasculitis induced by free fatty acids[92] or DIC[93] may also be a contributing factor.

## Leukostasis

White cells are less deformable than red cells, and myeloblasts are particularly rigid.[94] With increasing myeloblast counts in peripheral blood, leukostasis—small vessel plugging by myeloblasts, with or without fibrin microthrombi—occurs with increasing frequency.[95] In acute myeloid leukemia, transfusion to a hemoglobin level greater than 10 g/dl may increase the risk.[96] Clinical features arise principally from the brain and lungs;[95] purpura may also result from plugging of skin capillaries.[91]

## Paraproteinemias

Purpura and internal bleeding are commonly observed when large amounts of para-protein cause high levels of plasma or serum viscosity.[97] The paraproteins with the greatest effects on viscosity are IgM (due to its high molecular weight), and IgA and IgG3 (due to their tendency to form complexes). Hence, bleeding from hyperviscosity is most common in Waldenström's macroglobulinemia, and myeloma of types IgA and IgG3.[98,99] Neuro-logical and visual disturbances commonly coexist. Examination of the optic fundi usually shows marked venous dilatation and tortuosity; hemorrhages and papilledema may be present.

Bleeding and other clinical features usually respond rapidly to reduction in the paraprotein level and viscosity by plasma exchange.[97] It is thought that the hyperviscosity reduces blood flow and that this rheological obstruction causes stagnant hypoxia and vascular damage. Bleeding may also result from thrombocytopenia, and from interference by the paraproteins with platelet function and fibrin formation and polymerization.[100–102] The dis-turbances in clotting may be manifest by the presence of an abnormally long thrombin time.

## Proliferative Retinopathy

Studies using fluorescein angiography have shown that about 5 percent of diabetics and about 50 percent of patients with retinal vein thrombosis develop retinal capillary nonperfusion, which is followed by proliferation of new vessels in the retina and iris. These new vessels presumably arise as a response to ischemia. They are fragile and frequently cause intraocular hemorrhage, retinal detachment, and glaucoma. Urgent treatment by la-ser photocoagulation is required.

The cause of the initial nonperfusion of capillaries is uncertain, but increased blood viscosity has been demonstrated in patients with nonperfusion or proliferation complicat-ing retinal vein thrombosis[103,104] or diabetes. Abnormalities of coagulation and platelets were also found in such patients after retinal vein thrombosis.[105] Whether treatment of these blood disorders prevents neovascularization and hemorrhage is not known.

## IDIOPATHIC PURPURAS

## Simple Easy Bruising (Devil's Pinches)

Many women complain of easy bruising of the trunk and legs, especially during the reproductive period. Usually no cause is identified; some patients have mild platelet dysfunction, sometimes due to ingestion of drugs such as aspirin. Lackner and Karpatkin[106] recently studied 75 such patients with a normal platelet count and coagulation profile who had not recently taken aspirin or other antiplatelet drugs. Two groups were separated by platelet function studies; these groups were clinically identical. Forty-four patients had normal or increased platelet function; the other 31 had impaired platelet function, particu-larly aggregation induced by epinephrine and connective tissue. In each group, megathrom-bocytes were elevated in two-thirds of patients, and antiplatelet antibody was present in one-third. These findings raise the possibility of increased platelet turnover and immuno-logical disorder. Platelet defects are discussed further in Chapter 4. From the practical point of view, easy bruising is a cosmetic problem. If investigations do not reveal underly-ing disease, the patient should be reassured and advised to avoid taking aspirin.

## Progressive Pigmented Purpura (Idiopathic Capillaritis, Schamberg's Disease)

This is a chronic, progressive purpura of the lower limbs, resulting in pigmentation from hemosiderin deposition. The lesions are discoid and may spread to involve large areas of the leg, thighs, and even the trunk. Skin biopsy shows a lymphocytic infiltrate, in contrast to the granulocytic infiltrate of leukocytoclastic vasculitis. Immunological tests are negative. The cause is unknown, and there is no specific treatment.

## Autoerythrocyte Sensitization and Autosensitivity to Deoxyribonucleic Acid (DNA)

These unusual disorders, which are associated with psychiatric disturbances, are reviewed in Chapter 19.

## ACKNOWLEDGMENT

I am grateful to my colleagues, Drs. Charles Forbes and Colin Prentice, for their kind permission to reproduce photographs of their patients, as well as for teaching me about hemostasis.

## REFERENCES

1. Van Horn DL, Johnson SA: The mechanisms of thrombocytopenic bleeding. Am J Clin Pathol 46:204–213, 1966
2. Kitchens CS, Weiss L: Ultrastructural changes of endothelium associated with thrombocytopenia. Blood 46:567–578, 1975
3. Altura BM (ed): Vascular endothelium and basement membranes. Adv Microcirc 9:1–345, 1980
4. Jaffe EA, Minick CR, Adelman B, et al: Synthesis of basement membrane collagen by cultured human endothelial cells. J Exp Med 144:209–225, 1976
5. Mosher DF: Fibronectin, in Spaet TH (ed): Progress in Hemostasis and Thrombosis, vol. 5. New York, Grune & Stratton, 1980, pp 111–151
6. Weibel ER: On pericytes, particularly their existence on lung capillaries. Microvasc Res 8:218–236, 1974
7. Prokop DJ, Kivirikko KI, Tuderman L, et al: The biosynthesis of collagen and its disorders. N Engl J Med 301:13–23, 77–85, 1979
8. David G, Bernfield MR: Collagen reduces glycosaminoglycan degradation by cultured mammary epithelial cells: Possible mechanism for basal lamina formation. Proc Natl Acad Sci USA 76:786–790, 1979
9. Crosby WH: Wet purpura, dry purpura. JAMA 232:744–745, 1975
10. Hess AF: The involvement of the blood and blood vessels in infantile scurvy. Proc Soc Exp Biol Med 11:130–132, 1914
11. Leede C, Rumpel D: Zur Beurteilung des Rumpel-Leedeschen Scharlachphänomens. Munch Med Wochenschr 58:1673–1674, 1911
12. Gough KR: Capillary resistance to suction in hypertension. Br Med J 1:21–24, 1962
13. Kramar J: The determination and evaluation of capillary resistance—a review of methodology. Blood 20:83–93, 1962
14. Owen CA Jr, Bowie EJW, Thompson JH Jr: The Diagnosis of Bleeding Disorders (ed 2). Boston, Little, Brown, 1975, p 96

15. Borchgrevink CF: Tests for capillary fragility and resistance, in Bang NU, Beller FK, Deutsch E, et al (eds): Thrombosis and Bleeding Disorders. Theory and Methods. New York, Academic Press, 1971, pp 429–430

16. Bick RL, Fekete, LF: Hereditary hemorrhagic telangiectasia and associated thrombohemorrhagic defects in hemostasis. Blood 52(suppl 1):179, 1978 (abstract)

17. Blackburn EK: Long term treatment of epistaxis with estrogens. Br Med J 2:159–160, 1963

18. Harrison DFN: Familial haemorrhagic telangiectasia: 20 cases treated with systemic oestrogen. Q J Med ns 33:25–28, 1964

19. Saunders WH: Permanent control of nosebleeds in patients with hereditary hemorrhagic telangiectasia. Ann Intern Med 53:147–152, 1960

20. Laurian N, Kalmanovitch M, Shimberg R: Amniotic graft in the management of severe epistaxis due to hereditary hemorrhagic telangiectasia. J Laryngol Otol 93:589–595, 1979

21. Von Gemmingen G, Kierland RR, Opitz JM: Angiokeratoma corporis diffusum (Fabry's disease). Arch Dermatol 91:206–218, 1965

22. Wise D, Wallace HJ, Jellinek EH: Angiokeratoma corporis diffusum. Q J Med ns 31:177–206, 1962

23. McKusick VA: Heritable Disorders of Connective Tissue (ed 4). St Louis, CV Mosby, 1972

24. Beighton P: The Ehlers-Danlos Syndrome. London, Heinemann, 1970

25. Pope FM, Martin GR, Lichenstein JR: Patients with Ehlers-Danlos syndrome type IV lack type III collagen. Proc Natl Acad Sci USA 72:1314–1316, 1975

26. Estes JW: Platelet abnormalities in heritable disorders of connective tissue. Ann NY Acad Sci 201:445–450, 1972

27. Kashiwagi H, Riddle JM, Abraham JP, et al: Functional and ultrastructural abnormalities of platelets in Ehlers-Danlos syndrome. Ann Intern Med 63:249–254, 1965

28. Goodman RM, Smith EW, Paton D, et al: Pseudoxanthoma elasticum: A clinical and histopathological study. Medicine 42:297–334, 1963

29. Ross R, Failkow PJ, Altman LK: Fine structure alterations of elastic fibres in pseudoxanthoma elasticum. Clin Genet 13:213–223, 1978

30. Pyeritz RA, McKusick VA: The Marfan syndrome: Diagnosis and management. N Engl J Med 300:772–777, 1979

31. Priest RE, Moinuddin JF, Priest JH: Collagen of Marfan syndrome is abnormally soluble. Nature 245:264–266, 1973

32. Stefanini M, Baumgart ET: Purpura factitia. An analysis of criteria for its differentiation from auto-erythrocyte sensitization purpura. Arch Dermatol 106:238–241, 1972

33. Lovejoy FH Jr, Marcuse EK, Landrigan PJ: Two examples of purpura factitia. Clin Pediatr 10:183–184, 1971

34. Conrad ME: Purpura cyclops. Blood 24:316, 1964 (letter)

35. Tunstall Pedoe H, Lightman S: An unreported syndrome. Lancet 2:1429, 1981

36. Tunstall Pedoe H, Lightman S: Sucker-daddy (purpura cyclops). Lancet 1:632, 1982 (letter)

37. Barnes ND, Robertson NRC: Pediatrics. Lancaster, England, MTP Press, 1981

38. Franklin AW: Child Abuse. New York, Churchill Livingstone, 1978

39. Kempe HS, Kempe CH: Child Abuse. Cambridge, Mass, Harvard University Press, 1978

40. O'Doherty N: The Battered Child. Recognition in Primary Care. London, Baillière Tindall, 1982

41. Kempe CH: Pediatric implications of the battered baby syndrome. Arch Dis Child 46:28, 1971

42. Ounsted C, Oppenheimer J, Lindsay, J: Aspects of bonding failure: The psychopathology and psychotherapeutic treatment of families of battered children. Dev Med Child Neurol 16:447–456, 1974

43. Shiozawa S, Tanaka T, Miyahara T, et al: Age-related change in the reducible cross-link of human skin and aorta collagens. Gerontology 25:247–254, 1979

44. Shuster S, Black MM, McVitie E: Influence of age and sex on skin thickness, skin collagen and density. Br J Dermatol 93:639–643, 1975

45. Shuster S, Scarborough H: Senile purpura. Q J Med ns 30:33–40, 1961

46. Briselli MF, Ellman L: The template bleeding time in elderly individuals. Thromb Haemost 42:797–798, 1979

47. Feinstein RJ, Halprin KM, Penneys NS, et al: Senile purpura. Arch Dermatol 108:229–232, 1973

48. Wallerstein RO, Wallerstein RO Jr: Scurvy. Semin Hematol 13:211–218, 1976

49. Barnes MJ, Constable BJ, Morton LF, et al: Studies in vivo on the biosynthesis of collagen and elastin in ascorbic acid deficient guinea pigs. Biochem J 119:575–585, 1970

50. Wilson PA, McNicol GP, Douglas AS: Platelet abnormality in human scurvy. Lancet 1:975–978, 1967

51. Born GVR, Wright HP: Platelet adhesiveness in experimental scurvy. Lancet 1:477–478, 1967

52. Harrison MJG, Honour AJ: Hemostatic plug in experimental scurvy. Nature (Lond) 216: 1119–1120, 1967

53. Purcell IM, Constantine JW: Platelets and experimental scurvy. Nature (Lond) 235:389–391, 1972

54. Cox EV, Meynell MJ, Northam BE, et al: The anemia of scurvy. Am J Med 42:220–227, 1967

55. Scarborough H, Shuster S: Corticosteroid purpura. Lancet 1:93–94, 1960

56. Kyle RA, Bayrd EIO: Amyloidosis: Review of 236 cases. Medicine 54:271–299, 1975

57. Koch-Weser J: Coumarin necrosis. Ann Intern Med 68:1365–1367, 1968

57a. McGehee WG, Klotz TA, Epstein DJ, et al: Coumarin-induced necrosis in a patient with familial protein C deficiency. Blood 62:304a, 1983 (abstract)

58. Nalbandian RM, Beller FK, Kamp AK, et al: Coumarin necrosis of skin treated successfully with heparin. Obstet Gynecol 38:395–399, 1971

59. Owenby CL, Kainer RA, Tu AT: Pathogenesis of hemorrhage induced by rattlesnake venom: An electron microscopic study. Am J Pathol 76:401–414, 1974

60. Sotto MN, Langer B, Hoshino-Shimizu S, et al: Pathogenesis of cutaneous lesions in acute meningococcemia in humans: Light, immunofluorescent, and electron microscopic studies of skin biopsy specimens. J Infect Dis 133:506–514, 1976

61. Walker DH, Harrison A, Henderson F, et al: Identification of *Rickettsia rickettsii* in a guinea pig model by immunofluorescent electron microscopic techniques. Am J Pathol 86:343–358, 1977

62. DeBracco MME, Rimoldi MT, Cossio PM, et al: Argentine hemorrhagic fever: Alterations of the complement systems and anti-Junin-virus humoral response. N Engl J Med 299:216–221, 1978

63. Davis CE, Arnold K: Role of meningococcal endotoxin in meningococcal purpura. J Exp Med 140:159–171, 1974

64. Koster F, Levin J, Walker L, et al: Hemolytic-uremic syndrome after shigellosis. N Engl J Med 298:927–933, 1978

65. Spicer TE, Rau JM: Purpura fulminans. Am J Med 61:566–571, 1976

66. Robboy SJ, Mihm MC, Colman RW, et al: The skin in disseminated intravascular coagulation. Prospective analysis of 36 cases. Br J Dermatol 88:221–229, 1973

67. Hjort PF, Rapaport SI: The Shwartzman reaction: Pathogenetic mechanisms and clinical manifestations. Ann Rev Med 16:135–168, 1965

68. Forman EN, Abildgaard CF, Bolger JF, et al: Generalized Shwartzmann reaction: Role of the granulocyte in intravascular coagulation and renal cortical necrosis. Br J Haematol 16:507–515, 1969

69. Gaynor E, Bouvier C, Spaet TH: Vascular lesions: Possible pathogenetic basis of the generalized Shwartzmann reaction. Science 170:986–988, 1970

69a. Branson HE, Katz J, Marble R, et al: Inherited protein C deficiency and coumarin-responsible chronic relapsing purpura fulminans in a newborn infant. Lancet 2:1165–1168, 1983

69b. Marciniak E, Wilson HD, Marlar RA: Neonatal purpural fulminans as expression of homozygosity for protein C deficiency. Blood 62:303a, 1983 (abstract)

70. Fauci AS, Haynes BF, Katz P: The spectrum of vasculitis: Clinical, pathologic, immuno-logic and therapeutic considerations. Ann Intern Med 89:660–676, 1978

71. Sams WM Jr, Thorne G, Small P, et al: Leucocytoclastic vasculitis. Arch Dermatol 112:219–226, 1976

72. Wolff K, Winkelman RK (eds): Vasculitis. London, Lloyd-Luke, 1980

73. Braverman IM, Yen A: Demonstration of immune complexes in spontaneous and histamine-induced lesions and in normal skin of patients with leukocytoclastic angiitis. J Invest Dermatol 64:105–112, 1975

74. Von Gemmingen GB, Winkelmann RK: Osler's node of subacute bacterial endocarditis. Arch Dermatol 95:91–94, 1967

75. Rubenfield S, Min KW: Leukocytoclastic vasculitis in subacute bacterial endocarditis. Arch Dermatol 113:1073–1074, 1977

76. Winkelmann RK: Classification of vasculitis, in Wolff K, Winkelmann (eds): Vasculitis. London, Lloyd-Luke, 1980, pp 1–24

77. Waldenström J: Three new cases of purpura hyperglobulinemia: A study in long-lasting be-nign increase in serum globulin. Acta Med Scand 142(suppl 266):931–946, 1952

78. Capra JD, Winchester RJ, Kunkel HG: Hypergammaglobulinemic purpura. Studies on the unusual anti-γ-globulins characteristic of the sera of these patients. Medicine 50:125–138, 1971

79. Kyle RA, Gleich GJ, Bayrd ED, et al: Benign hypergammaglobulinemic purpura of Walden-ström. Medicine 50:113–123, 1971

80. Waldenström J: Incipient myelomatosis or "essential" hyperglobulinemia with fibrinogeno-penia—a new syndrome? Acta Med Scand 117:216–247, 1944

81. Cream JJ, Turk JL: A review of the evidence for immunocomplex depositions as a cause of skin disease in man. Clin Allergy 1:235–247, 1971

82. Brouet JC, Clauvel JP, Danon F, et al: Biologic and clinical significance of cryoglobulins. A report of 86 cases. Am J Med 57:775–788, 1974

83. Levo Y, Gureic PD, Kasuth HJ: Association between hepatitis B virus and essential mixed cryoglobulinemia. N Engl J Med 296:1501–1504, 1977

84. Ayoub EM, Hoyer J: Anaphylactoid purpura: Streptococcal antibody titers and $\beta_{IC}$-globulin levels. J Pediatr 75:193–196, 1969

85. Bywaters EGL, Isdale I, Kempton JJ: Schönlein-Henoch purpura: Evidence for a group A β-hemolytic streptococcal etiology. Q J Med ns 26:161–175, 1957

86. Trygstad CW, Stiehm ER: Elevated serum IgA globulin in anaphylactoid purpura. Pediatrics 47:1023–1028, 1971

87. De La Faille-Kuyper EH, Kater L, Kooker CJ, et al: IgA deposits in cutaneous blood vessel walls and in Henoch-Schönlein syndrome. Lancet 1:892–893, 1973

88. Tsai CC, Giangiacomo J, Zuckner J: Dermal IgA deposits in Henoch-Schönlein purpura and Berger's nephritis. Lancet 1:342–343, 1975 (letter)

89. Cream JJ, Gumpel JM, Peachey RDG: Schönlein-Henoch purpura in the adult. Q J Med 39:461–484, 1970

90. Meadow SR, Glasgow EF, White RHR, et al: Schönlein-Henoch nephritis. Q J Med ns 41:241–258, 1972

91. Kitchens CS: The anatomic basis of purpura, in Spaet TH (ed): Progress in Hemostasis and Thrombosis, vol. 5. New York, Grune & Stratton, 1980, pp 211–244

92. King EG, Wagner WW Jr, Ashbaugh DG, et al: Alterations in pulmonary microanatomy after fat embolism. Chest 59:524–530, 1971

93. King EG, Weily HS, Genton E, et al: Consumption coagulopathy in the canine oleic acid model of fat embolism. Surgery 69:533–541, 1971

94. Lichtman MA: Rheology of leukocytes, leukocyte suspensions and blood in leukemia: Possi-ble relationship to clinical manifestations. J Clin Invest 52:350–358, 1973

95. McKee LC Jr, Collins RD: Intravascular leukocyte thrombi and aggregates as a cause of morbidity and mortality in leukemia. Medicine 53:463–478, 1974

96. Harris AL: Leukostasis associated with blood transfusion in acute myeloid leukemia. Br Med J 1:1169–1171, 1978
97. Somer T: Hyperviscosity syndrome in plasma cell dyscrasias. Adv Microcirc 6:1–55, 1975
98. Preston E, Cooke KB, Foster ME, et al: Myelomatosis and the hyperviscosity syndrome. Br J Haematol 38:517–530, 1978
99. Tuddenham EGD, Whittaker JA, Bradley J, et al: Hyperviscosity syndrome in IgA multiple myeloma. Br J Haematol 27:67–76, 1974
100. Lackner H, Hunt V, Zucker MB, et al: Abnormal fibrin ultrastructure, polymerization and clot retraction in multiple myeloma. Br J Haematol 18:625–636, 1970
101. Pachter MR, Johnson SA, Neblett TR, et al: Bleeding, platelets and macroglobulinemia. Am J Clin Pathol 31:467–482, 1959
102. Perkins HA, Mackenzie MR, Fudenberg HH: Hemostatic defects in dysproteinemias. Blood 35:695–707, 1970
103. Lowe GDO, Trope G, McArdle BM, et al: Abnormal blood viscosity and haemostasis in chronic retinal vein thrombosis. Br J Haematol 51:327, 1982 (abstract)
104. Ring CP, Pearson TC, Sanders M, et al: Viscosity and retinal vein thrombosis. Br J Ophthalmol 60:397–410, 1976
105. Lowe GDO, Lowe JM, Drummond MM, et al: Blood viscosity in young male diabetics with and without retinopathy. Diabetologia 18:1–5, 1980
106. Lackner H, Karpatkin S: On the ''easy bruising'' syndrome with normal platelet count. Ann Intern Med 83:190–196, 1975
107. Jackson AM, Pollock AV: Skin necrosis after heparin injection. Br Med J 283:1087–1088, 1981

Oscar D. Ratnoff

# 19

## Psychogenic Bleeding

Nineteenth-century writers repeatedly suggested that some forms of bleeding might have a psychogenic origin. Our present-day organic orientation has dulled our recognition of this possibility. Several different hemorrhagic syndromes, however, do seem to be influenced or determined by emotional events.

### HEMOPHILIC SYNDROMES

Many, although not the majority, of patients with classic hemophilia (factor VIII "deficiency") or Christmas disease (factor IX "deficiency"), believe that episodes of bleeding may be precipitated by emotional stress such as the excitement generated by an anticipated event.[1,2] This anecdotal evidence is difficult to evaluate. Perhaps the stress and bleeding were coincidental but were thought to be related because the patient's disability interfered with a longed-for activity. Alternatively, emotional stresses may have altered the vascular bed in some unknown way, rendering the patient more susceptible to hemorrhage. Support for this possibility comes from studies of Jaques.[3] In his experiments, rabbits or rats that were treated with oral anticoagulants or parenteral heparin did not bleed spontaneously. Similarly treated animals that were subjected to a variety of stresses died from the results of spontaneous hemorrhage or from such vascular trauma as cardiac puncture that would not be lethal in the absence of stress.

### HYSTERICAL BLEEDING

In 1857, Magnus Huss[4] reported the case of a young servant girl that suggested strongly that bleeding might arise from emotional stresses. She was severely beaten on the head, after which she suffered seizures and became unconscious. Upon awakening, she bled through the scalp from a point that had not been injured. Thereafter, she bled additionally from the face, the ear, and the gastrointestinal tract. A year later, Huss studied her carefully during a hospital stay. Blood appeared to exude through the unbroken skin. She also had cutaneous ecchymoses, hemiparesis, and episodes of unconsciousness and convulsions. Huss observed that she could induce bleeding by picking a quarrel with another patient in order to induce the necessary emotional tension.

A few years later, the American neurologist S. Weir Mitchell[5] described a patient with ''a prolonged hysterical condition'' initiated by fright, who had painful ''extravasations'' of blood over a period of months. In this and several other cases, Mitchell linked the appearance of cutaneous bleeding to a ''nerve malady.'' His descriptions, unlike those of Huss, are not convincing to the modern reader, but a number of subsequent cases of ''hysterical bleeding'' seem more plausible.[6,7] Bleeding was sometimes observed through the intact skin, but the more common lesion was recurrent ecchymosis that was sometimes preceded by local erythema and prodromal sensations or pain. Both spontaneous bruising and remission of bleeding were induced by hypnosis. Some patients were said to have a spectrum of symptoms that included anxiety, nervousness, depression, and sexual disturbances, supporting the view that the bleeding tendency had an emotional basis. These reports were ignored by hematologists.

## AUTOERYTHROCYTE SENSITIZATION

In 1955, Gardner and Diamond,[8] who were apparently unaware of these earlier studies, described an unusual syndrome in 4 women. In each case, episodes of bleeding appeared within weeks or months of a physical injury. The patients experienced repeated episodes of bruising, usually on the extremities, accompanied by local pain and swelling and, in 2 of the patients, preceded by as long as 24 hours by pain, heat, or induration. Other evidence of a hemorrhagic tendency was described, including hematomas and gastrointestinal, urinary tract, and possibly central nervous system bleeding. Gardner and Diamond thought that the patients may have been sensitized to erythrocytic stroma during their initial injury and that subsequent extravasations, perhaps from unrecognized trauma, induced the cutaneous lesions. In support of this belief, they were able to reproduce the characteristic painful, inflammatory bruises by the intracutaneous injection of washed erythrocytes or erythrocytic stroma.

Since Gardner and Diamond's report, about 200 additional patients with ''autoerythrocyte sensitization'' have been recognized.[7,9] The patients have varied from 9 to 53 years of age at the time of onset of bruising; 95 percent of the cases have been in females. A story of injury or surgical trauma shortly before the onset of the syndrome was recounted by somewhat more than one-half of the patients we have seen. The patients have had recurrent bouts of bruising, nearly always in areas directly visible to them or readily seen in a mirror. Usually the bruises are preceded by painful stinging or tingling sensations at the site to be affected. These local sensations are sometimes accompanied by systemic symptoms such as headache, feverishness, or malaise. Within 1–2 hours, the patients become aware of local warmth, erythema, swelling, induration, tenderness, and pain. After a period ranging from a few hours to as long as three days, the area turns blue. Ecchymosis is usually superimposed upon the inflamed area, but in perhaps one-third cases it seems first to form a halo around the pink center, after which the whole area becomes purpuric. The bruises vary from 1 or 2 cm in diameter to an enormous size, encompassing, for example, the entire forearm. Most often, the bruises appear in crops over a period of days or weeks, after which there is a relative remission that may last for weeks or years. Some patients seem never to be free of bruises. Other evidence of a bleeding tendency may be present, of which menorrhagia is the most common, leading to a high incidence of hysterectomy, often at an early age.

Shortly after Gardner and Diamond's original report, it became evident that patients with autoerythrocyte sensitization may have deep emotional disturbances.[10] Typically, they have hysterical, martyristic, and masochistic character traits, obsessive behavior such as inordinate cleanliness or orderliness, depression, anxiety, and an inability to deal with their own hostile feelings. Sexual disturbances are frequently reported. Depression has been particularly impressive, leading to hospitalization or psychiatric care and to contemplated or attempted suicide. The patients display such overt conversion symptoms as paresis, hypesthesia, blindness, monocular diplopia, tunnel vision, aphonia, syncope, or seizures. Not surprisingly, they have had a wide range of somatic complaints, encompassing essentially all organ systems. These symptoms have led to an inordinate number of surgical procedures. Headache is commonplace and is often associated with visual disturbances, nausea, and vomiting. The patients' past history is rich in examples of both emotional and physical stresses. Often the patients have had a history of battering at the hands of a parent or spouse. Peculiarly, a number have related that they had close contact with someone with an amputated or traumatized extremity, often under harrowing circumstances.

The pathogenesis of autoerythrocyte sensitization is obscure. The lesions have been reproduced not only by erythrocytic stroma but also, in some instances, by hemoglobin, histamine, or even estrogenic hormones. As we have learned more of the emotional background of our patients, we have become increasingly unable to elicit ecchymotic responses to the intracutaneous injection of autologous blood, as though a positive skin test required the interaction of a patient and a physician who anticipated a positive result. A number of immunologic abnormalities have been described, but none seems to explain the syndrome. Current evidence suggests that the patients have "psychogenic purpura," but the possibility that the lesions are entirely or partially factitial is hard to eliminate.

Episodes of bleeding may recur over a period of only a few months or last for many years. Psychiatric therapy appears to be helpful only in younger patients. Treatment with a number of pharmacologic agents has been tried, with conflicting results.

## AUTOSENSITIVITY TO DEOXYRIBONUCLEIC ACID (DNA)

A syndrome strikingly similar to autoerythrocyte sensitization was described by Levin and Pinkus[11] in a 40-year-old woman in whom cutaneous ecchymoses could be reproduced by the intracutaneous injection of buffy coat or calf thymus DNA. Levin and Pinkus ascribed the disorder to autosensitivity to DNA. The author is aware of seven additional cases.[9] In all but one of these seven, emotional disturbances reminiscent of those observed in autoerythrocyte sensitization were present. The existence of autosensitivity to DNA as a distinctive entity is therefore not yet certain.

## FACTITIAL BLEEDING

The diagnostic challenge of autoerythrocyte sensitization and autosensitivity to DNA pales in comparison to the difficulties encountered in recognizing the various forms of factitial purpura.[9,12,13] Three types can be delineated: deliberate self-injury, simulation of a bleeding diathersis, and the induction of a bleeding tendency by the self-administration of anticoagulant agents.

Self-flagellation results in the formation of ecchymoses or hematomas that may be difficult to distinguish from those brought about by disease. Sometimes the linear distribution of a series of ecchymoses suggests that the patient has beaten himself with some object. In other patients, abrasions may be detected over apparently typical bruises. Obviously, patients with this syndrome have severe emotional problems, but they may present a facade that may hide the factitial nature of the disease from the physician. Other patients have induced circumscribed petechiae by applying suction to the skin with the lips; the lesions necessarily are within reach of the mouth. Still other patients have apparently induced hematuria, epistaxis, or vaginal bleeding by self-inflicted injury.

More difficult to recognize is the simulation of bleeding. In such cases, the patient may describe hemoptysis, hematemesis, hematuria, or menorrhagia and may even provide physical evidence for these phenomena. Careful observation may reveal the feigned nature of the symptoms. One young patient observed in Cleveland deliberately cut her finger and allowed the blood to drip into the urine.

The psychobiology of patients who simulate bleeding seems to vary from case to case, but most of the reported cases have been in males who are said to "chronic factitial disorder with physical symptoms." The term Munchausen's syndrome has been applied to this variety of factitial disease, but this name has unseemly moralistic implications that may blind the physician to the serious nature of the patient's psychiatric difficulties.

Rarely, bleeding is apparently a means to create factitial anemia. The patients may phlebotomize themselves to almost an unbelievable degree—for example, until the hemoglobin concentration is 1.5 g/dl.[14] Needless to say, such individuals require psychiatric as well as hematologic care.

The syndrome of surreptitious administration of anticoagulants is more frequently recognized than self-injury or simulated bleeding.[15,16] This usually takes the form of ingestion of oral anticoagulants such as Dicumarol or warfarin. Recently, a few have injected heparin to induce bleeding. The patients have had ready access to medication, nearly always because they are in medically related professions. Curiously, the patients usually consult their physicians, seeking an explanation for the sudden and unexpected appearance of ecchymoses, hematuria, melena, menorrhagia, or epistaxis. The diagnosis is readily established by demonstrating the presence of the anticoagulant—nowadays usually warfarin—in the patient's plasma. The immediate therapy for the patient taking oral anticoagulants is the administration of vitamin $K_1$, for example, 25 mg intramuscularly or intravenously. All that may be needed for those who inject heparin is isolation from further access to medication. Most individuals who self-administer anticoagulant agents are women who have serious emotional problems. In men, who make up a minority of patients, self-administration of oral anticoagulants has been used to avoid the draft or to obtain narcotics.

The deliberate self-administration of anticoagulants must be distinguished from the cases in which these agents have been dispensed by the pharmacist or administered by hospital personnel in error or, grimly, have been given with murderous intent. In one interesting Cleveland case, the patient took her husband's Dicumarol to treat her arthritis. She claimed great relief of pain, but came to us because of the sudden outbreak of bruising.

The various forms of factitial purpura are associated with severe emotional disturbances not dissimilar to those of autoerythrocyte sensitization. The affected patients, like those with autoerythrocyte sensitization, have histories replete with psychological and physical trauma.[15] Great care must be exercised in confronting the patient with the diagnosis.

The patient may quickly seek another physician who is less perspicacious or, tragically, he or she may attempt suicide. Obviously, psychiatric care is of the greatest urgency.

Syndromes of factitial bleeding must be distinguished from those of battering. The battered child is usually much younger than the patient with factitial bleeding, and careful examination may reveal telltale abrasions over the ecchymoses.

## RELIGIOUS STIGMATA

Over the last 7 centuries, individuals have been described who have bled through the skin, usually while in states of religious ecstacy.[9] The first person who is said to have experienced the religious stigmata was St. Francis in 1224. Most but not all stigmatics have been women. The disorder has been reported in individuals of various faiths whose bleeding has been appropriate to their beliefs. In Roman Catholics, the stigmata have taken the form of episodic bleeding from the palms and soles and from either the right or left anterior chest wall. Sometimes, bleeding from the brow occurs, as if from a crown of thorns. Although associated with religious fervor, the stigmata have not been recognized as of miraculous origin by most ecclesiastic authorities. Observations in some modern stigmatics suggest that they have the same panoply of psychiatric problems and manifestations as patients with autoerythrocyte sensitization. Whether the lesions are self-induced has been debated. In a stigmatized individual we studied, not a Roman Catholic, the patient raised this issue, but inconclusively, after her lesions disappeared upon her conversion to another religion.

## REFERENCES

1. Mattson A, Gross S: Social and behavioral studies on hemophilic children and their families. J Pediatr 68:952–964, 1966
2. Chilcote RR, Baehner RL: Atypical bleeding in hemophilia: Application of the conversion model to the case study of a child. Psychosom Med 42(suppl):221–230, 1980
3. Jaques LB: Anticoagulant Therapy. Pharmacologic Principles. Springfield, Ill, Charles C Thomas, 1965
4. Huss M: Cas de maladies rare. II Hémophilie. V série, tome 10. Arch Gen Med 2:165–195, 1857.
5. Mitchell SW: On certain forms of neuralgia accompanied with muscular spasms and extravasations of blood and on purpura as a neurosis. Am J Med Sci 68:116–122, 1869
6. Jacobi E: Psychogene Spontanblutungen der Haut. Archiv Psychiatr Nervenkr 88:631–645, 1929
7. Ratnoff OD, Agle D: Psychogenic purpura: A re-evaluation of the syndrome of autoerythrocyte sensitization. Medicine 47:475–500, 1968
8. Gardner FH, Diamond LK: Autoerythrocyte sensitization. A form of purpura producing painful bruising following autosensitization to red blood cells in certain women. Blood 10:675–690, 1955
9. Ratnoff OD: The psychogenic purpuras: A review of autoerythrocyte sensitization, autosensitization to DNA, ''hysterical'' and factitial bleeding, and the religious stigmata. Semin Hematol 17:192–213, 1980
10. Ratnoff OD: Bleeding Syndromes. Springfield, Ill, Charles C Thomas, 1960

11. Levin MB, Pinkus H: Autosensitivity to desoxyribonucleic acid (DNA). Report of a case with inflammatory skin lesions controlled by chloroquine. N Engl J Med 264:533–537, 1961
12. Forbes CD, Prentice CRM: Vascular and non-thrombocytopenic purpuras, in Bloom AL, Thomas DP (eds): Haemostasis and Thrombosis. New York, Churchill-Livingstone, 1981, pp 268–278.
13. Abram HS, Hollender MH: Factitious blood disease. South Med J 67:691–696, 1974
14. Barosi G, Morandi S, Cazzola M, et al: Abnormal splenic uptake of red cells in long-lasting iron deficiency anemia due to self-induced bleeding (factitious anemia). Blut 37:75–82, 1978
15. Agle DP, Ratnoff OD, Spring GK: The anticoagulant malingerer. Psychiatric studies in three patients. Ann Intern Med 73:67–72, 1970
16. O'Reilly RA, Aggeler PM: Covert anticoagulant ingestion: Study of 25 patients and review of world literature. Medicine 55:389–399, 1976

# Index

Prostaglandins *(continued)*
  in chronic renal disease, 477
  cyclooxygenase deficiency and, 154
Prostaglandin synthesis, in thrombotic
    thrombocytopenic purpura, 131
Prostate cancer
  bleeding in, 336, 357
  factor XI inhibitors in, 358
Prostatectomy, bleeding after, 342, 387
Prosthetic devices
  coagulant factors and, 400
  thrombohemorrhagic complications of, 400–402
Protease inhibitors, 324
Protein C, 9, 32, 41, 415
  role of vitamin K in synthesis, 7, 32, 42
Protein C inhibitor deficiency, 9, 282, 420, 536, 537
Protein deficiency, in final common clotting
    pathway, 55
Protein S, 42
Protein factor 4, in platelet granules, 82–83
Proteinuria, in thrombotic thrombocytopenic
    purpura, 130
Prothrombin
  activitation of, 27, 30–32
  in coagulation, 28
  measurement of, 3, 57
  purification of, 2
  role of vitamin K in synthesis, 7, 30
Prothrombin complex concentrates, for factor VIII
    antibody patients, 206–207, 274
  thrombotic complications, 300–301
Prothrombin consumption, PF3 activity and,
    146–147
Prothrombin conversion
  factor Xa in, 31
  platelet role in, 93
Prothrombin deficiency
  hereditary, 208
  in liver disease, 451–454
Prothrombin, inhibitor to, 281
Prothrombin time, 28, 52–53, 327, 335–336,
    352–353, 355–357
  in control of oral anticoagulant therapy,
    487–488
  defined, 52
  in factor VII, factor V, or factor X deficiency,
    55–56
  sensitivity of, 52–53
Pseudohemophilia, 49
*Pseudomonas aeruginosa,* DIC and, 304
Pseudothrombocytopenia, 96
Pseudotumors
  hemophilic blood cysts as, 184–185
  pathology of, 184–185
  treatment of, 185
Pseudo-von Willebrand's disease, 256–257
Pseudoxanthoma elasticum, 45, 532

Psychogenic bleeding, 45, 549–553
PTA, *see* Plasma thromboplastin antecedent, Factor
    XI
PTT, *see* Partial thromboplastin time
Pulmonary embolism, 8, 308–309
Purpura
  allergic or anaphylactoid, 539–542
  amyloidosis and, 536
  anoxic, 540–542
  atrophic, 534–536
  from drugs and chemicals, 536
  factitial, 551–553
  Henoch-Schönlein, 539–540
  hypergammaglobululinemic, 538–539
  idiopathic, 542–543
  idiopathic thrombocytopenic, *see* Idiopathic
    thrombocytopenic purpura
  from infections, 367–375, 536–537
  mechanical, 533
  in newborns, 427
  progressive pigmented, 543
  senile, 534
  simple, 542
  in vasculitis, 538
Purpura fulminans, 305–306, 374, 419–420, 537
Pyelonephritis, hemophilia and, 191

Qualitative platelet disorders, relationships in,
    144–145
Quantitative platelet disorders, relationships in,
    96–143
Quinidine-dependent thrombocytopenia, 127
Quinine-dependent thrombocytopenia, 127

Razoxane, 110
Reactive thrombocytosis, 138–139
Rebound thrombocytosis, 139
Rectal bleeding, 187
Religious stigmata, 553
Renal allograft rejection, platelet aggregation in, 481
Renal bleeding, management of, 190–192
Renal disease, *see* Kidney disease
Renal failure
  bleeding in, 191, 478–482
  platelet transfusions in, 481
Renal function tests, 189–190
Renal hemodialysis, in renal failure, 401
Renal pelvis, expanding hemophilic pseudotumor of,
    190
Renal tract, fibrinolytic inhibitors and, 215–216
Renal tract bleeding, obstruction in, 190
Renal transplantation
  fibrinogen-related antigens following, 309
  rejection reaction, 309
  thrombocytopenia and, 481

Sulfinpyrazone, in thrombotic thrombocytopenic
    purpura, 131
Sulindac, 496
Surgical hemorrhage, 342, 379–382
    coagulation factor deficiencies in, 386–387
    DIC-type syndromes in, 386–387
    drugs as cause of, 385–386
    in hemophilia, 179
    hemostasis in, 579–582
    platelet functional defects and, 383–385
    thrombocytopenia in, 383–384
    vascular defects, 382–383
Surreptitious anticoagulant administration, 552
Syphilis, congenital, 432
Syringomyelia, cavitation due to, 188
Systemic lupus erythematosus, *see* Lupus
        erythematosus
    HLD-D antigen in, 118
    inhibitors against, 278–280
Systemic vasculitis, clinical features of, 530

Taipan snake venom, 57
Tanned red cell hemagglutination inhibitor, 328
TAR syndrome, 111, 159, 430, 436
Teeth, bleeding at, 45, 192
Telangiectasias, distinction from hereditary
        hemorrhagic telangiectasia, 530
Therapeutic abortion, DIC and, 418
Thiazides
    neonatal thrombocytopenia and, 435
    thrombocytopenia and, 111
Thrombasthenia, laboratory data in, 64, 149
Thrombin, 2–7
    in coagulation, 28
    generation of, 2–7, 30–32, 455
    in platelet aggregation, 61
Thrombin-sensitive protein, 83
Thrombin time, 53, 335–336, 352, 355–357,
    460–461
Thrombocythemia, essential, 140–141, 361
    gastrointestinal bleeding in, 45
Thrombocytopenia, 45, 96–143. *See also*
        Thrombocytopenic purpura, Leukemia, etc.
    with abnormal blood vessels, 133–134
    with absent radii, 111, 159, 430–431
    acute viral-induced, 135–136
    alcohol-induced, 111, 137
    allergy-induced, 136
    alpha-storage pool disease and, 104
    antepartum medications and, 435
    antibody-medicated, 361
    anticoagulants in, 97
    and aplastic anemia, 106–107, 430, 462
    with artificial surfaces, 133–134
    autoimmune, 114–121, 434
    bacterial endotoxin in, 370–372
    Bernard-Soulier syndrome, 104

bone marrow examination in, 105–106
cancer and, 360–362
cardiopulmonary bypass and, 388–399
causes of, 48–49
chemotherapy, 107
and chronic idiopathic thrombocytopenic purpura,
    115, 118–119
clot retraction, 63
in cirrhosis, 462
congenital amegakaryocytosis and, 111
in congenital syphilis, 432
corticosteroid therapy in, 116
cyclic, 107
in cytomegalic inclusion disease, 432
with decreased megakaryocytes, 106, 111–113
decreased platelet survival and, 122, 133–135
defined, 367
diagnosis of, 433
in DIC, 292, 369, 388
diethylstilbestrol-associated, 111
in Down's syndrome, 431
drug-induced, 107–110, 435
    antibody-mediated, 123–127, 361
exchange transfusion in neonate, 432
Fanconi's anemia and, 106, 431
Glanzmann's, *see* Glanzmann's thrombasthenia
gold induced, 126–127
gray platelet syndrome, 104
hearing defect and, 104
hemolytic anemia with, 122
in hemolytic-uremic syndrome, 132–133, 308,
    473, 477
hereditary, 104, 430
in herpes simplex, 432
heparin-induced, 125, 361
in hepatitis, 462
in Hodgkin's disease, 122
from hypothermia, 137–138
immune mechanisms in, 371, 431–435
increased megakaryocytes and, 113
increased platelet utilization in, 129–136
with ineffective thrombopoiesis, 136
with infections, 135–136, 367–372
with isovaleric acidemia, 456
in kidney disease, 104, 478
in lupus erythematosus, 122
May-Hegglin anomaly in, 102–103, 432
measles vaccine, 369
Mediterranean macrothrombocytopenia, 104
with megakaryocytic hypoplasia in newborn, 430
with megaloblastic disorders, 136–137
menorrhagia and, 45
with methylmalonic acidemia, 436
mithramycin and, 360
Montreal platelet syndrome and, 104
murine cytomegalovirus infection and, 369
in neonates, 121–122, 128–129, 430–438
in noncardiac surgery, 383